28/2/87

Renal function and disease in the elderly

Renal function and disease in the elderly

Edited by

Juan F. Macias Nuñez
Associate Professor of Medicine, Hospital Clinico Universitario, University of Salamanca, Spain

and

J. Stewart Cameron
Professor of Renal Medicine, Renal Unit, Guy's Hospital Medical School, London, UK

Butterworths
London Boston Durban Singapore Sydney Toronto Wellington

First published, 1987

British Library Cataloguing in Publication Data
Renal function and disease in the elderly.
1. Geriatrics 2. Kidneys — Diseases
I. Macias Nuñez, Juan F. II. Cameron, J. Stewart
618.97'661 RC952.9

ISBN 0-407-00395-9

Library of Congress Cataloging-in-Publication Data
Renal function and disease in the elderly
Includes bibliographies and index.
1. Geriatric nephrology. I. Macias Nuñez, Juan F.
II. Cameron, J. Stewart (John Stewart) [DNLM:
1. Kidney—physiopathology.
2. Kidney Diseases—in old age.
WJ 300 R3916]
RC903.R486 1986 618.97'61 86-13709
ISBN 0-407-00395-9

Typeset by Gatehouse Wood Ltd., Sevenoaks, Kent.
Printed by Butler & Tanner Ltd., Frome, Somerset.

Contents

Contributors

José M. Alcazar
Hospital 1° de Octubre, Universidad Complutense, Madrid, Spain

Sharon Anderson
Laboratory of Kidney and Electrolyte Physiology, Brigham and Women's Hospital, Boston, Massachusetts, USA

Luis Hernando Avendaño
Department of Medicine, Universidad Autónoma de Madrid, Madrid, Spain

Manuel Urrutia Avisrror
Department of Urology, University of Salamanca, Salamanca, Spain

W. Kline Bolton
Department of Medicine, University of Virginia School of Medicine, Charlottesville, Virginia, USA

Barry M. Brenner
Laboratory of Kidney and Electrolyte Physiology, Brigham and Women's Hospital, Boston, Massachusetts, USA

John C. Brocklehurst
Department of Geriatric Medicine, University of Manchester, Manchester, UK

J. Stewart Cameron
Renal Unit, Guy's Hospital Medical School, London, UK

José L. Cangiano
Hypertension Section, Veterans Administration Hospital, San Juan, Puerto Rico

Alberto Cantaluppi
Division of Nephrology and Dialysis, Ospedale Maggiore Policlinico, Milan, Italy

Sisinio de Castro del Pozo,
Department of General Pathology, University of Salamanca, Salamanca, Spain

Sabri Challah
EDTA Registry, St Thomas's Hospital, London, UK

Samarendra L. Choudhury
Geriatric Department, Chester City Hospital, Chester, UK

Jose L. Rodruiguez Commes
Department of Nephrology, Hospital Clinico Universitario, University of Salamanca, Spain

Alfonso Domínguez-Gil
Department of Pharmacy, Clinical Hospital, University of Salamanca, Salamanca, Spain

Anastasius S. Dontas
Department of Medicine, Accident Hospital, Kifissia, Greece

David Galinsky
Geriatric Department, Soroka University Hospital, Ben-Gurion University of the Negev, Beer Sheva, Israel

Manuel J. García
Department of Pharmacy, Clinical Hospital, University of Salamanca, Salamanca, Spain

Jeffrey L. Glickman
Division of Nephrology, University of Virginia School of Medicine, Charlottesville, Virginia, USA

Juan Montero Gomez
Department of Urology, University of Salamanca, Salamanca, Spain

Giorgio Graziani
Division of Nephrology and Dialysis, Ospedale Maggiore Policlinico, Milan, Italy

Pedro Gil Gregorio
Geriatric Department, Hospital Cruz Roja, Madrid, Spain

Glen W. Hartman
Mayo Clinic, Rochester, Minnesota, USA

Juan Corrales Hernandez
Department of Clinical Pathology, University of Salamanca, Salamanca, Spain

Keith E. Holley
Department of General Pathology, Mayo Clinic, Rochester, Minnesota, USA

Carmen G. Iglesias
Department of Epidemiology, Mayo Clinic, Rochester, Minnesota, USA

Donald L. Kaiser
Department of Medicine, University of Virginia School of Medicine, Charlottesville, Virginia, USA

Saulo Klahr
Department of Medicine, Renal Division, Washington University School of Medicine, St Louis, Missouri, USA

Francisco Guillén Llera
Geriatric Department, Hospital Cruz Roja, Madrid, Spain

José M. López Novoa
Department of Nephrology, Fundación Jiménez Diaz, Madrid, Spain

Maurice McLachlan
Department of Radiology, The Cheshire Hospital, Keene, New Hampshire, USA

Manuel Martínez-Maldonado
Medical Service, Veterans Administration Hospital, San Juan, Puerto Rico

Yitzhak Meller
Orthopaedic Department, Soroka University Hospital, Ben-Gurion University of the Negev, Beer Sheva, Israel

Timothy W. Meyer
Laboratory of Kidney and Electrolyte Physiology, Brigham and Women's Hospital, Boston, Massachusetts, USA

Inmaculada Montañes
Department of Experimental Medicine and Surgery, Hospital Provincial, Madrid, Spain

Richard Moore
Department of Bacteriology, Hammersmith Hospital, London, UK

Brian M. Murray
Department of Medicine, State University of New York at Buffalo, New York, USA

Amparo S. Navarro
Department of Pharmacy, Clinical Hospital, University of Salamanca, Salamanca, Spain

Juan F. Macias Nuñez
Department of Nephrology, Hospital Clinico Universitario, University of Salamanca, Salamanca, Spain

Claudio Ponticelli
Division of Nephrology and Dialysis, Ospedale Maggiore Policlinico, Milan, Italy

Leopoldo Raij
Department of Medicine, University of Minnesota Medical School, Minneapolis, Minnesota, USA

José L. Rodicio
Hospital 1° de Octubre, Universidad Complutense, Madrid, Spain

Antonio Bondia Roman
Hospital Clinico Universitario, University of Salamanca, Salamanca, Spain

Jose M. Tabernero Romo
Department of Nephrology, University of Salamanca, Salamanca, Spain

Luis M. Ruilope
Hospital 1° de Octubre, Universidad Complutense, Madrid, Spain

Assumpta Serra-Cardús
Department of Nephrology, Hospital de Badalona, 'Germans Trias i Pujol', Badalona, Barcelona, Spain

Shraga Shany
Clinical Biochemistry Unit, Soroka University Hospital, Ben-Gurion University of the Negev, Beer Sheva, Israel

Nathan W. Shock
Scientist Emeritus, Gerontology Research Center, National Institute of Aging, Francis Scott Key Medical Center, Baltimore, Maryland, USA

David Taube
Renal Unit, Dulwich Hospital, London, UK

José A. Sanchez Tomero
Department of Nephrology, Hospital Clinico Universitario, Salamanca, Spain

Vicente E. Torres
Division of Nephrology and Internal Medicine, Mayo Clinic, Rochester, Minnesota, USA

Vassilios D. Tzias
Department of Medicine, Accident Hospital, Kifissia, Greece

Preface

Why write a book on renal function and renal disease in old people?

Although nephrology itself, and later paediatric nephrology, are now established features of the medical scene, little attention has been paid hitherto to the renal problems of older and elderly populations. This is surprising, since even in the so-called developed world the proportion of older individuals is still slowly rising, particularly the very old; and the elderly population requires a disproportionately large amount of medical supervision and expenditure.

Figure 1 shows the elderly population of England and Wales during the past 130 years, up to 1981, and *Figure 2* shows projections of the proportion of elderly up to 2001 for Spain. By 2001, those over 65 will comprise almost one-sixth of the total population. In the USA, already more than 40 million individuals are over the age of 65. In some other countries such as the UK, the total of over-65s has already peaked at 18 per cent of the population, with a very slight decline in numbers projected during the following decades (*Figure 1*). The proportion of *very* elderly, however, will continue to rise beyond 2001, when it may be expected to flatten out with about 1.5 per cent of the total population over 85 years of age (*Figure 1*). In the USA, this means no fewer than 3.6 million individuals!

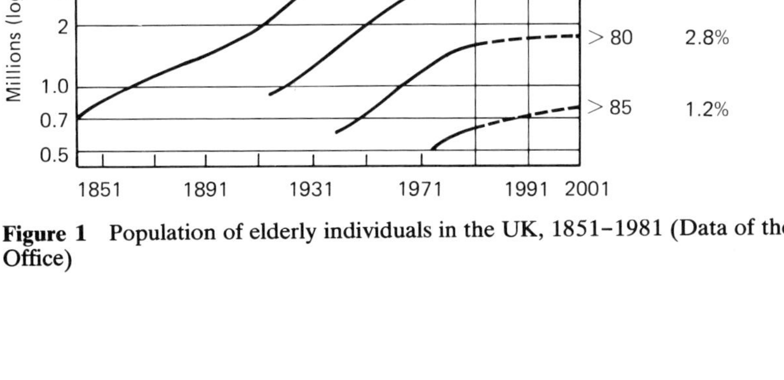

Figure 1 Population of elderly individuals in the UK, 1851–1981 (Data of the Registrar General's Office)

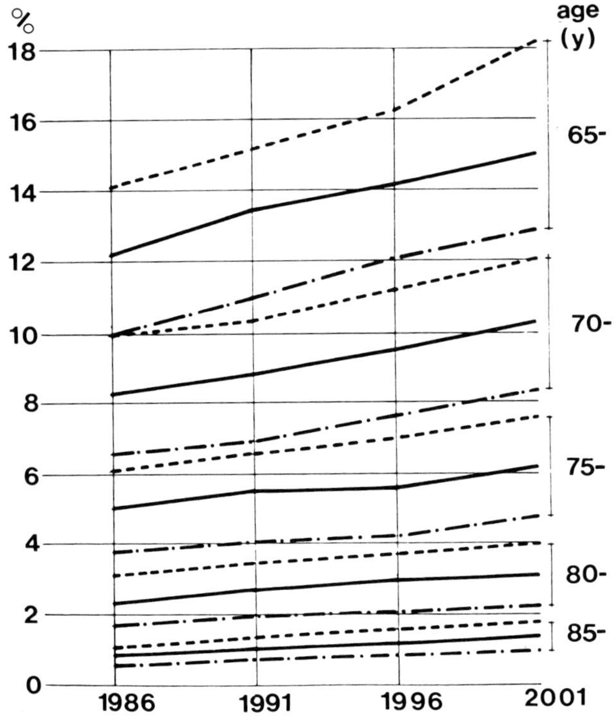

Figure 2 Projected proportions of total population of various age bands for 1986–2001 in Spain (- · - · -, men; ----, women; —, both)

In addition, as will become evident on reading this book, the incidence of many forms of renal disease, including such common entities as obstructive uropathy, interstitial nephritis and glomerulonephritis, becomes greater with age. The data for death from glomerulonephritis in the South-East and South-West Thames Region of the UK are shown in *Table 1:* the very high incidence of fatal glomerular disease in the elderly is immediately obvious. The death rate for glomerulonephritis, although it has fallen gradually in most Western countries for a century now, may even be increasing among the old (*Figure 3*).

Table 1 Death rates from nephritis and nephrosis (ICD 580–584) at various ages, South-East and South-West Thames Regions of the UK, 1980

	South-East	*South-West*
Overall:		
males	108	90
females	103	88
By age:	*Both regions, both sexes*	
0–14 yr	10	
15–44	50	
45–64	470	
> 65	5120	

Base population, 7 200 000; rates per million population per year.
(Source: Registrar General's Reports, 1980)

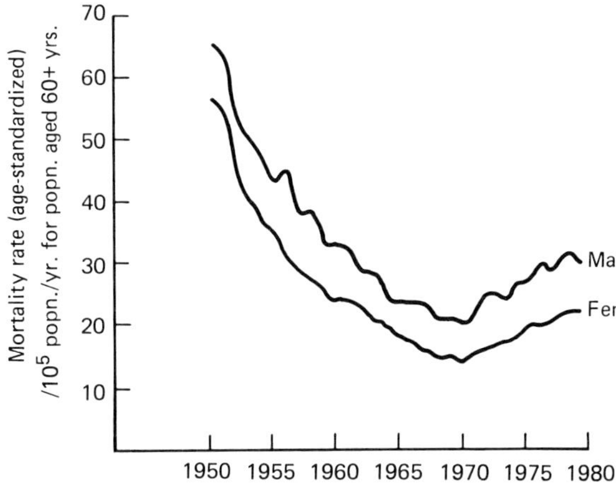

Figure 3 Death rates for nephritis and nephrosis (ICD 580–584) in the UK, 1950–80, for individuals more than 60 years of age (From Sorahan, T., Kotoszynska, R. and Adams, R.G. (1982). Trends in mortality from nephritis and nephrosis. *Lancet,* **1,** 567; reproduced with permission)

A theme which runs through all the chapters of this book is that older individuals, whether newly retired or very aged, have the right to expect the same attention and resources as their younger compatriots, even though no monetary return in national terms can be expected from this action; indeed, a great increase in health expenditure is made necessary by acceptance of this principle. The humanitarian and cultural advantages of preserving a healthy older population hardly needs stressing, but even though the majority of developed countries have accepted this responsibility tacitly or actively, nevertheless resources for the aged often fall well below those available to younger populations, and there is substantial underdiagnosis of renal disease in the elderly.

It is often forgotten by those not regularly concerned with their care just how long the aged can be expected to survive. At birth, the Japanese — world leaders in longevity — may expect, if female, to survive to 80 years of age on average and, if male, 76.5 years. Similar figures are found in Sweden and Switzerland, the leaders among European countries. The life expectancy of Americans (71.45 years at birth in 1973) is less than one might expect of this wealthy country. *Table 2* gives the data from England and Wales for the expected lifespan of those already aged, who are of course a selected population who have already survived the hazards of birth,

Table 2 Average life expectancy at various ages, England and Wales, 1981

	Estimated survival			
	Male		*Female*	
Age (yr)	*Life expectancy* (yr)	∴ *expected age at death* (yr)	*Life expectancy* (yr)	∴ *expected age at death* (yr)
65	12.4	77.4	16.4	81.4
70	10.9	80.9	14.4	84.4
75	7.4	82.4	9.8	87.8
80	6.8	86.8	8.7	88.7
85	4.6	89.6	5.6	90.6

(Source: Registrar General's Tables, 1981)

infancy, childhood and maturity. It is self-evident that expected survival decreases with age, but the extent of the years to come for those already aged 65, 70 or 80 years may surprise some readers. Our aim should be to ensure that old people with renal disease survive to enjoy any potentially 'lost' years in good health, wherever possible.

These figures of course apply to the lucky few who live in developed countries with adequate nutrition, housing and environment for the majority of citizens. At the other pole, life expectancy at birth remains below or around 40 years of age in India and many African countries, as it was in Sweden, the UK and the USA as recently as 1840. *Table 3* gives the population structure by age for different parts of the world. In the less developed world, the major impact of the increase in the numbers of the elderly is yet to come, but its appearance may be expected to be faster when it happens than in the so-called developed world.

Table 3 Population structure by age for different areas of the world

		Per cent of total population, age (yr)		
	Year	*0–14*	*15–64*	*> 65*
Whole world	1950	35	59.6	5.5
	1975	36	58.3	5.7
Developed countries	1950	27.9	64.6	7.6
	1975	25.0	64.5	10.5
Underdeveloped countries	1950	38.7	57.0	4.4
	1975	40.4	55.8	3.8
Europe	1950	25.4	65.9	8.7
	1975	23.9	63.8	12.3

(Source: *United Nations Concise Report on the World Population Situation in 1977.* New York, UNO)

Some may argue that the medical problems of the elderly are really the same as those of younger individuals, and that little is to be gained by attempting to highlight special medical problems of the aged. We believe that the contents of this book demonstrate the error of this attitude, even if we neglect to take into account the very different practical, social and psychological problems in the elderly. For instance, one is struck by the ease with which the elderly develop water and electrolyte imbalance in the presence of mild restriction or adverse conditions, leading to a number of clinical pictures ranging from behavioural alterations to acute renal failure. It is also important to recognize other changes of the normal aging process, such as low renin and aldosterone levels, in order to avoid superfluous searching for underlying pathology in the normal aged.

The biological and practical importance of the fall-off in some—but not all—renal functions with age hardly needs emphasis here. To what extent this process is inevitable, and whether or not it may be open to manipulation, has been the subject of much debate. Central to these discussions is whether or not data obtained in aging laboratory animals, whose kidneys differ structurally and functionally from the human kidney, can be applied to man. This important topic is dealt with in several chapters of this book.

While no one yet suggests that geriatric nephrology become a speciality like paediatric nephrology, we hope that this volume will redress the balance in thinking which we perceive to be out of equilibrium to the detriment of the aged.

We are particularly glad that Dr Nathan W. Shock, who provided so much of the basic functional data on the aging kidney, has contributed an introduction to the book, and record with regret that the end of a long struggle with illness deprived us of the contribution which Solomon Papper had agreed to make; this is a loss to us all.

JUAN F. MACIAS
Salamanca, Spain
J. STEWART CAMERON
London, England

Introduction

The kidney: a model for the study of aging in a physiological system

Nathan W. Shock

The kidney has been a most effective model for the study of aging in normal human subjects. This is due in part to the development of the clearance techniques by Homer Smith and his colleagues which made it possible to obtain quantitative estimates of discrete renal functions in normal human subjects (Smith, Goldring and Chasis, 1938). Clearances of inulin and creatinine provided reliable estimates of glomerular filtration rates, and estimates of effective renal plasma flow could be made from determinations of the clearance of diodrast or sodium para-aminohippurate (PAH). Furthermore, determinations of the maximum excretory capacity (T_m) for diodrast and the maximum resorptive capacity for glucose (T_m glucose) provided additional information on age differences in the ability of a physiological system to respond to stress.

Systematic measurements of these functions in normal human subjects of different ages, carefully screened to exclude any with clinical or laboratory evidence of cardiovascular or renal disease, provided the basic data needed for the emerging science of gerontology which looked upon aging and senescence as a normal part of the life-cycle rather than as a disease process. In short, thanks to studies made on normal subjects of different ages, aging became a part of physiology rather than pathology.

Thus cross-sectional studies on subjects in whom no evidence for renal disease could be detected offered the first data which showed clearly a systematic change in physiological function with increasing age, i.e. a gradual reduction in glomerular filtration rate, effective renal plasma flow, maximum excretory role for diodrast (Davies and Shock, 1950) or para-aminohippurate (PAH) (Miller, McDonald and Shock, 1950) and maximum capacity to reabsorb glucose (Miller, McDonald and Shock, 1952).

The studies also showed a marked range of values among subjects of the same chronological age. Some 70-year-old subjects performed as well as the average 60-year-old. Thus the individuality of aging was clearly demonstrated (Shock, 1952).

The kidney also provided the vehicle to test hypotheses about the effects of aging on the responsiveness of physiological adaptive mechanisms. For example, it was possible to show that with advancing age the sensitivity of renal tubules to endogenously administered pitressin was diminished. Young subjects responded to a standard intravenous dose of pitressin with a greater resorption of glomerular filtrate than did the old subjects (McDonald, Solomon and Shock, 1951). Thus age differences in physiological responses to normal stimuli could be demonstrated in intact humans.

Longitudinal studies in which measurements were repeated on the same subjects at one- to two-year intervals over a period of 25 years showed that although glomerular filtration rates, estimated from creatinine clearance in individual subjects, tended to follow a downward trend in most subjects as they aged (65 and over), individuals often differed in the pathway they followed (Rowe *et al.*, 1976). Some subjects maintained uniform glomerular filtration rates even into advanced old age. Pathways of aging showed marked individual differences (Lindeman, Tobin and Shock, 1984).

The kidney served as the proving ground for many studies which provide the basis for current knowledge about the effects of aging on many other organ systems. Studies on the kidney led the way.

References

DAVIES, D.F. and SHOCK, N.W. (1950). Age changes in glomerular filtration rate, effective renal plasma flow, and tubular excretory capacity in adult males. *Journal of Clinical Investigation,* **29,** 496–507

LINDEMAN, R.D., TOBIN, J. and SHOCK, N.W. (1984). Longitudinal studies on the rate of decline in renal function with age. Paper presented at the meeting of the Ninth International Congress of Nephrology, Los Angeles, CA, June 1984

MCDONALD, R.K., SOLOMON, D.H. and SHOCK, N.W. (1951). Aging as a factor in the renal hemodynamic changes induced by a standardized pyrogen. *Journal of Clinical Investigation,* **30,** 457–462

MILLER, B.J., MCDONALD, R.K. and SHOCK, N.W. (1950). The effect of bacitracin on renal function. *Journal of Clinical Investigation,* **29,** 389–395

MILLER, J.H., MCDONALD, R.K. and SHOCK, N.W. (1952). Age changes in the maximal rate of renal tubular reabsorption of glucose. *Journal of Gerontology,* **7,** 196–200

ROWE, J.W., ANDRES, R., TOBIN, J.D., NORRIS, A.H. and SHOCK, N.W. (1976). The effect of age on creatinine clearance in men: a cross-sectional and longitudinal study. *Journal of Gerontology,* **31,** 155–163

SHOCK, N.W. (1952). Age changes in renal function. In *Cowdry's Problems of Aging,* 3rd edn, edited by A.I. Lansing. Baltimore, MD, Williams and Wilkins

SMITH, H.W., GOLDRING, W. and CHASIS, H. (1938). The measurement of the tubular excretory mass, effective blood flow, and filtration rate in the normal human kidney. *Journal of Clinical Investigation,* **17,** 263

Chapter 1

Anatomic structural and vascular changes in the aging kidney

Maurice McLachlan

[*This chapter is dedicated to my good friend, the late John Hodson*]

'This condition of the kidney . . . is as characteristic of age as is the shrunken shank and tottering gait.' (Councilman, 1919)

'The problem which we have now to consider is one of the most alluring and the most baffling in pathology — alluring, perhaps, by its very subtlety.' (Allbutt, 1915)

Introduction

This chapter examines changes in renal morphology which accompany aging. It deals for the most part with those changes which affect the nephron and the renal vessels. In an extensive literature on the subject, sharp distinction is not always made between the results of aging and those of hypertension, particularly in the small arteries and arterioles. Opinion, nevertheless, although still divided, has in the past three decades moved closer to unanimity. Heptinstall (1974) reviewed some of the difficulties. Definitions of hypertension vary; conclusions at necropsy must at times be based on incomplete clinical information; conclusions at biopsy must generally be based on small, possibly unrepresentative samples. Opinion which rests so heavily on necropsy material suffers other disadvantages. Selective mortality, the argument that longevity depends on special characteristics, is one; the possibility of secular variation and of variation between cohorts, which undermines many investigations of the effects of aging, is another (Rowe *et al.*, 1976; Rowe, 1977). Moreover, although chronological age, paradoxically, may not be the best index of aging, there appears to be none better. With these cautionary remarks, the chapter begins. Despite the haze, despite the objects that obscure the view, it is still possible, with reasonable clarity, to chart the landscape and to examine, here and there, minute details of its complex topography.

Gross morphology

In early descriptions (Furno, 1909; Councilman, 1919) the typical senile kidney is said to be small and smooth in outline, 'a starved, but not a corrupt kidney . . . sufficient for the smaller life of an elderly man' (Allbutt, 1915). At necropsy, when renal disease has been excluded, only about 12 or 14 per cent of kidneys in the elderly are coarsely scarred; over half are smooth or manifest only a fine granularity

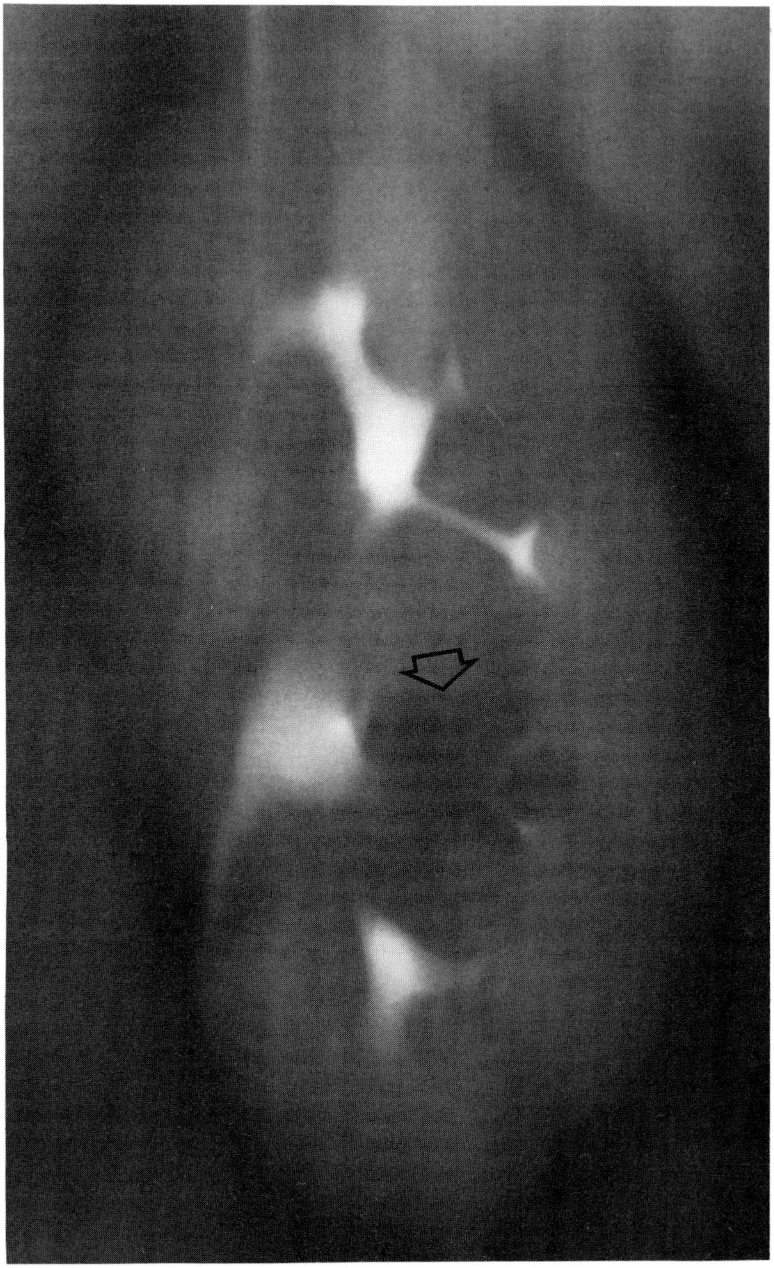

Figure 1.1 Tomography of the left kidney of a 59-year-old man during intravenous urography. It is normal in size, with normal calyces, but shows some irregularity of its surface and increased amounts of fat in its sinus (arrow). Most elderly kidneys are smooth in outline or only finely scarred

of their surface (McKeown, 1965; Griffiths *et al.*, 1976). Even with the inclusion of a few hypertensive subjects, the results are similar (Howell and Piggot, 1948). Unlike pyelonephritic scarring, which is associated with caliectasis and is usually seen at the poles (Hodson, 1959, 1968), these scars occur at all sites in the kidney, with no deformity of calyces, and are readily confused with fetal lobation on intravenous urograms (Griffiths *et al.*, 1976; *Figure 1.1).*

Necropsy evidence also suggests that the weight of the adult human kidney remains fairly constant until the fifth decade of life; between then and the eighth decade its weight diminishes by about one-fifth (Roessle and Roulet, 1932; deLeon, Garcia and deJesus, 1933; Wald, 1937). The decline in renal dimensions is less well documented in life. It may be greater than post-mortem evidence implies. At intravenous urography, renal length may diminish by as much as 2 cm between the fifth and eighth decades (McLachlan and Wasserman, 1981; *Figure 1.2*). This

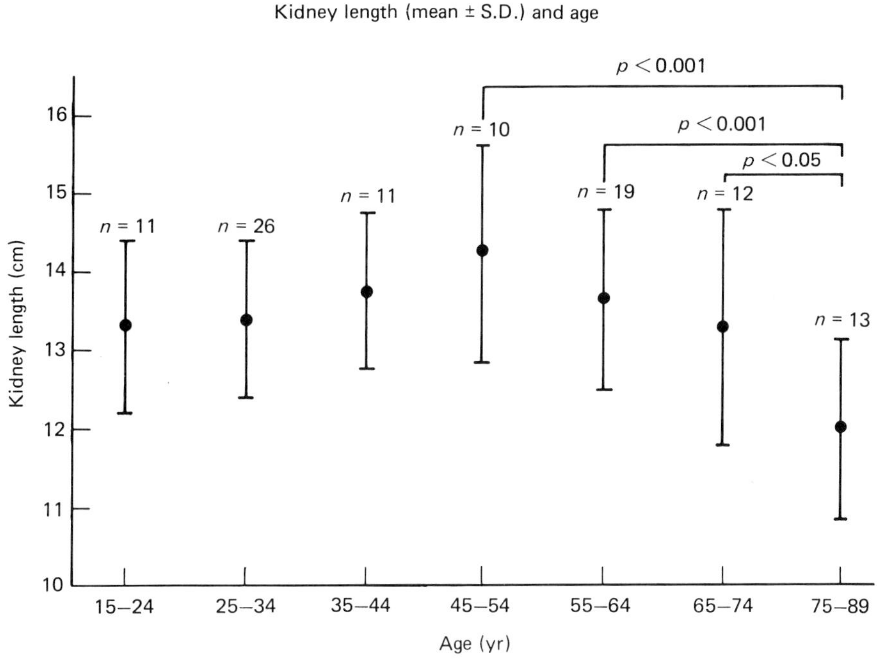

Figure 1.2 Measurements of renal length, obtained from intravenous urograms, grouped according to age. The decline after the middle years exceeds that expected from necropsy evidence. Numbers of subjects and significant differences are indicated (From McLachlan and Wasserman, 1981, by permission of the Editors, *British Journal of Radiology*)

represents a loss of volume of about 40 per cent, twice that recorded at necropsy. Evidence from computerized tomography (*Figure 1.3*) is similar. McLachlan and Kaplan (1981 and unpublished) measured transverse renal area in apparently healthy, normotensive adults who were examined for reasons unrelated to the urinary tract (*Figure 1.4*). The decline which they recorded after the age of 70 suggests a reduction in volume of about one-third. Measurements of cortical thickness obtained by similar techniques (Ishikawa *et al.*, 1981) also imply a reduction in renal size considerably greater than post-mortem evidence indicates.

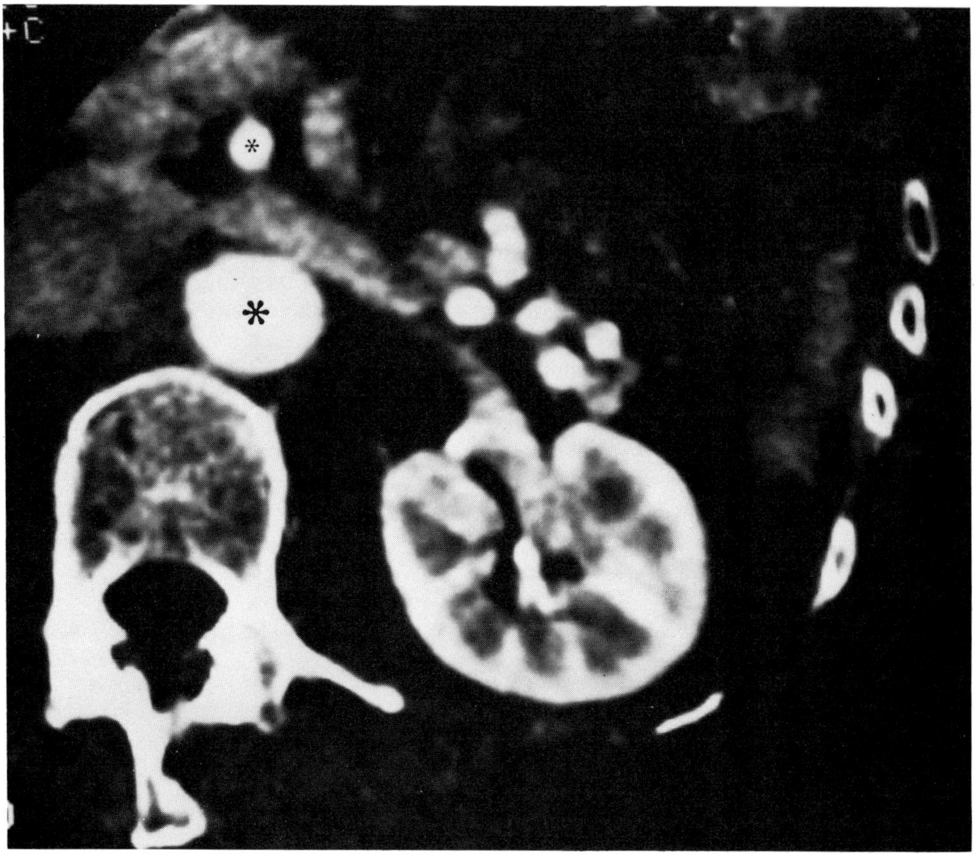

Figure 1.3 Computerized tomography of the left kidney of a 64-year-old man after rapid intravenous injection of radiographic contrast medium. Cortex, medulla and the contents of the renal sinus are well displayed. The technique allows accurate estimates of the proportion of the kidney occupied by these components in life. The aorta (large asterisk) and superior mesenteric artery (small asterisk) are densely opacified. The left renal vein is shown running between them to join inferior vena cava

The loss of substance, even in the absence of coarse scarring, is not uniform. It affects cortex slightly more than medulla. This was shown by Dunnill and Halley (1973) by point-counting techniques in sliced kidneys removed after death due to trauma. It has subsequently been confirmed by post-mortem renal angiography (Griffiths *et al.*, 1976; McLachlan *et al.*, 1977) and, more recently, by computerized tomography *in vivo* (Ishikawa *et al.*, 1981). As the cortex becomes thinner, glomeruli tend to become more crowded together (Oliver, 1952; McLachlan *et al.*, 1976). However, some variation in cortical substance is not age related. Dunnill and Halley (1973), in the adult kidneys which they examined, recorded a fourfold difference in the fraction of cortical volume occupied by tissue other than glomeruli and tubules; it varied independently of age. Perhaps for this reason, crowding of glomeruli may not be obvious on routine histological specimens (Goyal, 1982). In the medulla, on the other hand, interstitial tissue increases with age, fibrosis becoming especially marked after the seventh decade, when it may lead to atrophy of the pyramids (Keresztury and Megyeri, 1962). The development of interstitial fibrosis probably results from diminishing concentrations of acid mucopolysaccharides in the medulla; cortical concentrations do not change (Inoue *et al.*, 1970).

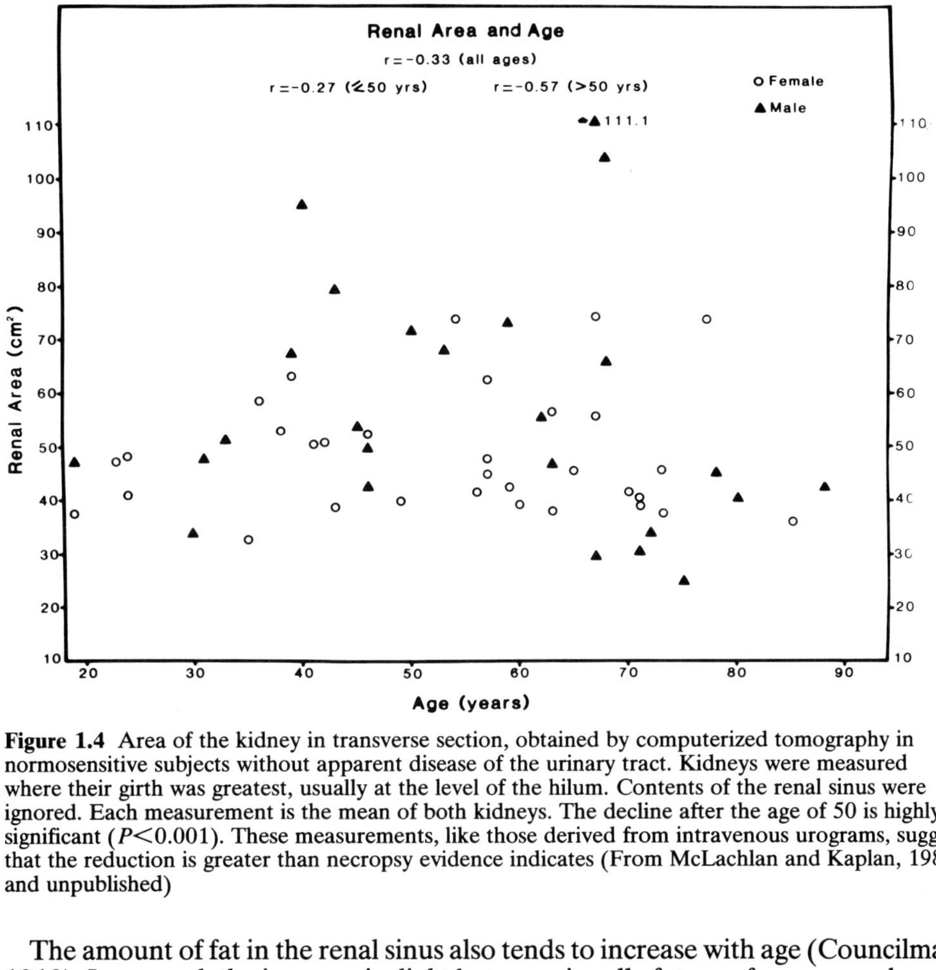

Figure 1.4 Area of the kidney in transverse section, obtained by computerized tomography in normosensitive subjects without apparent disease of the urinary tract. Kidneys were measured where their girth was greatest, usually at the level of the hilum. Contents of the renal sinus were ignored. Each measurement is the mean of both kidneys. The decline after the age of 50 is highly significant ($P<0.001$). These measurements, like those derived from intravenous urograms, suggest that the reduction is greater than necropsy evidence indicates (From McLachlan and Kaplan, 1981 and unpublished)

The amount of fat in the renal sinus also tends to increase with age (Councilman, 1919). In general, the increase is slight but occasionally fat may form as much as 17 per cent of the post-mortem weight of the kidney (Griffiths, Cartwright and McLachlan, 1975). The fat is usually apparent on computerized tomography (McLachlan and Kaplan, 1981 and unpublished; *Figure 1.5*), which has also confirmed (Hattery *et al.*, 1977) what the observations of morbid anatomists and surgeons (Councilman, 1919; Fahr, 1925; Braasch and Hendrick, 1944; Kissane, 1974) have long indicated: simple cysts are common in the aging kidney. They are unusual before the fifth decade, but increase in frequency and size thereafter (Laucks and McLachlan, 1981). The tendency for apparently functionless material to accumulate within the kidney as it ages, together with changes in the nephron which are discussed later, make renal dimensions derived from intravenous urograms imperfect indices of the amount of functioning renal tissue (Friedman *et*

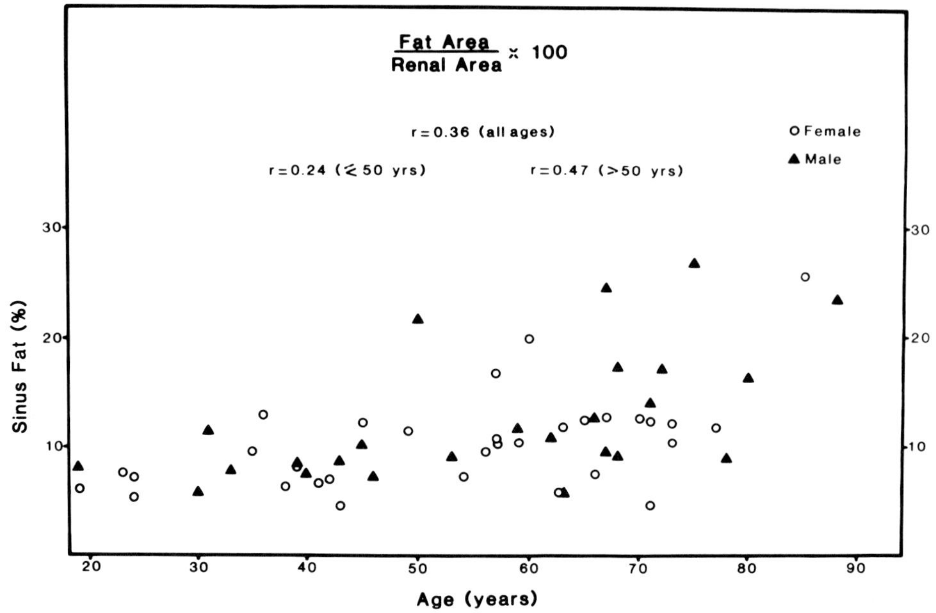

Figure 1.5 Area of fat in the renal sinus, measured from transverse sections of the kidney obtained by computerized tomography, expressed as a percentage of renal area measured in the same level. Subjects are the same as those discussed in *Figure 1.4*. The proportion of fat increases with age ($P<0.01$) (From McLachlan and Kaplan, 1981 and unpublished)

al., 1972; McLachlan *et al.*, 1976). Despite these developments, which might be expected to make the kidney a more rigid structure, aging does not appear to affect its capacity to distend in response to an osmotic load (McLachlan and Wasserman, 1981).

Changes in the vessels

Age-related changes in the histopathology of renal vessels (*Figure 1.6*) have been well documented since the early descriptions by Moritz and Oldt (1937). Bell (1950) described them in detail. In small arteries, interlobular in size, there is a progressive thickening of the intima, consisting mainly of elastic tissue. This is associated with atrophy of the media, which becomes almost entirely absent when intimal thickening is greatest. In pre-arterioles, terminal arteries from which afferent arterioles arise, the intima becomes thickened by the subendothelial deposition of hyaline and collagen fibres. Changes in the arterioles are similar, although fibrous material is present less commonly. Nevertheless, despite these careful descriptions, some confusion exists. Darmady, Offer and Woodhouse (1973) comment on how the literature varies in defining arteriosclerosis; intimal proliferation, hyalinization, hypertrophy and fibrosis, either singly or in combination, are all included within its boundaries. For vessels larger than arterioles, there is fairly general agreement: progressive reduplication of elastic tissue and thickening of the intima are predominantly age related (McKeown, 1965; Darmady, Offer and Woodhouse, 1973) and precede the subendothelial deposition of hyaline material in afferent arterioles (Bell, 1950; Oliver, 1952; Smith, 1955).

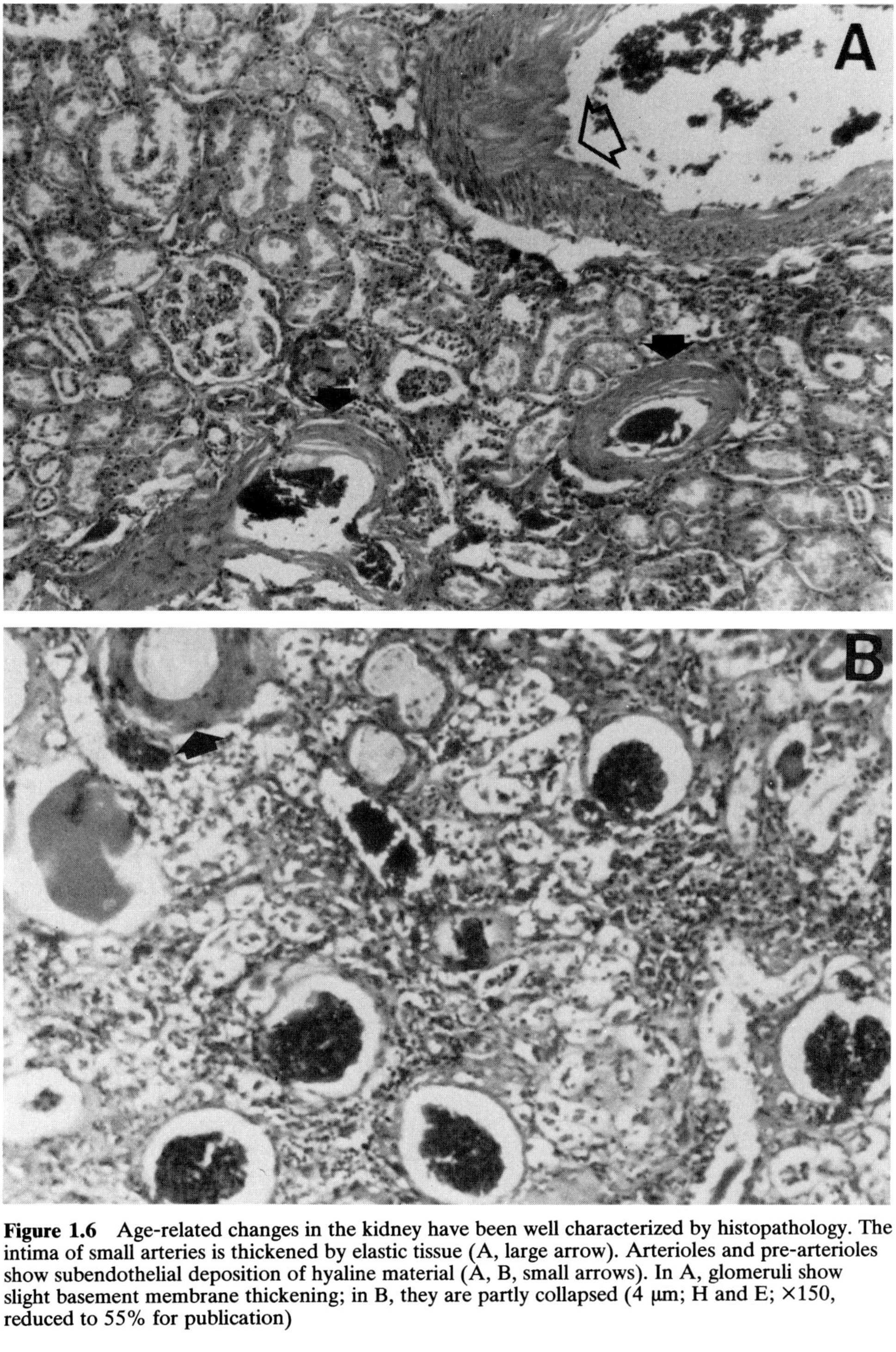

Figure 1.6 Age-related changes in the kidney have been well characterized by histopathology. The intima of small arteries is thickened by elastic tissue (A, large arrow). Arterioles and pre-arterioles show subendothelial deposition of hyaline material (A, B, small arrows). In A, glomeruli show slight basement membrane thickening; in B, they are partly collapsed (4 μm; H and E; ×150, reduced to 55% for publication)

At this level, authorities disagree. Williams and Harrison (1937) considered afferent arteriolosclerosis to be 'mainly the result of hypertension, increasing age being a less important factor than in the case of the larger renal arteries'. However, Bell (1950) left little doubt about where he stood: 'renal arteriolosclerosis is . . . an age change which develops independently of hypertension'. His opinion was based on nearly 18 000 necropsies. Smith (1955) was almost as emphatic and this view now appears to prevail (Heptinstall, 1974). Hypertension merely accelerates the change (Bell, 1950). The efferent arterioles were also considered in detail by Smith (1955) who concluded that, in the absence of diabetes mellitus, sclerosis at this site too was a phenomenon of aging.

Changes appear in small arteries as early as the second decade, but the most pronounced begin after the age of 30; arteriolar changes occur later (Bell, 1950; Smith, 1955; *Tables 1.1* and *1.2*). The pre-arterioles examined by Bell (1950)

Table 1.1 Grades of sclerosis in small arteries by age group (Data from Bell, 1950)

	Subjects (%)			
	Grade			
Age (yr)	*0*	*1*	2	*3*
10–19	71	29	0	0
20–29	46	42	12	0
30–39	26.5	53	11.7	8.8
40–49	8.6	56.9	24.1	10.4
50–59	0	58.8	22.8	18.4
60–69	0	34.9	39.5	25.5
70–79	0	18.5	32.1	49.4
80 and over	0	12.9	45.1	42

Table 1.2 Grades of arteriolosclerosis by age group (Data from Bell, 1950)

	Subjects (%)				
	Grade				
Age (yr)	*0*	*1p**	*1*	2	*3*
10–19	100	0	0	0	0
20–29	88.5	7.7	3.8	0	0
30–39	79.4	17.6	0	0	3
40–49	72.4	17.2	8.6	0	1.7
50–59	71	18.4	8.8	1.8	0
60–69	62.8	22.1	11.6	3.5	0
70–79	50.6	28.4	17.3	2.4	1.2
80 and over	51.6	19.3	25.8	3.2	0

*Occasional hyaline deposits.

occupied an intermediate position, being affected less frequently than small arteries but more frequently than arterioles. From the time of first appearance of the lesions, progression appears to occur fairly steadily and Bell (1950) could find no small artery which was entirely normal after the age of 50. However, this may not always be the case. Over one-third of subjects studied by Bell (1950) who were over 70 years old had normal pre-arterioles. In their meticulous micro-angiographic

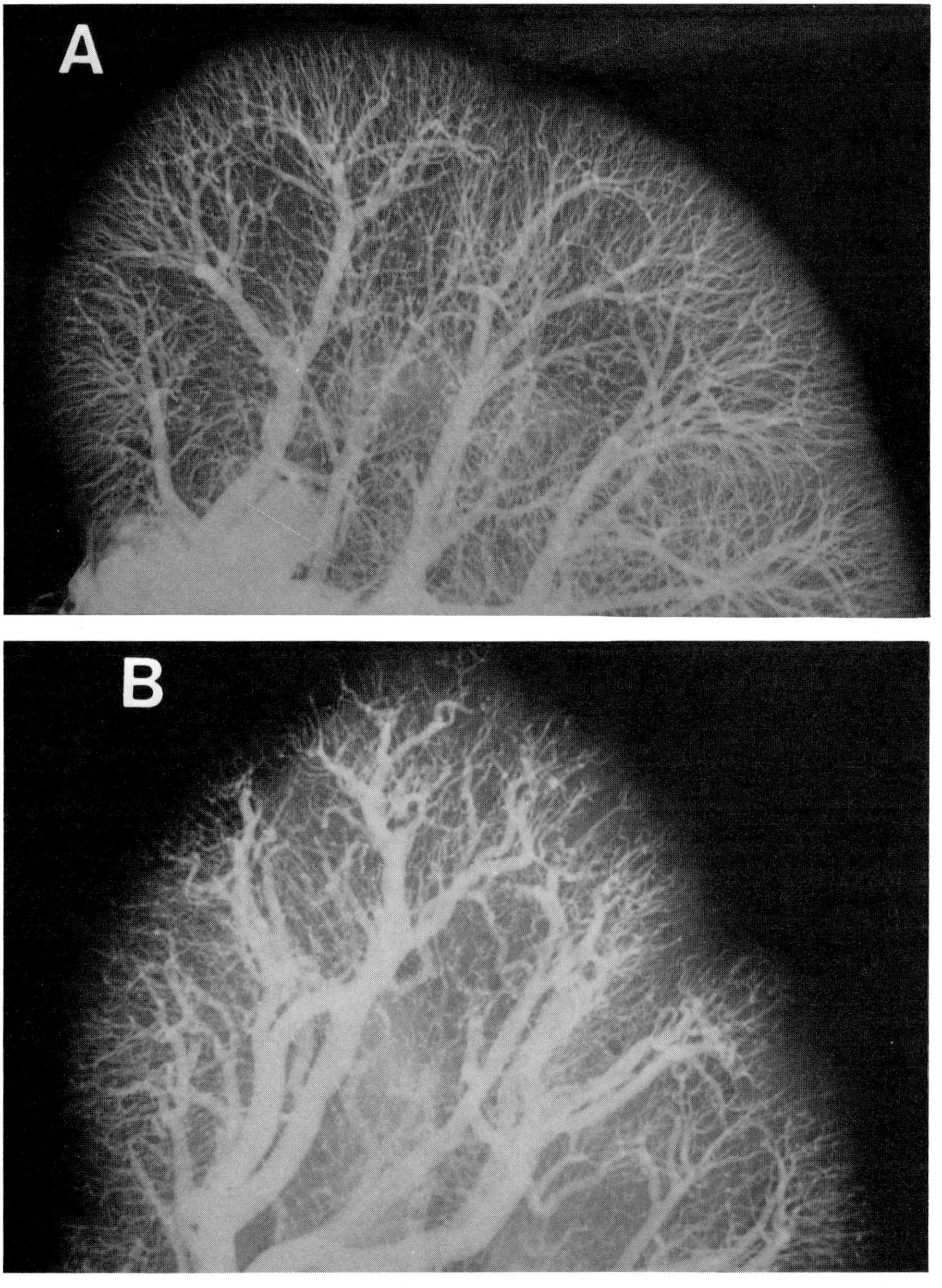

Figure 1.7 Post-mortem renal angiography in a 20-year-old man (A) and 73-year-old woman (B). Vessels to the level of interlobular arteries are demonstrated. The older kidney, which is scarred, shows poor opacification of small arteries and more tortuosity. Vascular change is generally greatest in the most peripheral arteries and at the poles, although scarring is not. Changes precede those observed histologically in arterioles

examination of the aging normotensive kidney, Ljungqvist and Lagergren (1962), who recorded increasing tortuosity ('spiralling') of the afferent arterioles, noted no differences between the ages of 60 and 79.

Post-mortem angiography (*Figure 1.7*) has been used by two groups of investigators (Davidson, Talner and Downs, 1969; Griffiths *et al.*, 1976) to examine semiquantitatively the more proximal renal vessels, up to the level of interlobular arteries. In kidneys removed from normotensive subjects, they observed angiographic abnormality of interlobular and arcuate arteries when the arterioles were histologically normal. They recorded the most severe changes in the most peripheral arteries, particularly those at the poles. However, they found no correlation between age and severity of vascular change in subjects more than 50 years old. Significant differences became apparent only when young and elderly subjects were compared. Observations in angiograms obtained in life are similar (Hollenberg *et al.*, 1969). The vascular changes appear to be structural rather than the result of spasm. In their examination of more than 200 potential kidneys donors, Hollenberg *et al.* (1974) demonstrated a reduction in the extent to which acetylcholine or sodium-loading could induce renal vasodilatation as age advanced.

Changes in the nephron

Glomeruli become fewer as the kidney ages. Moore (1931), in a widely quoted investigation, concluded that the mature adult kidney contained between 600 000 and 1.2 million glomeruli. He recorded one-half or two-thirds as many in subjects dying in the seventh decade of their lives. His technique, which included maceration of kidney tissue, did not allow him to examine histology. Many of the subjects he studied died from diseases which may affect the kidney; 6 of the 18 adults suffered from chronic pulmonary tuberculosis. Dunnill and Halley (1973) applied stereological techniques (Elias and Hennig, 1967; Weibel, 1969; Underwood, 1970; Elias, Hennig and Schwartz, 1971) to histological sections from kidneys obtained after accidental death. They documented a reduction in glomerular number of about 25 per cent, beginning, in accord with the results of Moore (1931), towards the end of the fourth decade of life, but only 4 of their 9 adults were more than 40 years old. Other work by similar techniques (McLachlan *et al.*, 1977) in larger numbers of elderly subjects confirmed that glomeruli tend to become fewer in number with age (*Figure 1.8*). Rather higher numbers of glomeruli were recorded, about 1.3 million on average, but with wide variation between individuals. In the sixth and seventh decades of life, the number of glomeruli varied more than threefold. This is not accounted for by the development of new glomeruli, which do not appear to be formed after birth (Vimtrup, 1928; Dunnill and Halley, 1973; McLachlan *et al.*, 1977).

Changes in the morphology of the aging nephron have been extensively characterized by histopathology (Oliver, 1952; Darmady, Offer and Woodhouse, 1973; *Figure 1.6*). The basement membrane of glomeruli and tubules becomes thicker and reduplicated. Tubular cells undergo fatty degeneration. After the third decade of life, glomerular sclerosis begins. Glomeruli collapse or are completely replaced by hyaline material. Oliver (1952) described hyalinization extending into the tuft from the afferent arteriole, similar to the changes observed in hypertension (McManus and Lupton, 1960). He concluded that this hyalinization preceded their disappearance, sclerosis replacing the glomerular tufts or, by occlusion, causing

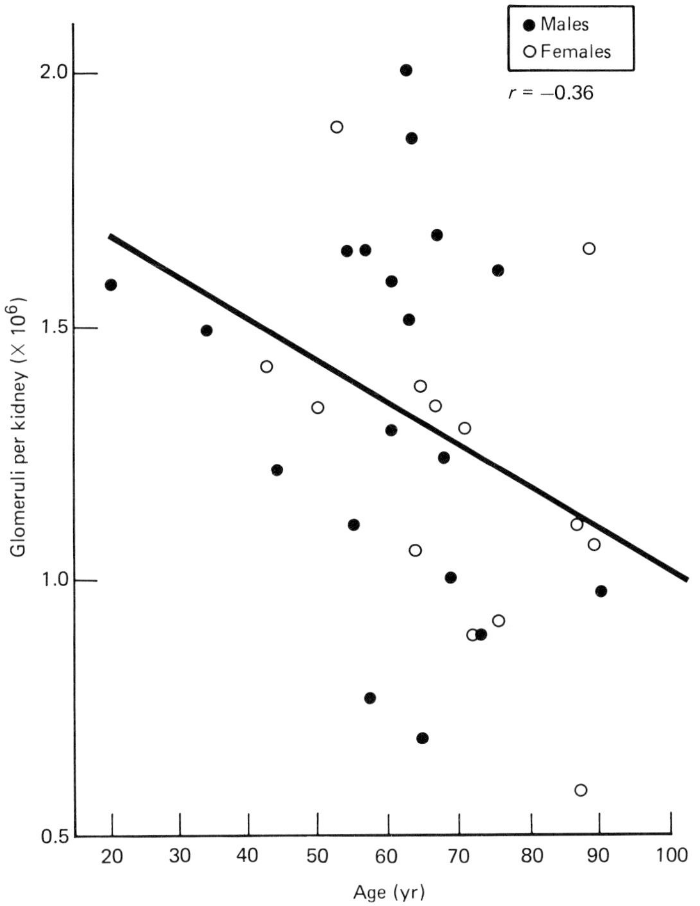

Figure 1.8 Glomeruli become fewer with age, but correlation is poor ($P<0.05$), with large differences between individuals (From McLachlan *et al.*, 1977, by permission of the Editors, *Journal of Pathology*)

their collapse. The proportion of hyalinized, obliterated glomeruli in the adult kidney tends to increase with age, particularly in men, but it varies widely (*Figure 1.9*). In subjects over the age of 50, the proportion ranges from 1 to 30 per cent (Kaplan *et al.*, 1975; McLachlan *et al.*, 1977) and is unrelated to the total number of glomeruli (McLachlan, unpublished). Presumably it depends on rates of obliteration and disappearance. Micro-angiography has provided striking evidence that obliteration of juxtamedullary nephrons, but not those sited more peripherally, establishes a direct continuity between afferent and efferent arterioles (Ljungqvist and Lagergren, 1962; Takazakura *et al.*, 1972; *Figure 1.10*).

Studies by electron microscopy are more limited. Darmady, Offer and Woodhouse (1973), who encountered difficulties due to post-mortem autolysis, examined the tubules. They concluded that the thickness of basement membrane varied greatly, with some nephrons showing little or no increase. Moreover, the thickening was not uniform, even within a single nephron. Recently, Steffes *et al.* (1983) have applied stereological methods (Elias and Hennig, 1967; Weibel, 1969; Underwood, 1970; Elias, Hennig and Schwartz, 1971) to electron micrographs of

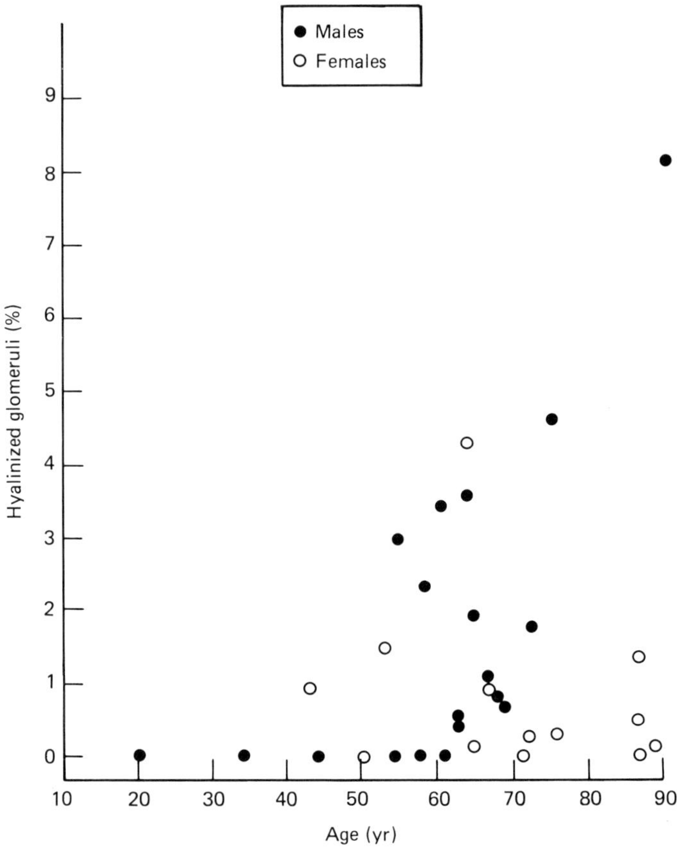

Figure 1.9 The proportion of completely hyalinized glomeruli tends to increase with age, but variation between individuals is wide. The number of these glomeruli is here expressed as a percentage of total glomerular number in each kidney. They are slightly more common in men, in whom a significant correlation with age exists ($r = 0.64$; $P < 0.01$) (From McLachlan *et al.*, 1977, by permission of the Editors, *Journal of Pathology*)

glomeruli obtained by open biopsy in healthy kidney donors. They observed increasing thickness of the glomerular basement membrane until the fourth decade, but no further increase thereafter. However, though they examined well over 100 normal kidneys, a disproportionately small number came from these older groups.

Electron microscopy has been more extensively applied in animals. Thickening of basement membrane has been shown to occur with aging in the glomerulus of a strain of golden hamster (McNelly and Dittmer, 1976) and the glomerulus and tubule of the Sprague–Dawley rat (Ashworth, Erdmann and Arnold, 1960; Couser and Stilmant, 1975, 1976; Haley and Bulger, 1983). canning electron microscopy, by documenting an age-related increase in the number of podocyte microvilli, suggests that this also occurs in at least one strain of mice (Johnson and Barrows, 1980). These observations in animals support evidence in the human kidney, but it is worth emphasizing that, even between strains of mice, changes in the nephron differ in their degree (Hackbarth and Harrison, 1982).

The most distal portions of the nephron have received less attention. Histology

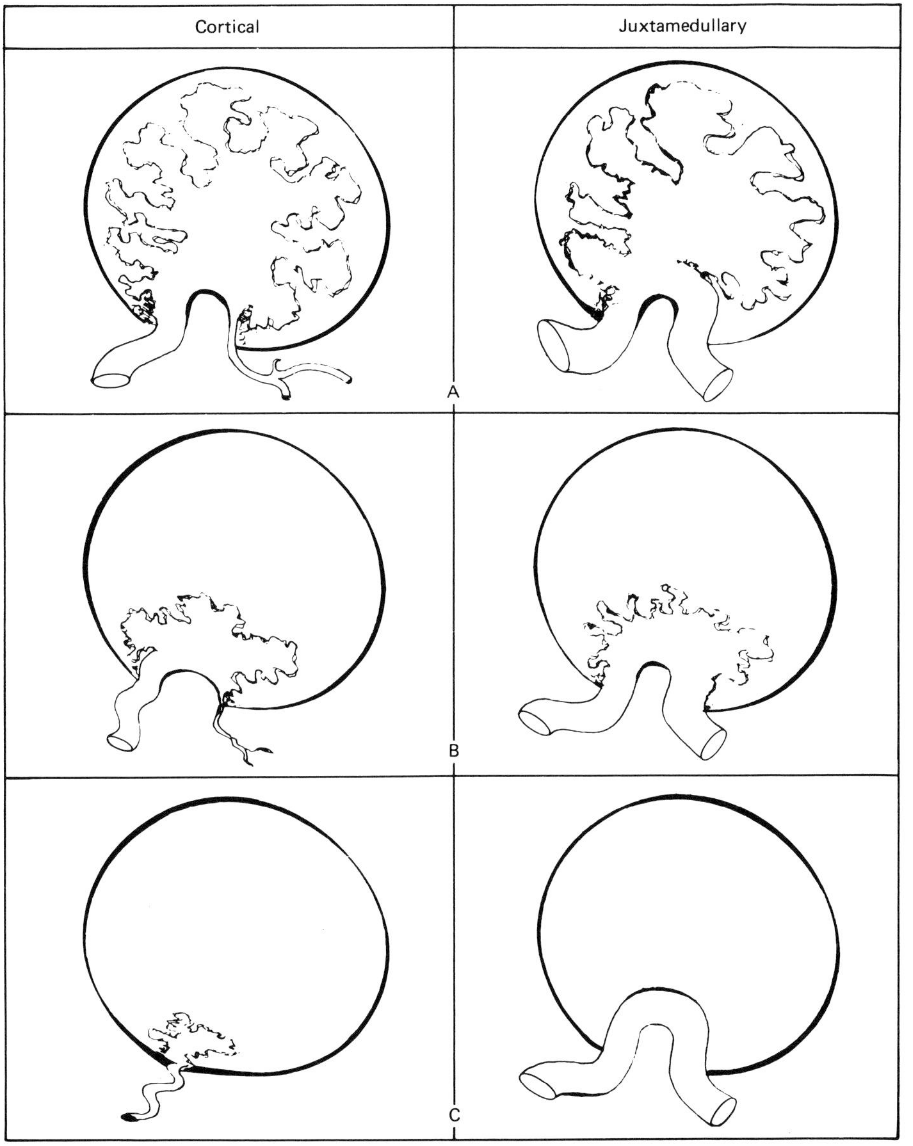

Figure 1.10 Micro-angiography demonstrates important differences in the vascular consequences of glomerular degeneration in juxtamedullary (right) and the more peripheral nephrons (left). Changes are shown progressing from top to bottom (A–C). In healthy peripheral nephrons the afferent arteriole forms glomerular capillaries which then join to become efferent arterioles; in juxtamedullary nephrons glomerular capillaries more closely resemble side branches of a continuous afferent–efferent arteriolar unit. When peripheral glomeruli degenerate, afferent arterioles end blindly; degeneration of juxtamedullary glomeruli results in direct communication between afferent and efferent arterioles (After Ljungqvist and Lagergren, 1962 and Takazakura *et al.*, 1972)

demonstrates dilatation of collecting tubules (Keresztury and Megyeri, 1962). Microdissection, despite the difficulties produced in the elderly kidney by medullary fibrosis, has not only confirmed this ectasia but has provided graphic demonstration of diverticula arising from distal and convoluted tubules (Darmady, Offer and Woodhouse, 1973; Baert and Steg, 1977). These become more common with age, 15 or 20 sometimes arising from a single nephron, and probably result from weakening of the tubular basement membrane (Darmady, Offer and Woodhouse, 1973). Some (Baert and Steg, 1977) have considered them to be precursors of simple renal cysts. In general, however, they retain their tubular connection, varying from 'little more than side pouches to pedunculated sacs' (Darmady, Offer and Woodhouse, 1973). Many contain histological evidence of casts, epithelial debris and organisms, leading Darmady, Offer and Woodhouse (1973) to propose them as likely sources of recurrent urinary tract infection. These changes in the distal nephron could then help explain the association between bacteriuria and diminished tubular function in the elderly (Dontas *et al.*, 1966; Dontas, Marketos and Papanayiotou, 1972; Alwall, 1978). If diverticula 'act as a focal point from which infection might spread to the surrounding tissue' (Darmady, Offer and Woodhouse, 1973), they could provoke medullary fibrosis and, by mechanisms discussed later, the glomerular obsolescence with which bacteriuria appears to be associated (Curtis, 1968).

In addition to subjective assessment, many changes in morphology of the nephron have been carefully quantified. Glomerular and tubular dimensions have been measured after microdissection, in attempts to establish to whatt extent the aging nephron degenerates as a unit. The results are conflicting. Oliver and MacDowell (1961) exhaustively examined 3 kidneys obtained after accidental death in the fourth decade of life. They demonstrated a highly significant correlation between the dimensions of glomeruli and proximal convoluted tubules. However, Oliver (1952) concluded that in later life 'there is little correlation between the size of glomerulus and tubule', adding, for emphasis, 'the tubule of the nephron does not constantly degenerate after glomerular destruction'. He described hypertrophy with hyperplasia of the proximal tubules of glomeruli which were normal in size, atrophied or even destroyed. More distal parts of the nephron were much less affected. Darmady, Offer and Woodhouse (1973) applied similar techniques to material drawn from over 100 subjects, including the newborn and the extremely old, who died 'acute or relatively sudden death'. They arrived at different conclusions. After the third or fourth decade, the volume of the glomeruli and proximal tubules diminished at the same rate, from which the authors concluded that 'renal function, although reduced, is still in balance'. They saw no tubular hyperplasia or hypertrophy and no aglomerular tubules. The differences between these two groups of scrupulous observers have not yet been reconciled.

Wide variation between individuals may provide an explanation. McLachlan *et al.* (1977) examined age-related changes in glomerular shape. In histological preparations they related the length of the perimeter of the glomerular tuft to its cross-sectional area. With aging, this ratio changed, reflecting a loss of glomerular lobulation. However, although obvious differences existed when young and old kidneys were compared, glomerular shape varied greatly in subjects aged 50 and over, in whom there was no significant correlation between this shape factor and age. In the 3 adult kidneys studied by Oliver and MacDowell (1961; *Table 1.3*), there was a twofold difference in mean glomerular volume between individuals; the difference in mean tubular volume, although less, was still considerable. Within

Table 1.3 Dimensions of the normal nephron (Data from Oliver and MacDowell, 1961)

Subject *Age* (yr)	*Sex*	*Glomerular volume* (mm^3) *Range*	*Mean*	*Proximal tubular volume* (mm^3) *Range*	*Mean*
32	F	0.0030–0.0191	0.0083	0.034–0.128	0.077
34	M	0.0055–0.0271	0.0133	0.036–0.105	0.069
40	M	0.0111–0.0301	0.0177	0.076–0.123	0.100

individual kidneys, variation was even greater. Glomerular volume varied as much as sixfold and proximal tubular volume only slightly less. Variation is similar in the immature kidney (Darmady *et al.*, 1964; Fetterman *et al.*, 1965; Darmady, Offer and Woodhouse, 1973), in which it does not appear to be due to artefact or to differences between zones. In the adult kidney, the dimensions of juxtamedullary nephrons are only twice those of the average nephron from a more peripheral site (Darmady, Offer and Woodhouse, 1973).

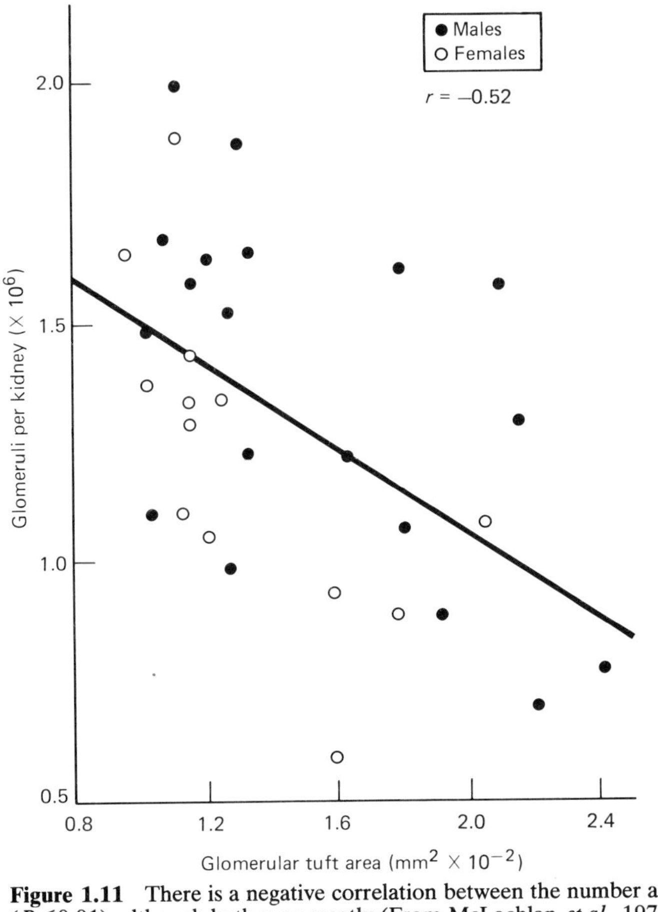

Figure 1.11 There is a negative correlation between the number and dimensions of glomeruli ($P<0.01$), although both vary greatly (From McLachlan *et al.*, 1977, by permission of the Editors, *Journal of Pathology*)

McLachlan *et al.* (1977) confirmed the variation in glomerular dimensions between individuals and demonstrated a significant negative correlation between glomerular size and glomerular number (*Figure 1.11*). This need not imply that glomeruli undergo hypertrophy as they become fewer, although the aging kidney does retain a capacity to enlarge after contralateral nephrectomy (Boner, Sherry and Rieselbach, 1972; Dossetor, 1975; Ekelund and Göthlin, 1976). No one appears to have attempted to correlate glomerular number and dimensions in young healthy adults. It is likely, however, that a kidney which maintained its functional integrity with relatively small numbers of relatively large glomeruli would be vulnerable if it were to suffer obliterative disease of its afferent arterioles This may contribute to the higher rate of failure reported in apparently healthy kidneys transplanted from middle-aged and elderly subjects (Darmady, 1974), a report which has, however, not gone unchallenged (Matas *et al.*, 1976).

Investigators disagree about the cortical distribution of glomerular aging. Some have found degenerate glomeruli with equal frequency throughout the cortex (Ljungqvist and Lagergren, 1962; Kaplan *et al.*, 1975). Those (Ljungqvist and Lagergren, 1962; Takazakura *et al.*, 1972) who demonstrated important differences in the vascular changes accompanying glomerular degeneration in inner cortical and more superficial zones (*Figure 1.10*) did not suggest a selective loss of juxtamedullary nephrons, although this is implied. That suggestion was left to Darmady, Offer and Woodhouse (1973). They documented a reduction in number and tubular volume of these nephrons in the oldest subjects whom they studied, commenting that this ‘may be important in the reduction of the urinary concentrating mechanism in the elderly’. Although the diminution in number was slight, from 8 per cent of the total to 6 per cent, proximal tubular volume was halved (*Table 1.4*). Councilman (1919), on the other hand, referred to subcapsular atrophy, but a number of the kidneys on which he based his opinion almost certainly came from hypertensive subjects. Similar suggestions, also based on histological study at necropsy, but with more scrupulous selection, have been made more recently (Moore, 1964). Xenon washout studies in the adult normotensive kidney have demonstrated a reduction in rapid-component, ‘outer cortical’ flow rate with age, from which a selective obliteration of outer cortical nephrons has been inferred (Hollenberg *et al.*, 1974). The question remains unresolved.

Table 1.4 Juxtamedullary nephrons—changes with age (Data from Darmady, Offer and Woodhouse, 1973)

	Age (yr)	
	20	*84*
Proportion of total number (%)	8	6
Proximal tubular volume (mm^3)	0.136	0.061

Relationship between changes in the vessels and the nephron

Do these events in the nephron result from vascular changes or, in the phrase used by Oliver (1952), ‘primary abiotrophic involution’? References to the possibility of involution recur, particularly in the early literature. Some of that early post-mortem evidence deserves scrutiny; not all is without flaw. Furno (1909), when he described the smooth atrophic kidney which he claimed was typical ('rene tipico senile') may not have excluded those which were diseased. Councilman (1919) considered 'chronic atrophic nephropathy' to be characteristic, but half of the subjects he studied showed cardiac hypertrophy. More recent authorities have been able more completely to separate the events of aging from those of disease. Nevertheless, Williams and Harrison (1937), after their detailed histological examination of the renal vessels, concluded that the possibility of involutional changes remained, 'similar to those occurring in certain lower animals'. Papper and Vaamonde (1971) held a similar view, commenting on the difficulty of distinguishing renal 'atrophy secondary to atherosclerosis . . . from an intrinsic involutional process'. Darmady, Offer and Woodhouse (1973) noted that events in the vessels did not precede but accompanied the reduction in nephron mass and deduced that some mechanism other than vascular change was responsible.

Oliver (1952), too, was prepared to concede that involution might occur, but argued from his own histological evidence that aging of the kidney resulted from aging of its vessels. He considered that much of the work by early morbid anatomists left 'great uncertainty in the mind of the reader'. For 'his personal satisfaction', he examined histologically the kidneys of 75 individuals over the age of 70. Although he recognized 'possible variation in personal interpretation', he was emphatic that 'every one of these kidneys showed an arteriosclerosis sufficient in his estimation to account for all the atrophic and degenerative changes that were present in the parenchyma'. By their nature, these subjective assessments could not separately consider the appearances of the nephron and the vessels.

Similar comments may be applied to studies by micro-angiography (Ljungqvist and Lagergren, 1962; Takazakura *et al.*, 1972), in which events in the small vessels and the glomerulus are assessed together. Attempts have been made to quantify changes in the nephron and the vessels by methods which differ and which minimize subjective bias. McLachlan *et al.* (1977) assessed changes in the renal vessels semiquantitatively by post-mortem angiography, which allowed evaluation to the level of interlobular arteries, and by histology. They related these observations to glomerular numbers, calculated by stereological methods (Elias and Hennig, 1967; Weibel, 1969; Underwood, 1970; Elias, Hennig and Schwartz, 1971). Glomerular numbers tended to decline as vascular changes became more marked, but correlation was poor and no better than correlation with age. The degree of vascular change was not related to glomerular size or to the proportion of glomeruli which were completely hyalinized. One rather tenuous argument may be advanced in favour of a relationship between vascular change and glomerular obliteration by hyalinization. When sexes are compared, hyalinized glomeruli (Kaplan *et al.*, 1975; McLachlan *et al.*, 1977) and arteriolosclerosis (Smith, 1955) are both more common in the elderly male kidney. The case is not proven. The 'very high correlation between aging and atherosclerosis' (Papper and Vaamonde, 1971) makes it difficult to exclude involution of the nephron as an event occurring independently of vascular change.

Other forms of vascular occlusion occur; the nephron may deteriorate in other ways. Moore (1964), after an extensive examination of material obtained at necropsy, concluded that superficial cortical scarring was produced by micro-emboli from plaques of aortic atherosclerosis. Moreover, a reduction in renal content of heparan sulphate in the aging kidney suggests that microthrombus formation may be less effectively inhibited (Murata and Horiuchi, 1978).

Obliteration of nephrons may follow tubular obstruction by interstitial fibrosis in the medulla, an event which, although related to aging, does not depend on changes in the vessels (Helpap, 1933; Keresztury and Megyeri, 1962). This appears to provide the basis for early descriptions which imply a tubular degeneration preceding more proximal atrophy (Furno, 1909; Kaufman, 1911; Councilman, 1919). Glomerular involution also occurs in childhood, in kidneys which are apparently healthy (Emery and Macdonald, 1960). Some have even speculated that focal glomerular sclerosis, generally regarded as a disease of unknown aetiology, is a form of renal aging (Bolton, Westervelt and Sturgill, 1978).

Involution of nephrons occurs in other species. The rat has been studied most extensively. As in man, glomerular numbers decline (Arataki, 1926; Moore and Hellman, 1930), but there is much evidence to suggest that changes in the nephron precede changes in the vessels (Kennedy, 1957; Andrew and Pruett, 1957; Bras, 1969; Sworn and Fox, 1974). Tubular and glomerular basement membrane thickens, blockage of tubular lumen follows hyperplasia of tubular cells; in turn, without vascular change, glomeruli become sclerosed (Saxton and Kimball, 1941; Kennedy, 1957; Andrew and Pruett, 1957; Ashworth, Erdmann and Arnold, 1960; Bras, 1969; Sworn and Fox, 1974; Haley and Bulger, 1983). High protein diets appear to provoke these lesions, the amount of protein required becoming less with age (Saxton and Kimball, 1941; Kennedy, 1957; Bras, 1969) (see Chapter 3). Immunofluorescence and electron microscopy (Couser and Stilmant, 1975, 1976) have demonstrated mesangial deposits of macromolecular material, mainly IgM, attributed to impaired clearing of globulin which has accumulated as a result of age-related increase in glomerular permeability. The collagen content of glomerular basement membrane increases (Kalant *et al.*, 1977) and its amino acid composition alters (Hoyer and Spiro, 1978).

Aging of the rat kidney shows itself in other ways. Specific activities of membrane-bound (O'Bryan and Lowenstein, 1974) and microsomal and mitochondrial enzymes (Grinna and Barber, 1972) in the kidney are reduced. Renal concentrations of polyamines decline (Ferioli and Comolli, 1974). In the mouse (Burich, 1975; Johnson and Barrows, 1980) and hamster (McNelly and Dittmer, 1976) similar changes occur. Involution of nephrons is described in the dog (Councilman, 1919; Oliver, 1952). A large body of evidence may be adduced to support the contention that aging affects the mammalian kidney well before sclerosis is apparent in its vessels. Moreover, in the aging rat, there are suggestions that juxtamedullary nephrons are selectively affected (Casellas and Mimran, 1979; McLachlan and Boylan, 1980). Evidence from animals cannot, however, be applied uncritically to support similar arguments in man. In rats (O'Bryan and Lowenstein, 1974) and in mice (Hackbarth and Harrison, 1982), major differences exist even between strains. These and similar considerations have led some to cautious conclusions (O'Bryan and Lowenstein, 1974; Haley and Bulger, 1983) and others to rigorous comparisons of strains (Burek, 1978; Masoro, 1980) (see Chaper 8).

Structure and function: possible relationships

This section (see also Chapters 2–8) examines some of these changes in structure in the light of age-related changes in function and, where possible, attempts to relate the two. In the words of Oliver and MacDowell (1961), it examines 'structural–functional equivalents'. It does not attempt to discuss functional changes in detail; that discussion follows in other chapters. Nor does it intend to imply that every alteration in function has a basis in structure. For example, it ignores the potential effect on renal function of age-related reduction in plasma-renin activity and aldosterone (Flood *et al.*, 1967; Crane and Harris, 1976) and tubular response to vasopressin (Epstein and Hollenberg, 1976). Nevertheless, even very recent opinion suggests that the explanation for at least one functional change that accompanies aging, the decline in concentrating capacity, should be sought within the kidney (Phillips *et al.*, 1984).

Lewis and Alving (1938), in their extensively quoted paper, first demonstrated the change in concentrating capacity. Attention has since been largely directed to functional events in the proximal nephron. Most of these studies were performed by Shock and his co-workers, who initially documented a decline in inulin clearance and transport maximum of iodopyracet (Diodrast) (Davies and Shock, 1950). These observations were subsequently reinforced and extended (Miller, McDonald and Shock, 1952; Miller and Shock, 1953; Adler *et al.*, 1968). Most important, the decline in glomerular filtration rate which they demonstrated in their cross-sectional investigations has been confirmed in longitudinal studies (Rowe *et al.*, 1976). Because glomerular and tubular function appeared to decrease at the same rate, Shock and his colleagues argued that the aging nephron fails as a unit. This view is supported by observations which show the reduction in size of glomerulus and proximal tubule proceeding hand in hand as age advances (Darmady, Offer and Woodhouse, 1973). Papper (1973) favoured the 'intact nephron hypothesis' (Bricker, Morrin and Kime, 1960) as an explanation for the decline; with the passage of time fewer and fewer competent nephrons remain. With function depending on the survival of these more robust nephrons, it becomes less necessary to argue that glomerulus and tubule degenerate together in the others, which by this reasoning contribute at most only minimally to function.

However, the reduction in glomerular filtration rate is not linear; in both cross-sectional and longitudinal studies (Lewis and Alving, 1938; Davies and Shock, 1950; Adler *et al.*, 1968; Hollenberg *et al.*, 1974; Epstein and Hollenberg, 1976; Rowe *et al.*, 1976) it is most profoundly reduced after the fifth or sixth decade, 10 or 20 years after glomerular loss begins (Moore, 1931; Dunnill and Halley, 1973). In renal disease, it is usually considered that the number of nephrons must be halved before function is affected, a reduction apparently unusual in the aging kidney (Moore, 1931; Dunnill and Halley, 1973); remaining nephrons probably undergo compensatory hypertrophy (Bricker, Morrin and Kime, 1960) (see Chapter 3). The negative correlation between glomerular number and dimensions (McLachlan *et al.*, 1977) suggests that the aging kidney too is capable of compensatory hypertrophy, which could account for the initial, relatively slow decline in glomerular function before the later, more abrupt fall. Differences between kidneys in this capacity for hypertrophy, possibly depending on the condition of their vessels, could explain the large differences in glomerular dimensions (McLachlan *et al.*, 1977). Wide functional variation in the elderly (Lewis and Alving, 1938; Davies and Shock, 1950; Rowe *et al.*, 1976) might then depend on these differences or differences in glomerular number. Because no information is yet available about the relationship between glomerular number and dimensions in the young kidney, only speculation is possible; nephrons in a normal kidney may, at one extreme, be relatively small and numerous or, at the other extreme, relatively large and few. The great variation in the dimensions and number of nephrons in apparently healthy kidneys (Moore, 1931; Oliver and MacDowell, 1961; Dunnill and Halley, 1973; McLachlan *et al.*, 1977) allows of this as a likely possibility.

Rowe, Shock and DeFronzo (1976) concluded that the decline in concentrating capacity could not be ascribed to reduction in glomerular filtration rate. They argued that the development of continuity between the afferent and efferent arterioles of juxtamedullary nephrons (Ljungqvist and Lagergren, 1962; Takazakura *et al.*, 1972) altered countercurrent mechanisms by elevating medullary blood flow. They referred to xenon washout studies by Hollenberg *et al.* (1974) purporting to show that outer cortical blood flow is less well maintained than blood flow in inner cortex and medulla. Continuity between juxtamedullary afferent and efferent arterioles, which could explain these alterations in blood flow, probably results from degeneration of juxtamedullary nephrons (Ljungqvist and Lagergren, 1962; Takazakura *et al.*, 1972). Because selective loss of these nephrons before the shorter-looped peripheral nephrons would itself explain the reduction in concentrating capacity (Darmady, Offer and Woodhouse, 1973), it may not be necessary to invoke changes in medullary blood flow. Even if both groups of nephrons were to deteriorate at the same rate, the effect on juxtamedullary nephrons, which probably comprise about 10 per cent or less of the total (Darmady, Offer and Woodhouse, 1973), would be much greater. Structural changes in the distal tubules and collecting ducts, with the development of diverticula as a source of urinary tract infection (Darmady, Offer and Woodhouse, 1973; Baert and Steg, 1977), could account for a relationship between bacteriuria and declining concentrating capacity (Dontas *et al.*, 1966; Dontas, Marketos and Papanayiotou, 1972; Alwall, 1978). Fibrosis in the medullary interstitium (Helpap, 1933; Keresztury and Megyeri, 1962) may follow infection and contribute to that functional decline. The structural changes are sufficiently large and varied to provide ample support for those who contend that the explanation for the decline in concentrating capacity lies within the kidney (Phillips *et al.*, 1984).

Conclusions

Davies and Shock (1950) attempted to relate their evidence of functional decline in the aging kidney to the morphological information available to them. They concluded that 'we do not yet have the crucial data to decide what mechanisms are involved'. Since then, important studies of morphology have appeared. Darmady, Offer and Woodhouse (1973), by careful microdissection, have presented powerful evidence that the aging nephron degenerates as a unit, despite earlier argument by Oliver (1952). Their work, and meticulous micro-angiographic examinations (Ljungqvist and Lagergren, 1962; Takazakura *et al.*, 1972), strongly suggest that the long-looped juxtamedullary nephrons degenerate earlier than shorter-looped nephrons more peripherally situated. Microdissection has also revealed distal tubular ectasia and, with organisms, diverticula (Darmady, Offer and Woodhouse, 1973; Baert and Steg, 1977), which may account for an association between impaired concentrating capacity and bacteriuria.

The aging nephron may be able to hypertrophy as its numbers decline (McLachlan *et al.*, 1977). At the very least, there is evidence that the aging kidney retains a capacity to enlarge after nephrectomy (Boner, Sherry and Rieselbach, 1972). By histopathological studies based on a lifetime of scrupulous observation (Bell, 1950), vascular changes which are the result of aging have, in large degree, been carefully unravelled from those which are due to hypertension; sclerosis of arterioles appears to be primarily an event of aging, although hypertension may make it worse. It follows change in small arteries. The weight of historical opinion favours, as a cause of glomerular degeneration, these vascular changes, rather than involution (Oliver, 1952). And yet a doubt persists, unstilled in over half a century. If 'primary abiotrophic involution' can affect other mammalian kidneys, if, for example, dietary manipulation can provoke glomerular degeneration (e.g. Kennedy, 1957), why should the kidney of man be granted an unusual immunity?

References

ADLER, S., LINDEMAN, R.D., YIENGST, M.J., BEARD, E. and SHOCK, N.W. (1968). Effect of acute acid loading on urinary acid excretion by the aging human kidney. *Journal of Laboratory and Clinical Medicine,* **72,** 278–289

ALLBUTT, C.T. (1915). In *Diseases of the Arteries including Angina Pectoris,* pp. 309–373. London; Macmillan

ALWALL, N. (1978). Population studies on non-obstructive urinary tract infection in non-pregnant women: importance of method and material. *Acta Medica Scandinavica,* **203,** 95–105

ANDREW, W. and PRUETT, D. (1957). Senile changes in the kidneys of Wistar Institute rats. *American Journal of Anatomy,* **100,** 51–69

ARATAKI, M. (1926). On the postnatal growth of the kidney, with special reference to the number and size of the glomeruli (albino rat). *American Journal of Anatomy,* **36,** 399–436

ASHWORTH, C.T., ERDMANN, R.R. and ARNOLD, N.J. (1960). Age changes in the renal basement membrane in rats. *American Journal of Pathology,* **36,** 165–179

BAERT, L. and STEG, A. (1977). Is the diverticulum of the distal and collecting tubules a preliminary stage of the simple cyst in the adult? *Journal of Urology,* **118,** 707–710

BELL, E.T. (1950). In *Renal Disease,* pp. 331–346. Philadelphia; Lea and Febiger

BOLTON, W.K., WESTERVELT, F.B. and STURGILL, B.C. (1978). Nephrotic syndrome and focal glomerular sclerosis in aging man. *Nephron,* **20,** 307–315

BONER, G., SHERRY, J. and RIESELBACH, R.E. (1972). Hypertrophy of the normal human kidney following contralateral nephrectomy. *Nephron,* **9,** 364–370

BRAASCH, W.F. and HENDRICK, J.A. (1944). Renal cysts, simple and otherwise. *Journal of Urology,* **51,** 1–10

BRAS, G. (1969). Age-associated kidney lesions in the rat. *Journal of Infectious Disease,* **120,** 131–135

BRICKER, N.S., MORRIN, P.A.F. and KIME, S.W. (1960). The pathologic physiology of chronic Bright's disease. *American Journal of Medicine,* **28,** 77–98

BUREK, J.D. (1978). *Pathology of Aging Rats.* West Palm Beach, Florida; CRC Press

BURICH, R.L. (1975). Effects of age on renal function and enzyme activity in male C57BL/6 mice. *Journal of Gerontology,* **30,** 539–545

CASELLAS, D. and MIMRAN, A. (1979). Aglomerular pathways in intrarenal microvasculature of aged rats. *American Journal of Anatomy,* **156,** 293–299

COUNCILMAN, W.T. (1919). The conditions presented in the heart and kidneys of old people. In *Contributions to Medical and Biological Research,* dedicated to Sir William Osler, pp. 918–928. New York; Hoeber

COUSER, W.G. and STILMANT, M.M. (1975). Mesangial lesions and focal glomerular sclerosis in the aging rat. *Laboratory Investigation,* **33,** 491–501

COUSER, W.G. and STILMANT, M.M. (1976). The immunopathology of the aging rat kidney. *Journal of Gerontology,* **31,** 13–22

CRANE, M.G. and HARRIS, J.J. (1976). Effect of aging on renin activity and aldosterone excretion. *Journal of Laboratory and Clinical Medicine,* **87,** 947–959

CURTIS, J.R. (1968). M.D. thesis, University of London. Quoted by Curtis, J.R. (1978). Ageing kidney. *Lancet,* **2,** 316

DARMADY, E.M. (1974). Transplantation and the ageing kidney. *Lancet,* **2,** 1046–1047

DARMADY, E.M., OFFER, J., PRINCE, J. and STRANACK, F. (1964). The proximal convoluted tubule in the renal handling of water. *Lancet,* **2,** 1254–1257

DARMADY, E.M., OFFER, J. and WOODHOUSE, M.A. (1973). The parameters of the ageing kidney. *Journal of Pathology,* **109,** 195–207

DAVIDSON, A.J., TALNER, L.B. and DOWNS, M. (1969). A study of the angiographic appearances of the kidney in an aging normotensive population. *Radiology,* **92,** 975–983

DAVIES, D.F. and SHOCK, N.W. (1950). Age changes in glomerular filtration rate, effective renal plasma flow, and tubular excretory capacity in adult males. *Journal of Clinical Investigation,* **29,** 496–507

DONTAS, A.S., MARKETOS, S.G. and PAPANAYIOTOU, P. (1972). Mechanisms of renal tubular defects in old age. *Postgraduate Medical Journal,* **48,** 295–303

DONTAS, A.S., PAPANAYIOTOU, P., MARKETOS, S., PAPANICOLAOU, N. and ECONOMOU, P. (1966). Bacteriuria in old age. *Lancet,* **2,** 305–306

DOSSETOR, R.S. (1975). Renal compensatory hypertrophy in the adult. *British Journal of Radiology,* **48,** 993–995

DUNNILL, R.S. and HALLEY, W. (1973). Some observations on the quantitative anatomy of the kidney. *Journal of Pathology,* **110,** 113–120

EKELUND, L. and GÖTHLIN (1976). Compensatory renal enlargement in older patients. *American Journal of Roentgenology,* **127,** 713–715

ELIAS, H. and HENNIG, A. (1967). Stereology of the human renal glomerulus. In *Quantitative Methods in Morphology,* edited by E.R. Weibel and H. Elias, pp. 130–166. Berlin; Springer

ELIAS, H., HENNIG, A. and SCHWARTZ, D.E. (1971). Stereology: applications to biomedical research. *Physiological Reviews,* **51,** 158–200

EMERY, J.L. and MACDONALD, M.S. (1960). Involuting and scarred glomeruli in the kidneys of infants. *American Journal of Pathology,* **36,** 713–723

EPSTEIN, M. and HOLLENBERG, N.K. (1976). Age as a determinant of renal sodium conservation in normal man. *Journal of Laboratory and Clinical Medicine,* **87,** 411–417

FAHR, TH. (1925). Benigne (einfache) Nierensklerose (Reine arteriosklerotische Nierenveranderung.) In *Handbuch der Speziellen pathologischen Anatomie u. Histologie,* vol. VI/1, pp. 374–375, edited by F. Henke and O. Lubarsch. Berlin; Springer

FERIOLI, M.E. and COMOLLI, R. (1974). Changes of liver and kidney polyamine levels during ageing. *Experimental Gerontology,* **10,** 13–15

FETTERMAN, G.H., SHUPLOCK, N.A., PHILIPP, F.J. and GREGG, H.S. (1965). The growth and maturation of human glomeruli and proximal convolutions from term to adulthood. *Pediatrics,* **35,** 601–619

FLOOD, C., GHERONDACHE, C., PINCUS, G., TAIT, J.F., TAIT, S.A.S. and WILLOUGHBY, S. (1967). The metabolism and secretion of aldosterone in elderly subjects. *Journal of Clinical Investigation,* **46,** 960-966

FRIEDMAN, S.A., RAIZNER, A.E., ROSEN, H., SOLOMON, N.A. and SY, W. (1972). Functional defects in the aging kidney. *Annals of Internal Medicine,* **76,** 41–45

FURNO, A. (1909). Ricerche anatomo-pathologiche intorno al rene atrofico senile. *La Sperimentale,* **63,** 99–129

GOYAL, V.K. (1982). Changes with age in the human kidney. *Experimental Gerontology,* **17,** 321–331

GRIFFITHS, G.J., CARTWRIGHT, G.O. and McLACHLAN, M.S.F. (1975). Estimation of renal size from radiographs: is the effort worthwhile? *Clinical Radiology,* **26,** 249–256

GRIFFITHS, G.J., ROBINSON, K.B., CARTWRIGHT, G.O. and McLACHLAN, M.S.F. (1976). Loss of renal tissue in the elderly. *British Journal of Radiology,* **49,** 111–117

GRINNA, L.S. and BARBER, A.A. (1972). Age-related changes in membrane lipid content and enzyme activities. *Biochimica et Biophysica Acta,* **288,** 347–353

HACKBARTH, H. and HARRISON, D.E. (1982). Changes with age in renal function and morphology in C57BL/6, CBA/HT6, and B6CBAF$_1$ mice. *Journal of Gerontology,* **37,** 540–547

HALEY, D.P. and BULGER, R.E. (1983). The aging male rat: structure and function of the kidney. *American Journal of Anatomy,* **167,** 1–13

HATTERY, R.R., WILLIAMSON, B., STEPHENS, D.H., SHEEDY, P.F. and HARTMAN, G.W. (1977). Computed tomography of renal abnormalities. *Radiologic Clinics of North America,* **15,** 401–418

HELPAP, K. (1933). Über aufsteigende Schrumpfniere durch Sklerose des Nierenmarks. *Virchows Archiv fur pathologische Anatomie,* **288,** 383–392

HEPTINSTALL, R.H. (1974). *Pathology of the Kidney,* pp. 121–162. Boston; Little, Brown

HODSON, C.J. (1959). Radiological diagnosis of pyelonephritis. *Proceedings of the Royal Society of Medicine,* **52,** 669–672

HODSON, C.J. (1968). Radiological diagnosis of renal involvement. In *Urinary Tract Infection*, edited by F. O'Grady and W. Brumfitt, pp. 108–112. London; Oxford University Press

HOLLENBERG, N.K., ADAMS, D.F., SOLOMON, H.S., RASHID, A., ABRAMS, H.L. and MERRILL, J.P. (1974). Senescence and the renal vasculature in normal man. *Circulation Research*, **34**, 309–315

HOLLENBERG, N.K., EPSTEIN, M., BASCH, R.I. and MERRILL, J.P. (1969). 'No man's land' of the renal vasculature. An arteriographic and hemodynamic assessment of the interlobar and arcuate arteries in essential and accelerated hypertension. *American Journal of Medicine*, **47**, 845–854

HOWELL, T.H. and PIGGOT, A.P. (1948). The kidney in old age. *Journal of Gerontology*, **3**, 124–128

HOYER, J.R. and SPIRO, R.G. (1978). Studies on the rat glomerular basement membrane: age-related changes in composition. *Archives of Biochemistry and Biophysics*, **185**, 496–503

INOUE, G., SAWADA, T., FUKUNAGA, Y. and YOSHIKAWA, M. (1970). Levels of acid mucopolysaccharides in aging human kidneys. *Gerontologia*, **16**, 261–265

ISHIKAWA, I., ONOUCHI, Z., SAITO, Y., KITADA, H., SHINODA, A., USHITANI, K., TABUCHI, M. and SUZUKI, M. (1981). Renal cortex visualization and analysis of dynamic CT curves of the kidney. *Journal of Computer Assisted Tomography*, **5**, 695–701

JOHNSON, J.E. and BARROWS, C.H. (1980). Effects of age and dietary restriction on the kidney glomeruli of mice: observations by scanning electron microscopy. *Anatomical Record*, **196**, 145–151

KALANT, N., SATOMI, S., WHITE, R. and TEL, E. (1977). Changes in renal glomerular basement membrane with age and nephritis. *Canadian Journal of Biochemistry*, **55**, 1197–1206

KAPLAN, C., PASTERNACK, B., SHAH, H. and GALLO, G. (1975). Age-related incidence of sclerotic glomeruli in human kidneys. *American Journal of Pathology*, **80**, 227–234

KAUFMAN, E. (1911). In *Lehrbuch der Speziellen pathologischen Anatomie*, pp. 815–818. Berlin; Reimer

KENNEDY, G.C. (1957). Effects of old age and over-nutrition on the kidney. *British Medical Bulletin*, **13**, 67–70

KERESZTURY, S. and MEGYERI, L. (1962). Histology of renal pyramids with special regard to changes due to ageing. *Acta Morphologica*, **11**, 205–215

KISSANE, J.M. (1974). In *Pathology of the Kidney*, edited by R.H. Heptinstall, pp. 51–68. Boston; Little, Brown

LAUCKS, S.P. and McLACHLAN, M.S.F. (1981). Aging and simple cysts of the kidney. *British Journal of Radiology*, **54**, 12–14

deLEON, W., GARCIA, A. and deJESUS, P.I. (1933). Normal weights of visceral organs in adult Filipinos. *Philippine Journal of Science*, **52**, 111–127

LEWIS, W.H. and ALVING, A.S. (1938). Changes with age in the renal function in adult men. *American Journal of Physiology*, **123**, 500–515

LJUNGQVIST, A. and LAGERGREN, C. (1962). Normal intrarenal arterial pattern in adult and ageing human kidney. *Journal of Anatomy, London*, **96**, 285–300

McKEOWN, F. (1965). *Pathology of the Aged*, pp. 171–204, London; Butterworths

McLACHLAN, M.S.F. and BOYLAN, L. (1980). Structural-functional relationships in the aging kidney. *Investigative Radiology*, **15**, 413

McLACHLAN, M.S.F., GAUNT, A., FULKER, M.J. and ANDERSON, C.K. (1976). Estimation of glomerular size and number from radiographs of the kidney. *British Journal of Radiology*, **49**, 831–835

McLACHLAN, M.S.F., GUTHRIE, J.C., ANDERSON, C.K. and FULKER, M.J. (1977). Vascular and glomerular changes in the ageing kidney. *Journal of Pathology*, **121**, 65–77

McLACHLAN, M.S.F. and KAPLAN, R. (1981). Aging and renal sinus fat. *American Journal of Roentgenology*, **137**, 200

McLACHLAN, M.S.F. and WASSERMAN, P. (1981). Changes in size and distensibility of the aging kidney. *British Journal of Radiology*, **54**, 488–491

McMANUS, J.F.A. and LUPTON, C.H. (1960). Ischemic obsolescence of renal glomeruli. *Laboratory Investigation*, **9**, 413–434

McNELLY, N.A. and DITTMER, J.E. (1976). Glomerular basement membrane width and proteinuria in the aging hamster kidney. *Experimental Gerontology*, **11**, 49–55

MASORO, E.J. (1980). Mortality and growth characteristics of rat strains commonly used in aging research. *Experimental Aging Research*, **6**, 219–233

MATAS, A.J., SIMMONS, R.L., KJELLSTRAND, C.M., BUSELMEIER, T.J. and NAJARIAN, J.S. (1976). Transplantation of the aging kidney. *Transplantation*, **21**, 160–161

MILLER, J.H., McDONALD, R.K. and SHOCK, N.W. (1952). Age changes in the maximal rate of renal tubular reabsorption of glucose. *Journal of Gerontology,* **7,** 196–200

MILLER, J.H. and SHOCK, N.W. (1953). Age differences in the renal tubular response to antidiuretic hormone. *Journal of Gerontology,* **8,** 446–450

MOORE, R.A. (1931). The total number of glomeruli in the normal human kidney. *Anatomical Record,* **48,** 153–168

MOORE, R.A. and HELLMAN, L.M. (1930). The effect of unilateral nephrectomy on the senile atrophy of the kidney in the white rat. *Journal of Experimental Medicine,* **51,** 51–57

MOORE, S. (1964). The relation of superficial cortical scars of the kidney to aortic atherosclerosis; a hypothesis of renal ischaemia. *Journal of Pathology,* **88,** 471–478

MORITZ, A.R. and OLDT, M.R. (1937). Arteriolar sclerosis in hypertensive and nonhypertensive individuals. *American Journal of Pathology,* **13,** 679–728

MURATA, K. and HORIUCHI, Y. (1978). Age-dependent distribution of acidic glycosaminoglycans in human kidney tissue. *Nephron,* **20,** 111–118

O'BRYAN, D. and LOWENSTEIN, L.M. (1974). Effect of aging on renal membrane-bound enzyme activities. *Biochimica et Biophysica Acta,* **339,** 1–9

OLIVER, J.R. (1952). In *Cowdry's Problems of Aging,* pp. 631–650. Baltimore; Williams and Wilkins

OLIVER, J. and MACDOWELL, M. (1961). The structural and functional aspects of the handling of glucose by the nephrons and the kidney and their correlation by means of structural–functional equivalents. *Journal of Clinical Investigation,* **40,** 1093–1112

PAPPER, S. (1973). The effects of age in reducing renal function. *Geriatrics,* **28,** 83–87

PAPPER, S. and VAAMONDE, C.A. (1971). In *Diseases of the Kidney,* edited by M.B. Strauss and L.G. Welt, pp. 735–768. Boston; Little, Brown

PHILLIPS, P.A., ROLLS, B.J., LEDINGHAM, J.G.G., FORSLING, M.L., MORTON, J.J., CROWE, M.J. and WOLLNER, L. (1984). Reduced thirst after water deprivation in healthy elderly men. *New England Journal of Medicine,* **311,** 753–759

ROESSLE, R. and ROULET, F. (1932). In *Mass und Zahl in der Pathologie,* pp. 63–66. Berlin; Springer

ROWE, J.W. (1977). Clinical research in aging: strategies and directions. *New England Journal of Medicine,* **297,** 1332–1336

ROWE, J.W., ANDRES, R., TOBIN, J.F., NORRIS, A.H. and SHOCK, N.W. (1976). The effect of age on creatinine clearance in men: a cross sectional and longitudinal study. *Journal of Gerontoloy,* **31,** 155–163

ROWE, J.W., SHOCK, N.W. and DeFRONZO, R.A. (1976). The influence of age on the renal response to water deprivation in man. *Nephron,* **17,** 270–278

SAXTON, J.A., Jr. and KIMBALL, GRACE C. (1941). Relation of nephrosis and other diseases of albino rats to age and to modifications of diet. *Archives of Pathology,* **32,** 951–965

SMITH, J.P. (1955). Hyaline arteriolosclerosis in the kidney. *Journal of Pathology and Bacteriology,* **69,** 147–168

STEFFES, M.W., BARBOSA, J., BASGEN, J.M., SUTHERLAND, D.E.R., NAJARIAN, J.S. and MAUER, S.M. (1983). Quantitative glomerular morphology of the normal human kidney. *Laboratory Investigation,* **49,** 82–86

SWORN, M.J. and FOX, M. (1974). Renal age changes in the rat compared with human renal senescence. An autoradiographic study. *Investigative Urology,* **12,** 140–145

TAKAZAKURA, E., SAWABU, N., HANDA, A., TAKADA, A., SHINODA, A. and TAKEUCHI, J. (1972). Intrarenal vascular changes with age and disease. *Kidney International,* **2,** 224–230

UNDERWOOD, E.E. (1970). *Quantitative Stereology.* Addison-Wesley; Reading, Massachusetts

VIMTRUP, B.J. (1928). On the number, shape, structure, and surface area of the glomeruli in the kidneys of man and mammals. *American Journal of Anatomy,* **41,** 123–151

WALD, H. (1937). The weight of normal adult human kidneys and its variability. *Archives of Pathology,* **23,** 493–500

WEIBEL, E.R. (1969). Stereological principles for morphometry in electron microscopic cytology. *International Review of Cytology,* **26,** 235–302

WILLIAMS, R.H. and HARRISON, T.R. (1937). A study of the renal arteries in relation to age and to hypertension. *American Heart Journal,* **14,** 645–658

Chapter 2

Glomerular filtration and renal blood flow in the aged

Luis Hernando Avendaño and José M. López Novoa

Renal blood flow and glomerular filtration rate in healthy humans

The renal circulation

General characteristics of the renal circulation

Although kidneys constitute only about 0.5 per cent of the human body mass, they receive about 20 per cent of the cardiac output. This rate of blood flow, which amounts to approximately 4 ml/min/g, is much greater than the one received by other organs ordinarily considered to be well perfused, such as heart, liver and brain. From this sizable blood flow (about 1 litre/min) only a small amount of urine is formed (less than 1 ml/min).

The blood that enters the kidney circulates through several areas with different characteristics. Thus the kidney can be divided into several microcirculatory networks, i.e. the glomerular microcirculation, the cortical peritubular microcirculation and the medullary network. It is important to be aware that there are physiological and pharmacological manoeuvres that can alter blood flow distribution between these areas without altering total renal blood flow.

Measurement of renal blood flow

Total renal blood flow is usually determined in humans by 'clearance techniques'. This determination is based upon the application of Fick's principle to the disappearance of an indicator substance from the blood passing through the kidney and its subsequent appearance in the urine. Assuming that this indicator substance is neither synthesized nor catabolized within the kidney, it is evident that its rate of disappearance from the plasma (DP) must be equal to the rate of urine appearance (UA). DP is equal to the difference in concentrations between the arterial (A_i) and venous (V_i) blood multiplied by the renal plasma flow (RPF):

$$\mathrm{DP} = (A_i - V_i) \times \mathrm{RPF} \quad (2.1)$$

UA is equal to the product of urinary concentration (U_i) by urinary flow rate (UF):

$$\mathrm{UA} = U_i \times \mathrm{UF} \quad (2.2)$$

Thus

$$(A_i - V_i) \times \mathrm{RPF} = U_i \times \mathrm{UF} \quad (2.3)$$

Rewriting this equation:

$$\mathrm{RPF} = U_i \times \mathrm{UF}/A_i - V_i \tag{2.4}$$

If the fraction of indicator removed by the arterial circulation is designated as the extraction ratio (E), equation (2.4) yields

$$\mathrm{RPF} = U_i \times \mathrm{UF}/E \times A_i \tag{2.5}$$

The indicator most frequently used to estimate RPF is para-aminohippuric acid (PAH) because its extraction rate in humans is between 0.7 and 0.9 when plasma concentrations are below the transport maximum (about 0.02 mg/ml). Plasma concentrations are maintained constant by means of a continuous infusion of PAH. In clinical practice, E is rarely measured and often assumed to be 1. Thus RPF is slightly underestimated. Formerly, it was assumed that the incomplete extraction of E_{PAH} in the human kidney was due to perfusion of 'inactive' tissue and PAH clearance was often referred to as 'effective renal plasma flow'. However, much of the flow supply to the medulla fails to perfuse pars recta segments of proximal tubules (which are the main nephron sites of PAH secretion). Furthermore, there is evidence that in experimental animals such as the dog, E_{PAH}, that is about 0.75 in normal conditions, falls below 0.5 under conditions of high renal blood flow (Earley and Friedler, 1965). Thus, determination of actual extraction ratio during experimental manoeuvres is necessary if precise measurement of RPF is desired. Renal blood flow (RBF) can be calculated from RPF by correcting for the haematocrit (HTC).:

$$\mathrm{RBF} = \mathrm{RPF}/1 - \mathrm{HTC} \tag{2.6}$$

where HCT is expressed in fractional form, about 0.45 in normal humans.

Because the clearance technique requires that patients have near normal urine flow rates and because the technique requires chemical analysis, several alternative methods for measuring total RBF have been developed. Those most used in humans are direct measurements of the dilution of indicators continuously infused in the renal artery and studies of uptake, transit time or washout kinetics of radioactive tracers.

By using clearance techniques, Smith (1943) reported that RPF in young people averaged 592 ± 153 ml/min/1.73 m^2 in women and 654 ± 163 in men (mean ± S.D.). In infants, RPF corrected by body weight is approximately one-half that of adults and increases progressively, reaching adult values by 3 years of age (McCrory, 1972). After the age of 30, RBF decreases progressively, and this fact will be the subject of a later section in this chapter.

Intrarenal distribution of renal blood flow

Analysis of RBF distribution into the kidney in man gives different figures depending on the technique used. As average, cortical blood flow represents 90–95 per cent of total RBF, or 6–8 ml/min/g. Distribution of renal cortical blood flow has been extensively investigated in several physiological and pathological situations, and it has been related with sodium balance. This hypothesis is based on the existence of at least two populations of nephrons with a different capacity to handle sodium. It was proposed that manoeuvres that distributed the flow towards inner nephrons, whose efferent arterioles form the medullary capillary network, the vasa recta, were associated with decreased sodium excretion due to the higher capacity of these nephrons to reabsorb sodium (Goodyear and Jaeger, 1955; Carriere *et al.*, 1966). Inversely, volume expansion would induce an increase in superficial cortical blood flow (Stein, Osgood and Ferris, 1972). This phenomenon has been widely studied and, although structural and functional heterogeneity of nephron population is established, the relationship between blood distribution and sodium excretion remains undefined (Beeuwkees, Ichikawa and Brenner, 1981).

Autoregulation of renal blood flow

A typical characteristic of the kidney is the phenomenon of autoregulation of RBF. Many organs are able to maintain blood flow rate relatively constant in the face of major changes in perfusion pressure. This property is termed 'autoregulation' and all organs do not show the same efficiency in this autoregulatory process, the brain and kidney being the most efficient. Kidneys are able to maintain RBF in a range of 20 per cent if pressure changes between 50 and 150 mmHg, a range which is termed 'autoregulatory range'. A similar phenomenon occurs with the glomerular filtration rate (Jones and Berne, 1964). Flow throughout the kidney depends on perfusion pressure and vascular resistance, and this is determined by the combined resistance due to the afferent and efferent arterioles (Thurau, 1964). However, the afferent arteriole seems to be the main locus of resistance changes (Thurau and Wober, 1962).

Since the changes in renal vascular resistance that accompany graded reductions in perfusion pressure are demonstrable in innervated, denervated and isolated kidneys, autoregulation of RBF is assumed to be mediated by mechanisms intrinsic to the kidney (Thurau, 1964) and to be independent of circulating humoral or neurogenic factors. Several theories have been proposed to account for this phenomenon. According to the *myogenic theory,* the capacity of arterial smooth muscle to contract depends on the vascular wall tension. Thus, an increase in arterial pressure, which initially will distend the vascular wall, will be followed by an active contraction of the resistance vessels, increase in resistance and the subsequent restoration of blood flow to levels similar to that previous to pressure increase. This theory, formulated by Bayliss (1902) has received recent experimental support (Robertson *et al.*, 1972), but cannot explain the mechanism by which changes in renal blood flow are sensed or the fine adjustment of arterial radius.

According to the *metabolic theory,* changes in blood flow through a tissue would alter oxygen tension, pH and/or concentration of metabolites which would alter vascular resistances. A number of substances have been suggested to play this role acting as vasodilators; among them are adenosine, adenine nucleotides, potassium, and Krebs-cycle intermediates. A decrease in RBF would increase the concentration of the hypothetical vasodilator, thus inducing smooth muscle relaxation and an increase in blood flow. Conversely, an increase in perfusion pressure and blood flow would diminish the concentration of this substance, inducing an increase in vascular resistance and a decrease in blood flow (Haddy and Scott, 1968).

A third theory is the role of *tubuloglomerular feedback.* According to this theory, changes in perfusion pressure would change salt delivery to the distal portion of the nephron that senses this alteration and induce a change in arteriolar constriction that reverts the change in perfusion flow. Renin secretion by the macula densa and local generation of angiotensin II seem to be involved in this mechanism (Gagnon *et al.*, 1970).

Although all of these hypotheses are supported by some experimental evidence, none of them can completely explain the autoregulatory phenomenon. Thus, it seems likely that several systems participate in the autoregulatory response, including myogenic, feedback, humoral and metabolic mechanisms, but the relative importance of each system remains to be defined.

Other mechanisms that regulate renal blood flow

In addition to autoregulatory mechanisms, the most important mechanisms that regulate renal blood flow are the renal innervation and the humoral substances with vasoactive action.

The kidney in man is a richly innervated organ. It receives both sympathetic and parasympathetic innervation, which are predominantly concentrated in the afferent and efferent arterioles of the glomerulus and the macula densa (Barajas, 1978). It has been proved that a sympathetic stimulation causes direct vasoconstriction of the arterioles, thus reducing renal blood flow (Di Salvo and Fell, 1971), and, in addition, induces the secretion of renin by the juxtaglomerular apparatus, thus producing a further vasoconstriction.

Vascular reactivity of the kidney to vasoactive substances is also notable. The kidney is among the most sensitive organs to angiotensin II or norepinephrine, which cause significant decreases of RBF even to doses which are ineffective in increasing arterial pressure. Glomerular arterioles seem to be the site of action of these hormones, although afferent vessels respond more strongly to norepinephrine, whereas efferent arterioles seem to be more sensitive to angiotensin II (Glick, Joyner and Gilmore, 1979).

Formation of glomerular ultrafiltrate

General characteristics of glomerular filtration

As previously stated, the normal human kidney receives a blood flow of about 1200 ml/min, which, assuming a haematocrit of 45 per cent, corresponds to 660 ml/min plasma flow. At the same time, the glomeruli form 125 ml/min of glomerular ultrafiltrate. Thus the filtration fraction defined as the ratio of the glomerular filtration rate to renal plasma flow is 125/660 = 0.19. This means that 19 per cent of the plasma entering the kidney is removed as filtrate.

Two main characteristics differentiate glomerular ultrafiltration from transcapillary exchange in other organs: (1) the glomerular filter exhibits an extraordinarily high permeability to water and small solutes; and (2) the glomerular filter is almost impermeable to proteins of the size of albumin and larger.

Glomerular filtration is a process determined by three factors: (1) the properties of both the filter and the molecules to be filtered; (2) the interactions between molecules and the filter; and (3) the balance of hydrostatic, osmotic and colloid osmotic forces across the filter, according to Starling's law.

Structure of the renal glomerular filter

The renal ultrafilter consists of three layers (*Figure 2.1*): (1) an inner layer of endothelial cells lining the lumen of the glomerular capillaries; (2) the basement membrane; and (3) the layer of epithelial cells (Tisher and Madsen, 1986).

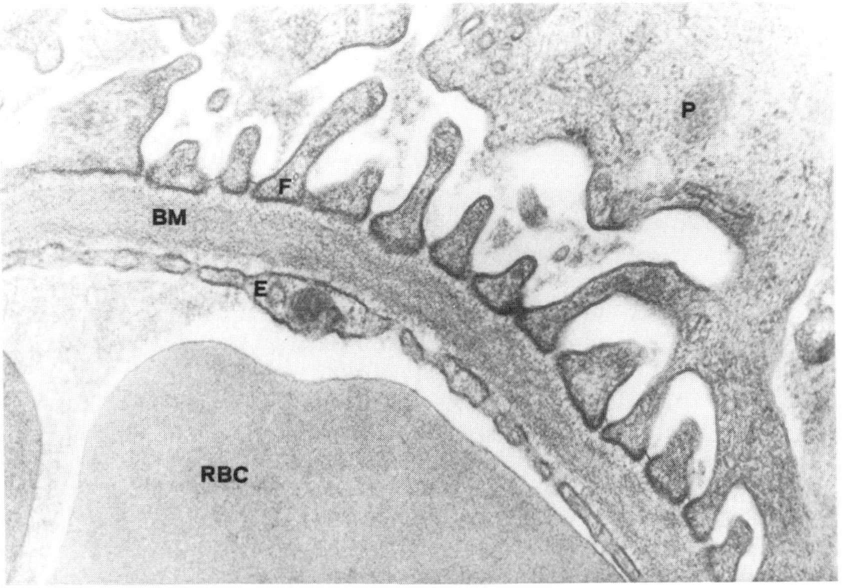

Figure 2.1 Electron micrograph of the glomerular barrier in a human glomerulus. The filtration pathway between the capillary lumen, in this case partially occupied by a red blood cell (RBC), and Bowman's space consists of (a) endothelial fenestrae in the endothelial cell body (E), (b) the glomerular basement membrane (BM), and (c) the filtration islets between the foot processes (F) of the pedicels (P) (Reproduced by courtesy of Dr A. Barat)

The endothelial cells are flat, with the nuclear zone protruding into the capillary light. Fenestrae or pores, which in the human kidney have a mean diameter of approximately 700 Å, are present in the attenuated endothelium (Jörgensen, 1966). The diaphragms have been observed to extend across these pores (Jörgensen, 1966). Clementi and Palade (1969) have suggested that the diaphragms are composed of a highly permeable protein–polysaccharide film, presenting no significant barrier to the passage even of large molecules.

The basement membrane is composed of a central dense layer, the lamina densa, and two thinner, more electron-permeable layers, the lamina rara interna and the lamina rara externa (Jörgensen, 1966). Thickness of the basement membrane averages about 3300 Å in adult humans. The width of the basement membrane is considerably less in infants than in adults, approaching the adult width by approximately 3 years of age (Vernier, 1964). No morphological evidence of the existence of pores in the basement membrane has been reported. Chemically, the three layers of glomerular basement membrane also show different composition: the lamina densa is composed of type IV collagen, whereas the lamina rara interna and externa are composed of proteoglycans and the attachment proteins laminin and fibronectin (Farquhar *et al.*, 1982).

Proteoglycans consist of a core protein of variable size to which one or more glucosamineglycan side chains are covalently bound. The special characteristics of proteoglycans are based on their glucosaminoglycan chains, formerly known as acid mucopolysaccharides, of which the major types are chondroitin sulphate, hyaluronic acid, keratan sulphate, heparan sulphate and heparin. All of them are composed of disaccharide repeating units made by hexuronic or iduronic acid and glucosamine or galactosamine (Farquhar, Lemkin and Stow, 1984).

In tissue, proteoglycans can be detected *in situ* with various cationic dyes, for example ruthenium red, alcian blue, safranin, colloidal iron or proteins (lysozyme or cationized ferritin). Using these techniques, proteoglycans were first detected in the rat glomerular basement membrane *in situ* by Caufield and Farquhar (1976), both in the lamina rara interna and externa. Proteoglycans were also isolated from glomerular basement membrane and its precise chemical composition analysed. The glucosamineglycans of these proteoglycans consisted mainly of heparan sulphate (Kanwar and Farquhar, 1980), whereas smaller amounts of other glycosamineglycans such as chondroitin sulphate and hyaluronic acid were also detected in glomerular basement membranes. However, it has been recently reported that chondroitin sulphate is present only in the mesangial matrix (Kanwar, Jakubowsky and Rosenzeig, 1983), whereas the precise location of hyaluronic acid is at present unknown.

Proteoglycans show some special properties which give them a special importance in the function and pathological changes of the glomerular filtration barrier. Thus, proteoglycans show the highest negative charge of all known biological macromolecules, which involve a series of characteristics such as their ability to repel anionic macromolecules, to bind cationic proteins and to bind divalent cations like ionized calcium (Farquhar, Lemkin and Stow, 1984). In aqueous solution, proteoglycans form polymeric networks of a viscous, gel-like consistency. Thus, they retard transport of macromolecules and diffusion of ions.

The available data indicate that basement membrane is formed by a gel of hydrated glycoprotein polymers. In such gels, the pathways for water and solute transport are constituted by the hydrated interior of the polymer matrix, in between the elongated, intertwining chains of the polymer (Laurent, 1966; Venkatachalam and Rennke, 1978). Thus, basement membrane seems to show a high hydraulic conductivity and a limited permeability to macromolecules, mainly to cationic ones, as will be detailed later in this chaper.

The epithelial layer is composed of a very specialized type of cell, the so-called 'podocytes', which are composed by a cell body and several cytoplasmic primary processes, from which individual foot processes or 'pedicels' project to come into contact with the lamina rara externa of the basement membrane of one or more glomerular capillary loops. Secondary and tertiary processes, that extend from the primary processes, can also give origin to the foot processes. It has been demonstrated in humans that immediately adjacent foot processes arise from different podocytes (Arakawa, 1971). In the normal glomerulus the distance between individual foot processes varies between 250 and 600 Å near the basement membrane. A thin membrane, termed the 'filtration slit membrane' (Latta, 1973) or 'slit diaphragm' (Rodewald and Karnovsky, 1974), bridges the gap between adjacent foot processes at a distance of approximately 600 Å of the basement membrane.

Both endothelial and epithelial cells are covered by a cell surface coat, whose thickness is about 120 Å in the endothelial cells and 800 Å in the podocytes (Latta, Johnston and Stanley, 1973). The epithelial and endothelial cell coats in glomeruli possess a strong net negative charge revealed by its interaction with polycationic reagents. Histochemical studies have demonstrated that carboxyl groups of sialic acid form the bulk of cell coat anionic radicals (Venkatachalam and Rennke, 1978). It has been recently demonstrated that, in addition to sialoglycoproteins, proteoglycans constitute an important part of polyanionic constituent of cell coat. They have been observed in the entire surface of the epithelial cells, mostly in the surfaces exposed to the urinary spaces. A lower amount was observed over the surface of the endothelial cells (Farquhar, Lemkin and Stow, 1984). Proteoglycans can also be detected in the rough endoplasmic reticulum and Golgi apparatus which probably represent the organelles responsible for their biosynthesis. Proteoglycans associated with endothelial and epithelial cell membranes show different antigenicity from those associated with glomerular basement membrane, suggesting that their composition is rather different (Farquhar, Lemkin and Stow, 1984).

According to ultrastructural tracer studies (Graham and Karnovsky, 1966), macromolecules are transferred across the glomerular filter through an extracellular pathway that consists of (1) the endothelial fenestrae, partially narrowed by the endothelial cell coat, (2) the glomerular basement membrane, (3) the filtration slit pore diaphragm, and (4) the filtration slits, filled with epithelial cell coat (see *Figure 2.1*).

Physical determinants of glomerular ultrafiltration

The mechanism of glomerular ultrafiltration is similar to that of tissue fluid formation in any other part of the organism. Thus, the rate of glomerular ultrafiltration is governed by the same driving forces that govern fluid movement across other capillaries: the imbalance between transcapillary hydraulic pressure (ΔP) and colloid osmotic pressure ($\Delta\pi$). This relationship may be expressed as

$$\mathrm{GFR} = K_f\,(\Delta P - \Delta\pi) \qquad (2.7)$$

where GFR is the glomerular filtration rate and K_f the ultrafiltration coefficient, an expression of the hydraulic permeability of the ultrafilter, expressed in ml/min mmHg. The magnitude of the transcapillary hydraulic pressure is large and equal to the difference between the capillary blood pressure (P_g) and the Bowman's space hydrostatic pressure (P_c). The gradient of colloido-osmotic pressure is due almost exclusively to the plasma oncotic pressure (π_g) since ultrafiltrate is virtually free of macromolecules (Eisenbach, Van Liew and Boyland, 1975). Thus, equation (2.7) can be rewritten as

$$\mathrm{GFR} = K_f\,(P_g - P_c - \pi_g) = K_f.\Delta P_f \qquad (2.8)$$

As defined by equation (2.8), GFR is proportional to the effective filtration force (ΔP_f) and depends on the characteristics of the filtration barrier represented by the filtrate coefficient K_f. Pappenheimer (1953) demonstrated that ultrafiltration coefficient depends on the intrinsic hydraulic permeability of the glomerular filter (K) and on the effective filtration surface (S_f). In turn, ΔP_f depends on glomerular haemodynamics.

The afferent arteriole is the only source of blood supply to the glomerular capillaries. The magnitude of blood inflow depends on the pressure gradient across the glomerular capillaries and the resistance of the glomerulus. However, in the glomerular circulation there are two sites of actively regulable resistances, the afferent and efferent arterioles. Thus, glomerular blood flow (GBF) is determined by the pressure gradient ($P_a - P_e$) across these two resistances (R_a and R_e) in series:

$$\mathrm{GBF} = (P_a - P_e)/(R_a \div R_e) \qquad (2.9)$$

Intraglomerular hydrostatic pressure depends on the transmission of the arterial pressure across the afferent arteriole and the dissipation of this gradient by the efferent arteriole. Thus, P_g is inversely proportional to the afferent resistance and directly proportional to the efferent resistance. It will be increased by manoeuvres that induce afferent vasodilatation or efferent vasoconstriction, and decreased by the opposite manoeuvres.

The magnitude of the pressures involved in glomerular filtration have been measured using micropuncture techniques in animals with glomeruli in the surface of the kidney, such as Munich–Wistar rats (Brenner, Troy and Daugharty, 1971), and there are reasons to believe that values are similar in other mammals, including the human being (Brenner, Dworkin and Ichikawa, 1986). Thus, for mean arterial pressure between 110 and 130 mmHg, P_g is 45 mmHg and P_c about 10 mmHg. Plasma protein oncotic pressure is about 20 mmHg, thus giving an effective filtration pressure of about 15 mmHg (Brenner, Dworkin and Ichikawa, 1986; Andreucci *et al.*, 1971). However, an unexpected finding in these studies was that effective filtration pressure (P_f) decreased from the values given for the afferent side of the glomerulus to zero at the efferent end of the glomerulus. This fact was explained by measurements of efferent and afferent plasma protein concentration which indicated that plasma colloid osmotic pressure increases from about 20 mmHg at the afferent end of the glomerular capillary to 35 mmHg by the efferent end, owing to the ultrafiltration of water and crystalloids, but not protein.

Thus, although capillary hydrostatic pressure falls only a little, the net ultrafiltration pressure declines from a maximum of about 15 mmHg at the afferent end to zero by the efferent end. This means that no significant filtration occurs in that part of the capillary, because $\Delta\pi = \Delta P$. This phenomenon is referred as *filtration pressure equilibrium* (Brenner, Dworkin and Ichikawa, 1986). Studies using a mathematical model of the process (Deen *et al.*, 1973) reveal that net ultrafiltration pressure declines in a nonlinear way. Thus, the formation of ultrafiltrate occurs most rapidly at the afferent end of the capillary network, and therefore glomerular capillary protein concentration and hence plasma colloid osmotic pressure increase more rapidly near the afferent end of the capillary.

The existence of filtration pressure equilibrium in the process of glomerular filtration introduces some qualitative and quantitative modifications not contemplated in the previously defined formulae. In those formulae, no dependence of GFR on RFB is evident. However, as depicted in *Figure 2.2*, changes in RBF importantly modify the effective ultrafiltration pressure. In this figure, in accordance with equation (2.8), GFR is proportional to K_f, which in the figure is represented by the area between ΔP and $\Delta\pi$. It can be observed that net ultrafiltration occurs only in a part of the capillary length (l). If a higher volume of fluid enters the capillary in a fixed time, as filtration occurs at a rate similar to the previous situation, in accordance with equation (2.8) colloid osmotic pressure would increase more slowly (line 2 in *Figure 2.2*) and net ultafiltration pressure, represented by the area between ΔP and $\Delta\pi$, would be higher than in line 1. Thus, GFR_2 would also be higher than GFR. Greater increases in glomerular blood flow would lead to filtration pressure disequilibrium (line 3) in which $\Delta\pi$ does not equal P_g.

Increases in glomerular blood flow not only affects net ultrafiltration pressure (ΔP_f) but also K_f. As can be observed in *Figure 2.2*, in line 2, net filtration occurs in a part of the glomerular capillary longer than in line 1 and, subsequently, in a wide surface. As previously stated, K_f depends on hydraulic permeability of the membrane, which is an intrinsic property of the glomerular filter, and on the effective ultrafiltration surface (s). Thus, increase in blood flow affects the

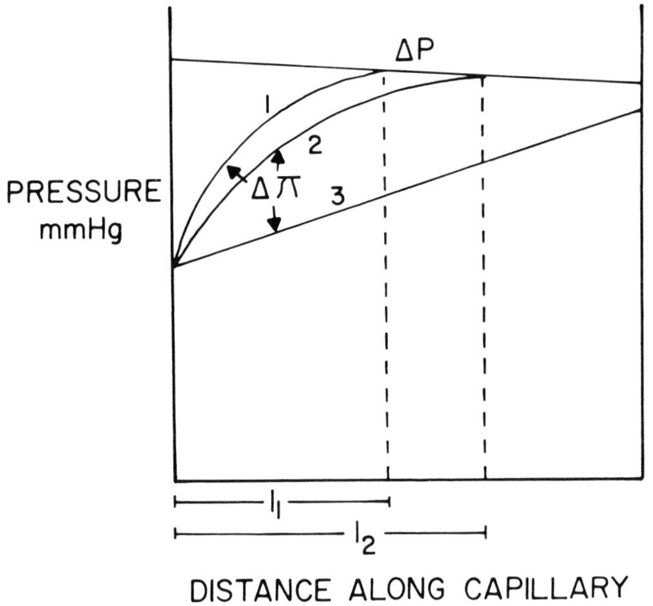

Figure 2.2 Determinants of glomerular filtration in three different situations of glomerular blood flow (see text for definition of symbols)

ultrafiltration coefficient by increasing *s*. All these theoretical predictions have received experimental support in the Munich–Wistar rat (Baylis and Brenner, 1978) and they are supposed to be valid for humans.

Autoregulation of glomerular filtration rate

As previously discussed, the kidney is able to maintain relatively constant its blood flow in spite of variations in arterial pressure above 80 mmHg to about 190 mmHg. This phenomenon, called autoregulation, also occurs for GFR (Shipley and Study, 1951) and, as demonstrated for RBF, it occurs in innervated, denervated and isolated kidneys (Shipley and Study, 1951). Robertson *et al.* (1972) have demonstrated that the maintenance of GFR and RBF, in spite of changes in mean arterial flow (MAF), depends on co-ordinated changes in afferent and efferent resistances, with maintenance of effective ultrafiltration pressure (ΔP_f) (Deen, Robertson and Brenner, 1974).

Measurement of glomerular filtration rate

The rate at which plasma is filtered in the glomerulus is usually measured in both humans and experimental animals by using clearance techniques. The clearance of a substance x (C_x) is defined as

$$C_x = U_x . \mathrm{UF} / P_x \qquad (2.10)$$

where U_x and P_x are the concentrations of x in urine and plasma, respectively, and UF is the urine flow.

If the substance is freely filtered in the glomerulus, i.e. its concentration in the ultrafiltrate is equal to that of plasma, the amount of x filtered by unit of time (F_x) will be

$$F_x = \mathrm{GFR} \,.\, P_x \tag{2.11}$$

The amount of substance x excreted in the urine by unit of time is equal to the product of urine flow and the urinary concentration of x (U_x). If substance x is neither reabsorbed nor excreted or metabolized in their passage throughout the tubules, then F_x will be excreted in the urine:

$$F_x = U_x .\, \mathrm{UF} \tag{2.12}$$

Thus

$$\mathrm{GFR} \,.\, P_x = U_x \,.\, \mathrm{UF} \tag{2.13}$$

Rearranging equation (2.13) gives

$$\mathrm{GFR} = (U_x .\, \mathrm{UF})/P_x = C_x \tag{2.14}$$

This equation means that the clearance of a substance which shows the properties previously described (to be freely filterable across the wall of glomerular capillary, to be biologically inert and to be neither secreted nor reabsorbed by the tubules) measures the GFR.

It is important to differentiate the rate of excretion of a substance (U_x. UF), which will vary in proportion to P_x, from the clearance of this substance (U_x . UF/P_x), which is independent of P_x.

Inulin is the substance most widely used for the measurement of GFR in both humans and experimental animals because it possesses all the attributes of an ideal marker for GFR (Levinsky and Levy, 1973). Other substances currently employed to estimate GFR include radioisotope-labelled EDTA and sodium iothalamate, which obviate chemical determinations. Although all these substances provide accurate measurements of GFR, they are exogenous and must be infused into the circulation to maintain stable and adequate plasma levels. Thus, in order to simplify the measurement, several other substances are used. The most commonly employed is creatinine. Urinary creatinine is almost entirely derived from the endogenous catabolism of muscle creatinine and phosphocreatinine. In humans, endogenous creatinine clearance closely approximates inulin clearance, in part as a result of compensatory errors (Brenner, Dworkin and Ichikawa, 1986). Urea, which has also been used as a marker for GFR measurement, shows major limitations because of the high degree of urea reabsorption by the renal tubules and the dependence of urea excretion on urine volume (Levinsky and Levy, 1973).

In order to avoid constant infusion to patients and its associated troubles, some alternative techniques have been developed for GFR measurement.

Israelit, Long and White (1973) have reported that constant plasma levels of sodium iothalamate labelled with ^{125}I were demonstrable for several hours after a single subcutaneous injection when a small amount of epinephrine was added to the test substance in order to slow its absorption. This allows measurement of GFR with almost steady plasma levels. Data obtained with this technique agree very well with those obtained with conventional techniques like inulin clearance. Also, the variation of the data obtained with iothalamate and this technique were within the limit of the classical techniques.

Another method consists of a rapid venous infusion of the test substance; after intravascular and extravascular equilibrium, plasma concentration of substance falls with time, and serial plasma samples in the middle of each urine collection period are needed to obtain accurate data. With this technique, ^{51}Cr–EDTA clearances agree very well with the inulin clearance rate (Chantler *et al.*, 1969), although ^{51}Cr–EDTA values were 10–15 per cent lower than that of inulin clearance.

In some instances the collection of urine is difficult, inaccurate or impracticable, making it necessary to develop some techniques which avoid urine collection. The simplest of these methods is the single slope plasma method. It is based on the fact that when a fixed dose (D) of a test substance is rapidly injected into a vein and plasma samples are taken at intervals, if the test substance is removed in an amount that is proportional to its plasma concentration, the apparent distribution volume of the substance can be calculated in a conventional manner by plotting the logarithm of the plasma concentration as a function of time and extrapolating the linear part of the curve back to zero time to obtain the effective initial activity of the plasma (P_0) at time $t = 0$. The apparent volume of distribution V(ml) is then given by the formula

$$V = D/P_0 \tag{2.15}$$

The half-period ($t_{\frac{1}{2}}$) of the linear portion of the previously described curve can be obtained graphically and the plasma clearance constant (K, min^{-1}) obtained by the relationship

$$K = 0.693/t_{\frac{1}{2}} \tag{2.16}$$

The apparent plasma clearance rate of the substance (PCR, ml/min) is then given by the equation

$$\text{PCR} = K.V \tag{2.17}$$

The PCR has the same value as the GFR if the test substance, in addition to being a valid marker to measure GFR, can only be removed by glomerular filtration. In other words, it must not be metabolized or otherwise removed from the circulation by an organ other than the kidney. It has been demonstrated that ^{51}Cr–EDTA accomplishes this condition because in anephric individuals its clearance rate is negligible (Chantler *et al.*, 1969).

The single plasma slope technique described above is based on the assumption that the indicator is rapidly and thoroughly distributed in a single compartment of volume V. Evidently this is a gross simplification because we know that there are at least two different compartments, intravascular and extravascular spaces, in which the test substance is distributed. To solve this problem, Sapirstein *et al.* (1955) and Matthews (1957) have developed a two-compartment open model as follows:

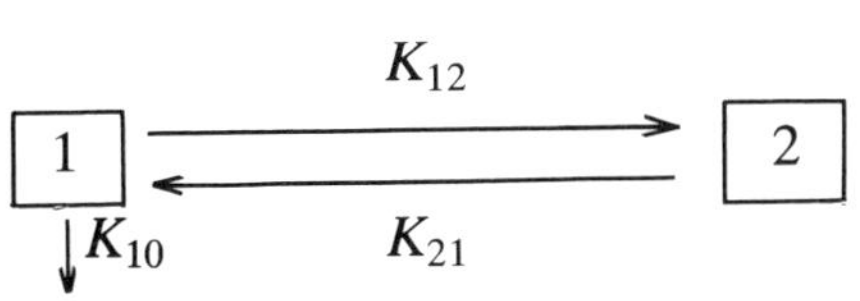

This model is based on the assumption of the distribution of the test substance between two compartments, compartment 1 (which represents roughly the plasma) and compartment 2, approximately the extravascular fluid, with rate constants K_{12} and K_{21}. The rate constant K_{10} depends on the renal clearance. In this model the concentration of the test substance (C) in compartments 1 and 2 in function of time are given by the equations

$$C_1 = \frac{K_{21} - b_1}{(b_2 - b_1)} \exp(-b_1 t) \div \frac{K_{21} - b_2}{(b_1 - b_2)} \exp(-b_2 t) \quad (2.18)$$

$$C_2 = \frac{K_{12}}{(b_2 - b_1)} [\exp(-b_1 t) - \exp(-b_2 t)] \quad (2.19)$$

where b_1 and b_2 are constants with the following characteristics:

$$b_1.b_2 = K_{10}.K_{21} \quad (2.20)$$

and

$$b_1 \div b_2 = K_{10} \div K_{21} \div K_{12} \quad (2.21)$$

Provided that the rate constants b_1 and b_2 differ in a significant manner and that the time span is enough, the plasma curve can be fitted to a double exponential function of time of the form

$$C_1 = A\exp(-b_1 t) \div B\exp(-b_2 t) \quad (2.22)$$

This curve can be analysed graphically or by means of computer techniques to yield parameters A, B and b_2. These values are then substituted in the formula developed by Sapirstein *et al.* (1955) to obtain plasma clearance (or renal clearance if the test substance has the conditions previously stated):

$$\text{Clearance} = \frac{D}{A/b_1 \div B/b_2} \quad (2.23)$$

The single compartment analysis previously explained assumes that, after mixing is completed, K_{21}» K_{21}, and subsequently $b1$»b_2. Thus, the first term in equations (2.18) and (2.22) can be ignored. Also, the single compartment analysis is equivalent to equation (2.23), in which the first term in the denominator is removed. This overestimates the clearance by 15–25 per cent (Chantler *et al.*, 1969; Granerus and Aurell, 1981).

The two-compartment model is also a simplified scheme, because it implies that the test substance is distributed between only two compartments, with rapid and homogeneous mixing within each compartment. The actual phenomenon is not like that, especially in the cases of patients with oedema or ascites, in which there is a third space with dynamic characteristics different from intravascular or 'normal' interstitial fluid.

An approach which solves these limitations is the stochastic method, which has been extensively used in circulatory studies (Zierler, 1963). According to this approach, plasma clearance (C) is given by the formula

$$C = \frac{D}{\int_0^\infty C(t)\, dt} \quad (2.24)$$

The mean transit time ($\bar{t}$) is defined by

$$\bar{t} = \frac{\sum C_i . t_i}{\sum C_i} \quad (i = 0 - \infty) \quad (2.25)$$

The application of this general principle to the renal clearance calculation was performed by Nosslin (1965). He described that the curve for $C(t)$ can be fitted to the sum of two exponential functions. Since in equation (2.24) the denominator is equivalent to the area under the concentration–time curve, and the area under an exponential curve is equal to $A.\bar{T}$ or A/b, it can be deduced that the denominator in equation (2.23) is the area of a concentration–time curve represented by a double exponential curve. This assumption means that, in practice, few data points (blood samples) are required to fit the curve, which can be extrapolated to infinity once becoming mono-exponential, so that the period of observation must not be too prolonged. Again in the case of oedematous patients this is not true, and the concentration–time curves require for adequate fitting an additional exponential component, which involves a longer observation period if the area of the curve is not to be grossly underestimated.

If the first term in the denominator in equation (2.23) is neglected, the number of blood samples is reduced to those necessary to define the slope of the mono-exponential part of the curve, but this fact overestimates the clearance rate. However, the overestimation is a constant fraction of the true value of GFR, which can be calculated by multiplying the value obtained with the mono-exponential curve method by 0.80.

In addition, the stochastic method allows us to estimate the error arising from the use of a venous instead of arterial blood sample. This error can be obviated by multiplying the obtained value by 1.11. Combined correction factors (about 0.9) yield values of ^{51}Cr–EDTA clearances without urine collection, which agrees with the inulin clearance values within 10 per cent. In addition, this method is more reproducible than the inulin and creatinine standard clearance method (Chantler *et al.*, 1969), with the exception of patients with oedema or a third space, cases in which a longer period of sampling is required and the urine collection method is preferable. In these cases, the subcutaneous or intramuscular single injection method previously reported can be used in order to obtain steady plasma levels.

In the average sized adult male, the clearance of inulin averages 130 ml/min and remains remarkably constant from day to day in spite of wide variations in exercise or water or sodium intake (Brenner, Dworkin and Ichikawa, 1986).

Selectivity of the glomerular filtration barrier

As previously stated, a special characteristic of the glomerular ultrafilter is that it exhibits a high permeability to water and small solutes, but it is impermeable to proteins. Several factors influence the filtration or not of macromolecules, including molecular size, molecular shape or configuration and molecular charge. In addition, filtration is also influenced by such haemodynamic variables as renal plasma flow. However, the most important influences are molecular size and charge.

Measurable restriction to filtration of neutral globular substances does not occur until effective radius (Stokes–Einstein radius) exceeds 20 Å. Beyond this radius, fractional clearances decrease progressively with increasing size, approaching zero at radii greater than about 42 Å (Arturson, Groth and Grotte, 1971; Chang *et al.*, 1976; Bohrer, Baylis and Humes, 1978). In addition to molecular size, charge also influences substantially the filtration of macromolecules. The fractional clearance of proteins is substantially lower than that of neutral dextran of comparable molecular size and this discrepancy cannot be explained by tubular reabsorption. Experimental studies have confirmed that polyanions show a restricted passage across the glomerular ultrafilter if compared with neutral macromolecules of similar size, whereas polycations show a facilitated transport (Chang *et al.*, 1975; Bohrer, Baylis and Humes, 1978). It is important to note that most of the circulating proteins are polyanions. The influence of molecular charge on glomerular filtration seems to be based on its interaction with the anionic group present in the cell coat of endothelial and epithelial cells, and in the basement membrane (Kanwar and Farquhar, 1980), as previously described. It is also important to point out that the alteration of these fixed charges in several pathologies, such as glomerulonephritis or in the aging kidney, plays an important role in proteinuria that characterizes these pathological or aging states. This process is extensively described in other chapters of this book.

Renal blood flow and glomerular filtration in the aged

Effect of age on renal efficiency

'Death follows on account of the insufficiency of the excretory process, therefore the limit of life is a matter of excretion. Old age is considered by many to be a chronic, incurable disease, associated in large part with, or caused by a diminution in kidney function' (Rappleye and Foxboro, 1918). If, in 1985, not everybody will agree with this statement, published nearly 70 years ago, that the kidney's efficiency deteriorates progressively with aging apart from any interfering disease, it has been well reported in the literature. Changes in renal function with advancing years had been studied by many investigators, with many different methods, and the almost invariable conclusion was that renal function decreases with aging.

In the last years of the nineteenth century authors, especially the French (Ballet, 1881; see also Vallery-Radot and Delafontaine, 1930), emphasized the extreme frequency of morphologic renal lesions in the elderly. From the beginning of the twentieth century enquiries into the functional conditions of the kidneys in late life, using the relatively crude test then available — amount of urea in blood, concentrating ability, urea clearance (Musser and Philips, 1930; Lewis and Alving, 1938; Binet, Laroche and Mathé, 1952) — concluded that all these functions alter with age.

In the 1940s, the use of more sophisticated procedures measuring effective renal plasma flow and glomerular filtration rate on the basis of clearance techniques confirmed the gradual reduction in renal function with advancing years observed in the previous studies. Davies and Shock (1950) demonstrated a linear decrease of average inulin and iodopyracet (Diodrast) clearances beyond the age of 30 with a drop of 46 per cent in inulin clearance, from 122 to 65 ml/min, between the ages of 20 and 90 years. Iodopyracet clearance dropped from 613 to 290 ml/min between the ages of 20 and 90 years (53%).

Those findings were confirmed with other techniques (Olbrich *et al.*, 1950; McDonald, Solomon and Shock, 1951; Mitchell and Valk, 1953) and interpreted as depending on the arteriosclerosis present in the aged population responsible for the decrease in renal parenchyma on the basis of a restricted blood supply.

When renal function was studied in patients with urinary obstruction, either from benign prostatic hyperplasia, prostatic adenocarcinoma or vesical neck stricture (Mitchell and Valk, 1953), considered more representative of the older general population due to the high incidence of prostatism in this group, no significant differences in glomerular filtration rate or effective plasma flow were found in aged patients with or without urinary obstruction.

More recently, Brenner, Meyer and Hostetter (1982) advanced a comprehensive hypothesis that attempts to account for the progressive deterioration in kidney function seen in normal aging and many different renal diseases (see Chapter 3).

Once the decline in glomerular filtration rate with age after maturity had been shown in a number of cross-sectional and longitudinal analyses (Wesson, 1969; Barratt and Chantler, 1975; Rowe *et al.*, 1976a) (*Figure 2.3*), in recent years several papers have been published on the best method to estimate GFR in the elderly and to establish age-adjusted normative standards. This is necessary, since the decrease in creatinine excretion with age (Kampmann *et al.*, 1974) (*Figure 2.4; Table 2.1*) makes necessary the use of certain corrections or a nomogram constructed from the data obtained for the different age groups (*Figure 2.5*).

Serum creatinine has been widely adopted as a screening method for clinical renal function evaluation; however, serum creatinine determinations in large groups of healthy persons have shown no significant change with age despite the considerable

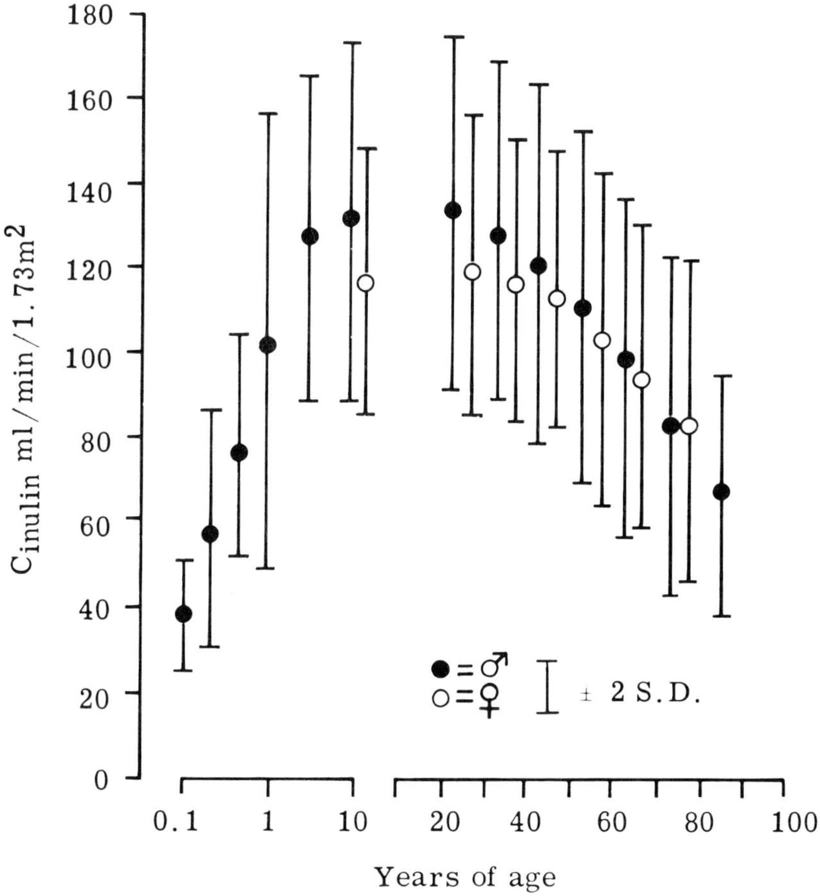

Figure 2.3 Changes in glomerular filtration rate with age in male (filled symbols) and female (open symbols) subjects (After collected data of Wesson, 1969, and Barratt and Chantler, 1975)

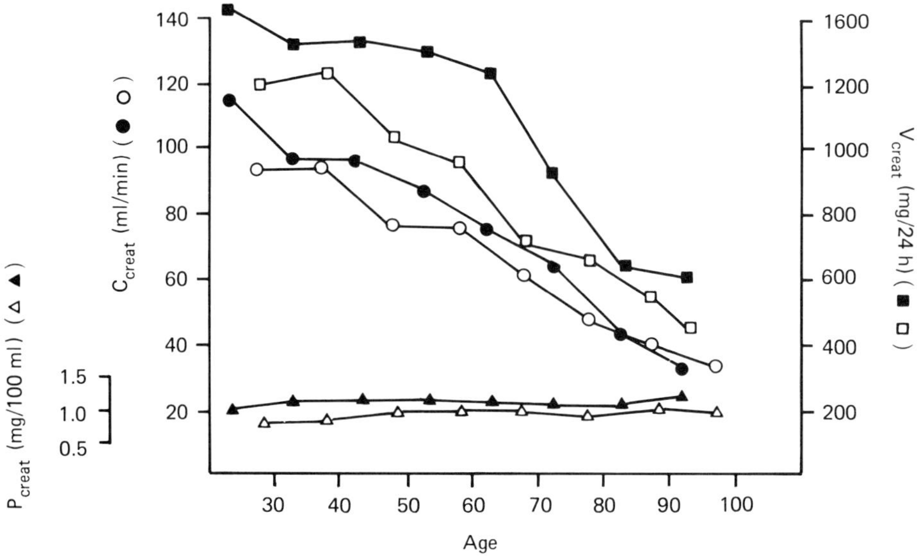

Figure 2.4 Changes in excretion and clearance creatinine with age in male (filled symbols) and female (open symbols) subjects (Data from Kampmann *et al.*, 1974)

decrease in GFR demonstrated in the elderly. The finding of unaltered serum creatinine in the aged in spite of decreased GFR indicates a decrease in endogenous creatinine production with age, demonstrated by a fall in urinary creatinine per kg body weight in the elderly (Balusu *et al.*, 1970) and related to a greater reduction in lean body mass than in total body weight (Forbes and Reina, 1970). Therefore, the use of serum creatinine values as the principal parameter in the measurement of GFR in clinical work implies the risk of overestimation in old patients; thus a correction must be introduced. Multiplying the value for the age group to which the patient belongs, by the body weight in kg, and dividing by the serum creatinine value in mg/100 ml, offers a rather approximate estimation of the patient's creatinine

Table 2.1 Creatinine clearance at different ages in different countries

	Source		
Age (yr)	*Denmark* Siersback-Nielsen *et al.* (1971); Kampmann *et al.* (1974) (ml/min/1.73 m^2)	*France* Laine *et al.* (1977) (ml/min/1.73 m^2)	*Spain* Macias *et al.* (1981) (ml/min/1.73 m^2)
20–29	110	107	
30–39	97	104	126*
40–49	88	100	
50–59	81	95	
60–69	72	86	91†
70–79	64	77	
80–89	47	73	
90–99	34		

*Age 20–50 yr.
†Age 60–79 yr.

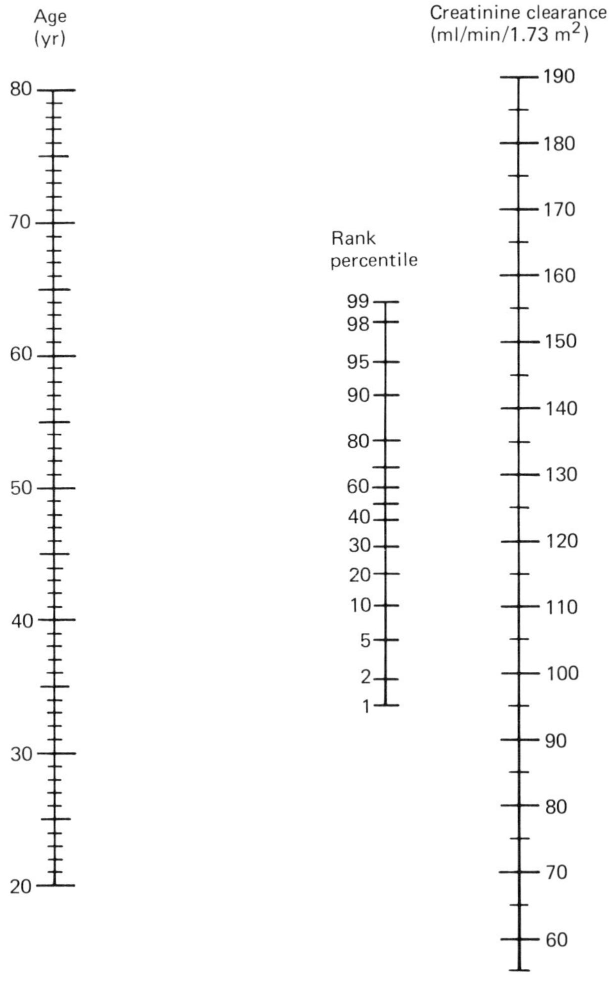

Figure 2.5 Nomogram for determination of age-adjusted percentile rank in creatinine clearance (From Rowe *et al.*, 1976b, reproduced with permission)

clearance in ml/min. The use of a nomogram (*Figure 2.5*) is less precise but quicker (Kampmann *et al.*, 1974; Rowe *et al.*, 1976b).

Other formulae have been developed to predict creatinine clearance (C_{cr}) from serum creatinine (S_{cr}) in adults, including a correction for age and body weight (Cockcroft and Gault, 1976):

$$C_{cr} = \frac{(140-\text{age})\ (\text{kg body weight})}{72 \times S_{cr}\ (\text{mg}/100\ \text{ml})}$$

This formula gives a correlation coefficient between predicted and mean measured creatinine clearance of 0.83, not greater than between paired clearances.

These formulae seem to be sufficiently precise for daily use, but the method employing an oral overload of creatinine in the day of clearance is said to give more pharmacokinetic information (Miric *et al.*, 1982).

Since the endogenous creatinine clearance directly measured or calculated overestimates the GFR at all ages, especially in the elderly, and inulin clearances are lengthy, troublesome and involve the use of an indwelling catheter, other methods have been suggested. Macias *et al.* (1981) consider ^{51}Cr–EDTA clearance to be an accurate determination not requiring urine collection and one which can readily be made, since the radiopharmaceutical is commonly available (although not in the USA, where ^{125}I iothalamate is used). They confirmed with this method the reduction of GFR with advancing years and the overestimation of using creatinine clearance.

The importance of adequate measurement of renal function in the aged patients, particularly those in need of surgery or medication with potential toxic drugs, needs great emphasis. The fact of decreasing function with increasing age is well established, but the wide range of values at all ages and the possible effects of associated pathologies preclude predictability of renal function on the basis of age alone.

The frequency of vascular changes is reflected in the fact that effective plasma flow is more decreased than glomerular filtration, with a significant rise in filtration fraction.

The influence of nitrogen intake and balance of blood urea or BUN make these parameters of limited value, even as a screening method for renal function in clinical work.

It is useful to be able to predict the GFR quickly without collecting urine when instituting therapy with potentially toxic drugs known to be excreted primarily by the kidneys, and this can be done either by predicting creatinine clearance as outlined above, or using ^{51}Cr–EDTA or some other radiopharmaceutical. ^{99}Tc–Sn–DPTA, with a short half-life (6 h), makes possible repeated examinations even at short intervals and with a negligible radiation dose (Klopper and Atkins, 1977).

The need to have an accurate knowledge of the GFR has been strengthened through the increasing use of potentially toxic drugs mainly excreted by the kidney (see Chapter 9). This refers primarily to drugs such as cardiac glycosides, antimicrobials, hypoglycaemic agents, sedatives, hypnotics, analgesics and diuretics, but might also apply to many other medicaments since the majority of drugs are excreted, at least in part, by the kidney. The rate of elimination of drugs is related in a major proportion to kidney function and depends on (1) renal blood flow — delivery of drugs to the kidney, (2) glomerular filtration rate — entry of drug into the tubule fluid, and (3) tubule transport of the drug — both entry and removal from tubule fluid (see Chapter 9).

The rate of removal of a medicament from the body is often expressed as its half-life, defined as the time required for the amount of drug in the body to decline by one-half; for most drugs this value increases as an inverse exponential function of GFR. It can also be stated as the depuration coefficient fraction of the total amount of the drug in the body excreted per hour, a quantity that bears a direct relationship to GFR.

In the normal population of adults, it is generally recommended that the need to reduce dosage of drugs or to lengthen the interval between doses only arises when the GFR is reduced 50 per cent at a time, where BUN and serum creatinine rise above normal values. In the elderly, as previously stated, the decline in lean body mass decreases endogenous production of creatinine and the aged patient, with serum creatinine in the normal range, might have a notable impairment of his GFR.

In consideration of these facts, to lessen adverse drug reactions in aged patients the following simple rules should be taken into consideration:

(1) Dosage of drugs and intervals between doses should be based on accurate timed measurement of GFR by clearance of Cr or a radiopharmaceutical, rather than on serum creatinine or urea level alone.
(2) Remember that renal function decreases with age and do not use drugs potentially toxic unless specific indication exists.
(3) When possible, the modifications of doses and regimen of administration should follow schedules previously evaluated in elderly patients.
(4) When available, monitoring drug level is of considerable help.

References

ANDREUCCI, V.E., HERRERA-ACOSTA, J., RECTOR Jr., F.C. and SELDIN, D.W. (1971). Effective glomerular filtration pressure and single nephron filtration rate during hydropenia, elevated ureteral pressure and active volume expansion with isotonic saline. *Journal of Clinical Investigation,* **50,** 2230–2234

ARAKAWA, M. (1971). A scanning electron microscopy of the human glomerulus. *American Journal of Pathology,* **64,** 457–466

ARTURSON, G., GROTH, T. and GROTTE, G. (1971). Human glomerular membrane porosity and filtration pressure: dextran clearance data analyzed by theoretical models. *Clinical Science,* **40,** 137–158

BALLET, G. (1881). Contribution à l'étude du rein sénile. *Revue de Médecine,* **221,** 451

BALUSU, L., HODGKINSON, A., NORDIN, B.E.L. and PEACOCK, D. (1970). Urinary excretion of calcium and creatinine in relation to age and body weight in normal subjects and patients with renal calculus. *Clinical Science,* **38,** 601–612

BARAJAS, L. (1978). Innervation of the renal cortex. *Federation Proceedings,* **37,** 1192–1201

BARRATT, T.M. and CHANTLER, C. (1975). Clinical assessment of renal function. In *Paediatric Nephrology,* edited by M.I. Rubin and T.M. Barratt, pp. 55–83. Baltimore; Williams and Wilkins

BAYLISS, W.M. (1902). On the local reactions of the arterial wall to changes in internal pressure. *Journal of Physiology (London),* **28,** 220–231

BAYLIS, C. and BRENNER, B.M. (1978). The physiologic determinants of glomerular ultrafiltration. *Reviews in Physiology, Biochemistry and Pharmacology,* **80,** 1–47

BEEUWKES, R. III, ICHIKAWA, I. and BRENNER, B.M. (1981). The renal circulation. In *The Kidney,* edited by B.M. Brenner and F.C. Rector, pp. 249–288. Philadelphia; Saunders

BINET, L., LAROCHE, C. and MATHÉ, G. (1952). Contribution à l'étude du rein sénile. *Presse Medicale,* **60,** 1211

BOHRER, M.P., BAYLIS, C. and HUMES, H.D. (1978). Permselectivity of the glomerular capillary wall. Facilitated filtration of circulating polycations. *Journal of Clinical Investigation,* **61,** 72–78

BRENNER, B.M., DWORKIN, L. and ICHIKAWA, I. (1986). Glomerular filtration. In *The Kidney,* 3rd edn, edited by B.M. Brenner and F.C. Rector, pp. 124–144. Philadelphia; Saunders

BRENNER, B.M., MEYER, T.W. and HOSTETTER, T.H. (1982). Dietary protein intake and the progressive nature of kidney disease. *New England Journal of Medicine,* **307,** 625–660

BRENNER, B.M., TROY, J.L. and DAUGHARTY, T.M. (1971). The dynamics of glomerular filtration in the rat. *Journal of Clinical Investigation,* **50,** 1776–1780

CARRIERE, S., THORBURN, G.D., O'MORCHOE, C.C.C. and BORGER, A.C. (1966). Intrarenal distribution of blood flow in dogs during hemorrhagic hypotension. *Circulation Research,* **19,** 167–179

CAULFIELD, J.P. and FARQUHAR, M.G. (1976). Distribution of anionic sites in glomerular basement membranes. Their possible role in filtration and attachment. *Proceedings of the National Academy of Sciences of the U.S.A.,* **73,** 1646–1649

CHANG, R.L.S., DEEN, W.M., ROBERTSON, C.R. and BRENNER, B.M. (1975). Permselectivity of the glomerular capillary wall. III Restricted transport of polyanions. *Kidney International,* **8,** 212–226

CHANG, R.L.S., DEEN, W.M., ROBERTSON, C.R. and BRENNER, B.M. (1976). Permselectivity of the glomerular capillary wall. Studies of experimental glomerulonephritis in the rat using neutral dextrans. *Journal of Clinical Investigation,* **57,** 1272–1286

CHANTLER, C., GARNETT, E.S., PARSONS, V. and VEALL, N. (1969). Glomerular filtration rate measurement in man by the single injection method using ^{51}Cr–EDTA. *Clinical Science,* **37,** 169–180

CLEMENTI, F. and PALADE, G.E. (1969). Intestinal capillaries. I. Permeability to peroxidase and ferritin. *Journal of Cell Biology,* **41,** 33–58

COCKCROFT, D.W. and GAULT, M.H. (1976). Prediction of creatinine clearance from serum creatinine. *Nephron,* **16,** 31–41

COMPER, W.D. and LAURENT, T.C. (1978). Physiological function of connective tissue polysaccharides. *Physiological Reviews,* **58,** 255–315

DAVIES, D.F. and SHOCK, N.W. (1950). Age changes in glomerular filtration rate, effective renal plasma flow, and tubular excretory capacity in adult males. *Journal of Clinical Investigation,* **29,** 496–507

DEEN, W.M., ROBERTSON, C.R. and BRENNER, B.M. (1974). Glomerular ultrafiltration. *Federation Proceedings,* **33,** 14–20

DEEN, W.M., TROY, S.L., ROBERTSON, C.R. and BRENNER, B.M. (1973). Dynamics of glomerular ultrafiltration in the rat IV. Determination of the ultrafiltration coefficient. *Journal of Clinical Investigation,* **52,** 1500–1508

DI SALVO, J. and FELL, G. (1971). Changes in renal blood flow during renal nerve stimulation. *Proceedings of the Society for Experimental Biology and Medicine,* **136,** 150–153

EARLY, L.E. and FRIEDLER, R.M. (1965). Studies on the mechanism of natriuresis accompanying increased renal flow and its role in the renal response to extracellular volume expansion. *Journal of Clinical Investigation,* **44,** 1857–1865

EISENBACH, G.M., VAN LIEW, J.B. and BOYLAND, J.W. (1975). Effect of angiotensin on the filtration of protein in the rat kidney: a micropuncture study. *Kidney International,* **8,** 80–84

FARQUHAR, M.G., GOMTOY, P.J., LEMKIN, M.D. and KANWAR, Y.S. (1982). Current knowledge of the functional architecture of the glomerular basement membrane. In *New Trends in Basement Membrane Research,* edited by K. Kuhn, H. Schone and R. Temple, pp. 9–29. New York; Raven Press

FARQUHAR, M.G., LEMKIN, M.C. and STOW, S.L. (1984). Role of proteoglycans in glomerular function and pathology. In *Nephrology,* edited by R.R. Robinson, pp. 510–600. New York; Springer

FORBES, G.B. and REINA, J.C. (1970). Adult lean body mass declines with age, some longitudinal observations. *Metabolism,* **19,** 653

GAGNON, J.A., KELLER, H.I., KOKOTIS, W. and SCHRIER, R.W. (1970). Analysis of role of renin–angiotensin system in autoregulation of glomerular filtration. *American Journal of Physiology,* **219,** 491–496

GLICK, R.L., JOYNER, W.L. and GILMORE, J.P. (1979). Reactivity of glomerular afferent and efferent arterioles in hypertension. *Kidney International,* **15,** 109–115

GOODYEAR, A.V.N. and JAEGER, C.A. (1955). Renal response to non-shocking hemorrhage in the dog. *American Journal of Physiology,* **180,** 69–75

GRAHAM, R.C. and KARNOVSKY, M.J. (1966). Glomerular permeability. Ultrastructural cytochemical studies using peroxidases as protein tracers. *Journal of Experimental Medicine,* **124,** 1123–1134

GRANERUS, G. and AURELL, M. (1981). Reference values for ^{51}Cr–EDTA clearance as a measure of glomerular filtration rate. *Scandinavian Journal of Clinical and Laboratory Investigation,* **41,** 611–616

HADDY, F.S. and SCOTT, S.B. (1968). Metabolically linked vasoactive chemicals in local regulation of blood flow. *Physiological Reviews,* **48,** 688–707

ISRAELIT, A.H., LONG, D.L. and WHITE, M.G. (1973). Measurement of glomerular filtration rate utilizing a single injection of ^{125}I-iothalamate. *Kidney International,* **4,** 346–349

JONES, R.D. and BERNE, R.M. (1964). Intrinsic regulation of skeletal muscle blood flow. *Circulation Research,* **14,** 126–138

JÖRGENSEN, F. (1966). *The Ultrastructure of the Normal Human Glomerulus.* Copenhagen; Ejnar Munksgaard

JÖRGENSEN, F. and BENTZON, M.W. (1968). The ultrastructure of the normal human membrane. *Laboratory Investigation,* **18,** 42–48

KAMPMANN, J., SIERSBAEK-NIELSEN, K., KRISTENSEN, M. and MÖLHOLM HANSEN, J. (1974). Rapid evaluation of creatinine clearance. *Acta Medica Scandinavica,* **196,** 517–520

KANWAR, Y.S. and FARQUHAR, M.G. (1980). Role of glycosaminoglycans in the permeability of glomerular basement membrane. *Federation Proceedings,* **30,** 334

KANWAR, Y.S., JAKUBOWSKY, M.L. and ROSENZEIG, L.J. (1983). Distribution of sulfated glycosaminoglycans in the glomerular basement membrane and mesangial matrix. *European Journal of Cell Biology,* **31,** 290–295

KLOPPER, J.F. and ATKINS, H.L. (1977). Measurement of glomerular filtration rate (letter). *The New England Journal of Medicine,* **296,** 284

LAINE, G., GOULLE, J.P., HOULBREQUE, P., GRUCHY, D. and LEBLANC, J. (1977). Clairance de la créatinine. Valeurs de référence en fonction de l'âge et du sex. *La nouvelle Presse Médicale,* **30,** 2690–2691

LATTA, H. (1973). Ultrastructure of glomerulus and the juxtaglomerular apparatus. In *Handbook of Physiology,* sec. 8, *Renal Physiology,* edited by J. Orloff and R.W. Berliner, pp. 1–29. Washington D.C.; American Physiological Society

LATTA, H., JOHNSTON, W.H. and STANLEY, T.M. (1973). Sialoglycoproteins and filtration barriers in the glomerular capillary wall. *Journal of Ultrastructural Research,* **51,** 354-359

LAURENT, T.C. (1966). *In vitro* studies on the transport of macromolecules through the connective tissue. *Federation Proceedings,* **25,** 1128–1134

LEVINSKY, N.G. and LEVY, M. (1973). Clearance techniques. In *Handbook of Physiology,* sec. 8, *Renal Physiology,* edited by J. Orloff and R.W. Berliner, pp. 103–118. Washington D.C.; American Physiological Society

LEWIS, W.H. and ALVING, A.S. (1938). Changes with age in the renal function in adult men. *American Journal of Physiology,* **123,** 500–515

MACIAS NUÑEZ, J.F., GARCIA IGLESIAS, C., TABERNERO ROMO, J.M., BONDIA, A., RODRIGUEZ COMMES, J.L., CORBACHO, M. *et al.* (1981). Estudio del filtrado glomerular en viejos sanos. *Revista Española de Geriatria y Gerontología,* **16**(2), 113–124

McCRORY, W.W. (1972). *Developmental Nephrology.* Cambridge, Mass.; Harvard University Press

McDONALD, R.K., SOLOMON, D.H. and SHOCK, N.W. (1951). Aging as a factor in the renal hemodynamic changes induced by a standardized pyrogen. *Journal of Clinical Investigation,* **30,** 457–462

MATTHEWS, C.M.E. (1957). The theory of tracer experiments with ^{131}I-labelled proteins. *Physics in Medicine and Biology,* **2,** 36–53

MIRIC, D., MIRIC, J., CONOVICI, L., MEMIN, Y. and VENET, R. (1982). Détermination simple de la fonction rénale du sujet âgé par absorption orale de créatinine. *Revue de Geriatrie,* **7,** 273–279

MITCHELL, A.D. and VALK, W.L. (1953). Renal function in the aged. *Geriatrics,* **8,** 263–266

MUSSER, J.H. and PHILIPS, A.W. (1930). A comparison of blood pressure, blood urea nitrogen, phenolsulphonephthalein and urine tests in the aged. *Journal of Laboratory and Clinical Medicine,* **15,** 633–637

NOSSLIN, B. (1965). Determination of clearance and distribution volume with the single injection technique. *Acta Medica Scandinavica,* **179,** suppl. 442, 97–101

OLBRICH, O., FERGUSON, M.H., ROBSON, J.S. and STEWART, C.P. (1950). Renal function in aged subjects. *Edinburgh Medical Journal,* **57,** 117–127

PAPPENHEIMER, J.R. (1953). Passage of macromolecules through capillary walls. *Physiological Reviews,* **33,** 387–423

RAPPLEYE, W.C. and FOXBORO, A.B. (1918). A study of the kidney function in senility. *Boston Medical and Surgical Journal,* **178,** 191–194

ROBERTSON, C.R., DEEN, W.M., TROY, J.L. and BRENNER, B.M. (1972). Dynamics of glomerular ultrafiltration in the rat. III Hemodynamics and autoregulation. *American Journal of Physiology,* **223,** 1191–1200

RODEWALD, R. and KARNOVSKY, M.J. (1974). Porous structure of the glomerular slit diaphragm in the rat and mouse. *Journal of Cell Biology,* **60,** 423–433

ROWE, J.W., ANDRES, R., TOBIN, J.D., NOMIS, A.H. and SHOCK, N.W. (1976a). The effect of age on creatinine clearance in men: a cross sectional and longitudinal study. *Journal of Gerontology,* **31,** 155–163

ROWE, J.W., ANDRES, R., TOBIN, J.D., NOMIS, A.H. and SHOCK, N.W. (1976b). Age-adjusted standards for creatinine clearance. *Annals of Internal Medicine,* **84,** 567–569

SAPIRSTEIN, L.A., VIDT, D.C., MANDEL, M.J. and HANUSEK, G. (1955). Volumes of distribution and clearances of intravenously injected creatinine in the dog. *American Journal of Physiology,* **181,** 330–336

SHIPLEY, R.E. and STUDY, R.S. (1951). Changes in renal blood flow, extraction of inulin, glomerular filtration rate, tissue pressure and urine flow with acute alteration of renal artery blood pressure. *American Journal of Physiology,* **167,** 676–688

SIERSBAEK-NIELSEN, K., MÖLHOLM HANSEN, J., KAMPMANN, J. and KRISTENSEN, M. (1971). Rapid evaluation of creatinine clearance. *Lancet,* **i,** 1133–1134

SMITH, H.W. (1943). *Lectures on the Kidney.* University Extension Division of University of Kansas, Lawrence, Kansas, p. 97

STEIN, J.M., OSGOOD, R.W. and FERRIS, T.F. (1972). Effect of volume expansion on distribution of glomerular filtrate and renal cortical blood flow in the dog. *American Journal of Physiology,* **223,** 984–990

THURAU, K. (1964). Renal hemodynamics. *American Journal of Medicine,* **36,** 698–719

THURAU, K. and WOBER, E. (1962). Zur Localization der Autoregulationen. Widerstands-änderungen in der Niere. *Pfluegers Archiv,* **274,** 553–566

TISHER, C.C. and MADSEN, K.M. (1986). Anatomy of the kidney. In *The Kidney,* 3rd edn, edited by B.M. Brenner and F.C. Rector, Jr., pp. 3–59. Philadelphia; Saunders

VALLERY-RADOT, P. and DELAFONTAINE, P. (1930). Le rein des viellards. *Presse Medicale,* **38,** 265–268

VENKATACHALAM, M.A. and RENNKE, H.G. (1978). The structural and molecular basis of glomerular filtration. *Circulation Research,* **43,** 337–347

VERNIER, R.L. (1964). Electron microscopic studies of the normal basement membrane. In *Small Blood Vessel Involvement in Diabetes Mellitus,* edited by Siperstein, M.D., Colwell, A.R. and Meyer, K. American Institute of Biological Sciences, Arlington

WESSON, L.G. (1969). Renal hemodynamics in physiological states. In *Physiology of the Human Kidney,* edited by Wesson, L.G., p. 96. New York; Grune and Stratton

ZIERLER, K.L. (1963). Equations for measuring blood flow by external monitoring of radioisotopes. *Circulation Research,* **16,** 309–321

Chapter 3

Mechanisms of age-associated glomerular sclerosis

Sharon Anderson, Timothy W. Meyer and Barry M. Brenner

Functional and structural glomerular changes in the aging kidney

The biological price of aging in many species includes renal functional and structural deterioration. In humans, the glomerular filtration rate (GFR) is low at birth, achieves adult levels by the end of the second year of life (Rubin, Bruck and Rapaport, 1949) and is maintained at approximately 140 ml/min/1.73 m^2 until the age of 30 (Davies and Shock, 1950). Thereafter, GFR declines in a roughly linear fashion, so that values in the eighth decade are only one-half to two-thirds those measured in young adults (Davies and Shock, 1950; Rowe *et al.*, 1976). Parallel changes in renal blood flow (RBF) occur, so that RBF is well maintained at about 350 ml/min until approximately the fourth decade, and then declines by about 10 per cent per decade. The decrement in renal perfusion associated with aging is most profound in the cortex; redistribution of flow from cortex to medulla may account for the slight increase in filtration fraction observed with advancing age (Wesson, 1969; Hollenberg *et al.*, 1974).

Studies in laboratory rats, whose age-related renal changes closely resemble an accelerated version of those in humans, suggest that another functional change in the aging kidney is an increase in glomerular basement membrane (GBM) permeability, leading to an increase in urinary protein excretion. Young rats excrete very little protein, which consists primarily of a sex-dependent α_2-microglobulin in the male and virtually no albumin. With aging, both the total amount of protein and the percentage of albumin rise sharply. Eventually, the full spectrum of serum proteins appears in the urine (Weaver, Gray and Schultz, 1975; Bolton *et al.*, 1976; Neuhaus and Flory, 1978). This progressive proteinuria heralds the development of age-associated glomerular structural injury.

In humans, renal mass increases from about 50 g at birth to over 400 g during the third and fourth decades, with a subsequent decline to under 300 g by the ninth decade. The loss of renal mass is primarily cortical, with relative sparing of the renal medulla (Tauchi, Tsuboi and Okutomi, 1971). Morphologic studies have confirmed that the decline in renal mass is accompanied by marked glomerular alterations (Elema and Arends, 1971; Tauchi, Tsuboi and Okutomi, 1971; Couser and Stilmant, 1975; Bolton *et al.*, 1976; Coleman *et al.*, 1977; McLachlan *et al.*, 1977). The number of glomeruli declines roughly in accord with the changes in renal weight, while the size of the remaining glomeruli increases (McLachlan, 1978; Goyal, 1982). With maturation and aging, important changes in glomerular shape also occur (McLachlan, 1978). The spherical glomerulus in the fetal kidney develops lobular indentations as it matures, which increases the surface area available for filtration. With aging, lobulation tends to diminish and the glomerular tuft perimeter length decreases relative to its area.

Studies using micro-angiopathic and histologic techniques have elucidated the sequence of glomerular structural changes with aging (McManus and Lupton, 1960; Ljungqvist and Lagergren, 1962; Takazakura *et al.*, 1972). Briefly summarized, the GBM undergoes progressive folding and then thickening. This stage is accompanied by glomerular simplification, with the formation of free anastomoses between a reduced number of glomerular capillary loops. Frequently, dilatation of the afferent arteriole near the hilum is seen at this stage. Eventually, the folded and thickened GBM condenses into hyaline material with collapse of the glomerular tuft. Degeneration of glomeruli in the renal cortex results in atrophy of the afferent and efferent arterioles, with eventual global sclerosis. However, a different pattern of change predominates in the arteriolar–glomerular units in the juxtamedullary area. In these units, sclerosis of the glomerular tuft is accompanied by the formation of a direct channel between afferent and efferent arterioles, resulting in the arteriolae rectae verae, or aglomerular arterioles (Ljungqvist and Lagergren, 1962; Takazakura *et al.*, 1972). Presumably, the formation of these direct channels contributes to the maintenance of medullary blood flow as cortical perfusion declines. These aglomerular arterioles are rarely found in kidneys from healthy young persons; their frequency increases both in aging kidneys and in kidneys from patients with intrinsic renal disease (Takazakura *et al.*, 1972).

The incidence of sclerotic glomeruli increases with advancing age. To the age of 40, sclerotic glomeruli comprise fewer than 5 per cent of the total. With increasing age thereafter, the incidence increases so that sclerosis involves 10–30 per cent of the total glomerular population by the eighth decade (Kaplan *et al.*, 1975; Kappel and Olsen, 1980). Accordingly, diminished glomerular lobulation and glomerular loss contribute to a reduction of the surface area available for filtration and thus to the observed age-related decline in GFR (McLachlan, 1978).

Dietary modification of age-related glomerular sclerosis

Progressive glomerular sclerosis, heralded by proteinuria, takes place in aging animals of many species (Saxton and Kimball, 1941; Guttman and Andersen, 1968; Elema *et al.*, 1971; Woodhead, Pond and Dailey, 1983) as well as humans. Attempts to elucidate the mechanisms responsible for age-related glomerular sclerosis have led to the identification of a number of factors which can be shown to modify the process in experimental animals (*Tables 3.1* and *3.2*). Of these, dietary manipulations have been the most dramatic and the most extensively studied.

The importance of nutrition in the aging process was first recognized by McCay, Crowell and Maynard (1935), who demonstrated that restriction of food intake increases the lifespan of laboratory rats. During the next 50 years, many investigators have offered evidence that food restriction slows the aging process, as manifested by (1) extension of the lifespan, (2) retardation of age-related physiologic processes, and (3) retardation of age-related disease processes in experimental animals (Masoro *et al.*, 1980). Saxton and Kimball (1941) noted that 'chronic nephrosis' was second in frequency only to chronic pneumonia in pathologic lesions found in aging rats, and that limitation of caloric intake resulted in fewer glomerular lesions. Female animals, which eat less and have smaller kidneys,

Table 3.1 Factors known to accelerate age-related proteinuria and glomerular sclerosis

Overfeeding (Kennedy, 1957; Koletsky, 1975; Shimamura, 1982)
High protein diet (Newburgh and Curtis, 1928; Blatherwick and Medlar, 1937; Saxton and Kimball, 1941)
High salt diet (Elema and Arends, 1971)
Male gender (Blatherwick and Medlar, 1937; Saxton and Kimball, 1941; Berg and Simms, 1960; Elema and Arends, 1975)
Androgen therapy (Sellers *et al.*, 1950; Linkswiler, Reynolds and Baumann, 1952)
Partial renal ablation (Kennedy, 1957; Wachtel, Cole and Rosen, 1966; Striker *et al.*, 1969; Meyer *et al.*, 1983a)
Renal irradiation (Guttman and Kohn, 1960; Wachtel, Cole and Rosen, 1966; Elema *et al.*, 1971)
Thyroid supplements (Berg, 1966)
Thymectomy (Guttman and Bailey, 1965)

Table 3.2 Factors known to ameliorate age-related proteinuria and glomerular sclerosis

Food restriction (Saxton and Kimball, 1941; Berg and Simms, 1960; Tucker, Mason and Beauchene, 1976; Johnson and Barrows, 1980; Everitt, Porter and Wyndham, 1982; Yu *et al.*, 1982)
Protein restriction (Saxton and Kimball, 1941; Bras and Ross, 1964; Johnson and Barrows, 1980; Feldman, McConnell and Knapka, 1982; Meyer *et al.*, 1983a; Spector *et al.*, 1985)
Sodium restriction (Elema and Arends, 1975)
Female gender (Blatherwick and Medlar, 1937; Saxton and Kimball, 1941; Berg and Simms, 1960; Elema and Arends, 1975)
Castration (Sellers *et al.*, 1950; Linkswiler, Reynolds and Baumann, 1952)
Adrenalectomy (Addis *et al.*, 1950)
Hypophysectomy (Everitt, Seedsman and Jones, 1980)

acquire renal lesions more slowly (Blatherwick and Medlar, 1937; Saxton and Kimball, 1941; Berg and Simms, 1960; Elema and Arends, 1975). Development of renal lesions in both sexes can be delayed by making food available on alternate days or by limiting the amount of food to one-half to two-thirds the amount consumed by animals fed *ad libitum* (Berg and Simms, 1960; Tucker, Mason and Beauchene, 1976; Johnson and Barrows, 1980; Everitt, Porter and Wyndham, 1982). In contrast, progression of glomerular sclerosis in rats is hastened when overeating is conditioned by heredity (Koletsky, 1975; Shimamura, 1982) or induced by hypothalamic injury (Kennedy, 1957). In rats with hereditary overeating, as in normal rats fed *ad libitum*, progression of glomerular injury may be retarded by restricting food intake (Shimamura, 1982).

Reduction of dietary protein content delays the development of age-related proteinuria and glomerular sclerosis even when total caloric intake is not restricted (Saxton and Kimball, 1941; Bras and Ross, 1964; Johnson and Barrows, 1980; Feldman, McConnell and Knapka, 1982; Meyer *et al.*, 1983a; Spector *et al.*, 1985). Although the most complete protection of the kidney is afforded by restricting protein intake to levels (4–6 per cent) low enough to limit body growth, significant protection is also afforded by reducing protein intake to a level (12 per cent) that does not impair growth (Everitt, Seedsman and Jones, 1980; Feldman, McConnell and Knapka, 1982).

It seems likely that haemodynamic alterations mediate these glomerular structural changes (Brenner, Meyer and Hostetter, 1982). While dietary intake of carbohydrates and fats have little effect on the kidney, renal size, structure and function are markedly influenced by protein intake. Kidney size increases in rats fed protein-rich diets (MacKay, MacKay and Addis, 1928) and in patients on chronic hyperalimentation receiving large amounts of amino acids intravenously (Cochran, Pagani and Barbaric, 1979). Renal blood flow and glomerular filtration rates rise acutely by 40–100 per cent in dogs fed a meal of meat, but not carbohydrate or fat (Shannon, Jolliffe and Smith, 1932; O'Connor and Summerill, 1976a). Micropuncture studies in rats have demonstrated that intravenous infusion of amino acids results in afferent and efferent arteriolar vasodilatation. The resultant increase in glomerular plasma flow, together with a small increase in glomerular capillary hydraulic pressure, account for the observed 43 per cent rise in single nephron GFR (SNGFR) (Meyer *et al.*, 1983b).

Recently, striking increases in GFR (Bosch *et al.*, 1983) and RBF (Avasthi *et al.*, 1985) have been reported to follow meat feeding in normal humans. The postprandial increase in RBF is unrelated to changes in cardiac output (Fronek and Stahlgren, 1968; Bosch *et al.*, 1983); thus, ingestion of protein, as opposed to other nutrients, appears to result in a preferential increase in renal perfusion that is accompanied by an increase in GFR. In turn, there is a relatively rapid excretion of water, electrolytes and nitrogenous wastes, so that urine flow doubles and excretion of urea, sodium, potassium and phosphorus increases by more than 200 per cent in the dog (O'Connor and Summerill, 1976b). When animals are maintained continuously on protein-rich diets, the mechanisms which increase RBF and GFR after individual protein meals lead, by cumulative effect, to sustained increases in GFR and RBF and to renal hypertrophy. Baseline GFR values have been found to be markedly higher in subjects eating conventional diets than in vegetarians (Bosch *et al.*, 1983). Shannon, Jolliffe and Smith (1932) observed that the basal pre-meal GFR in a dog maintained on daily meat feedings was twice that seen when the dog was maintained for 2 weeks on a diet rich in carbohydrate and fat. Similarly, the average GFR is some 40 per cent higher in rats maintained on 24–35 per cent protein diets than in rats fed 6 per cent protein chow (Schoolwerth *et al.*, 1975) or fed standard (24 per cent protein) chow on alternate days (Gehrig *et al.*, 1985). In a micropuncture study of rats fed a 40 per cent protein diet, Ichikawa *et al.* (1980) noted a 30 per cent increase in whole kidney and single nephron GFR as compared to animals pair-fed a 6 per cent protein diet. The higher SNGFR in rats fed the protein-rich diet resulted from afferent and efferent arteriolar vasodilatation, which increases glomerular plasma flow; the glomerular capillary ultrafiltration coefficient was also higher than in protein-restricted rats.

The mechanism by which protein ingestion increases renal perfusion and filtration remains unclear. The renal haemodynamic changes triggered by a meat meal can be reproduced by gastric instillation or intravenous infusion of amino acids (Pitts, 1944; Lee and Summerill, 1982; Meyer *et al.*, 1983b; Castellino, Coda and DeFronzo, 1985), but not by consumption of urea, sulphate or acid in amounts equivalent to those produced by catabolism of the meat (O'Connor and Summerill, 1976b, 1976c). Administration of somatostatin has recently been reported to block the increases in GFR and RBF otherwise seen following intravenous infusion of amino acids in humans (Castellino, Coda and DeFronzo, 1985) and in rats (Meyer *et al.*, 1983b), and GFR fails to rise after a protein load in growth-hormone deficient adults (Kleinman and Glassock, 1985). It seems likely, therefore, that amino acids trigger the release of a circulating hormone (or other intermediate effector), which in turn is responsible for increasing RBF and GFR.

It seems reasonable to assume that, whatever its mechanism, the renal haemodynamic response to protein feeding reflects evolutionary adaptation of the kidney to the excretory needs of animals whose protein intake was not constant. Such animals, presumably including our remote ancestors, obtained meals containing large amounts of protein at irregular intervals. The renal vasodilator mechanisms triggered by protein ingestion, by increasing RBF and GFR, would be expected to facilitate excretion of these large solute loads. With irregular access to protein, it is likely that RBF and GFR reside at low baseline levels during interprandial intervals. RBF and GFR should thus be more variable and, on average, lower in intermittent feeders than in animals with more nearly constant access to protein-rich food. Support for this concept comes from the recent report that GFR and RBF in rats fed every other day are lower on fasted days than on fed days, and that renal perfusion and filtration rates on both days are lower than in rats fed every day (Gehrig *et al.*, 1985).

We have suggested that the protein-rich diet characteristic of modern Western society might itself induce chronic renal hyperfiltration and hyperperfusion, and thereby contribute to the functional and structural deterioration of the aging kidney (Brenner, Meyer and Hostetter, 1982). According to this hypothesis, the excessive glomerular pressures and flows necessary to meet the demands of a multiple meal per day, protein-rich diet may contribute to eventual glomerular sclerosis. By itself, age-related glomerular sclerosis poses no threat to well-being. If, however, intrinsic renal disease or surgical loss of renal tissue adds to the glomerular burden imposed by *ad libitum* feeding, the course of glomerular sclerosis may be hastened appreciably. In this regard, although the incidence of primary renal disease in the elderly may not be significantly greater than in younger adults,* the frequency of acute renal failure and of renal disease associated with such systemic diseases as atherosclerosis, hypertension, cardiac failure, diabetes mellitus and malignancy most certainly increases with advancing age (Samiy, 1983).

Acceleration of progressive glomerular sclerosis when *ad libitum* feeding is combined with loss of renal mass

The simplest model of reduced nephron number is produced by surgical nephrectomy. Surgical reduction of renal mass leads to structural and functional hypertrophy of the residual nephrons (Hayslett, 1979), resulting in marked increases in the perfusion and filtration of remaining nephrons. Micropuncture studies in the rat have shown that reduction of renal mass results in afferent and efferent arteriolar vasodilatation, allowing an increase in glomerular plasma flow rate (Deen *et al.*, 1974; Hostetter *et al.*, 1981). Because the reduction in afferent arteriolar resistance is proportionately greater than the reduction in efferent arteriolar resistance, the glomerular capillary hydraulic pressure increases. Together, these increases in glomerular capillary plasma flow and hydraulic pressure account for the increased GFR in remnant nephrons. Hyperfiltration in remnant nephrons has generally been regarded as beneficial, since it minimizes the reduction in total GFR which would otherwise ensue.

Recent experimental observations, however, suggest that these changes are in fact 'maladaptive', in that sustained glomerular hypertension and hyperperfusion cause progressive glomerular structural damage. More than 50 years ago, Chanutin and Ferris (1932) demonstrated a syndrome of progressive azotaemia and eventual glomerular sclerosis following removal of three-quarters of the total renal mass in

*But see *Table 1* of the Preface (Eds).

the rat. The progressive morphologic changes seen in remnant glomeruli of rats with five-sixths renal ablation were later documented by Shimamura and Morrison (1975) and Purkerson, Hoffsten and Klahr (1976). Within 3 months after ablation, remnant glomeruli exhibited hypertrophy, accompanied by ultrastructural alterations including vacuolization of epithelial cells, deposition of osmophilic droplets in these cells, and foot process fusion. After 6 months, mesangial matrix expansion and denudation of cells from areas of basement membrane were evident. These ultrastructural alterations heralded progressive hyalinization and eventual sclerosis of remnant glomeruli.

The glomerular morphologic injury which follows reduction of renal mass is reflected by progressive proteinuria (Chanutin and Ferris, 1932; Meyer *et al.*, 1983a). Olson *et al.* (1982), in studies of glomerular processing of tracer macromolecules following extensive renal ablation, demonstrated that the proteinuria is due to defects in both the size-selective and charge-selective properties of the glomerular capillary wall.

The glomerular changes that eventuate in glomerular sclerosis in the rat remnant kidney are morphologically identical to those seen in the aging rat kidney; the only difference is the rapidity of glomerular structural deterioration. In the rat, the pace of glomerular structural injury, like the magnitude of remnant glomerular haemodynamic changes, increases in proportion to the amount of renal tissue removed. The modest increases in glomerular capillary pressures and flows following uninephrectomy are associated with moderate acceleration of the glomerular sclerosis seen in aging rats (Striker *et al.*, 1969; Meyer *et al.*, 1983a). With the marked elevations in pressures and flows that occur after more extensive (over 75 per cent) nephrectomy, structural alterations of remnant glomeruli may be seen within a few weeks (Hostetter *et al.*, 1981).

In the remnant kidney, manoeuvres which limit these increases in glomerular capillary pressures and flows retard the progressive sclerosis of the remaining kidney. Dietary protein restriction, which slows the pace of glomerular sclerosis in the aging kidney, has also been shown to retard glomerular injury in the remnant kidneys of animals with reduced renal mass. In a study of rats subjected to surgical removal of 90 per cent of the total renal mass, Hostetter *et al.* (1981) found that the SNGFR in remnant nephrons of animals fed standard (24 per cent protein) chow averaged more than twice normal by 1 week after ablation. This increment in SNGFR resulted from marked increases in the glomerular plasma flow rate and glomerular capillary hydraulic pressure. In contrast, glomerular capillary pressures and flows remained at near normal levels in similarly prepared rats fed a 6 per cent protein diet, despite equivalent ablation of renal tissue. Values for SNGFR were therefore considerably lower in these rats than in rats subjected to a similar degree of renal ablation but fed the standard diet.

Limitation of glomerular hyperfiltration and prevention of glomerular capillary hypertension and hyperperfusion by protein restriction were associated with preservation of glomerular structure. Within 2 weeks following ablation, remnant kidneys of animals fed standard chow showed protein reabsorption droplets in glomerular epithelial cells, attenuation of epithelial cell bodies, and focal fusion of foot processes. These epithelial cell changes were associated with lifting of endothelial cells from the inner aspect of the GBM and with increases in the mesangial area. Glomerular morphologic abnormalities were much less extensive in remnant kidneys of protein-restricted rats. In addition, proteinuria was limited in protein-restricted rats, suggesting preservation of the glomerular permselectivity barrier. Subsequent long-term studies have confirmed that dietary protein restriction delays the development of proteinuria and pathologic changes in remnant kidneys of rats and dogs subjected to less extensive renal ablation (El-Nahas *et al.*, 1983; Madden and Zimmerman, 1983; Meyer *et al.*, 1983a; Polzin *et al.*, 1984).

Glomerular capillary pressures and flows increase not only following renal ablation, but also when functioning nephron number has been reduced by intrinsic renal disease. Pathologic studies in diverse forms of human renal disease have revealed hypertrophy (presumably reflecting hyperfiltration) of the nephrons least damaged by the original disease process (Gottschalk, 1971). Studies in rats with 'post-salt' hypertension (Azar *et. al.*, 1977, 1978) and with mineralocorticoid-induced hypertension (Dworkin *et al.*, 1984) have also revealed a strong correlation between glomerular pathology and pre-existing glomerular capillary hypertension and hyperperfusion. As with renal ablation, lowering of glomerular capillary pressures and flows in rats with mineralocorticoid-induced hypertension by dietary protein restriction results in limitation of proteinuria and protection against glomerular injury (Dworkin *et al.*, 1984). Reduction of dietary protein intake has also been shown to retard the progression of nephrotoxic serum nephritis in rats (Farr and Smadel, 1939; Neugarten *et al.*, 1983) and the lupus-like nephropathy of the NZB/NZW mouse (Friend *et al.*, 1978), as well as the nephropathy of the rat with streptozotocin-induced diabetes (Wen, Benell and Moorthy, 1984). Dietary protein restriction lowers glomerular pressures and flows in diabetic rats (Zatz *et al.*, 1985); it is likely that the beneficial effects of protein restriction in these models are likewise due to limitation of hyperfiltration.

Conversely, manoeuvres which are known to increase glomerular pressures and flows accelerate the pace of experimental injury in such diverse forms of experimental renal disease as nephrotoxic serum nephritis, diabetes mellitus, puromycin aminonucleoside nephrosis and lupus-like nephropathy (Teodoru, Saifer and Frankel, 1959; Beyer *et al.*, 1977; Velosa *et al.*, 1977; Seyer-Hansen, 1978). Presumably, uninephrectomy adds to the haemodynamic burden of glomerular capillaries previously subjected to various injurious influences, thereby accelerating glomerular destruction.

Taken together, the foregoing observations in normal aging and in patients and animals with various forms of renal parenchymal disease, are consistent with the hypothesis that sustained hyperfiltration (or some haemodynamic determinant(s)

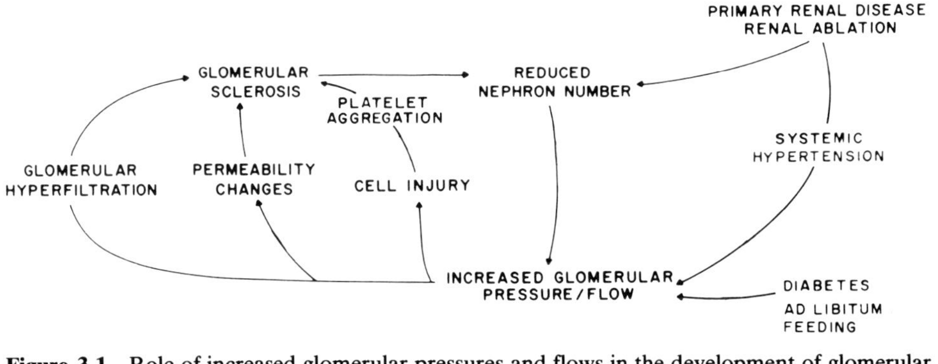

Figure 3.1 Role of increased glomerular pressures and flows in the development of glomerular sclerosis (see text for discussion)

thereof) is ultimately detrimental to glomerular structure and function. According to this scheme (*Figure 3.1*), reduction in functioning renal mass, systemic hypertension, conventionally treated diabetes and *ad libitum* feeding all lead to unrelenting renal vasodilatation. The resulting long-term elevations in glomerular pressures and flows promote hyperfiltration, impair the permselective properties of the glomerular wall and injure the component cells of the glomerulus. The resulting glomerular sclerosis exerts a positive feedback stimulus to compensatory hyperfiltration in less affected glomeruli, contributing in turn to their eventual destruction.

The mechanisms whereby increased glomerular pressures and flows alter glomerular structure are not clear. The increased glomerular transcapillary hydraulic pressure gradient may injure the capillary network by some mechanism analogous to the effects of hypertension on the systemic arterial vessels, presumably involving mechanical disruption of normal vascular integrity (Parving *et al.*, 1983). In the aging rat kidney, Elema and Arends (1975) noted that glomerular structural lesions always seemed to arise near the afferent arterioles, raising the possibility that some haemodynamic factor accompanied by increased local pressure was involved in the pathogenesis of the lesion. In this regard, it is important to point out that systemic hypertension is not a prerequisite for the glomerular sclerosis that accompanies aging or reduction in renal mass (Madden and Zimmerman, 1983; Meyer *et al.*, 1983a). Furthermore, it has been reported that pharmacologic control of systemic hypertension without reduction of glomerular capillary hypertension fails to afford protection to the glomeruli of rats with mineralocorticoid-induced hypertension (Dworkin, Feiner and Randazzo, 1985). Intraglomerular hypertension may induce mechanical injury to the glomerular endothelium. Denudation of the GBM has been noted following extensive renal ablation (Hostetter *et al.*, 1981). Endothelial damage may, in turn, result in exposure of circulating plasma proteins to GBM constituents, thereby activating local coagulation cascades. Capillary thrombosis has been demonstrated in glomeruli of remnant kidneys following renal ablation in rats. Heparin, warfarin, thromboxane synthetase inhibitors, and aspirin in combination with dipyridamole, have all been reported to retard glomerular injury in this model (Olson, 1984; Purkerson, Hoffsten and Klahr, 1976; Purkerson *et al.*, 1982, 1984, 1985), but the mechanism of the protective effect is unclear. Of note, each of these therapies was associated not only with anticoagulation, but also with significant lowering of systemic blood pressure. It is possible, therefore, that the efficacy of these agents is due not only to their anticoagulant properties, but to unrecognized beneficial effects on intrarenal haemodynamics.

Increased capillary pressures and flows may also damage the glomerulus by promoting increased movement of macromolecules through the glomerular wall and into the glomerular mesangium. Studies employing tracer macromolecules have shown that the progressive proteinuria occurring in remnant nephrons results from defects in both the charge- and size-selective properties of the glomerular capillary wall (Robson *et al.*, 1979; Olson *et al.*, 1982). The presence of albumin and of larger macromolecules in the urine of aging animals (Weaver, Gray and Schultz, 1975; Bolton *et al.*, 1976; Neuhaus and Flory, 1978) suggests that a similar defect develops during the aging process. It is unclear whether passage of macromolecules through the capillary wall and into the urinary space by itself aggravates glomerular injury. Damage to the filtration barrier has, however, been associated with increased deposition of tracer macromolecules in the mesangium both in the remnant kidney

(Olson *et al.*, 1982) and in other disease models (Sterzel *et al.*, 1982), and mesangial deposits of IgM in the aging rat kidney (Couser and Stilmant, 1975; Bolton *et al.*, 1976). An increase in mesangial 'trafficking' of macromolecules may in turn promote increases in mesangial matrix production and hypercellularity, leading eventually to glomerular sclerosis (Michael *et al.*, 1980; Sterzel *et al.*, 1982).

These observations in experimental animals raise an important clinical question: how much renal mass must be lost in humans to induce progressive glomerular disease, or to accelerate significantly age-related glomerular injury? An increased incidence of focal and segmental glomerular sclerosis has been reported in patients with unilateral renal agenesis (Kiprov, Colvin and McCluskey, 1982; Thorner *et al.*, 1984); but it is possible that these solitary kidneys, like the kidneys of patients with bilateral reduction in nephron number ('oligomeganephronia') (Fetterman and Habib, 1969; McGraw *et al.*, 1984), are congenitally abnormal. Long-term follow-up studies of patients undergoing uninephrectomy for unilateral renal disease or kidney transplant donation are required to establish the consequences of reducing nephron number in humans with an initially normal complement of nephrons. The success of living related donor transplantation makes particularly important the need to gather more precise information regarding the long-term consequences of uninephrectomy in humans.

Follow-up studies of renal transplant donors, who have been carefully screened to rule out pre-existing renal disease, are only now becoming available. From these studies, it appears that renal function is well maintained in the majority of donors for up to 3 decades post-donation (Vincenti *et al.*, 1983; Hakim, Goldszer and Brenner, 1984; Weiland *et al.*, 1984). However, recent studies of donors 10–30 years after nephrectomy have revealed significantly higher incidences of hypertension and proteinuria than in age- and sex-matched controls (Vincenti *et al.*, 1983; Hakim, Goldszer and Brenner, 1984; Ferran *et al.*, 1985). Of special concern are recent reports of biopsy proven glomerular sclerosis occurring in previously healthy donors (Chocair *et al.*, 1984) and in recipients of grafts from identical (monozygotic) twins, where immunologically mediated 'chronic rejection' can be ruled out with certainty (Dammin, 1981; Rivolta *et al.*, 1983). Clearly, further studies are required to assess the long-term sequelae of kidney donation, particularly in the younger donor who will presumably have longer exposure to glomerular hyperfiltration after nephrectomy.

The progression of human renal disease

Chronic renal insufficiency progresses to end-stage renal failure in patients, just as it does after renal ablation in rats. Virtually all patients with GFR values below about 30 ml/min will eventually require dialysis or transplantation, regardless of the original cause of reduced renal function. Time plots of the reciprocal of serum creatinine concentration suggest steady deterioration of nephron function at rates peculiar to each patient, but not characteristic of the underlying disease (Mitch *et al.*, 1976; Rutherford *et al.*, 1977). In some patients, the disease responsible for the initial renal injury remains active, but more frequently, renal function declines despite the initiating process having resolved spontaneously or been controlled therapeutically. For example, renal disease progresses in patients after acute poststreptococcal glomerulonephritis in the absence of ongoing immunologic injury to the kidney (Baldwin, 1982). Likewise, patients with bilateral cortical necrosis may temporarily recover stable, albeit reduced renal function, before proceeding to end-stage renal failure (Kleinknecht *et al.,* 1973). Recovery of renal function is frequently incomplete in acute renal failure of other aetiologies, and in some of these cases progressive loss of renal function also follows initial recovery (Finn, 1983). Patients with vesico-ureteric reflux who have developed significant impairment of renal function and proteinuria may progress to renal failure despite control of systemic hypertension, prevention of urinary tract infection and surgical correction of the reflux (Torres *et al.,* 1980; Cotran, 1982). Likewise, patients with analgesic nephropathy, sometimes said to exhibit stable renal insufficiency, in fact frequently progress to renal failure despite discontinuation of analgesic medications (Kincaid-Smith, 1980).

In addition to the foregoing examples, where diffuse nephron destruction by a disease process is presumed to increase the haemodynamic burden of the remaining normal nephrons, there are certain diseases which may of themselves increase the haemodynamic burden of an initially normal glomerular population. Patients with insulin-dependent (Type I) diabetes mellitus have markedly elevated values of GFR and RBF through the first decade of the disease (Mogensen, 1976). Equivalent hyperfiltration in rats with streptozotocin-induced diabetes has been shown to result from elevations of glomerular capillary pressures and flows similar to those seen in the remnant kidney (Hostetter, Troy and Brenner, 1981). These observations have prompted the suggestion that glomerular hyperperfusion in diabetes initiates a cycle of glomerular injury, causing exaggerated glomerular haemodynamic changes and leading, in turn, to accelerated glomerular destruction (Hostetter, Rennke and Brenner, 1982). The recent observation that juvenile diabetics whose glomerular filtration rates are markedly elevated at the time diabetes is diagnosed are more likely to progress to clinically overt proteinuria or diabetic nephropathy, lends further support to this hypothesis (Mogensen and Christensen, 1984).

We have suggested that the glomerular haemodynamic burden engendered by our modern protein-rich diet similarly contributes to the glomerular sclerosis of the aging kidney (Brenner, Meyer and Hostetter, 1982). The consequences of this process are summarized in *Figure 3.2.* The bottom panel depicts the nephron population that we may regard as typical of the healthy young rat, and presumably the healthy young human as well. SNGFR values for the entire glomerular population follow a narrow Gaussian distribution, with the mean value depicted by the dashed line. By eating our modern, hence biologically excessive, protein diet a small fraction of the glomeruli at the upper end of the function scale (the shaded area in the bottom panel) are considered to be burdened, due to the adaptive increases in pressures and flows that account for their relative hyperfiltration. Over time, these glomeruli develop progressive sclerosis and eventually fail so that, as shown in the middle panel, populations of non-functioning and poorly functioning nephrons emerge. In consequence, more normal glomeruli hyperfilter to accommodate the unrelenting high-protein diet in the face of fewer functioning nephrons. SNGFR values therefore widen considerably in distribution and in doing so, all operate at risk, as depicted by the marked expansion of the shaded area. This risk in low SNGFR nephrons reflects the high hydraulic pressures regularly seen in chronically injured glomeruli, whereas in higher SNGFR glomeruli, pressures and flows must both be elevated for hyperfiltration to occur.

Despite the heterogeneity in SNGFR values shown in the middle panel, the population is still largely Gaussian and the average SNGFR value is unchanged from that shown in the bottom panel. Since total nephron number remains constant, total GFR at this stage also remains at 100 per cent of the starting value. Eventually, we

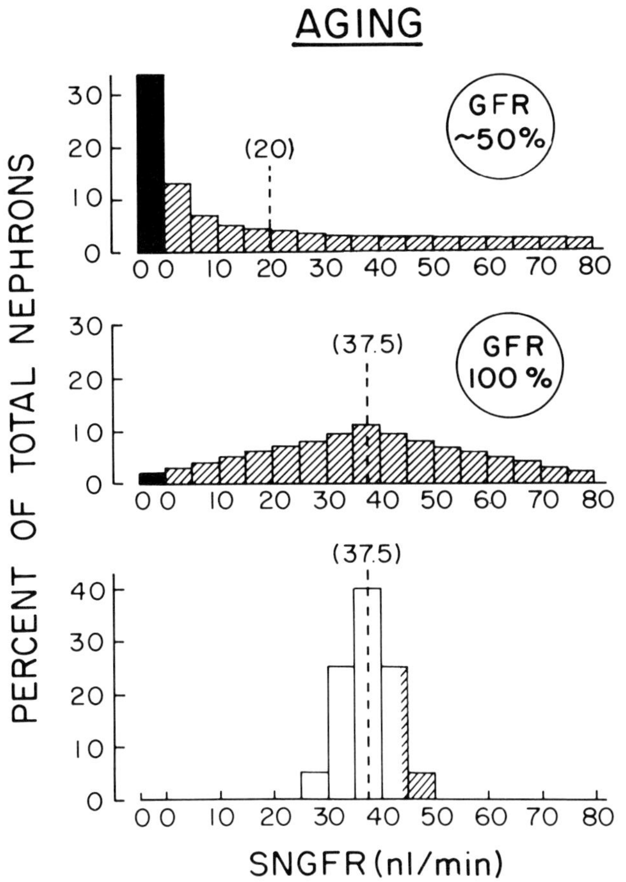

Figure 3.2 Age-related changes in single nephron glomerular filtration rate. SN, single nephron; GFR, glomerular filtration rate (see text for discussion) (From Brenner, 1985, reproduced with permission)

reach the stage depicted in the top panel, where the previously most burdened glomeruli have now ceased functioning, which yields a large population with SNGFR values essentially equal to zero (black bar, bracketed by zero values) and an increasing fraction of the total nephron population with SNGFR values below normal. Not surprisingly, therefore, total GFR must also decline, but in this example by only 50 per cent, since that is the magnitude of reduction in average nephron GFR. Certainly, it would seem prudent to consider therapeutic intervention before this stage is reached.

Therapeutic implications

If elevated glomerular capillary pressures and flows contribute to the progression of glomerular sclerosis in patients with aging or disease-induced renal insufficiency, therapies aimed at reducing glomerular hypertension and hyperperfusion may be effective in preserving renal function over the long term. One obvious therapy is restriction of dietary protein intake, implemented early in the course of glomerular adaptation. More than 30 years ago, Addis (1948) suggested that protein intake be restricted in patients with early renal insufficiency. His aim was to decrease the 'workload' of surviving nephrons in diseased kidneys to preserve their function. The subsequent development of dialysis and transplantation distracted attention from the effects of diet on renal disease. Recently, however, there has been renewed interest in the possibility that protein restriction may slow the typically progressive course of renal insufficiency (Mitch, 1984). Several investigators have suggested that reduction of dietary protein intake can slow the rate of decline in renal function, and postpone the necessity for dialysis and/or transplantation, in patients with chronic renal failure (Giordano, 1982; Maschio *et al.*, 1982; Mitch *et al.*, 1984). In these studies, reduction of dietary protein intake to 0.6 g protein/kg body weight/day, or to even lower levels with supplementation by essential amino acids or their nitrogen-free analogues, may favourably affect renal function with maintenance of positive nitrogen balance.

Early and aggressive therapy of systemic hypertension, perhaps to reduce diastolic pressure to levels below those now generally regarded as acceptable, may also confer protection against haemodynamically-mediated glomerular injury when functioning nephron number is reduced. While uncontrolled hypertension hastens the decline in GFR which accompanies both normal aging (Lindeman, Tobin and Shock, 1984) and chronic renal disease (Moyer *et al.*, 1958), long-term studies of the effect of strict blood pressure control on the progression of renal disease remain to be performed. Nevertheless, studies evaluating moderate blood pressure control over periods of up to 1 year have suggested that reduction of systemic blood pressure may slow renal functional deterioration in patients with renal insufficiency due to intrinsic renal disease or to essential hypertension (Bauer, 1984; Branca *et al.*, 1984; Nabel *et al.*, 1984), and recent prospective studies offer evidence that control of systemic hypertension slows the progression of renal disease in patients with Type I diabetes mellitus (Mogensen, 1981; Parving *et al.*, 1983). In this regard, reduction of systemic and glomerular pressures with the converting enzyme inhibitor enalapril has been reported to lessen glomerular structural injury in rats with renal ablation (Anderson *et al.*, 1985), and to limit the development of albuminuria in the hyperfiltering kidneys of rats with streptozotocin-induced diabetes (Zatz *et al.*, 1986).

These encouraging findings notwithstanding, a great deal clearly remains to be learned about the mechanisms responsible for glomerular injury in normal aging as well as in acquired renal disease. It is hoped that further experimental and clinical studies relating both nutritional and pharmacologic manoeuvres to glomerular function will ultimately enable us to prevent deterioration of renal function in patients who are at risk for progressive renal injury.

Acknowledgements

These studies were supported by U.S. Public Health Service Grant AM-19467. Dr Anderson is the recipient of an Individual National Research Service Award of the National Institutes of Health (S F32 AM 07206). Michelle Hardiman provided expert secretarial assistance.

References

ADDIS, T. (1948). *Glomerular Nephritis: Diagnosis and Treatment.* New York; Macmillan

ADDIS, T., MARMORSTON, J., GOODMAN, H.C., SELLERS, A.L. and SMITH, M. (1950). Effect of adrenalectomy on spontaneous and induced proteinuria in the rat. *Proceedings of the Society for Experimental Biology and Medicine,* **74,** 43–46

ANDERSON, S., MEYER, T.W., RENNKE, H.G. and BRENNER, B.M. (1985). Control of glomerular hypertension limits glomerular injury in rats with reduced renal mass. *Journal of Clinical Investigation,* **76,** 612–619

AVASTHI, P.S., GREENE, E.R., VOYLES, W.F. and FISHER, D.C. (1985). Postprandial renal hemodynamics in humans. *Kidney International,* **27,** 291A

AZAR, S., JOHNSON, M.A., HERTEL, B. and TOBIAN, L. (1977). Single-nephron pressures, flows and resistances in hypertensive kidneys with nephrosclerosis. *Kidney International,* **12,** 28–40

AZAR, S., JOHNSON, M.A., IWAI, J., BRUNO, L. and TOBIAN, L. (1978). Single nephron dynamics in 'post-salt' rats with chronic hypertension. *Journal of Laboratory and Clinical Medicine,* **91,** 156–166

BALDWIN, D.S. (1982). Chronic glomerulonephritis: nonimmunologic mechanisms of progressive glomerular damage. *Kidney International,* **21,** 109–120

BAUER, J.H. (1984). Role of angiotensin converting enzyme inhibitors in essential and renal hypertension. *American Journal of Medicine,* **77**(2A), 43–51

BERG, B.N. (1966). Effect of thyroxine on spontaneous nephrosis in the rat. *Proceedings of the Society for Experimental Biology and Medicine,* **121,** 198–203

BERG, B.N. and SIMMS, H.S. (1960). Nutrition and longevity in the rat. II. Longevity and onset of disease with different levels of food intake. *Journal of Nutrition,* **71,** 255–263

BEYER, M.M., STEINBERG, A.D., NICASTRI, A.D. and FRIEDMAN, E.A. (1977). Unilateral nephrectomy: effect on survival in NZB/NZW mice. *Science,* **198,** 511–513

BLATHERWICK, N.R. and MEDLAR, E.M. (1937). Chronic nephritis in rats fed high protein diets. *Archives of Internal Medicine,* **59,** 572–596

BOLTON, W.K., BENTON, F.R., MACLAY, J.G. and STURGILL, B.C. (1976). Spontaneous glomerular sclerosis in aging Sprague-Dawley rats. I. Lesions associated with mesangial IgM deposits. *American Journal of Pathology,* **85,** 277–302

BOLTON, W.K. and STURGILL, B.C. (1981). Ultrastructure of the aging kidney. In *Aging and Cell Structure,* edited by J.E. Johnson, Jr., Vol. 1, pp. 215–250. New York; Plenum

BOSCH, J.P., SACCAGGI, A., LAUER, A., RONCO, C., BELLEDONNE, M. and GLABMAN, S. (1983). Renal functional reserve in humans: effect of protein intake on glomerular filtration rate. *American Journal of Medicine,* **75,** 943–950

BRANCA, G.F., SATTA, A., FAEDDA, R., SOGGIA, G., OLMEO, N.A., VACCA, R. and BARTOLI, E. (1984). Effects of blood pressure control on the progression of renal insufficiency in chronic renal failure. *Panminerva Medica,* **25,** 215–218

BRAS, G. and ROSS, M.H. (1964). Kidney disease and nutrition in the rat. *Toxicology and Applied Pharmacology,* **6,** 247–262

BRENNER, B.M. (1985). Nephron adaptation to renal injury or ablation. *American Journal of Physiology,* **249,** F324–F337

BRENNER, B.M., MEYER, T.W. and HOSTETTER, T.H. (1982). Dietary protein intake and the progressive nature of kidney disease. *New England Journal of Medicine,* **307,** 652–660

CASTELLINO, P., CODA, B. and DEFRONZO, R.A. (1985). The effect of intravenous amino acid infusion on renal hemodynamics in man. *Kidney International,* **27,** 243A

CHANUTIN, A. and FERRIS, E.B. (1932). Experimental renal insufficiency produced by partial nephrectomy. I. Control diet. *Archives of Internal Medicine,* **49,** 767–787

CHOCAIR, P.R., SALDANHA, L.B., LUCON, A.M., GOES, G.M. and SABBAGA, E. (1984). Long term follow up of related kidney donors. Incidence of hypertension and proteinuria. *IXth International Congress of Nephrology,* 471A

COCHRAN, S.T., PAGANI, J.J. and BARBARIC, Z.L. (1979). Nephrology in hyperalimentation. *Radiology,* **130,** 603–606

COLEMAN, G.L., BARTHOLD, S.W., OSBALDISTON, G.W., FOSTER, S.J. and JONES, A.M. (1977). Pathological changes during aging in barrier-reared Fischer 344 male rats. *Journal of Gerontology,* **32,** 258–278

COTRAN, R.S. (1982). Glomerulosclerosis in reflux nephropathy. *Kidney International,* **21,** 528–534

COUSER, W.G. and STILMANT, M.M. (1975). Mesangial lesions and focal glomerular sclerosis in the aging rat. *Laboratory Investigation,* **33,** 491–501

DAMMIN, G.J. (1981). Transplantation in the 1950's. *Transplantation Proceedings,* **13,** 16–23

DAVIES, D.F. and SHOCK, N.W. (1950). Age changes in glomerular filtration rate, effective renal plasma flow and tubular excretory capacity in adult males. *Journal of Clinical Investigation,* **29,** 496–507

DEEN, W.M., MADDOX, D.A., ROBERTSON, C.R. and BRENNER, B.M. (1974). Dynamics of glomerular ultrafiltration in the rat. VII. Response to reduced renal mass. *American Journal of Physiology,* **277,** 556–562

DWORKIN, L.D, FEINER, H.D. and RANDAZZO, J. (1985). Evidence for hemodynamically mediated glomerular injury despite antihypertensive therapy in rats with desoxycorticosterone-salt (DOC-salt) hypertension. *Kidney International,* **27,** 189A

DWORKIN, L.D., HOSTETTER, T.H., RENNKE, H.G. and BRENNER, B.M. (1984). Hemodynamic basis for glomerular injury in rats with desoxycorticosterone-salt hypertension. *Journal of Clinical Investigation,* **73,** 1448–1461

ELEMA, J.D. and ARENDS, A. (1971). Functional overload as a possible cause for non-immune glomerular damage. Effect of nephrectomy and irradiation of the contralateral kidney. *Journal of Pathology,* **103,** 21–29

ELEMA, J.D. and ARENDS, A. (1975). Focal and segmental glomerular hyalinosis and sclerosis in the rat. *Laboratory Investigation,* **33,** 554–561

ELEMA, J.D., KOUDSTAAL, J., LAMBERTS, H.B. and ARENDS, A. (1971). Spontaneous glomerulosclerosis in the rat. Effect of nephrectomy and irradiation of the contralateral kidney. *Archives of Pathology,* **91,** 418–425

EL-NAHAS, A.M., PARASKEVAKOU, H., ZOOB, S., REES, A.J. and EVANS, D.J. (1983). Effect of dietary protein restriction on the development of renal failure after subtotal nephrectomy in rats. *Clinical Science,* **65,** 399–406

EVERITT, A.V., PORTER, B.D. and WYNDHAM, J.R. (1982). Effects of caloric intake and dietary composition on the development of proteinuria, age-associated renal disease and longevity in the male rat. *Gerontology,* **28,** 168–175

EVERITT, A.V., SEEDSMAN, N.J. and JONES, F. (1980). The effects of hypophysectomy and continuous food restriction, begun at ages 70 and 400 days, on collagen aging, proteinuria, incidence of pathology and longevity. *Mechanisms of Ageing and Development,* **12,** 161–172

FARR, L.E. and SMADEL, J.E. (1939). The effect of dietary protein on the course of nephrotoxic nephritis in rats. *Journal of Experimental Medicine,* **70,** 615–627

FELDMAN, D.B., McCONNELL, E.E. and KNAPKA, J.J. (1982). Growth, kidney disease, and longevity of Syrian hamsters (*Mesocricetus auratus*) fed varying levels of protein. *Laboratory Animal Science,* **32,** 613–618

FERRAN, N.L., DELANO, B.G., BEYER, M.M., URIBARRI, J. and FRIEDMAN, E.A. (1985). Hypertension and proteinuria post renal donation. *Kidney International,* **27,** 137A

FETTERMAN, G.H. and HABIB, R. (1969). Congenital bilateral oligonephronic renal hypoplasia with hypertrophy of nephrons (Oligoméganéphronie). Studies by microdissection. *American Journal of Clinical Pathology,* **52,** 199–207

FINN, W.F. (1983). Recovery from acute renal failure. In *Acute Renal Failure,* edited by B.M. Brenner and J.M. Lazarus, pp. 753–774, Philadelphia; Saunders

FRIEND, P.S., FERNANDES, G., GOOD, R.A., MICHAEL, A.F. and YUNIS, E.J. (1978). Dietary restrictions early and late effects on the nephropathy of the NZB × NZW mouse. *Laboratory Investigation,* **38,** 629–632

FRONEK, K. and STAHLGREN, L.H. (1968). Systemic and regional hemodynamic changes during food intake and digestion in nonanesthetized dogs. *Circulation Research,* **23,** 687–692

GEHRIG, J.J., Sr., MEYER, T.W., JAMISON, R.L., BAYLIS, C., TROY, J.L. and BRENNER, B.M. *et al.* (1985). Effect of intermittent feeding on renal function in conscious rats. *Kidney International,* **27,** 295A

GIORDANO, C. (1982). Protein restriction in chronic renal failure. *Kidney International,* **22,** 401–408

GOTTSCHALK, C.W. (1971). Function of the chronically diseased kidney: the adaptive nephron. *Circulation Research,* **28**(S1), 1–13

GOYAL, V.K. (1982). Changes with age in the human kidney. *Experimental Gerontology,* **17,** 321–331

GRAF, H., STUMMROLI, H.F., LUGER, A. and PRAGER, R. (1983). Effect of amino acid infusion on glomerular filtration rate. *New England Journal of Medicine,* **308,** 159–160

GUTTMAN, P.H. and ANDERSEN, A.C. (1968). Progressive intercapillary glomerulosclerosis in aging and irradiated beagles. *Radiation Research,* **35,** 45–60

GUTTMAN, P.H. and BAILEY, D.W. (1965). Potentiating effect of neonatal thymectomy on x-ray-induced intercapillary glomerulosclerosis. *Nature,* **207,** 539–540

GUTTMAN, P.H. and KOHN, H.I. (1960). Progressive intercapillary glomerulosclerosis in the mouse, rat, and Chinese hamster, associated with aging and x-ray exposure. *American Journal of Pathology,* **37,** 293–306

HAKIM, R.M., GOLDSZER, R.C. and BRENNER, B.M. (1984). Hypertension and proteinuria: long-term sequelae of uninephrectomy in humans. *Kidney International,* **25,** 930–936

HAYSLETT, J.P. (1979). Functional adaptation to reduction in renal mass. *Physiological Reviews,* **59,** 137–164

HOLLENBERG, N.K., ADAMS, D.F., SOLOMON, H.S., RASHID, A., ABRAMS, H.L. and MERRILL, J.P. (1974). Senescence and the renal vasculature in normal man. *Circulation Research,* **34,** 309–316

HOSTETTER, T.H., OLSON, J.L., RENNKE, H.G., VENKATACHALAM, M.A. and BRENNER, B.M. (1981). Hyperfiltration in remnant nephrons: a potentially adverse response to renal ablation. *American Journal of Physiology,* **241,** F85–F93

HOSTETTER, T.H., RENNKE, H.G. and BRENNER, B.M. (1982). The case for intrarenal hypertension in the initiation and progression of diabetic and other glomerulopathies. *American Journal of Medicine,* **72,** 375–380

HOSTETTER, T.H., TROY, J.L. and BRENNER, B.M. (1981). Glomerular hemodynamics in experimental diabetes mellitus. *Kidney International,* **19,** 410–415

ICHIKAWA, I., PURKERSON, M.L., KLAHR, S., TROY, J.L., MARTINEZ-MALDONADO, M. and BRENNER, B.M. (1980). Mechanism of reduced glomerular filtration rate in chronic malnutrition. *Journal of Clinical Investigation,* **65,** 982–988

JOHNSON, J.E. and BARROWS, C.H., Jr. (1980). Effects of age and dietary restrictions on the kidney glomeruli of mice: observations by scanning electron microscopy. *Anatomical Record,* **196,** 145–151

KAPLAN, C., PASTERNACK, B., SHAH, H. and GALLO, G. (1975). Age-related incidence of sclerotic glomeruli in human kidneys. *American Journal of Pathology,* **80,** 227–234

KAPPEL, B. and OLSEN, S. (1980). Cortical interstitial tissue and sclerosed glomeruli in the normal human kidney, related to age and sex. A quantitative study. *Virchows Archiv A,* **387,** 271–277

KENNEDY, G.C. (1957). Effects of old age and over-nutrition on the kidney. *British Medical Bulletin,* **13,** 67–70

KLEINMAN, K.S. and GLASSOCK, R.J. (1985). GFR fails to increase following protein ingestion in growth hormone deficient adults. *Kidney International,* **27,** 296A

KINCAID-SMITH, P. (1980). Analgesic abuse and the kidney. *Kidney International,* **17,** 250–260

KIPROV, D.D., COLVIN, R.B. and McCLUSKEY, R.T. (1982). Focal and segmental glomerulosclerosis and proteinuria associated with unilateral renal agenesis. *Laboratory Investigation,* **46,** 275–281

KLEINKNECHT, D., GRÜNFELD, J.P., GOMEZ, P.C., MOREAU, J.F. and GARCIA-TORRES, R. (1973). Diagnostic procedures and long-term prognosis in bilateral renal cortical necrosis. *Kidney International,* **4,** 390–400

KOLETSKY, S. (1975). Pathologic findings and laboratory data in a new strain of obese hypertensive rats. *American Journal of Pathology,* **80,** 129–142

LEE, K.L. and SUMMERILL, R.A. (1982). Glomerular filtration rate following administration of individual amino acids in conscious dogs. *Quarterly Journal of Experimental Physiology,* **67,** 459–465

LINDEMAN, R.D., TOBIN, J.D. and SHOCK, N.W. (1984). Association between blood pressure and the rate of decline in renal function with age. *Kidney International,* **26,** 861–868

LINKSWILER, H., REYNOLDS, M.S. and BAUMANN, C.A. (1952). Factors affecting proteinuria in the rat. *American Journal of Physiology,* **168,** 504–508

LJUNGQVIST, A. and LAGERGREN, C. (1962). Normal intrarenal arterial pattern in adult and ageing human kidney. A micro-angiographical and histological study. *Journal of Anatomy,* **96,** 285–300

McCAY, C.M., CROWELL, M.F. and MAYNARD, L.A. (1935). The effect of retarded growth upon the length of life span and upon the ultimate body size. *Journal of Nutrition,* **10,** 63–79

MacKAY, E.M., MacKAY, L.L. and ADDIS, T. (1928). Factors which determine the renal weight. V. The protein intake. *American Journal of Physiology,* **86,** 459–465

McGRAW, M., POUCELL, S., SWEET, J. and BAUMAL, R. (1984). The significance of focal segmental glomerulosclerosis in oligomeganephronia. *International Journal of Pediatric Nephrology,* **5,** 67–72

McLACHLAN, M.S.F. (1978). The ageing kidney. *Lancet,* **2,** 143–146

McLACHLAN, M.S.F., GUTHRIE, J.S., ANDERSON, C.K. and FULKER, M.J. (1977). Vascular and glomerular changes in the ageing kidney. *Journal of Pathology,* **121,** 65–78

McMANUS, J.F.A. and LUPTON, C.H., Jr. (1960). Ischemic obsolescence of renal glomeruli. The natural history of the lesions and their relation to hypertension. *Laboratory Investigation,* **9,** 413–434

MADDEN, M.A. and ZIMMERMAN, S.W. (1983). Protein restriction and renal function in the uremic rat. *Kidney International,* **23,** 217A

MASCHIO, G., OLDRIZZI, L., TESSITORE, N., D'ANGELO, A., VALVO, E., LUPO, A. *et al.* (1982). Effects of dietary protein and phosphorus restriction on the progression of early renal failure. *Kidney International,* **22,** 371–376

MASORO, E.J., YU, B.P., BERTRAND, H.A. and LYND, F.T. (1980). Nutritional probe of the aging process. *Federation Proceedings,* **39,** 3178–3182

MEYER, T.W., HOSTETTER, T.H., RENNKE, H.G., NODDIN, J.L. and BRENNER, B.M. (1983a). Preservation of renal structure and function by long term protein restriction in rats with reduced renal mass. *Kidney International,* **23,** 218A

MEYER, T.W., ICHIKAWA, I., ZATZ, R. and BRENNER, B.M. (1983b). The renal hemodynamic response to amino acid infusion in the rat. In *Transactions of the Association of American Physicians* (Washington, 1983), Vol. 96, pp. 76–83. Baltimore; Waverly Press

MICHAEL, A.F., KEANE, W.F., RAIJ, L. and VERNIER, R.L. (1980). The glomerular mesangium. *Kidney International,* **17,** 141–154

MITCH, W.E. (1984). The influence of diet on the progression of renal insufficiency. *Annual Review of Medicine,* **35,** 249–264

MITCH, W.E., WALSER, M., BUFFINGTON, G.A. and LEMANN, J., Jr. (1976). A simple method for estimating progression of chronic renal failure. *Lancet,* **2,** 1326–1328

MITCH, W.E., WALSER, M., STEINMAN, T.I., HILL, S., ZEGER, S. and TUNGSANGA, K. (1984). The effect of a keto acid–amino acid diet supplement to a restricted diet on the progression of chronic renal failure. *New England Journal of Medicine,* **311,** 623–629

MOGENSEN, C.E. (1976). Renal function changes in diabetes. *Diabetes,* **25,** 872–879

MOGENSEN, C.E. (1981). Long-term antihypertensive treatment (over six years) inhibiting the progression of diabetic nephropathy. *Acta Endocrinologia,* **242,** Suppl., 31–32

MOGENSEN, C.E. and CHRISTENSEN, C.K. (1984). Predicting diabetic nephropathy in insulin-dependent patients. *New England Journal of Medicine,* **311,** 89–93

MOYER, J.H., HEIDER, C., PEVEY, K. and FORD, R.V. (1958). The effect of treatment on the vascular deterioration associated with hypertension, with particular emphasis on renal function. *American Journal of Medicine,* **24,** 177–192

NABEL, E.G., KUGELMASS, A., ZINS, G., PHIPPS, E. and DZAU, V.J. (1984). Does blood pressure control alter renal function in refractory hypertension? *Circulation,* **70,** Suppl. II, II–213A

NEUGARTEN, J., FEINER, H.D., SCHACHT, R.G. and BALDWIN, D.S. (1983). Amelioration of experimental glomerulonephritis by dietary protein restriction. *Kidney International,* **24,** 595–601

NEUHAUS, O.W. and FLORY, W. (1978). Age-dependent changes in the excretion of urinary proteins by the rat. *Nephron,* **22,** 570–576

NEWBURGH, L.H. and CURTIS, A.C. (1928). Introduction of renal injury in the white rat by the protein of the diet: dependence of the injury on the duration of feeding, and on the amount and kind of protein. *Archives of Internal Medicine,* **42,** 801–821

O'CONNOR, W.J. and SUMMERILL, R.A. (1976a). The effect of a meal of meat on glomerular filtration rate in dogs at normal urine flows. *Journal of Physiology,* **256,** 81–91

O'CONNOR, W.J. and SUMMERILL, R.A. (1976b). The excretion of urea by dogs following a meal of meat. *Journal of Physiology,* **256,** 93–102

O'CONNOR, W.J. and SUMMERILL, R.A. (1976c). Sulphate excretion by dogs following ingestion of ammonium sulphate or meat. *Journal of Physiology,* **260,** 597–607

OLSON, J.L. (1984). Role of heparin as a protective agent following reduction of renal mass. *Kidney International,* **25,** 376–382

OLSON, J.L., HOSTETTER, T.H., RENNKE, H.G., BRENNER, B.M. and VENKATACHALAM, M.A. (1982). Altered glomerular permselectivity and progressive sclerosis following extreme ablation of renal mass. *Kidney International,* **22,** 112–126

PARVING, H-H., ANDERSEN, A.R., SMIDT, U.M., CHRISTIANSEN, J.S., OXENBØLL, B. and SVENDSEN, P.A. (1983). Diabetic nephropathy and arterial hypertension: the effect of antihypertensive treatment. *Diabetes,* **32,** Suppl. 2. 83–87

PARVING, H-H. and GYNTELBERG, F. (1973). Transcapillary escape rate of albumin and plasma volume in essential hypertension. *Circulation Research,* **32,** 643–651

PITTS, R.F. (1944). The effects of infusing glycin and of varying the dietary protein intake on renal hemodynamics in the dog. *American Journal of Physiology,* **142,** 355–365

POLZIN, D.J., OSBORNE, C.A., HAYDEN, D.W. and STEVENS, J.B. (1984). Influence of reduced protein diets on morbidity, mortality, and renal function in dogs with induced chronic renal failure. *American Journal of Veterinary Research*, **45**, 506–517

PURKERSON, M.L., HOFFSTEN, P.E. and KLAHR, S. (1976). Pathogenesis of the glomerulopathy associated with renal infarction in rats. *Kidney International*, **9**, 407–417

PURKERSON, M.L., JOIST, J.H., GREENBERG, J.M., KAY, D., HOFFSTEN, P.E. and KLAHR, S. (1982). Inhibition by anticoagulant drugs of the progressive hypertension and uremia associated with renal infarction in rats. *Thrombosis Research*, **26**, 227–240

PURKERSON, M.L., JOIST, J.H., YATES, J. and KLAHR, S. (1984). Role of hypertension and coagulation in the glomerulopathy of rats with subtotal renal ablation. *IXth International Congress of Nephrology*, 359A

PURKERSON, M.L., JOIST, J.H., YATES, J., VALDES, A., MORRISON, A. and KLAHR, S. (1985). Inhibition of thromboxane synthesis ameliorates the progressive kidney disease of rats with subtotal renal ablation. *Proceedings of the National Academy of Science*, **82**, 193–197

RIVOLTA, E., PONTICELLI, G., IMBASCIATI, E. and VEGETO, A. (1983). De novo focal glomerular sclerosis in an identical twin renal transplant recipient. *Transplantation*, **35**, 328–331

ROBSON, A.M., MOR, J., ROOT, E.R., JAGER, B.V., SHANKEL, S.W., INGELFINGER, J.R. *et al.* (1979). Mechanism of proteinuria in nonglomerular renal disease. *Kidney International*, **16**, 416–429

ROWE, J.W., ANDRES, R., TOBIN, J.D., NORRIS, A.H. and SHOCK, N.W. (1976). The effect of age on creatinine clearance in men: a cross-sectional and longitudinal study. *Journal of Gerontology*, **31**, 155–163

RUBIN, M.I., BRUCK, E. and RAPAPORT, M. (1949). Maturation of renal function in childhood: clearance studies. *Journal of Clinical Investigation*, **28**, 1144–1162

RUTHERFORD, W.E., BLONDIN, J., MILLER, J.P., GREENWALT, A.S. and VAVRA, J.D. (1977). Chronic progressive renal disease: rate of change of serum creatinine concentration. *Kidney International*, **11**, 62–70

SAMIY, A.H. (1983). Renal disease in the elderly. *Medical Clinics of North America*, **65**, 463–480

SAXTON, J.A., Jr. and KIMBALL, G.C. (191). Relation of nephrosis and other diseases of albino rats to age and to modifications of diet. *Archives of Pathology*, **32**, 951–965

SCHOOLWERTH, A.C., SANDLER, R.S., HOFFMAN, P.M. and KLAHR, S. (1975). Effects of nephron reduction and dietary protein content on renal ammoniogenesis in the rat. *Kidney International*, **7**, 397–404

SELLERS, A.L., GOODMAN, H.C., MARMORSTON, J. and SMITH, M. (1950). Sex differences in proteinuria in the rat. *American Journal of Physiology*, **163**, 662–667

SEYER-HANSEN, K. (1978). Renal hypertrophy in experimental diabetes: a comparison to compensatory hypertrophy. *Diabetologia*, **14**, 325–328

SHANNON, J.A., JOLLIFFE, N. and SMITH, H.W. (1932). The excretion of urine in the dog. IV. The effect of maintenance diet, feeding, etc., upon the quantity of glomerular filtrate. *American Journal of Physiology*, **101**, 625–638

SHIMAMURA, T. (1982). Relationship of dietary intake to the development of glomerulosclerosis in obese Zucker rats. *Experimental and Molecular Pathology*, **36**, 423–434

SHIMAMURA, T. and MORRISON, A.B. (1975). A progressive glomerulosclerosis occurring in partial five-sixths nephrectomized rats. *American Journal of Pathology*, **79**, 95–106

SPECTOR, D., HILL, G., DiCIANI, N., TELLER, D. and SACKTOR, B. (1985). Low protein but not low sulphate diet inhibits proteinuria in aging rats. *Kidney International*, **27**, 251A

STERZEL, R.B., LOVETT, D.H., STEIN, H.D. and KASHGARIAN, M. (1982). The mesangium and glomerulonephritis. *Klinische Wochenschrift*, **60**, 1077–1105

STRIKER, G.E., NAGLE, R.B., KOHNEN, P.W. and SMUCKLER, E.A. (1969). Response to unilateral nephrectomy in old rats. *Archives of Pathology*, **87**, 439–442

TAKAZAKURA, E., SAWABU, N., HANDA, A., TAKADA, A., SHINODA, A. and TAKEUCHI, I. (1972). Intrarenal vascular changes with age and disease. *Kidney International*, **2**, 224–230

TAUCHI, H., TSUBOI, K. and OKUTOMI, J. (1971). Age changes in the human kidney of the different races. *Gerontologia*, **17**, 87–97

TEODORU, C.V., SAIFER, A. and FRANKEL, H. (1959). Conditioning factors influencing evolution of experimental glomerulonephritis in rabbits. *American Journal of Physiology*, **196**, 457–460

THORNER, P.S., ARBUS, G.S., CELERMAJER, D.S. and BAUMAL, R. (1984). Focal segmental glomerulosclerosis and progressive renal failure associated with a unilateral kidney. *Pediatrics*, **73**, 806–810

TORRES, V.E., VELOSA, J.A., HOLLEY, K.E., KELALIS, P.P., STICKLER, G.B. and KURTZ, S.B. (1980). The progression of vesicourteteral reflux. *Annals of Internal Medicine*, **92**, 776–784

TUCKER, S.M., MASON, R.L. and BEAUCHENE, R.E. (1976). Influence of diet and feed restriction on kidney function of aging male rats. *Journal of Gerontology*, **31**, 264–270

VELOSA, J.A., GLASSER, R.J., NEVINS, T.E. and MICHAEL, A.F. (1977). Experimental model of focal sclerosis. II. Correlation with immunopathologic changes, macromolecular kinetics, and polyanion loss. *Laboratory Investigation*, **36**, 527–534

VINCENTI, F., AMEND, W.J.C., Jr., KAYSEN, G., FEDUSKA, N., BIRNBAUM, J., DUCA, R. *et al.* (1983). Long-term renal function in kidney donors. Sustained compensatory hyperfiltration with no adverse effects. *Transplantation*, **36**, 626–629

WACHTEL, L.N., COLE, L.J. and ROSEN, V.J. (1966). X-ray-induced glomerulosclerosis in rats: modification of lesion by food restriction, uninephrectomy, and age. *Journal of Gerontology*, **21**, 442–448

WEAVER, R.N., GRAY, J.E. and SCHULTZ, J.R. (1975). Urinary proteins in Sprague-Dawley rats with chronic progressive nephrosis. *Laboratory Animal Science*, **25**, 705–710

WEILAND, D., SUTHERLAND, D.E.R., CHAVERS, B., SIMMONS, R.L., ASCHER, N.L. and NAJARIAN, J.S. (1984). Information on 628 living-related kidney donors at a single institution, with long-term follow-up in 472 cases. *Transplantation Proceedings*, **16**, 5–7

WEN, S.F., BENELL, N.M. and MOORTHY, A.V. (1984). Effects of low protein diet on experimental diabetic nephropathy. *IXth International Congress of Nephrology*, 363A

WESSON, L.G. (1969). *Physiology of The Human Kidney*. New York; Grune and Stratton

WOODHEAD, A.D., POND, V. and DAILEY, K. (1983). Aging changes in the kidneys of two poecilid fishes, the guppy *Poecilia reticulatus* and the Amazon molly *P. formosa*. *Experimental Gerontology*, **18**, 211–221

YU, B.P., MASORO, E.J., MURATA, I., BERTRAND, H.A. and LYND, F.T. (1982). Life span study of SPF Fischer 344 male rats fed *ad libitum* or restricted diets: longevity, growth, lean body mass and disease. *Journal of Gerontology*, **37**, 130–141

ZATZ, R., DUNN, B.R., MEYER, T.W., ANDERSON, S., RENNKE, H.G. and BRENNER, B.M. (1986). Prevention of diabetic glomerulopathy by pharmacological amelioration of glomerular capillary hypertension. *Journal of Clinical Investigation*, **77**, 1925–1930

ZATZ, R., MEYER, T.W., RENNKE, H.G. and BRENNER, B.M. (1985). Predominance of hemodynamic rather than metabolic factors in the pathogenesis of diabetic glomerulopathy. *Proceedings of the National Academy of Sciences*, **82**, 5963–5967

Chapter 4

Physiology and disorders of water balance and electrolytes in the elderly

Juan F. Macias Nuñez, Antonio Bondia Roman and Jose L. Rodruiguez Commes

Introduction

Although the aging kidney is able to maintain an acceptable water and electrolyte balance in conditions of health, its resources to adapt to any restriction of these elements is limited. Because of this, it is necessary for all surgeons and physicians treating elderly patients to be able to recognize this reduced capacity before undertaking any therapeutic decision related to fluid replacement, diuretic prescription, or salt and water restriction.

This chapter will deal with the specific aspects that the normal aging process has on the kidney with regard to water and electrolyte control, and the deleterious effect that ignorance of these changes may have for the elderly patient's outcome. The first part of the chapter is a summary of some fundamentals of the normal physiology necessary to better understand the changes occurring with age. Then, the special characteristics shown by the aging kidney with respect to these elements will be discussed. Finally, a section is devoted to the diagnosis, treatment and prevention of the pathology as a result of deficient care and mishandling of the elderly in relation to water and electrolytes.

Summary of the normal physiology of the kidney

Proximal tubule

This segment is heterogeneous with respect to structure and function, exhibiting some special characteristics along its length. First, we will summarize the commonest steps involved in water and electrolyte transport.

Sodium reabsorption is an active phenomenon carried out against a concentration gradient which can be inhibited by ouabain (Burg, 1976). In the mechanisms by which sodium is transported from the tubular lumen to the peritubular vessels, the first is the passive movement of sodium from the lumen to the interior of the tubular cell. The majority of the sodium, once within the cell, is transported to the paracellular space. Because the interior of the cell is electronegative, and sodium concentration is higher outside the cell than within it, additional force is needed to transport sodium from the cell to the paracellular space. The energy for this transport is provided by a sodium ATPase-dependent pump. Due to the generated osmotic gradient, water follows sodium to the paracellular space. Consequently, as water accumulates into the basocellular space, the increase of hydrostatic pressure releases water from the basocellular to the peritubular space. There is a small degree of backflow to the tubular lumen that is minimized by the tight junctions. Water and electrolytes enter the peritubular vessels because of the oncotic pressure of the intravascular proteins.

The presence and reabsorption of compounds normally present in the glomerular ultrafiltrate, such as bicarbonate, glucose and amino acids (Burg, 1976; Schrier and Anderson, 1980) are responsible for a relatively significant amount of the reabsorbed sodium. It has been well documented that sodium and non-electrogenic solutes (sugars, amino acids) share a common system of transport (10–20 per cent of the reabsorbed sodium). The energy required for this common system to work is derived from the electrochemical gradient generated by active sodium reabsorption (Sacktor, 1982).

Chloride enters passively into the cell because of an electrochemical concentration gradient (Sullivan and Grantham, 1982). The latter force is not enough to fully balance the opposing gradient. Other mechanisms must become involved at this level. Although they are not completely known, it is possible that part of the chloride enters the cell combined with sodium as a neutral salt (Pitts, 1976). From the cell, being favoured by an electrochemical gradient, chloride is passively transported to the peritubular space.

Potassium is reabsorbed actively from the lumen against an electrochemical and concentration gradient, since potassium is an intracellular ion and the interior of the cell is positive with respect to the tubular lumen (Grantham, 1986; Gabow and Peterson, 1980; Adrogue and Martinez-Maldonado, 1982). The active reabsorption of potassium is based on the property of the biological membranes to maintain the intracellular/extracellular potassium proportion (Morgan, 1979). Potassium is expelled from the cell to maintain the intracellular/extracellular concentration. The intracellular potassium is replenished either by peritubular or luminal membrane (the latter is more permeable and its contribution is most significant). In this way, a net reabsorption of potassium is produced without the existence of a gradient between tubular lumen and peritubular fluid.

Approximately 60–80 per cent of the *water* filtered by the glomerulus is reabsorbed passively in the proximal tubule following sodium transport (Burg, 1986; Jamison and Kriz, 1982). The osmotic gradient is largely responsible for the reabsorption of proximal tubular fluid. In the proximal tubule, the reabsorption process is isosmotic, which means that there is no concentration or dilution of the tubular fluid in this segment.

Loop of Henle

The descending limb is highly permeable to water but quite impermeable to sodium, potassium and chloride. However, there is some passage of these electrolytes in both directions (from the lumen to the peritubular space and vice versa), but this is of limited quantitative importance (Morgan, 1979).

As tubular fluid flows downward in the descending limb, the osmolarity of the fluid equilibrates with the osmolarity of the medullary interstitium. It is likely that this equilibrium is achieved by both the incoming solutes from the interstitium to the lumen, and by the passage of water from the lumen to the interstitium. About 20 per cent of the water present in the descending limb has previously passed from the lumen to the interstitium before returning to the lumen of the descending limb (Thier, 1981; Jamison and Kriz, 1982).

The ascending limb exhibits completely different characteristics from those in the descending limb: it is impermeable to water and highly permeable to sodium and urea. In the thin ascending limb, sodium moves passively from the lumen to the interstitium by means of a concentration gradient (Burg, 1976; Schrier and Anderson, 1980). As fluid ascends in the thin ascending limb, electrolytes pass to the interstitium but water remains in the lumen. As a result, water in the ascending limb is devoid of electrolytes. This is the process of free water formation. Tubular fluid is diluted because electrolytes pass from the lumen and water accumulates within in. Because of this, the ascending limb and the early part of the distal convoluted tubule have been named the diluting segment.

As previously described, the ascending limb is impermeable to water. Because of this, fluid leaving the ascending limb has an osmolarity of 100 mosmol/l (Maude, 1977; Morgan, 1979) and an important percentage of free water is formed in this segment of the nephron.

In the thick ascending limb of Henle's loop there occurs another change in the membrane properties. Chloride is transported actively from the lumen to the interstitium against an electrochemical gradient. This segment of Henle's loop maintains a low water permeability. The energetic mechanism responsible for the active transport of chloride is inhibited by ouabain and frusemide (Burg, 1976; Pitts, 1976; Morgan, 1979; Schrier and Anderson, 1980; Sullivan and Grantham, 1982). Sodium follows chloride passively, although the possibility of some active sodium transport cannot be completely excluded. Although the amount of potassium reaching the ascending limb of Henle's loop is very low, its movement resembles that of sodium.

There is a passive entrance of potassium from the interstitium to the descending limb. This potassium comes from the medullary collecting tubules. This is the process of potassium recycling which resembles the process of urea recycling. Potassium movement is not influenced by sodium or hydrogen ion transport (Morgan, 1979; Gabow and Peterson, 1980).

Distal convoluted tubule

The distal convoluted tubule is lumen negative. The degree of negativity increases in magnitude along its length. This segment has the capability of *active sodium reabsorption* against an electrochemical concentration gradient (Adrogue and Martinez-Maldonado, 1982). The early part of the distal convoluted tubule exhibits similar properties to those of the thick ascending limb of Henle's loop and therefore tubular fluid continues to be diluted. The late segment of the distal convoluted tubule is less permeable to sodium. Sodium reabsorption is influenced by aldosterone and, in any case, the total capacity for sodium reabsorption in this segment is limited. The nature of *chloride* reabsorption is distinct in each segment of the distal convoluted tubule. In the early part, chloride is reabsorbed actively. As chloride moves along the tubular length, its reabsorption gradually becomes passive.

The negative gradient present in this part of the tubule accounts for the secretion of potassium and hydrogen ions rather than for active sodium reabsorption (Morgan, 1979). Potassium is reabsorbed and secreted along the distal tubule. The fluid that reaches the distal tubule is virtually free of potassium; 90 per cent of the filtered potassium has been reabsorbed in previous segments. The process of *potassium secretion* is passive due to the great permeability of the membrane to potassium and to the intratubular electronegativity (Grantham, 1986; Pitts, 1976; Gabow and Peterson, 1980; Adrogue and Martinez-Maldonado, 1982).

The existence of an energetic pump at the peritubular site of the cell that introduces potassium into the tubular cell has been recently proven. The intracellular concentration of potassium is elevated in the cell by means of this pump. Potassium diffuses from the cell to the lumen and its passage from the peritubular space to the cell is stimulated by aldosterone (Gabow and Peterson, 1980).

A small quantity of potassium is reabsorbed against both an electrochemical and concentration gradient (the interior of the cell is electronegative and potassium is an intracellular ion). The energy required for this active transport is provided by an ATP-dependent pump. Approximately 75 per cent of the potassium eliminated in the urine comes from the secretion that occurs in the distal convoluted tubule. As the distal convoluted tubule is rather impermeable to water, the reabsorption of water is not important at this site.

Collecting duct

The amount of sodium reabsorbed in the collecting duct is 3 per cent of the total present in glomerular filtrate. Although the *quantity* of sodium that is handled by the collecting duct is almost negligible, it is of paramount importance. This segment adjusts the amount of sodium reabsorbed or excreted, depending on the physiological requirements of salt. The collecting duct is also responsible for the excretion of sodium present in the urine (Burg, 1976; Schrier and Anderson, 1980). The gradient against which sodium is reabsorbed in this segment is very high. An active means of transport is therefore required which is modulated by aldosterone. In some circumstances, sodium can be secreted in this segment of the nephron, and there is some evidence that natriuretic hormone can be involved in this action. This segment is lumen negative and chloride may be passively reabsorbed, but an active transport under special circumstances can be achieved (Burg, 1976; Sullivan and Grantham, 1982). Potassium is secreted and reabsorbed in superficial cortical collecting tubules. In states of potassium overload, the collecting tubules of the deep nephrons are able to excrete the excess of potassium, and to reabsorb the potassium reaching this segment in situations of potassium depletion.

Water is passively reabsorbed under the influence of antidiuretic hormone and transepithelial osmotic gradient. Water passes through the cellular tubular membrane down an osmotic gradient. The osmolarity inside the cell is lower than in both the lumen and peritubular space. Because of this, water cross the lateral membrane to the basolateral space and through the lateral membrane to the interstitium and peritubular vessels (Burg, 1986; Jamison and Kriz, 1982). In this segment, water can be almost completely reabsorbed under conditions of water restriction, making urine concentration very high.

Concentration and dilution mechanisms

The same mechanisms are responsible for both the concentration and the dilution of urine: the generation and maintenance of a hyperosmolar interstitium. It is necessary to take into account that two different processes are involved. The first starts in the ascending limb of Henle's loop. This process makes the interstitium hypertonic due to both the transport of electrolytes from the lumen to the interstitium and the low water permeability of this segment. The second process protects the interstitial medullary gradient which is generated by the special characteristic of permeability in Henle's loop. The vasa recta maintains the osmolar gradient. The permeability of the collecting tubules to water, controlled by the antidiuretic hormone, must be considered when regarding the final urinary concentration. The absence of antidiuretic hormone makes the collecting tubules impermeable to water. Under conditions of antidiuretic hormone absence, there is no water diffusion from the lumen to the interstitium. Consequently, abnormally high amounts of water remain within the tubular lumen, diluting the final urine. For the concentration and dilution mechanisms to function properly, the close anatomical relationship between Henle's loop, the medullary collecting tubule, vasa recta, their parallel course and the hairpin loop anatomy of the medullary vessels (vasa recta) are crucial.

As we have previously seen, in the ascending limb of the loop, chloride and sodium are transported from the lumen to the interstitium, while water remains in the interior of the tubular lumen. Therefore, the fluid that moves upwards in the ascending limb gradually becomes more and more diluted. The interstitium becomes hyperosmolar as a result of the above process. The concentration gradient that can be achieved at any point along the ascending limb of Henle's loop is 200 mosmol/l lower than its horizontal level on the interstitium and the descending limb. This is known as the *single effect.* This means that, regardless, the osmolarity of the tubular fluid at any point of the ascending limb must be 200 mosmol lower than the osmolarity existing at the same horizontal level of the interstitium and descending limb of Henle's loop (*Figure 4.1*).

The tubular fluid entering the descending limb is 300 mosmol/l because the reabsorption in the proximal tubule is iso-osmotic to plasma. As fluid moves downwards in the descending limb it becomes more and more concentrated, until at the bend the concentration level reaches that of 1200 mosmol/l. It is clear that as tubular content flows upwards in the ascending limb it is diluted and a gradient of 200 mosmol/l is established. Thus, if we consider that the intratubular osmolarity at another point beyond the bend is 800, its corresponding horizontal level in the interstitium and descending limb is 1000 mosmol/l (*Figure 4.1*). In successive steps the intratubular content is diluted. The intratubular osmolarity is at 100 when the fluid leaves the thick limb of Henle's loop.

All in all, although the gradient that can be achieved at any point is 200, the osmolarity is considerably higher at the end of the descending limb, 1200 mosmol/l, than when fluid enters it, 300 mosmol/l. The 200 mosmol/l gradient results are multiplied due to the countercurrent flow. This system is known as the *countercurrent multiplier.*

Probably the passive diffusion of urea from the medullary collecting tubule to the interstitium plays an important role in the generation of medullary hyperosmolarity. The thick ascending limb of Henle's loop, the distal tubule and the cortical portion of the medullary collecting tubules are impermeable to urea. The medullary portion of the collecting ducts is permeable to urea. Because of this, the intraductal concentration of urea increases as tubular fluid flows through this segment. When tubular fluid reaches the medullary section of the collecting duct its luminal concentration is very high. As a result the urea passively crosses to the interstitium towards a concentration gradient. From the interstitium, part of the urea passively enters the descending and thin ascending limb of Henle's loop. Some amount of urea diffuses from the interstitium to the vasa recta. The trapping of important quantities

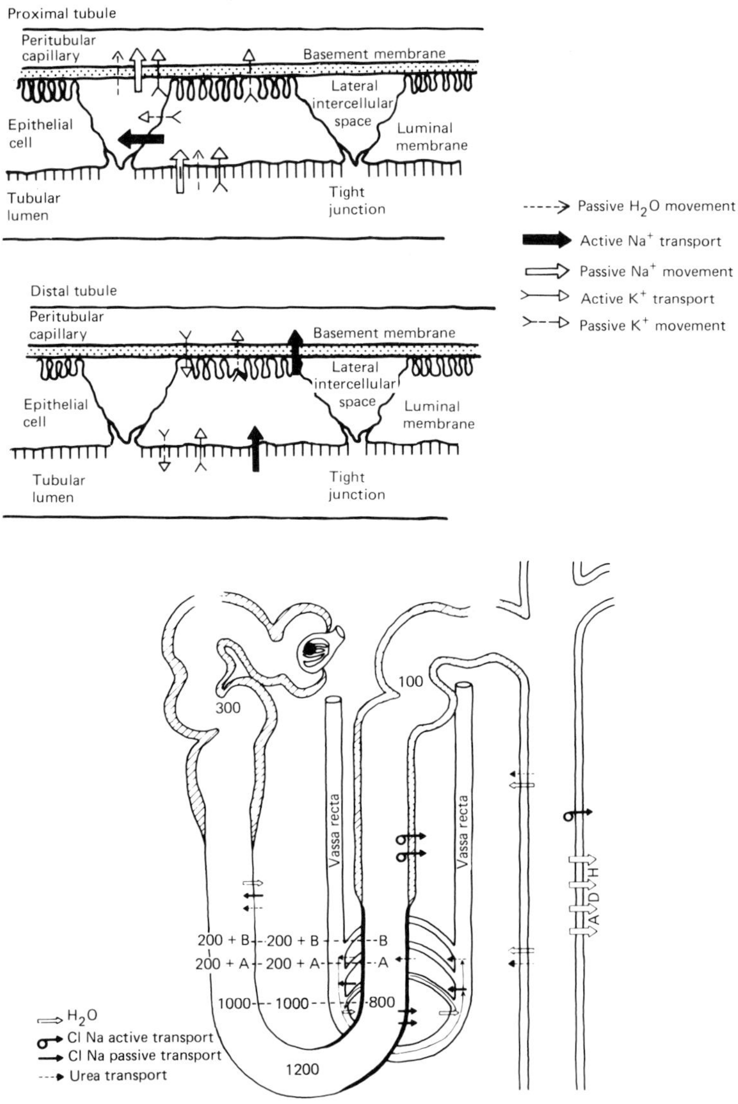

Figure 4.1 Representation of a normal nephron

of urea in the interstitium is possible because of the medullary recirculation and the countercurrent interchange mechanism (Jamison and Hall, 1983).

It is obvious that solutes cannot indefinitely accumulate in the medullary interstitium and they must be adequately removed, in order to preserve the interstitial hyperosmolarity. The removal of solutes and water is accomplished owing to the special structural arrangement of the hairpin of Henle's loop and of the medullary vessels (vasa recta). Blood enters the capillary loop with an osmolarity of 300 mosmol/l. Water passively diffuses from the vessels to the hypertonic interstitium and solutes move from the interstitium to the vascular lumen. As blood moves deeper into the medulla its osmolarity gradually increases. In the ascending limb of the vasa recta the overall movement of water and solutes changes. Solutes diffuse into the medullary interstitium and water is diluted as it flows into the vessels. When blood leaves the ascending limb its osmolarity is about 325 mosmol/l.

The vasae rectae do not only interchange with interstitial tissue, but also the descending and ascending vasa recta interchange with each other. In this manner a diffusion gradient is established and the ascending vasa recta gives up solutes to the descending vessels. The movement of both water and solutes across the vasa recta is passive in nature. These vessels do not generate the hyperosmolar medullary gradient: their action is limited to preserve the medullary interstitial gradient. The mechanisms mentioned above are known as *countercurrent exchanger* (Jamison and Kriz, 1982; Marsh, 1983).

By means of these co-ordinated events, the vasae rectae prevent the organism from unnecessary spillage of water and electrolytes. These vessels combine to provide the adequate conditions to incorporate and to remove the excessive interstitial amount of solutes and water that could interfere with the maintenance of the steady-state interstitial gradient. Any alteration in the renal blood flow to the medullae, either in excess or defect, impairment or functional alteration of Henle's loop, interstitial fibrosis, or the presence of any factor interfering with the normal steady-state gradient, will substantially alter the urinary concentration or dilution, or both functions (Jamison, 1981).

Thirst

Thirst is governed by hypothalamic ventromedial and anterior nuclei, anatomically very closely situated to the nucleus involved in the synthesis and release of antidiuretic hormone. In this manner, water elimination is preserved and water intake balances to maintain the normal steady state. On the other hand, when there is an excess of water, thirst disappears and the secretion of antidiuretic hormone stops, favouring the renal water elimination (Berl and Chaimowitz, 1983). The more powerful physiological stimulus for thirst is the decrease in total body water and a discrete increase in plasma osmolarity. This is the way that osmoreceptors control thirst. This control is very sensitive to modest changes (1–2 per cent) in the extracellular fluid osmolarity and minimal intracellular dehydration.

Apart from the osmotic stimulus, thirst is produced by non-osmotic stimuli. The contraction of the extracellular volume is the most important factor producing thirst non-osmotically. This is the case in bleeding, vomiting, diarrhoea, ascites, accumulation of fluids in the gastrointestinal tract (ileus) and, in general, in any situation in which the effective plasma volume is reduced. Some electrolytic imbalances such as hypokalaemia and hypercalcaemia stimulate thirst (Fitzsimons, 1976; Thier, 1981).

It is possible that angiotensin II mediates the dipsogenic response acting upon structures located in the wall of the third ventricle and through neurogenic mechanisms (Berl and Chaimowitz, 1983; Fitzsimons, 1985; Robertson and Berl, 1986).

Antidiuretic hormone

The antidiuretic hormone is a nonapeptide, synthesized in the ribosomes of the supra-optic nucleus; 10–20 per cent of antidiuretic hormone is immediately released in response to many stimuli, while the remaining 80–90 per cent is slowly released. Antidiuretic hormone acts by attaching to specific receptors located in the basolateral membrane of the collecting tubular cells. The union of antidiuretic hormone to its specific receptors activates adenyl cyclase which catalyses the conversion of ATP to cAMP, which then increases the permeability of the tubular luminal membrane to water. Antidiuretic hormone, in physiological dose, increases the permeability to water of the cortical and medullary segments of the collecting tubule and the permeability to urea of the deep medullary and papillary segments of the collecting tubule. The release of antidiuretic hormone is influenced by osmotic and, to a lesser extent, volumetric factors (Weitzman, 1979).

The existence of an osmoreceptor in the anterior hypothalamic nucleus which controls the release of antidiuretic hormone is well known from Verney's experiment. When plasma osmolarity increases, there is a prompt liberation of this hormone to the systemic circulation. The osmotic threshold is about 280 mosmol/kg of water in young people. This threshold can be modified by starvation and by hypokalaemia. Non-osmotic factors not only increase the sensitivity, but also diminish the osmotic threshold for the release of antidiuretic hormone (Berl and Chaimowitz, 1983).

The low pressure baroceptors of the left atrium, aortic arc and carotid sinus (high pressure receptors) and great veins account for the release of antidiuretic hormone in the presence of volume decrease. There are many reflexes which interfere with antidiuretic hormone release, such as pain, tiredness, noise, emotion, hypoxaemia, hyperthermia and cortisol, and some pharmacological agents—indomethacin, morphine, nicotine, tolbutamide, barbiturates, cyclophosphamide, beta-blockers and clofibrate—which increase the release of antidiuretic hormone. Hypokalaemia, hypercalcaemia, reserpine and alpha-adrenergic blockers inhibit antidiuretic hormone liberation. The role played by oestrogens, glucocorticoids and prostaglandins in modulating the release of antidiuretic hormone is still undefined (Morgan, 1979; Berl and Chaimowitz, 1983).

Both osmotic and non-osmotic factors act synergically in the majority of physiological conditions. Changes in plasma osmolarity ranging between 1 and 2 per cent have a comparable effect in antidiuretic hormone secretion of that of 8–10 per cent in plasma volume (Weitzman, 1979; Berl and Chaimowitz, 1983).

Peculiarities of the aging kidney regarding sodium, potassium and water management

Sodium

There is some discrepancy among researchers regarding the ability of the aging kidney to excrete sodium. Some suggest that the capacity of the aging kidney to excrete a sodium overload, either under basal conditions or during volume expansion, diminishes with age (Yamada *et al.*, 1979; Hiraide, 1981; Bengele, Mathias and Alexander, 1981; Hackbarth and Harrison, 1982; Myers *et al.*, 1982). One study has not shown a difference in regard to age in the renal handling of sodium (Karlberg and Tolagen, 1977). Nevertheless, the observation of a diminished renal capacity to conserve sodium with age is consonant with the clinical observation that high natriuresis and sodium depletion are frequently found in geriatric wards (Epstein and Hollenberg, 1976; Macias *et al.*, 1978, 1980).

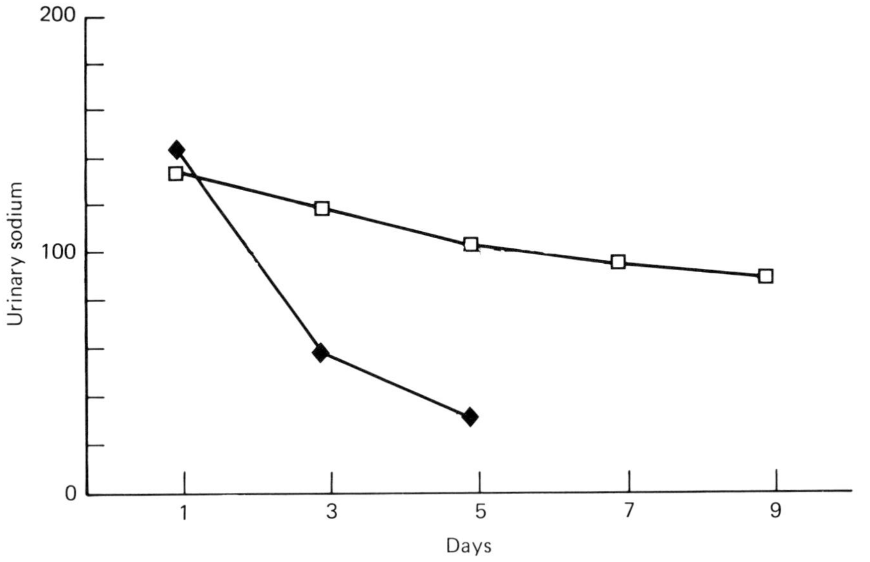

Figure 4.2 Results of the renal capacity to adapt to a 50 mEq salt restriction (□, elderly; ◆, young). The aging kidney was unable to reach sodium balance in 9 days. The young reached sodium balance in 5 days

The renal and hormonal response to a mild salt restriction differs substantially between young and elderly well-nourished healthy people (*Figure 4.2*). We studied 2 groups of healthy volunteers: young (mean age 24 ± 6) and aged (mean age 73 ± 4) under basal conditions and following a 50 mEq salt diet.

Basal sodium handling

In basal conditions, plasma sodium levels were similar in both populations (*Table 4.1*). As glomerular filtration rate (GFR), measured as inulin clearance, was lower in the aged, the amount of filtered sodium was also lower than in the young. In spite of the lower sodium tubular load, 24 h urinary sodium output and fractional

Table 4.1 Sodium handling

	Plasma sodium		*UNa.V*		*FE Na(%)*	
	Y	*E*	*Y*	*E*	*Y*	*E*
1	140.0	137.3	124.8	114.0	0.7	1.3
2	137.3	138.6	51.1	121.1	0.9	1.0
3	137.3	138.6	70.7	129.1	1.0	1.1
4	142.6	142.6	103.6	139.1	1.0	1.1
5	140.0	142.5	14.7	126.0	0.5	2.6
6	140.0	140.0	33.4	164.0	1.5	2.4
Mean	139.5	139.9	66.4	165.5*	0.93	1.58*
S.D.	2.0	2.2	42.0	97.6	0.33	0.71

Y, young; E, elderly; FE Na(%), fractional excretion of sodium; UNa.V, urinary sodium output per 24 h after a 50 mEq salt diet.
* $P<0.05$.

excretion of sodium were significantly higher in the elderly (*Table 4.1*). This means that the renal tubule of the elderly is unable to retain sodium adequately. Plasma, urinary aldosterone and plasma renin were lower either lying down or following 2 h of deambulation in the old than in the young group.

Diminished response to a low salt intake

Regarding the capacity of the aging kidney to *adapt to a low salt intake,* it is clearly *blunted.* Young people reached sodium balance in 5 days, whereas the elderly were not able to reach sodium balance, in spite of a mean loss of 1.4 kg of body weight in 9 days of 50 mEq salt diet (*Figure 4.2*). Salt restriction was discontinued at the ninth day in the aged group because their body weight was significantly diminished with respect to the beginning of the restrictive period (*Table 4.2*), although blood pressure was unchanged.

Table 4.2 Changes in body weight

	Young			Elderly		
	Normal diet	*Salt restrict*	*Δ−B.wt*	*Normal diet*	*Salt restrict*	*Δ−B.wt*
1	55.0	55.0	0.0	55.6	55.4	−0.2
2	83.0	82.0	−1.0	89.3	87.4	−1.9
3	51.7	51.2	−0.5	67.0	64.9	−2.1
4	71.0	69.4	−1.6	76.6	74.1	−2.5
5	84.0	83.1	−0.9	68.2	67.1	−1.1
6	54.0	52.5	−1.5	67.7	67.7	0.0
Mean	66.4	65.5	−0.9	70.7	69.4	−1.3*
S.D.	14.9	14.7	0.3	11.3	10.7	0.3

*$P<0.05$.

Several factors could account for renal sodium losses in the aged: obstructive uropathy, urinary infections, surreptitious diuretic intake and pyelonephritis (Brocklehurst and Hanley, 1979). Nevertheless, these conditions are not present in most elderly subjects who exhibit a defect in renal sodium handling. There may also be unexplained losses of salt in healthy elderly people (Narins, 1970; Sunderam and Mankikar, 1983).

Sodium loading

To determine the site in the nephron of the aging kidney responsible for the defect, we measured sodium excretion when patients were challenged with a saline overload. This test is able to discriminate the functional capacity of the 'proximal nephron' from the 'distal nephron'—ascending limb of Henle's loop (Macias *et al.*, 1978). It is clear from results shown in *Figure 4.3* and *Table 4.3* that the 'proximal nephron' behaved similarly in the young and the elderly. When the 'distal nephron' was considered, a clear-cut different in the handling of sodium in the elderly, in respect to the young, could be seen. This alteration has been found in 85 per cent of the tested population of healthy elderly persons. The diminished capacity to reabsorb sodium by the ascending limb of Henle's loop of healthy elderly persons has two direct important consequences:

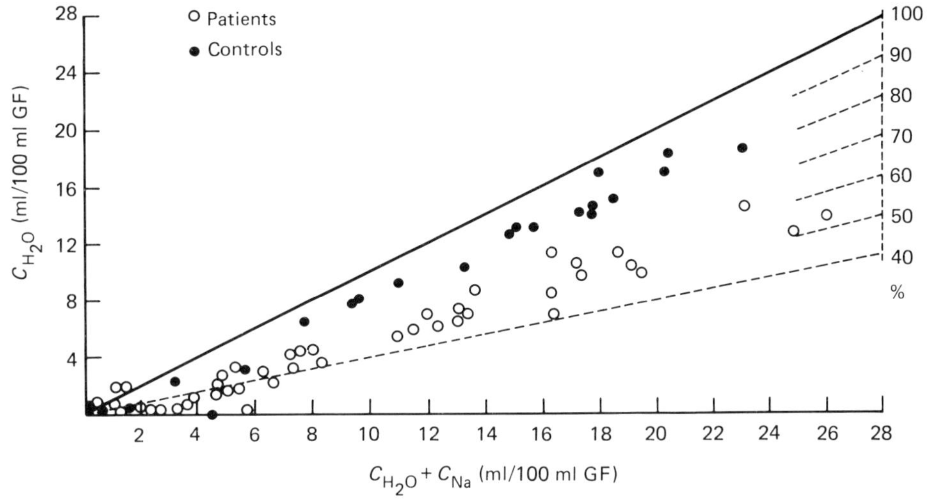

Figure 4.3 Graphic representation of the segmental capacity to reabsorb sodium by 'proximal' and 'distal' nephrons of young and elderly (referred to as 'patients') (From Macias *et al.*, 1978, reproduced with permission)

Table 4.3 Segmental study of the renal handling of sodium in young and healthy elderly individuals

C_{Na}		*Proximal nephron*		*Distal nephron*	
Y	*E*	*Y*	*E*	*Y*	*E*
4.20	3.41	23.03	6.34	81.76	46.20
3.30	7.17	17.80	18.60	81.40	61.45
1.38	8.53	17.97	19.10	92.32	53.50
1.87	16.00	15.07	34.40	87.59	53.40
2.28	8.25	15.79	23.12	85.56	64.31
2.63	8.64	13.48	16.00	80.48	46.00
8.32	7.50	27.12	17.37	69.37	56.82
1.39	4.80	9.93	16.28	86.00	70.50
2.42	9.39	10.58	19.42	72.12	51.64
5.01	12.79	32.07	33.05	84.37	61.30
	4.52		11.11		70.08
	3.02		14.60		79.50
			Mean values		
3.20	6.52*	18.28	18.86	82.95	59.10*
±	±	±	(standard deviation)	±	±
2.12	2.35	7.15	5.91	6.27	7.90

Y, young; E, elderly; C_{Na}, sodium clearance.
*$P > 0.05$ between elderly and young groups.

(1) The amount of sodium arriving at more distal segments of the nephron (distal convoluted and collecting tubules) increases.
(2) The capacity to concentrate the medullary interstitium is also diminished. As a consequence, elderly subjects would exhibit increased sodium excretion and inability to maximally concentrate the urine.

Blood and urinary aldosterone levels are significantly reduced in the elderly, in basal conditions and after salt restriction (*Table 4.4*). These results have been confirmed by other authors (Flood *et al.*, 1967; Sambhi, Crane and Genest, 1973; Crane and Harris, 1976; Epstein and Hollenberg, 1976). The tubular response to the administration of aldosterone, as assessed from the fall in sodium excretion, is

Table 4.4 Aldosterone

	Normal diet				*Salt restriction*			
	Blood		*Urine*		*Blood*		*Urine*	
	Y	*E*	*Y*	*E*	*Y*	*E*	*Y*	*E*
1	14.0	2.5	12.0	4.6	30.0	12.0	46.5	7.8
2	13.0	2.5	4.7	2.7	26.0	4.0	7.7	7.5
3	13.0	3.9	6.9	2.0	34.0	4.2	28.5	6.0
4	38.0	11.0	28.0	9.4	38.5	12.0	55.5	10.5
5	18.0	2.5	4.8	4.5	28.0	7.5	30.0	16.8
6	21.5	11.0	9.2	2.0	27.0	12.0	9.5	9.0
Mean	19.6	5.56†	10.95	4.2†	30.58*	8.6†	29.3*	9.6†
S.D.	9.6	4.2	8.8	2.8	4.8	3.9	19.6	3.8

*$P<0.05$ between normal diet and salt restriction.
†$P<0.05$ between young (Y) and elderly (E).

attenuated with age (Ceruso *et al.*, 1970). Plasma renin is also lower in the elderly than in the young population (*Table 4.5*), which has also been proved by other laboratories (Weidmann *et al.*, 1977). *Low aldosterone level* and the diminished sodium reabsorption in the *ascending limb of Henle's loop can account for the renal* sodium losses in the healthy aged population.

Other possible factors involved in renal sodium handling are diminished glomerular filtration rate and renal blood flow (Davies and Shock, 1950; Sourander, 1983). However, both of these changes tend to reduce renal sodium losses, so that increased excretion cannot be attributed to these factors.

Equally unlikely is that the inability to conserve sodium normally is related to excess prostaglandin production in the elderly. These substances act on the distal segments of the nephron (Strandhoy *et al.*, 1974) presumably to inhibit sodium reabsorption (Lee, Patak and Mookerjee, 1976). However, indomethacin, an

Table 4.5 Renin

	Normal diet				*Salt restriction*			
	Rest		*Walk*		*Rest*		*Walk*	
	Y	*E*	*Y*	*E*	*Y*	*E*	*Y*	*E*
1	3.80	0.23	7.50	0.27	8.33	0.24	7.56	0.5
2	2.47	0.96	2.60	1.10	3.17	4.46	5.97	9.6
3	9.70	1.23	13.50	1.53	14.70	3.63	16.30	6.0
4	1.06	1.80	5.80	2.37	2.37	1.40	6.00	5.2
5	3.03	0.26	3.63	0.27	5.00	0.24	8.00	0.4
6	7.26	0.29	9.20	0.36	7.30	0.53	9.60	0.9
Mean	4.55	0.79†	7.06*	0.98†	6.20*	1.75†	8.10*	3.77†
S.D.	3.26	0.60	4.00	0.85	4.70	1.80	4.20	3.77

*$P<0.05$ between rest and walk.
†$P<0.05$ between young (Y) and elderly (E).

inhibitor of prostaglandin synthesis, has no effect on the reabsorption of sodium in the ascending limb of Henle's loop of elderly subjects (Macias *et al.*, 1980). Therefore, it seems unlikely that prostaglandins play any major role in the high natriuresis seen in healthy elderly subjects. Despite the tendency for exaggerated natriuresis in the elderly, total body sodium is not significantly decreased with age (Weidmann *et al.*, 1977; Cox and Shalaby, 1981; Fülöp *et al.*, 1985).

Of interest is the fact that, in contrast to the tendency to lose sodium via the kidney, the erythrocytic sodium content is increased in the aged population (Naylor, 1970; Nagaki and Teraoka, 1976; Cumberbatch and Morgan, 1981). In other tissues, such as skeletal muscle, intracellular sodium seems to vary with age, although the data obtained was in a population not older than 57 years (Campana *et al.*, 1971). The high erythrocytic levels of sodium in the aged have been related to any alteration in the capacity for ionic transport by the red cell membrane (Naylor, 1970; Cox and Shalaby, 1981; Cumberbath and Morgan, 1981). This alteration can account for the high sodium and low potassium content of the red cells (Cox and Shalaby, 1981). The cause of this alteration has been attributed to an effect of aging

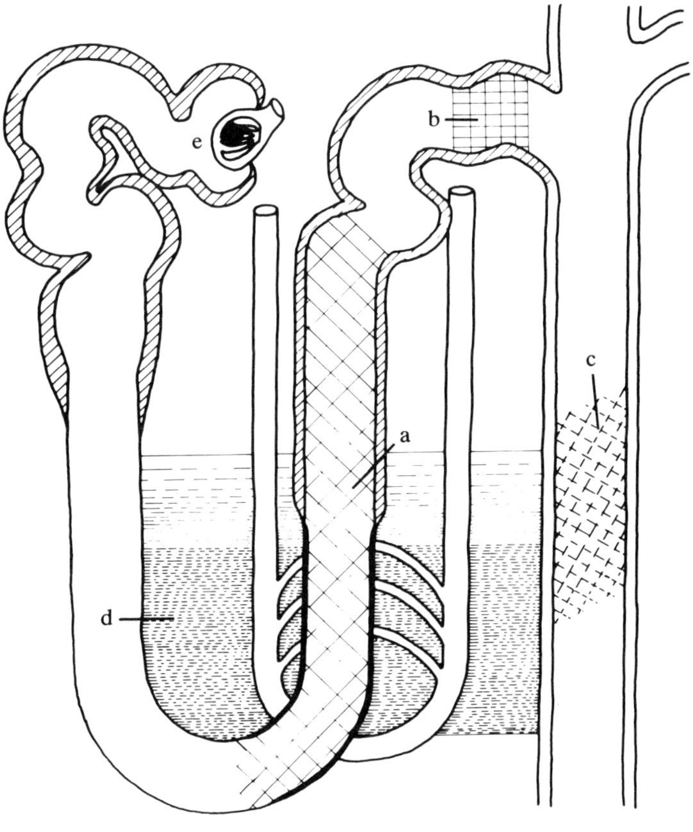

Figure 4.4 Highlighted areas represent the major segments of the nephron of the aging kidney responsible for impairment of water, electrolytes, concentration and dilution mechanisms. These segments are: (*a*) ascending limb of Henle's loop; (*b*) segment of the distal tubule where aldosterone exerts its action upon sodium reabsorption; (*c*) zones of the collecting tubule sensitive to antidiuretic hormone action; (*d*) interstitial fibrosis. There is also a certain degree of glomerular sclerosis (*e*) responsible for GFR diminution with age

itself, in altering membrane synthesis or metabolic membrane support (Naylor, 1970). Others claim that a functional defect of Na–K–ATPase-dependent pump is present (Ibrahim *et al.*, 1978). In the brain of old rats there is no decrease in Na–K–ATPase activity (La Manna *et al.*, 1983), and others have shown that, with age, the number of units able to extract sodium from the cell diminishes (Cumberbath and Morgan, 1981). The Na–K–ATPase activity of the renal medulla of old rats has been shown to be reduced (Bengele *et al.*, 1983), and while a Na–K–ATPase deficit may contribute to a loss of sodium in various models, it is not clear that it is important in the salt-losing defect in elderly human beings.

Other factors, such as interstitial fibrosis, peritubular forces and sexual hormones, could contribute to the defect. However, definitive evidence is lacking for these (Epstein and Hollenberg, 1979). In summary, the ascending limb of Henle's loop and tubular segments where aldosterone exerts its effect (Ceruso *et al.*, 1970) are primarily responsible for the impairment in renal sodium handling by the aging kidney (*Figure 4.4*).

Potassium

Plasma potassium

Plasma potassium in the aged does not significantly differ from that of the young population (Videbaek and Ackermann, 1953), a finding that has been confirmed by various studies (Dall, Paulose and Fergusson, 1971; Burini *et al.*, 1973). Under normal conditions, potassium in plasma among the elderly is normal, but when diuretics are taken, the elderly develop hypokalaemia more rapidly than do the young (Dall, Paulose and Fergusson, 1971; Sunderam and Mankikar, 1983).

Erythrocyte potassium

It is generally accepted that intra-erythrocytic potassium is a reasonable reflection of intracellular potassium content (Videbaek and Ackermann, 1953), and a significant *decrease of the intra-erythrocytic potassium* has been confirmed in the elderly (Kromhout *et al.*, 1977; Hiraide, 1981; Young, 1983) despite a normal plasma potassium, while there is only one study in which the erythrocytic potassium was found to be elevated as compared to the young (Nagaki and Teraoka, 1976).

Total body potassium and altered membrane handling of K^+

Isotopic analysis of total body potassium content has uncovered a significant difference between the young and the aged. Total exchangeable body potassium measurements using an isotopic dilution procedure with radiolabelled potassium 42-α, potassium 43 or whole body potassium detection of potassium 40 have been in agreement that there is a *lower potassium content in the body of the elderly* as compared to the young (Allen, Anderson and Langham, 1960; Forbes and Reina, 1970; Molaschi and Molaschi, 1974; Cohn *et al.*, 1976; Lye *et al.*, 1976; Rajagopalan *et al.*, 1980; Hiraide, 1981; Lye, 1981; Cox and Shalaby, 1981; Young, 1983). The total mean potassium in the elderly of 2500 mEq is approximately one-fifth less than in the young (3000 mEq).

Since 85 per cent of potassium is deposited in the muscle, efforts to explain the different content of potassium have focused on this tissue, principally in relation to the diminution of the muscular tissue that occurs with age (Allen, Anderson and

Langham, 1960; Forbes and Reina, 1970; Kromhout *et al.*, 1977; Rajagopalan *et al.*, 1980; Lye, 1981). When correction of total body potassium content is made using the lean body mass as a point of reference, the difference between young and elderly is even more pronounced (Lye, 1981). When potassium supplements are given to the healthy elderly, the intra-erythrocytic deficit of potassium vanishes, but total body potassium deficit remains unchanged. This finding could mean: (1) that the intra-erythrocytic potassium content is not an accurate method to assess total body potassium content; (2) that the muscular cells of the elderly are relatively impermeable to potassium; or (3) that the elderly possess a reduced number of muscular cells which are already potassium replenished (Kromhout *et al.*, 1977). This last observation is supported by the fact that the tissue potassium found in muscular biopsies remains constant throughout life (Campana *et al.*, 1971; Moller *et al.*, 1983).

Other theories have been proposed to explain potassium depletion in the aged. One of them claims that an *alteration of the cell membrane* may be responsible for a potassium loss from and sodium gain by the cell. Support for this comes from studies performed in the red cell of the elderly (Naylor, 1970; Nagaki and Teraoka, 1976; Cumberbatch and Morgan, 1981), demonstrating a high content of sodium in these cells. The demonstration that muscle potassium may be normal, despite aging, is against this view. Conceivably, an alteration of the erythrocyte membrane could be specific for those cells and not be present in any other cells, but proof for both are lacking.

It has also been suggested that the cause for both low calcium and potassium levels are the *nutritional deficiencies,* the hormonal alteration and/or reduction in physical activity (Cohn *et al.*, 1976). Daily potassium intake ranges between 60 and 150 mEq/day in the healthy young population. In the UK and the USA, potassium intake is lower in the old than in young populations, being on the average less than 60 mEq/day (Dall, Paulose and Fergusson, 1971; Davies, Hastrop and Bender, 1973; Abdulla *et al.*, 1979b). This low potassium ingestion is attributed to the inclination that the elderly have to eat more carbohydrates (sweets and cakes) instead of fresh fruit, meat or fish that offer a higher potassium content (Dall and Gardiner, 1971; Davies, Hastrop and Bender, 1973). Low potassium intake may be responsible for the low erythrocytic potassium content (Kromhout *et al.*, 1977; Barbagallo, Disciacca and Pardo, 1979; Hiraide, 1981) and could explain why there is correction of the defect after potassium administration (Kromhout *et al.*, 1977).

Table 4.6 Renal handling of potassium

	Plasma potassium		*UK.V*		*FE K(%)*	
	Y	*E*	*Y*	*E*	*Y*	*E*
	3.70	3.60	45.70	23.20	7.32	10.50
	3.50	3.90	51.10	25.20	9.50	5.40
	3.70	3.50	50.50	22.50	5.60	10.50
	3.10	3.50	47.10	44.20	12.80	14.10
	3.60	3.70	36.80	37.20	7.50	14.80
	3.70	3.70	27.80	30.60	8.90	11.00
Mean	3.60	3.60	43.20	30.5*	8.60	9.30
S.D.	0.24	0.16	9.10	9.70	3.10	3.40

Y, young; E, elderly; UK.V, urinary potassium output per 24 h; FE K(%), fractional excretion of potassium.
*$P<0.05$.

The final possibility of a tendency to potassium deficiency is an inability of the kidney to conserve potassium. We have observed that the *renal excretion of potassium is significantly lower* in the aged population than in the young (*Table 4.6*). However, when corrected for the reduced GFR, fraction excretion of potassium shows a trend to be greater in the elderly than in young (*Table 4.6*). Possibly, as the number of functioning nephrons is decreased with age, the elimination of potassium per single nephron is higher in the aged. Whether this is or is not responsible for the low erythrocyte potassium in the aged is unknown.

Water

Water equilibrium is achieved through a balance between water intake and water disposal. This balance is controlled by the regulation of thirst, neurohypophyseal function and the renal capacity for water excretion. Thirst and the intake of liquids diminish with age (Goldman, 1981). When healthy active elderly volunteers are water restricted for 24 h, the threshold for thirst is found to be increased and water intake reduced in respect to a control group of younger subjects. Despite the reduction in water intake and thirst, a considerable increase in blood osmolality, plasma sodium concentration and in circulating vasopressin occurred (Phillips *et al.*, 1984).

The lack of thirst development in the elderly despite an increase in plasma tonicity remains unexplained. Dryness of the mouth and a decrease of taste with age may contribute to the diminution of the thirst observed in the aged (Hugonot, Dubos and Mathes, 1978). Another mechanism for diminished thirst in the elderly may be an alteration in mental capacity (Seymour *et al.*, 1980) or cortical cerebral dysfunction (Miller *et al.*, 1982). It has also been theorized that a reduction in the sensitivity of the osmoreceptors responsible for thirst regulation may play a role in the water-handling alterations in elderly persons. A contrary view has arisen from the studies of Helderman *et al.* (1978).

In these studies an increase in the sensitivity of the osmoreceptors that regulate vasopressin release was observed. Thirst diminution may also result from an inappropriate response to hypovolaemia. Age diminishes the sensitivity of the baroreceptors (Rowe *et al.*, 1982). Therefore, stimulation of thirst requires a severe hypovolaemia and/or hypotension (Robertson, 1984). It should be pointed out, however, that there is no difference in the plasma concentration of vasopressin between the young and the elderly before or following water deprivation.

Urinary concentration

Aging reduces the capacity of the concentration mechanism (Dontas, Marketos and Papanayioutou, 1972). This capacity diminishes 5 per cent with every 10 years of age (Lewis and Alving, 1938). The aetiology of this process is not clear. Small differences between the amount of liquid taken by young and elderly subjects cannot completely explain the differences in solutes and urinary elimination observed during water deprivation (Rowe, Shock and De Fronzo, 1976). This diminution of the concentration ability has been related to the decrement in glomerular filtration rate that occurs with age. It is assumed that as the number of functioning nephrons decreases with age, the remainder are subjected to osmotic diuresis which impairs the ability to concentrate urine (Lindeman, Van Buren and Raisz, 1960; Kleeman, 1972). Despite this, some data do not reveal a close relationship between the reduction of glomerular filtration rate and the capacity to concentrate urine in the elderly (Rowe, Shock and De Fronzo, 1976).

Increased medullary blood flow could contribute to the impairment of renal concentration capacity (Takazakura *et al.,* 1972; Hollenberg *et al.,* 1974). Nevertheless, data substantiating this suggestion are not available. Inappropriately low ADH is not, as already discussed, a factor in the genesis of the defect. The defect in sodium chloride reabsorption in the ascending limb of the loop of Henle can also contribute to a decrease in the capacity to concentrate urine seen in the aged.

Urinary dilution

There are only a few reports dealing with the capacity of the aging kidney to dilute urine, but it has been found to be decreased (Phillips *et al.*, 1984; Editorial, 1984). The functional impairment of the diluting segment described earlier in this chapter seems to account for the diminution of the capacity to dilute urine observed in the aged (Macias *et al.,* 1978).

Plasma volume

Total body water is slightly diminished with age, so that only 54 per cent of total body weight is water (Edelman and Leibman, 1959). The loss seems to be predominantly intracellular (Edmonds, Jasani and Smith, 1975). Cross-sectional and longitudinal studies have revealed that plasma and blood volume do not alter as a result of age in healthy adults (Cohn and Shock, 1949; Chien, Usami and Simmons, 1966), although Wórum *et al.* (1984) found that elderly women have significantly higher plasma volume than the young. We have found that plasma and blood volume measurements using radiolabelled albumin do not differ between young and elderly healthy volunteers. Males have a higher plasma volume than females, regardless of age (*Table 4.7*).

Table 4.7 Plasma volume

	Young		*Elderly*	
	M (ml/m^2)	*F* (ml/m^2)	*M*(ml/m^2)	*F (ml/m^2)*
1	1575	1381	1282	1275
2	1591	1341	1802	1568
3	1693	1481	1403	1520
4	1610	1455	1275	1510
5	1307	1341	1843	1325
6	1471	1457	1542	1553
7	1258	1332	1357	1559
8	1601	1211	1471	1694
9		1318	1444	1306
10			1528	1453
11			1587	1243
12			1660	972
13				1187
14				1403
Mean	1516.17	1368.56*	1513.25	1397.71*
S.D.	±184.25	±85.4	±155.24	±191.33

*$P<0.05$ between males (M) and females (F).

In patients with psychiatric pathology, an alteration of the intracellular, extracellular and total body water has been found. The deterioration of verbal learning is associated with an increase in body water, intracellular and extracellular fluid and exchangeable sodium and potassium in relation to dry body weight. The diminution in verbal ability is associated with a shifting of water from the extracellular to the intracellular compartments and diminution of the interchangeable sodium in relation to lean body weight (Cox and Orme, 1973).

Diagnosis, treatment and prevention of electrolyte and water disturbances in the elderly

Sodium

Hyponatraemia

Hyponatraemia (plasma sodium lower than 130 mEq/l) is frequently found in elderly patients. Acute and chronically ill geriatric patients have a higher incidence of hyponatraemia than the general hospitalized population. The incidence of hyponatraemia is 11 per cent in acute and 22 per cent in chronic elderly hospitalized patients. This incidence is significantly higher than in the general hospitalized population (Kleinfeld, Casimir and Borra, 1979; Sunderam and Mankikar, 1983). Hyponatraemia has been explained on the basis of the incidence in the aged population of specific pathology, and also medical mismanagement or misreading of the situation especially in relation to fluid balance. Thus, heart failure, liver cirrhosis (Forbes and Reina, 1970; McCarthy, 1982), digestive losses such as diarrhoea, vomiting and uncontrolled diabetes mellitus with severe hyperglycaemia and subsequent osmotic polyuria (Ledoux, Corvol and Milliez, 1977; Azevedo, 1981) are common causes of hyponatraemia among the elderly.

The use and abuse of laxatives and diuretics is a common cause of hyponatraemia. Restriction of oral salt intake and the administration of hypotonic or non-electrolyte-containing solutions are another common cause of hyponatraemia. Other causes of hyponatraemia may include urinary tract infections or acute and chronic tubulo-interstitial disease. In males, the post-obstructive diuresis of lower urinary tract obstruction can be a cause of hyponatraemia. Inappropriate secretion of antidiuretic hormone syndrome is also a frequent cause of a major hyponatraemia in the aged (Ledoux, Corvol and Milliez, 1977; Kleinfeld, Casimir and Borra, 1979). Furthermore, cerebrovascular accidents, lung disease, paraneoplasic syndrome, chlorpropamide and clofibrate intake are also common in the elderly subject.

The differential diagnosis of the inappropriate secretion of antidiuretic hormone must carefully take into account that the blood level of antidiuretic hormone in the healthy elderly is sometimes in the upper part of the normal range or even slightly above it when compared to the young population. In view of this, the diagnosis cannot be made based on antidiuretic hormone measurement alone. The syndrome of inappropriate secretion of antidiuretic hormone is characterized by a urinary osmolality that exceeds that of plasma, when plasma osmolality is clearly under 270 mosmol/kg and plasma sodium concentration is clearly below 130 mEq/l. This should be differentiated from the *commonest cause* of hyponatraemia seen in the elderly due to the defect in tubular reabsorption of the aging kidney (Macias *et al.*, 1978, 1980).

Clinical history and physical examination are important in combination with blood and urinary tests for electrolytes and osmolarity levels. The most frequent clinical findings leading to hyponatraemia in the elderly are loss of appetite for a few days, diarrhoea and vomiting or profuse sweating, without thirst. It must be remembered that the threshold for thirst in the elderly is higher than in younger persons.

In the elderly a state of disorientation consisting of one or many of these symptoms may occur in addition to loss of memory, tiredness, transient hemiparesis, neuromuscular weakness and difficulties in motor co-ordination. Upon physical examination, signs of volume depletion including postural hypotension are occasionally present. A blood test may show low sodium levels, and normal or modestly raised osmolarity. A high urinary sodium output, in spite of low blood sodium, usually over 100 mEq/l is present (Yamori *et al.*, 1982). Administration of water or electrolyte-free solutions in excess may induce dilutional hyponatraemia. The association of hyponatraemia to an underlying disease worsens the prognosis, regardless of its aetiology (Sunderam and Mankikar, 1983).

Hypernatraemia may also be seen in the elderly, in the majority of instances, related to hypertonic dehydration (Jana and Romano-Jana, 1973) caused by the greater loss of water than of salt or by a lack of water intake, rather common among the elderly due to a decrease in natural thirst. The most common symptom of hypernatraemia is mental confusion and disorientation.

Prophylaxis and treatment of disorders involving sodium

Close follow-up of elderly patients before and after surgical operations or on diuretic treatment, and in any situations in which even a transient loss of appetite is present, is of paramount importance. Similarly, when water and electrolyte losses such as from diarrhoea, vomiting and excessive sweating in hot climates are found, these losses must be replaced immediately to prevent the electrolyte imbalance and acute renal failure which can supervene. In our experience, 2 litres of liquid with 6–9 g of salt per day are enough to prevent these situations arising or becoming worse. When diuretics are needed, salt should not be eliminated entirely from the diet to avoid large deficits. It is necessary to be sure that the elderly drink the amount of water and other liquids prescribed. Because, rather frequently, the elderly patients do not feel appetite for salt or water, it is best to give them 200 ml of liquids (1 glass) per hour during the day. If only liquids are prescribed, it is likely that the patient will ignore taking them. Salt should be added to foods; when foods are refused, salt solutions should be provided.

If patients refuse or are unable to eat or drink, they should be parenterally treated with no delay. If the degree of dehydration is severe, a central venous pressure catheter must be used to measure the haemodynamic state and administer salt solutions. Central venous pressure must be kept around 8–10 cm H_2O. The infusion rate should not result in marked elevation of central venous pressure, for the danger of congestive failure is great in elderly patients. As a general rule, a rate of no more than 70 drops/min is enough to replace water and electrolytes in these patients. Persistence of oliguria once central venous pressure is maintained between 8 and 10 cm of water for at least 1 h may indicate the need for further therapy on the development of renal insufficiency.

If it is necessary to fast and avoid oral intake in elderly patients the day before surgery, it would be advisable to give 2 litres of normal isotonic saline intravenously.

In the postoperative period, the hydroelectrolytic balance should be carefully monitored. Electrolyte-free solutions should not be routinely prescribed after surgery, without knowledge of the blood electrolytes concentration.

If the syndrome of inappropriate secretion of antidiuretic hormone is present, restriction of oral water ingestion with negative balance of water is enough to treat the syndrome (Ledoux, Corvol and Milliez, 1977). When hyponatraemia is severe and acute and central nervous system dysfunction such as coma is present, hypertonic saline may be necessary. This should not exceed 300 mEq/l (twice normal); the use of stronger solutions such as 8.4 per cent sodium bicarbonate or sodium chloride is dangerous and unnecessary.

Potassium

Hypokalaemia

The most common finding *regarding potassium handling in old people is hypokalaemia.* Hypokalaemia is present in 11 per cent of the elderly patients seen in the emergency room, regardless of the reasons for the visit (McCarthy, 1982). Hypokalaemia may result from extrarenal losses of potassium and/or through the kidney. Diuretics, surgical wounds, interstitial nephropathy, diarrhoea, vomiting, malabsorption, laxatives, diabetes mellitus or diabetes insipidus may provoke hypopotassaemia (Karlberg and Tolagen, 1977; Cox and Shalaby, 1981; Azevedo, 1981; McCarthy, 1982). Symptoms of hypopotassaemia are due to intracellular potassium depletion. When potassium depletion is present, the fall of 1 mEq/l in plasma potassium concentration represents a deficit of 20 per cent of intracellular potassium.

Potassium depletion leads to neuromuscular alterations that may be characterized by reduced intellectual capacity, postural hypotension and muscular weakness. In more advanced states, arrythmias, adynamia and superficial breathing will appear. Depression is frequently seen in states of chronic potassium depletion; thus, depression in the elderly may be the consequence of hypokalaemia (Davies, Hastrop and Bender, 1973).

Hypokalaemia is commonly associated with a high plasma bicarbonate concentration. Intolerance to carbohydrates may also be seen. In severe cases electrocardiographic abnormalities such as QT interval widening, ST depression, T-wave flattening, U-wave and diverse arrhythmias may be present (Karlberg and Tolagen, 1977). Elderly patients on digitalis treatment are particularly prone to develop hypokalaemia-related arrhythmias. These patients become sensitive to the effect of digitalis, and intoxication with that agent is a frequent problem (Dall, Paulose and Fergusson, 1971).

Hyperkalaemia is rather unusual in the elderly unless they are on renal failure. Hyperkalaemia is provoked when old animals are given a chronic potassium load (Bengele, 1983). This should be considered when treating old patients in chronic renal failure. Occasionally, hyperkalaemia of extreme degree will be found in patients taking potassium-sparing diuretics such as amiloride, triamterene or spironolactone.

Prophylaxis and treatment of disorders involving potassium

The commonest cause of hypokalaemia in the elderly is the use of diuretics. Prevention of hypokalaemia can be achieved by concomitant administration of potassium supplements. When hypokalaemia is severe, potassium-sparing diuretics may be required in addition to potassium supplements. Low potassium intake among the elderly is also a factor in the development of hypokalaemia. A major problem is the consumption of predominantly carbohydrate diet deficient in potassium (Davies, Hastrop and Bender, 1973; Abdulla *et al.*, 1979b). To correct this lack of dietary potassium, elderly patients should be encouraged to consume dairy products, fresh fruit, cereals, nuts, coffee and chocolate. It has been proposed that a potassium-rich diet (100 mEq/day) can prevent the need for potassium supplements and/or potassium-sparing diuretics in the elderly who are receiving diuretics (Henschke, Spence and Cape, 1981).

Oral potassium supplements must be given in the form of chloride compounds, always considering that they are potentially ulcerogenic. Despite the presence of a potassium deficit in the elderly, potassium supplements should not be given routinely because these supplements have been ineffective in restoring the total body potassium content (McLennan, Lye and May, 1977; Kromhout *et al.*, 1977; Ibrahim *et al.*, 1978). Moreover, unless the serum potassium is below 2.5 mEq/l or symptoms occur, the need for potassium supplements is not clear. When hypokalaemia is present, potassium oral supplements must be prescribed in doses that have been proved effective in normalizing plasma potassium levels (20–40 mEq/day). In special circumstances, such as oedematous states, it has been suggested that potassium oral supplements are unable to restore plasma levels because urinary potassium elimination is almost equal to the oral amount of potassium administered (Dow, Polak and Rao, 1972). In most severe cases, or when oral administration is not feasible, digestive intolerance is present; potassium must be administered intravenously and careful plasma potassium and electrocardiographic monitoring are necessary under these circumstances.

Potassium-sparing diuretics (amiloride, triamterene and spironolactone) are useful in the prophylaxis of hypokalaemia when used with other diuretics (McFarlane and Kennedy, 1973; McCarthy, 1982). For example, amiloride (5 mg/day) administered with thiazide will maintain normal potassium levels particularly in the elderly. It must be emphasized that a potassium-rich diet may be all that is required to prevent hypokalaemia (Henschke, Spence and Cape, 1981).

Finally, potassium supplements and potassium-sparing diuretics must be administered with caution to diabetic patients, because in these patients the extrarenal control of potassium metabolism is impaired and severe hypopotassaemia may result. Moreover, hyporeninaemic hypoaldosteronism may be present in the elderly and make them susceptible to hyperkalaemia.

Water

Dehydration

Dehydration is common in the elderly. It results from diminished water intake or excessive losses through the lungs, skin, kidney and gastrointestinal tract. Water intake may be reduced with age because of (1) confusion, (2) inability to recognize thirst and/or to be able to reach a source to placate it, and (3) immobilization due to apathy or physical limitations (Brocklehurst and Hanley, 1979). The elderly who are suffering from mental confusion or are bedridden are most likely to experience pure water depletion or dehydration. They are also plagued by diseases that cause thirst diminution such as trauma and acute cerebrovascular accidents. While the cause of hypodipsia without hypothalamic or pituitary gland lesions is not well known (Miller *et al.*, 1982) iatrogenic processes such as deficient post-surgical replacement, drugs which increase apathy or stuporous states, should be readily identified and corrected.

Pure water depletion can also be seen in respiratory infectious diseases, excess alcohol intake and solute overload leading to hyperosmolarity (Leaf, 1984; Fitzsimons, 1976; Lye, 1984; Phillips *et al.*, 1984). Water depletion causes headaches, trembling, weakness, mental confusion, lethargy and hyperthermia. Oliguria and acute renal failure may also occur. Dehydration can be severe enough to induce delirium, maniacal behaviour, convulsions and a comatose state.

Thirst, which is always an early symptom of dehydration in young patients, may be attenuated, diminished or even absent in the elderly. Physical examination may reveal skin and tongue dryness. The natural skin turgor may be a last sign, but the skin-fold sign is not always easy to evaluate in elderly patients as a result of loss of subcutaneous fat. A more important sign of dehydration is dryness of axillae and groins. The collapse of veins and systemic or postural hypotension seen with salt depletion are absent in dehydration. Tachycardia may be present if hyperthermia exists (Hugonot, Dubos and Mathes, 1978; Lye, 1984).

Laboratory tests may appear normal early in dehydration, but as it worsens, the haematocrit will increase. The increase may not be significant if anaemia is present in the elderly, a fact that must be taken into consideration when evaluating changes due to dehydration. Plasma sodium is increased as a result of water loss. The level of blood sodium is valuable in differentiating between water (high) and salt (low) depletion. The concentration of proteins in plasma rises as long as hyponatraemia was not present previously. Blood urea is usually increased, as is urinary urea excretion. The urinary urea/blood urea rate is higher than 10. This is a useful finding to differentiate between oliguria due to acute renal failure and that due to dehydration. Under these conditions, urine sodium is usually less than 70 mEq/l in our experience. In more severe dehydration, urinary sodium output may be 10 mEq/l or not detectable at all (Phillips *et al.*, 1984).

Prophylaxis and treatment of disorders involving water

Water depletion is always a sign of deficient care either when the elderly are hospitalized or at home (Himmelstein, Jones and Woolhandler, 1983). For elderly patients who temporarily refuse food and drink (depression, febrile illnesses and occasionally loss of appetite), it has been useful in our experience to administer 2 litres of liquids per day as a prophylactic approach to avoid dehydration. If the patient is seen when already dehydrated, the following equation can be used to calculate the volume of water required:

$$\text{Water deficit} = \text{Calculated total body water} - \text{Calculated actual body water}$$

$$\text{Water deficit} = (0.5 \,.\, \text{Body weight}) - 140 \,.\, (0.5 \,.\, \text{body weight})/\text{Plasma sodium concentration}$$

This calculation assumes that normal plasma sodium is 140 mEq/l and total body water is 50 per cent of body weight in kilograms. Body weight is the weight of the patient at the time of evaluation (Covey and Arieff, 1978).

Replacement therapy should be corrected by the administration of one-half the deficit in the first 24 h, followed by the other half in the next 24 h. If dehydration cannot be treated orally, the same amount of water should be given intravenously using 5 per cent dextrose solutions (Lye, 1984).

References

ABDULLA, M., JAGERSTAD, M., NORDEN, A., THULIN, T. and SVENSSON, S. (1979a). Nutrition and old age. Sodium. *Scandinavian Journal of Gastroenterology,* **14,** 138–142.

ABDULLA, M., JAGERSTAD, M., THULIN, T., SVENSSON, S. and NORDEN, A. (1979b). Nutrition and old age. Potassium. *Scandinavian Journal of Gastroenterology,* **14,** 143–147

ADROGUE, H.J. and MARTINEZ-MALDONADO, M. (1982). Compendio de fisiologia renal. In *Tratado de Nefrologia,* edited by M. Martinez-Maldonado and J.L. Rodicio, pp. 54–72. Barcelona; Salvat Editores

ALLEN, T.H., ANDERSON, E.C. and LANGHAM, W.H. (1960). Total body potassium and gross body composition in relation to age. *Journal of Gerontology,* **15,** 348–357

AZEVEDO, F. (1981). Percepcion de la sed, deshidrataciones y alteraciones del equilibrio de electrolitos. In *Iniciacion en Geriatria y Gerontologia,* Vol. I, edited by F.J. Herrero, pp. 221–227. Barcelona; Ferrer Internacional

BARBAGALLO, G., DISCIACCA, A. and PARDO, A. (1979). Potassium depletion in aged patients: an evaluation through red-blood cell potassium determination. *Age and Ageing,* **8,** 190–195

BENGELE, H.H., MATHIAS, R.S. and ALEXANDER, E.A. (1981). Impaired natriuresis after volume expansion in the aged rat. *Renal Physiology,* **4,** 22–29

BENGELE, H.H., MATHIAS, R., PERKINS, J.H., McNAMARA, E.R. and ALEXANDER, E.A. (1983). Impaired renal and extrarenal adaptation in old rats. *Kidney International,* **23,** 684–690

BERL, T. and CHAIMOWITZ, C. (1983). Water and sodium metabolism. In *Textbook of Nephrology,* edited by S.G. Massry and R.J. Glassock, pp. 3.6–3.12. Baltimore; Williams and Wilkins

BROCKLEHURST, J.C. and HANLEY, T. (1979). *Fundamentals of Geriatrics,* 1st edn, pp. 195–214. Barcelona; Toray, S.A.

BURG, M.B. (1976). The renal handling of sodium chloride. In *The Kidney,* edited by B.M. Brenner and F.C. Rector, pp. 272–298. Philadelphia; Saunders

BURG, M.B. (1986). Renal handling of sodium, chloride, water, aminoacids and glucose. In *The Kidney,* 3rd edn, edited by B.M. Brenner and F.C. Rector, pp. 145–176. Philadelphia; Saunders

BURINI, R., DASILVA, C.A., RIBEIRO, M.A.C. and CAMPANA, A.O. (1973). Concentracão de sodio e de potassio no soro e plasma de individuos normais. Influencia da idade, do sexo e do sistema de colheita do sange sobre os resultados. *Revista de Hospitale Clinico da Facultad do Medicina de Sao Paulo,* **28,** 9–14

CAMPANA, A.O., DE ANDRADE, D.R., GAZONI, E., BURINI, R.C. and NEVES, D.P. (1971). Water, fat, sodium, potassium and chloride content of skeletal muscle in 'normal' subjects. *Revista Brasileira de Pesquisas Medicas e Biologicas,* **4,** 409–415

CERUSO, D., SQUADRITO, G., QUARTARONE, M. and PARISI, M. (1970). Comportamento della funzionalità renale e degli elettroliti ematici ed urinari dopo aldosterone in soggetti anziani. *Giornale di Gerontologia,* **18,** 1–6

CHIEN, S., USAMI, S. and SIMMONS, R.L. (1966). Blood volume and age: repeated measurements on normal men. *Journal of Applied Physiology,* **21,** 583–588

COHN, J.E. and SHOCK, N.W. (1949). Blood volume studies in middle-aged and elderly males. *American Journal of Medical Sciences,* **217,** 388–391

COHN, S.H., VASWANI, A., ZANZI, I., ALOIA, J.F., ROGINSKY, M.S. and ELLIS, K.J. (1976). Changes in body chemical composition with age measured by total body neutron activation. *Metabolism,* **25,** 85–96

COVEY, C.M. and ARIEFF, A.I. (1978). Disorders of sodium and water metabolism and their effects on the central nervous system. In *Sodium and Water Homeostasis,* edited by B.M. Brenner and J.H. Stein, pp. 212–241. New York; Churchill Livingstone

COX, J.R. and ORME, J.E. (1973). Body water, electrolytes and psychological test performance in elderly patients. *Gerontologica Clinica,* **15,** 203–208

COX, J.R. and SHALABY, W.A. (1981). Potassium changes with age. *Gerontology,* **27,** 340–344

CRANE, M. and HARRIS, J.J. (1976). Effect of aging on renin activity and aldosterone excretion. *Journal of Laboratory and Clinical Medicine,* **87,** 947–959

CUMBERBATCH, M. and MORGAN, D.B. (1981). Relations between sodium transport and sodium concentration in human erythrocytes in health and disease. *Clinical Science,* **60,** 555–564

DALL, J.L.C. and GARDINER, H.S. (1971). Dietary intake of potassium by geriatric patients. *Gerontologia Clinica,* **13,** 119–124

DALL, J.L.C., PAULOSE, S. and FERGUSSON, J.A. (1971). Potassium intake of elderly patients in hospital. *Gerontologia Clinica,* **13,** 114–118

DAVIES, D.F. and SHOCK, N.W. (1950). Age changes in glomerular filtration rate, effective renal plasma flow, and tubular excretory capacity in adult males. *Journal of Clinical Investigation,* **29,** 496–507

DAVIES, L., HASTROP, K. and BENDER, A.E. (1973). Potassium intake of the elderly. *Modern Geriatrics,* **4,** 482–488

DONTAS, A.S., MARKETOS, S. and PAPANAYIOUTOU, P. (1972). Mechanisms of renal tubular defects in old age. *Postgraduate Medical Journal,* **48,** 295–303

DOW, P.F., POLAK, A. and RAO, R. (1972). Fate of potassium supplements in six outpatients receiving long term diuretic for oedematous disease. *Lancet,* **2,** 721–724

EDELMAN, I.S. and LEIBMAN, J. (1959). Anatomy of body water and electrolytes. *American Journal of Medicine,* **27,** 256–260

EDITORIAL (1984). Thirst and osmoregulation in the elderly. *Lancet,* **2,** 1017–1018

EDMONDS, C.J., JASANI, B.M. and SMITH, T. (1975). Total body potassium and body fat estimation in relationship to height, sex, age, malnutrition and obesity. *Clinical Science and Molecular Medicine,* **48,** 431–440

EPSTEIN, M. and HOLLENBERG, N.K. (1976). Age as a determinant of renal sodium conservation in normal man. *Journal of Laboratory and Clinical Medicine,* **87,** 411–417

EPSTEIN, M. and HOLLENBERG, N.K. (1979). Renal 'salt wasting' despite apparently normal renal, adrenal and central nervous system function. *Nephron,* **24,** 121–126

FITZSIMMONS, J.T. (1976). The physiological basis of thirst. *Kidney International,* **10,** 3–11

FITZSIMMONS, J.T. (1985). Physiology and pathology of thirst and sodium appetite. In *The Kidney, Physiology and Pathophysiology,* Vol. 2, edited by D.W. Seldin and G. Giebisch, pp. 885–901. New York; Raven Press

FLOOD, C., GERONDACHE, C., PINCUS, G., TAIT, J.F., TAIT, S.A.S. and WILLOUGHBY, S. (1967). The metabolism and secretion of aldosterone in elderly subjects. *Journal of Clinical Investigation,* **46,** 960–966

FORBES, G.B. and REINA, J.C. (1970). Adult lean body mass declines with age: some longitudinal observations. *Metabolism,* **19,** 653–663

FÜLÖP, T., WÓRUM, I., CSONGOR, J., FÓRIS, G. and LEÖVEY, A. (1985). Body composition in elderly people. *Gerontology,* **31,** 6–14

GABOW, P.A. and PETERSON, L.N. (1980). Disorders of potassium metabolism. In *Renal and Electrolyte Disorders,* edited by R.W. Schrier, pp. 185–196. Boston; Little, Brown

GOLDMAN, R. (1981). Modern ideas about the renal function in the elderly. In *Geriatrics for the Practitioner,* edited by A.N.J. Reinders Folmer and J. Shouten, pp. 157–166. Amsterdam; Excerpta Medica

GRANTHAM, J.J. (1986). Renal transport and control of potassium excretion. In *The Kidney,* 3rd edn, edited by B.M. Brenner and F.C. Rector, pp. 299–317. Philadelphia; Saunders

HACKBARTH, H. and HARRISON, D.E. (1982). Changes with age in renal function and morphology in C57BL/6, CBA, and B6CBAF1 mice. *Journal of Gerontology,* **37,** 540–547

HELDERMAN, J.H., VESTAL, R.E., ROWE, J.W., TOBIN, J.D., ANDRES, R. and ROBERTSON, G.L. (1978). The response of arginine vasopressin to intravenous ethanol and hypertonic saline in man: the impact of aging. *Journal of Gerontology,* **33,** 39–47

HENSCHKE, P.J., SPENCE, J.D. and CAPE, R.D.T. (1981). Diuretics and the institutional elderly: a case against routine potassium prescribing. *Journal of the American Geriatrics Society,* **29,** 145–150

HIMMELSTEIN, D.U., JONES, A.A. and WOOLHANDLER, S. (1983). Hypernatremic dehydration in nursing home patients: an indicator of neglect. *Journal of the American Geriatric Society,* **31,** 466–471

HIRAIDE, K. (1981). Alterations in electrolytes with aging. *Nihon University Journal of Medicine,* **23,** 21–31

HOLLENBERG, N.K., ADAMS, D.F., SOLOMON, H.S., RASHID, A., ABRAMS, H.L. and MERRILL, J.P. (1974). Senescence and the renal vasculature in normal man. *Circulation Research,* **34,** 309–316

HUGONOT, R., DUBOS, G. and MATHES, G. (1978). Étude experimental des troubles de la soif du viellard. *La Revue de Gériatrie,* Sept. 4, 179–191

IBRAHIM, I.K., RITCH, A.E.S., McLENNAN, W.J. and MAY, T. (1978). Are potassium supplements for the elderly necessary? *Age and Ageing,* **7,** 165–170

JAMISON, R.L. (1981). Urine concentration and dilution. In *The Kidney,* 2nd edn, edited by B.M. Brenner and F.C. Rector, pp. 495–550. Philadelphia; Saunders

JAMISON, R.L. and HALL, D.A. (1983). The renal excretion of urea. In *Textbook of Nephrology,* edited by S.G. Massry and R.J. Glassock, pp. 1.51–1.52. Baltimore; Williams and Wilkins

JAMISON, R.L. and KRIZ, W. (1982). *Urinary Concentrating Mechanisms.* New York; Oxford University Press

JANA, D.K. and ROMANO-JANA, L. (1973). Hypernatremia psychosis in the elderly: case reports. *Journal of the American Geriatrics Society,* **21,** 473–477

KARLBERG, B.E. and TOLAGEN, K. (1977). Relationships between blood pressure, age, plasma renin activity and electrolyte excretion in normotensive subjects. *Scandinavian Journal of Clinical and Laboratory Investigation,* **37,** 521–528

KLEEMAN, C.R. (1972). Water metabolism. In *Clinical Disorders of Fluid and Electrolyte Balance,* edited by M.H. Maxwell and C.R. Kleeman, p. 697. New York; McGraw-Hill

KLEINFELD, M., CASIMIR, M. and BORRA, S. (1979). Hyponatremia as observed in a chronic disease facility. *Journal of the American Geriatrics Society,* **27,** 156–161

KROMHOUT, D., BROBERG, U., CARLMARK, B., KARLSSON, S., NISELL, O. and REIZENSTEIN, P. (1977). Potassium depletion and ageing. *Comprehensive Therapeutics,* **3,** 32–37

LA MANNA, J.C., DOULL, G., McCRACKEN, K. and HARIK, S.I. (1983). (Na^+–K^+)-ATPase activity and oubain-binding sites in the cerebral cortex of young and aged Fischer-344 rats. *Gerontology,* **29,** 242–247

LEAF, A. (1984). Dehydration in the elderly. *New England Journal of Medicine,* **311,** 791–792

LEDOUX, F., CORVOL, P. and MILLIEZ, P. (1977). L'hyponatrémie du sujet agé. *La Revue du Practicien,* **27,** 3073–3076

LEE, J.B., PATAK, R.V. and MOOKERJEE, B.K. (1976). Renal prostaglandins and the regulation of blood pressure and sodium and water homeostasis. *American Journal of Medicine,* **60,** 798–816

LEWIS, W.H. and ALVING, A.S. (1938). Changes with age in the renal function of adult men. Clearance of urea, amount of urea nitrogen in the blood, concentrating ability of kidneys. *American Journal of Physiology,* **123,** 505–515

LINDEMAN, R.D., VAN BUREN, H.C. and RAISZ, L.G. (1960). Osmolar renal concentrating ability in healthy young men and hospitalized patients without renal disease. *New England Journal of Medicine,* **262,** 1396–1409

LYE, M. (1981). Distribution of body potassium in healthy elderly subjects. *Gerontology,* **27,** 286–292

LYE, M. (1984). Electrolyte disorders in the elderly. In *Clinics in Endocrinology and Metabolism,* edited by B. Morgan, pp. 377–398. London; Saunders

LYE, M., MAY, T., HAMMICK, J. and ACKERY, D. (1976). Whole-body and exchangeable potassium measurements in normal elderly subjects. *European Journal of Nuclear Medicine,* **1,** 167–171

McCARTHY, S.T. (1982). Body fluid, electrolytes and diuretics. *Current Medical Research and Opinion,* **7,** 87–95

McFARLANE, J.P.R. and KENNEDY, R.D. (1973). Clinical experience with amiloride in the elderly. *Acta Cardiologica,* **28,** 365–374

MACIAS NUÑEZ, J.F., GARCIA-IGLESIAS, C., BONDIA-ROMAN, A., RODRIGUEZ-COMMES, J.L., CORBACHO-BECERRA, L., TABERNERO-ROMO, J.M. *et al.* (1978). Renal handling of sodium in old people: a functional study. *Age and Ageing,* **7,** 178–181

MACIAS NUÑEZ, J.F., GARCIA-IGLESIAS, C., TABERNERO-ROMO, J.M., RODRIGUEZ-COMMES, J.L., CORBACHO-BECERRA, L. and SANCHEZ-TOMERO, J.A. (1980). Renal management of sodium under indomethacin and aldosterone in the elderly. *Age and Ageing,* **9,** 165–172

McLENNAN, W.J., LYE, M.D.W. and MAY, T. (1977). The effect of potassium supplements on total body potassium levels in the elderly. *Age and Ageing,* **6,** 46–50

MARSH, D.J. (1983). Urinary concentration and dilution. In *Textbook of Nephrology,* edited by S.G. Massry and R.J. Glassock, pp. 1.59–1.64. Baltimore; Williams and Wilkins

MAUDE, D.L. (1977). *Kidney Physiology and Kidney Disease.* Philadelphia; Lippincott

MILLER, P.D., KREBS, R.A., NEAL, B.J. and McINTYRE, D.O. (1982). Hypodipsia in geriatric patients. *American Journal of Medicine,* **73,** 354–356

MOLASCHI, M. and MOLASCHI, E.S. (1974). Correlazione tra metabolismo del potassio, funzionalita renale ed invecchiamento nell'uomo. *Giornale di Gerontologia,* **22,** 241–250

MOLLER, P., AVVESTRASND, A., BERGSTROM, J. and FURST, P. (1983). Electrolytes and free amino acids in leg skeletal muscle of young and elderly women. *Gerontology,* **29,** 1–8

MORGAN, T. (1979) Renal physiology. In *Nephrology,* edited by J. Hamburger, J. Cosnier and J.P. Grunfeld, pp. 59–100. New York; Wiley–Flammarion

MYERS, J., MORGAN, T., WAGA, S. and MANLEY, K. (1982). The effect of sodium intake on blood pressure related to the age of the patients. *Clinical and Experimental Pharmacology and Physiology,* **9,** 287–289

NAGAKI, J. and TERAOKA, M. (1976). Age and sex differences of sodium and potassium concentration in red blood cells. *Clinica Chimica Acta,* **66,** 453–455

NARINS, R.G. (1970). Post-obstructive diuresis: a review. *Journal of the American Geriatric Society,* **18,** 925–936

NAYLOR, G.J. (1970). The relationship between age and sodium metabolism in human erythrocytes. *Gerontologia,* **16,** 217–222

PHILLIPS, P.A., ROLLS, B.J., LEDINGHAM, D.M., FORSLING, M.L., MORTON, J.J., CROWE, M.J. *et al.* (1984). Reduced thirst after water deprivation in healthy elderly men. *New England Journal of Medicine,* **311,** 753–759

PITTS, R.F. (1976). Mechanisms of reabsorption and excretion of ions and water. In *Physiology of the Kidney and Body Fluids,* pp. 90–127. Chicago; Yearbook

RAJAGOPALAN, B., THOMAS, G.W., BEILIN, L.J. and LEDINGHAM, J.G.G. (1980). Total body potassium falls with age. *Clinical Science,* **59,** 427s–429s

ROBERTSON, G.L. (1984). Abnormalities of thirst regulation. *Kidney International,* **25,** 460–469

ROBERTSON, G.L. and BERL, T. (1986). Pathophysiology of water metabolism. In *The Kidney,* 3rd edn, edited by B.M. Brenner and F.C. Rector, pp. 385–432. Philadelphia; Saunders

ROWE, J.W., MINAKER, K.L., SPARROW, D. and ROBERTSON, G.L. (1982). Age-related failure of volume-pressure-mediated vasopressin release. *Journal of Clinical Endocrinology and Metabolism,* **54,** 661–664

ROWE, J.W., SHOCK, N.W. and DE FRONZO, R.A. (1976). The influence of age on the renal response to water deprivation in man. *Nephron,* **17,** 270–278

SACKTOR, B. (1982). Na^+ gradient-dependent transport systems in renal proximal tubule brush border membrane vesicles. In *Membrane and Transport,* Vol. 2, edited by E. Martonosi. New York; Plenum

SAMBHI, M.P., CRANE, M.G. and GENEST, J. (1973). Essential hypertension: new concepts about mechanisms. *Annals of Internal Medicine,* **79,** 411–424

SCHRIER, R.W. and ANDERSON, R.J. (1980). Renal sodium excretion, edematous disorders, and diuretic use. In *Renal and Electrolyte Disorders,* edited by R.W. Schrier, pp. 65–80. Boston; Little, Brown

SEYMOUR, D.G., HENSCHKE, P.J., CAPE, R.D.T. and CAMPBELL, A.J. (1980). Acute confusional states and dementia in the elderly: the role of dehydration/volume depletion physical illness and age. *Age and Ageing,* **9,** 137–146

SOURANDER, L. (1983). The kidney. In *Geriatrics,* edited by D. Platt, pp. 202–221. Berlin; Springer

STRANDHOY, J.W., OTT, C.E., SCHNEIDER, E.G., WILLIS, L.K., BECK, N.P., DAVIS, B.B. *et al.* (1974). Effects of prostaglandins E1 and E2 on renal sodium reabsorption and Starling forces. *American Journal of Physiology,* **53,** 389–392

SULLIVAN, L.P. and GRANTHAM, J.J. (1982). Mechanisms of salt and water reabsorption. In *Physiology of the Kidney,* pp. 119–132. Philadelphia; Lea and Febiger

SUNDERAM, S.G. and MANKIKAR, G.D. (1983). Hyponatremia in the elderly. *Age and Ageing,* **12,** 77–80

TAKAZAKURA, E., SAWABU, N., HANDA, A., TAKADA, A., SHINDDA, A. and TAKEUCHI, J. (1972). Intrarenal vascular change with age and disease. *Kidney International,* **2,** 224–230

THIER, S.O. (1981). The kidney. In *The Biological Principles of Disease,* edited by Ll.H. Smith and S.O. Thier, pp. 814–837. Philadelphia; Saunders

VIDEBAEK, A. and ACKERMANN, P.G. (1953). The potassium content of plasma red cells in various age groups. *Journal of Gerontology,* **8,** 63–64

WEIDMANN, P., CHATEL, R., SCHIFFMAN, A., BACHMANN, E., BERETTA-PICCOLI, C., REUBI, F.C. *et al.* (1977). Interrelations between age and plasma renin, aldosterone and cortisol, urinary catecholamines, and the sodium/volume state in normal man. *Klinische Wochenschrift,* **55,** 725–733

WEITZMAN, R.E. (1979). Factors regulating the secretion and metabolism of arginine vasopressin (antidiuretic hormone). In *Hormonal Function and the Kidney,* edited by B.M. Brenner and J.H. Stein, pp. 146–168. New York; Churchill Livingstone

WÓRUM, I., FÜLÖP, T., CSONGOR, J., FÓRIS, G. and LEÖVEY, A. (1984). Interrelation between body composition and endocrine system in healthy elderly people. *Mechanisms of Aging and Development,* **28,** 315–324

YAMADA, T., ENDO, T., ITO, K., NAGATA, H. and IZUMIYAMA, T. (1979). Age-related changes in endocrine and renal function in patients with essential hypertension. *Journal of the American Geriatric Society,* **27,** 286–292

YAMORI, Y., KIHARA, M., FUJIKAWA, J., SOH, Y., NARA, Y., OHTAKA, M. *et al.* (1982). Dietary risk factors of stroke and hypertension in Japan. Part I: Methodological assessment of urinalysis for dietary salt and protein intakes. *Japanese Circulation Journal,* **46,** 933–938

YOUNG, V.R. (1983). Protein and aminoacid metabolism and nutrition during human aging. In *Geriatrics,* Vol. 2, edited by D. Platt, pp. 393–416. Heidelberg; Springer

Chapter 5

Hypertension in the elderly: pathophysiology and its implications for treatment

José L. Cangiano and Manuel Martínez-Maldonado

Introduction

This chapter should be read in conjunction with Chapter 12 which it complements. Some aspects of treatment are dealt with in both chapters, but not necessarily in an identical fashion.

Hypertension is a major and frequent problem that affects the adult population (United States Public Health Hospital Cooperative Study Group, 1972). In the USA the prevalence of hypertension in adults before age 60 is 20 per cent; between the ages of 60 and 65 it is 30 per cent and over the age 65 it may be as high as 40 per cent (Department of Health, 1966). It has long been recognized that hypertension results in an increased cardiovascular morbidity and mortality. Stroke, congestive heart failure, angina pectoris, myocardial infarction and renal failure are frequent complications of hypertension (Ostfeld *et al.*, 1974). The risk of cardiovascular disease increases with age in hypertensive subjects (Kannel and Brand, 1985) (see Chapter 12). Over 50 per cent of the mortality after age 65 is caused by cardiac and cerebrovascular diseases (Gubner, 1962; Colandrea *et al.*, 1970). In addition, chronic disability which impairs quality of life may result from these cardiovascular diseases.

A recent decline in cardiovascular morbidity and mortality has been achieved by judicious and rational antihypertensive treatment. Nevertheless, several misconceptions about the treatment of hypertension in the elderly patient have resulted in considerable neglect of the management of hypertension in these individuals. In this chapter we review the pathophysiological characteristics of the aging process as related to hypertension; based on this background, we will propose a safe and effective therapeutic regimen for the management of hypertension in the elderly.

Pathophysiological characteristics

Advancing age affects the anatomy and physiology of the cardiovascular system. Structural and functional changes are observed in the arteries and cerebrocardiorenal parenchymas. Arterial intimal thickening is a common finding (French *et al.*, 1963; Gerrity and Cliff, 1981). The endothelial surface may appear irregular with an increased number and accumulation of subendothelial cells which may be derived from the vessel wall and blood (Haudenschild, Prescott and Chobanian, 1981). In the arterial media, collagen content increases and elastin is replaced by lipid infiltration followed by thickening and atheromatous formation with calcification of the wall. There is loss of elasticity and compliance with elongation, tortuosity and obstruction of arteries. As wall to lumen ratio increases with the aging process, the resistance of vessels increases. Regardless of age, similar changes occur with hypertension. These observations have led to the hypothesis that these vascular changes may be accelerated by a hypertensive process. The aortic wall distends during systole and recoils during diastole, maintaining a small difference between systolic and diastolic pressures. The aging process diminishes aortic wall compliance, widening the pulse pressure and producing a rise in pressure for a given change in volume. Loss of the aortic capacity of maintaining a small pressure difference may result in isolated systolic hypertension, particularly in the aged. In addition, arterial wall rigidity blunts the responsiveness of the aortic and carotid sinus baroreceptors to changes in blood pressure. The insensitivity of baroreceptors impairs cardiac acceleration during hypotension and cardiac slowing in response to acute increases in blood pressure (Gribbin *et al.*, 1971; Minaker, Rowe and Sparrow, 1980).

Regional haemodynamics

Cardiac

The influence of advancing age on left ventricular function and cardiac haemodynamics has been extensively investigated. The function of the left ventricle as a pump is determined by (1) the filling or preload, measured as the end diastolic volume, (2) the afterload or impedance of ejection of blood, and (3) the onotropic or contractile state of the ventricular muscle. At rest, invasive studies have shown a decline of cardiac output and stroke volume (Strandell, 1976; Messerli *et al.*, 1983), with no variations in heart rate (Strandell, 1964). Brandfronbrener, Landowne and Schock (1955) observed a 50 per cent decrease in cardiac index as age increased from 20 to 80 years of age. However, the population studied was afflicted with disease or other medical conditions which may affect cardiac performance. Participants of the Baltimore Longitudinal Study of Aging (Gerstenblith *et al.*, 1977), who were free of organic heart disease, had mild hypertrophy as noted by increasing thickness of systolic and diastolic left ventricular wall by echocardiography. However, cardiac output measured by radionuclide scanning did not vary over an age range of 30–80 years. Similarly, Proper and Wall (1972) reported no age-associated changes in cardiac output and stroke volume. Preload does not change significantly with age in healthy individuals; afterload is modestly increased at rest, mostly due to a higher systolic pressure (Tarazi and Levy, 1982). As a consequence, a mild left ventricular hypertrophy occurs probably as an adaptive mechanism to maintain normal wall stress.

There is general agreement that the cardiovascular response to exercise is seriously affected by advancing age. As early as 1929, Master and Oppenheimer described a limitation in exercise tolerance in elderly individuals. At maximal workload, heart rate, stroke volume, cardiac output and oxygen uptake were lower. Left and right ventricular end diastolic and pulmonary artery pressures are elevated (Rodeheffer *et al.*, 1980; Vantosh *et al.*, 1980) and the peripheral vascular resistance is higher during exercise. The end result is an inability to increase the left ventricular ejection fraction (Port *et al.*, 1980).

The mechanisms which have been implicated to explain the abnormal response to exercise in the elderly are (1) a diminished action of the Frank–Starling mechanism,

(2) a decreased contractility of the myocardium, and (3) an increased afterload.

Echocardiographic studies have shown that the Frank–Starling mechanism is not altered in the older individual (Weisfeldt, 1980). In addition, isometric contraction of the myocardium remains intact, but its contractile response to catecholamines is markedly diminished (Lakatta *et al.*, 1975). The latter abnormality is attributed to a generalized deficiency of the sympathetic system in the elderly (*vide infra*). Anatomic and functional changes may occur in the conduction system, muscle fibres and valves and in the peripheral arteries. Metabolic changes can also occur in the cardiac musculature. Of great interest is the decline in myofibrillar ATPase (Alpert, Gale and Taylor, 1967). However, the physiologic significance of these changes is unknown.

Most investigators agree that the main factor which limits the increase in the left ventricular ejection fraction during exercise is the vascular impedance or afterload which is determined by the size and compliance of the aorta, and the pressure waves reflected by the peripheral resistance vessels. Several indexes have been used to determine aortic compliance in the elderly. Tarazi (1984) has found a close correlation between the ratio of pulse pressure to stroke volume (PP/SV, mmHg rise in pressure per ml of ejected blood) and the index derived from pulse pressure tracings. With exercise, systolic pressure increases in the presence of a poorly compliance aortic wall and a greater vasodilatory response and as a result afterload increases (Julius *et al.*, 1967). The increase in cardiac work which ensues is almost proportional to the elevation of systolic pressure. Myocardial oxygen supply is therefore impaired and symptoms of cardiac anoxia may develop. Ultimately, signs and symptoms of congestive heart failure may develop. *Table 5.1* summarizes the main changes that occur at rest and exercise in the elderly individual.

Table 5.1 Alterations and consequences of hypertension at rest and during exercise in the elderly

Anatomic and functional alterations		*Haemodynamic consequences*	
AT REST			
Myocardial contractility	↓	Left ventricular stroke volume	↓
Left ventricular stiffness	↑	Cardiac output	↓
Afterload	↑	Systolic blood pressure	↑
		Total peripheral resistance	↑
		Ejection time	↑
DURING EXERCISE			
Myocardial contractility	↓	Maximal cardiac output	↓↓
Heart rate	↓	Left ventricular end diastolic pressure	↓
Left ventricular stiffness	↑	Systolic blood pressure	↑↑
Afterload	↑	Systemic vascular resistance	↑
Adrenergic receptors	↓	Maximal O_2 consumption	↓

↑, increased; ↓, decreased; ↓↓, greatly decreased; ↑↑, greatly increased.

During the early phase of essential hypertension, cardiac output is high and total peripheral resistance is normal or low. The young and the older patients with sustained essential hypertension exhibit an increase in total peripheral resistance. Cardiac output remains normal or is reduced in the older hypertensive patients. A small group of elderly patients may present with a hyperkinetic circulation and increased cardiac output (Ibrahim *et al.*, 1975). Topol, Traill and Fortuin (1985) studied a subgroup of elderly patients with hypertension who demonstrated severe concentric cardiac hypertrophy by echocardiography, a small left ventricular cavity and supernormal indexes of systolic function. These patients are best treated with beta-blockers. It is clear then that subgroups of elderly hypertensive patients may be identified using echocardiographic techniques. The importance of classifying them may help to delineate a more rational therapeutic approach.

Renal

Senescence also affects the renal anatomy and function. Total and cortical renal mass, the number and surface area of glomeruli, and the proximal tubule length and volume decrease with age (Dunill and Halley, 1973). These changes are primarily a consequence of vascular abnormalities in the kidneys. The cortex is principally affected and there is relative sparing of the renal medulla (Darmady, Offer and Woodhouse, 1973). The great majority of arterioles and glomeruli in the juxtamedullary region show no alterations, but glomeruli in the cortical area may become sclerosed (Takazakura *et al.*, 1974).

As a consequence of these anatomical changes, effective renal plasma flow is reduced; the most dramatic decrease observed is after the age of 50 years (Miller, McDonald and Shock, 1951). As renal blood flow decreases, the renal vascular resistance progressively increases (Miller, McDonald and Shock, 1952) and glomerular filtration rate falls. This reduction in glomerular filtration has important clinical implications in the aged. For example, drugs that are excreted by the kidneys must be used with extreme caution in elderly patients.

Cerebral

The cerebral vessels also suffer major changes with aging. Narrowing of the lumen of cerebral arteries by the process of sclerosis is commonly observed. Hypertension accelerates the formation of atheromatous plaques that damage the integrity of vessels (Kannel *et al.*, 1976). Thrombotic occlusions and cerebral infarction are their sequelae. In addition, hypertension results in the formation of micro-aneurysms in small cerebral arteries. These are located principally in basal ganglia, internal capsule, pons and subcortical white matter (Ross Russell, 1963). These lesions have been reported in 15 per cent of elderly normotensive subjects and in 71 per cent of elderly hypertensives (Cole and Yates, 1967). Rupture of these aneurysms may result in extensive destruction of brain tissue.

The anatomic changes that occur with age in the brain may reduce cerebral blood flow and increase cerebral vascular resistance. However, cerebral blood flow is under an autoregulatory mechanism which maintains a constant flow despite wide fluctuations in blood pressure. In elderly individuals the range of autoregulation narrows and shifts to a higher level of mean pressure. A similar change occurs in hypertensive patients regardless of age. As a result, a sudden fall of blood pressure in aged hypertensives may bring profound changes in cerebral blood flow and the development of a stroke. It is recommended that blood pressure reduction in this group of patients may be carried out slowly and with extreme caution.

Neurohumoral alterations

Renin–angiotensin–aldosterone system

Advancing age displays major changes in the endocrine and neurogenic functions. Systems which control blood pressure such as the renin–angiotensin–aldosterone system and the sympathoadrenal medullary system are clearly affected. It is possible that other vasoactive systems such as the prostaglandin and the kallikrein–kinin systems may also be affected, but these have not been studied in depth with aging.

The renin–angiotensin–aldosterone system shows marked variations through the lifetime of an individual. Plasma renin and aldosterone levels are high during infancy and decrease rapidly as adult age is reached. A persistent decline in plasma renin activity, angiotensin II and aldosterone is observed with age in normotensive subjects (Crane and Harris, 1976). However, racial differences in renin secretion have been reported; at all ages, black people have substantially lower levels of renin activity.

Several theories have been advanced to explain the low renin state in elderly subjects. Among them are (1) thinning of renal cortex and renal atrophy, (2) hyposensitivity to circulating catecholamines, possibly related to a decrease in the number or a reduced sensitivity of beta-adrenergic receptors, and (3) a physiologic response to the gradual increase in systemic blood pressure.

In addition to a low renin state, the capacity to increase renin and aldosterone secretion following sodium restriction or furosemide administration is markedly impaired in the elderly subject (Weidmann *et al.*, 1975). This abnormal response to volume contraction makes them more vulnerable to hypovolaemia and hypotension.

Sympathetic system

The sympathetic system is also affected with age. Circulating catecholamines can arise from the adrenal medulla or from the peripheral nerves. A qualitative or quantitative difference in the degree of dysfunction of these two systems has not been described. Nevertheless, most studies have focused on the influence of age on the sympathetic nervous system rather than in the function of the adrenal medulla. Several investigators have shown that plasma norepinephrine concentrations increase with age; no change in plasma epinephrine was observed (Ziegler, Lake and Kopin, 1976; Rowe and Troen, 1980). The higher norepinephrine levels may indicate a heightened sympathetic tone. This possibility is strengthened by the demonstration that the number of adrenergic receptors and their binding affinity and sensitivity are decreased (Schoken and Roth, 1977; Vestal, Wood and Shand, 1979). Nevertheless, recent studies on the kinetics of norepinephrine have shown a reduced clearance from the circulation in older subjects (Esler *et al.*, 1981), indicating that higher norepinephrine levels cannot be ascribed solely to increased sympathetic tone.

As mentioned before, baroreceptor sensitivity is reduced with aging. This perturbation is largely due to rigidity of the arterial wall and/or intrinsic alteration of the receptors. The capacity to produce bradycardia and peripheral vasodilatation is impaired when acute increases in pressure occur. During hypotension, the reflex vasoconstrictor response and tachycardia is blunted to a greater extent in the elderly as compared to the young (Niarchos and Laragh, 1980). These abnormalities make the elderly subject much more sensitive to changes in posture and hypotensive drugs.

It has been proposed that there is a causal relationship between plasma norepinephrine levels, baroreceptor sensitivity and blood pressure elevation. In fact, a recent study supports the hypothesis that, in aged individuals, an impairment of baroreflex sensitivity may cause a sympathetic activation with an associated increase in plasma norepinephrine levels resulting in elevation of blood pressure (Shimada *et al.*, 1985).

Secondary hypertension

The most common forms of hypertension in the elderly are shown in *Table 5.2*. In an older patient, secondary hypertension is suspected in the presence of a sudden, severe elevation of blood pressure in a previously normotensive patient or in one with mild or moderate hypertension who has been responsive to treatment.

Table 5.2 Common types of hypertension in the elderly

(A) Systolic hypertension
- (1) Arteriosclerosis
- (2) Increased cardiac output
  - (i) Anaemia
  - (ii) Paget's disease with arteriovenous fistula
  - (iii) Thyrotoxicosis

(B) Systolic and diastolic hypertension
- (1) Essential hypertension
- (2) Secondary hypertension
  - (i) Renal:
    renal artery stenosis;
    acute renal failure;
    chronic renal failure;
    renal cell tumour;
    renal cysts;
    obstructive uropathy
  - (ii) Endocrine:
    adrenal cortex
      primary aldosteronism;
    adrenal medulla
      pheochromocytoma;
    hyperparathyroidism;
    oestrogens
  - (iii) Non-steroidal anti-inflammatory drugs

Renal artery stenosis is the most common correctable lesion producing hypertension. It is encountered in about 4 per cent of the hypertensive population and its prevalence is 1 per cent or less in the elderly; it is more frequent in males (Hunt and Strong, 1973). It can produce hypertension *de novo* or can aggravate a pre-existing mild or moderately severe essential hypertension of long duration. Renovascular hypertension usually refers to partial or total occlusion of one or both renal arteries or branches. Ischaemia distal to the lesion may result in activation of the renin–angiotensin system and sustained severe hypertension. In the elderly, the obstructive lesion is virtually always secondary to an atherosclerotic plaque that reduces the lumen by 50 per cent or more. Renovascular hypertension should be clinically suspected in patients with (1) diastolic blood pressure greater than 120 mmHg, (2) a recent onset of hypertension or a recent worsening of previously controlled hypertension, (3) the presence of a systolic–diastolic or systolic bruit heard best in the epigastrium, upper abdominal quadrants or flank region, (4) the presence of a grade III or IV hypertensive retinopathy, or (5) the presence of spontaneous hypokalaemic alkalosis, and hypertension resistant to optimal treatment. In the elderly, however, the major indication for an extensive work-up for renovascular hypertension is refractoriness of blood pressure to an optimal antihypertensive regimen.

Renal parenchymal disease is associated with secondary hypertension in the elderly. It is unlikely that acute glomerulonephritis, collagen disease with renal involvement and congenital disorders may be present in this age group. More frequently, chronic renal insufficiency in the elderly may arise as a manifestation of obstructive uropathy, interstitial nephritis or a previously undetected progressive renal disorder. Furthermore, hypertension, *per se,* can inflict damage to the kidneys and alter renal function, contributing further to a vicious cycle. Recently, much emphasis has been placed on the association of non-steroidal anti-inflammatory drugs to permanent kidney damage (Kimberly *et al.,* 1978). The use of these agents is widespread in elderly patients and makes them a large group at risk.

When hypertension and renal insufficiency co-exist, a careful evaluation of renal function is needed. Analysis of kidney size, presence or absence of masses, evidence of obstruction, etc., may be done by sonography (see Chapters 11 and 19). Invasive procedures may do more harm than good and should be carefully evaluated before they are utilized. In most cases, the degree of renal insufficiency can be evaluated by serial blood levels of urea, creatinine and electrolytes. This evaluation enables the clinician to take proper care, select appropriate medication, and adjust doses of drugs that are eliminated by the kidney.

Primary aldosteronism is a rare clinical entity that occurs in less than 1 per cent of the hypertensive population. It is produced by excessive aldosterone production in a solitary benign tumour in the zona glomerulosa of the adrenal gland (Conn's syndrome) or as a result of bilateral adrenal gland hyperplasia. It affects women more than men, usually between the ages of 30 and 50 years; occasionally it has been reported in elderly patients (Conn, 1977). The spectrum of clinical manifestations varies from hypertension alone, to a constellation of symptoms and signs. Blood pressure elevation is usually mild or moderately severe. Symptoms are related to hypokalaemia and hypomagnesaemia. In advanced cases, the symptoms consist of frontal headaches, periodic muscular paralysis, tetany, polyuria and polydipsia (nephrogenic diabetes insipidus) and paraesthesiae.

Spontaneous hypokalaemic alkalosis is the most distinct laboratory feature of this syndrome. This abnormality is usually accompanied by a diminished capacity to concentrate the urine. The urine shows an acid pH ('paradoxical aciduria') that contributes to the alkalosis. Specific gravity is low or fixed and it does not increase in response to the administration of vasopressin. In addition, increased aldosterone levels produce volume expansion which suppresses renin release.

The laboratory criteria for the diagnosis of primary aldosteronism include low plasma renin concentration and very high aldosterone levels which are not suppressible by salt loading. Moreover, no change in aldosterone concentration is observed during upright posture. When aldosteronism is the result of adrenal hyperplasia, upright posture aldosterone will rise dramatically (Ganguly *et al.,* 1973). Measurements of aldosterone levels in samples obtained from the adrenal veins may also help to differentiate a tumour from hyperplasia. The presence of lateralization of aldosterone levels strongly suggest an aldosterone-producing tumour. Computed tomography measurements may also be useful in the diagnosis and localization of aldosterone-producing adenomas (White *et al.,* 1980).

Pheochromocytoma is another rare cause of hypertension, being observed in less than 0.5 per cent of the hypertensive population. It may occur at any age, but the greatest frequency is in the fourth and fifth decades. Approximately 99 per cent of the tumours occur in the abdomen and 85–90 per cent are located in the adrenal gland (Manger and Gifford, 1977). Symptoms are protean. The classical manifestations are labile hypertension and paroxysmal episodes of severe, pulsatile headaches, palpitations, syncope, excessive perspiration, flushing, pallor and tremulousness. Vasovagal attacks, anxiety episodes and postmenopausal vasomotor crises may mimic symptoms of pheochromocytoma. Similarities of these conditions may make it difficult to distinguish among them. The diagnosis of pheochromocytoma should also be entertained in patients with perioperative paroxysmal hypertension.

A 24-hour urine collection, the determination of catecholamines and their metabolites, metanephrine and vanillylmandelic acid, can establish the diagnosis. Urinary metanephrine determination is the most sensitive and specific test. The incidence of false negative results can be as low as 4 per cent (Wolf *et al.*, 1973). Another useful and accurate determination for the diagnosis of pheochromocytoma is the plasma catecholamine levels. Newer radioenzymatic assays permit separation of norepinephrine, epinephrine and dopamine. Notwithstanding, there are many factors which may alter these levels, including diuretics, exercise, smoking and volume contraction. Similarly, plasma catecholamines are twice as high at age 70 than in young patients (Christensen, 1973). These conditions are unlikely to raise norepinephrine levels above 1000 pg/ml, whereas pheochromocytoma elevates them clearly over those levels. Pharmacologic suppression of catecholamines with clonidine might prove a very useful test to differentiate elevation of plasma catecholamines caused by anxiety or aging from elevation due to a tumour. Clonidine does not decrease norepinephrine levels arising from an adrenomedullary tumour (Bravo *et al.*, 1981). Finally, localization of the tumour can be made by ultrasonogram or body computerized tomography scan (Stewart *et al.*, 1978).

Primary hyperparathyroidism is a common disease in the elderly, since 25–50 per cent of all cases occur between the ages of 60 and 90. Hypertension may accompany hyperparathyroidism in 30–50 per cent of cases. The classic manifestations of recurrent kidney stones, bone lesions and gastrointestinal disturbances do not occur as frequently in the elderly population. Many of the presenting symptoms are also associated with advancing years and senility. For instance, mental and neuromuscular complications are described more frequently in this age group. Other presenting symptoms in these patients may be accelerated osteoporosis and atraumatic fractures.

The serum calcium levels are often lower in older than younger individuals (Mannix *et al.*, 1980). Modest elevations of serum calcium to levels between 11 and 12 mg/dl may result in substantial mental alterations; the cause-and-effect relationship can be inferred from the marked improvement in mental status as the hypercalcaemia is corrected. Mild elevation of serum calcium concentration can occur in patients on thiazide diuretics. This should be taken into consideration when ordering and interpreting serum calcium levels. Diuretics, on the other hand, may help to unmask the hypercalcaemia of primary hyperparathyroidism. Other laboratory hallmarks observed in primary hyperparathyroidism are an elevated serum immunoreactive parathyroid hormone, low serum phosphate and elevated or high normal serum chloride. Interpretation of elevated PTH levels should consider that hormone levels increase with age and in the presence of renal insufficiency.

Administration of oestrogens to postmenopausal women may result in elevation of blood pressure. In addition, they may induce glucose intolerance, thrombo-embolic episodes and possibly increase the risk of developing uterine cancer. A community study showed a higher systolic pressure in women aged 50–59 years using oestrogens as compared to their matched controls, non-users of oestrogens (Pfeffer, 1978). Another study showed a highly significant association between hypertension and oestrogens in women using contraceptives (Stern *et al.*, 1976). The rise in blood pressure evolves within 6 months of therapy, and upon discontinuation of the drug, blood pressure returns to normal levels.

Non-steroidal anti-inflammatory drugs (NSAIDs) are commonly used in the elderly for the treatment of musculoskeletal and arthritic conditions. Experimental and clinical data have shown that these agents do not produce hypertension *de novo,* but may aggravate a pre-existing hypertension in the presence or absence of antihypertensive medications (Lopez-Ovejero *et al.*, 1978). Careful monitoring of blood pressure should be carried out whenever elderly subjects use NSAIDs.

Pseudo-hypertension, although uncommon in the elderly, must be ruled out (Messerli, Ventura and Anrodeo, 1985).

Treatment of hypertension in the elderly (see also Chapter 12)

Value and goals of therapy

The reports of the Veterans Administration Cooperative Study Group (1967, 1970), the Hypertension Detection and Follow-up Program Cooperative Group (1979a, b, 1985) and the Australian National Blood Pressure Study Management Committee (1979, 1980) have marshalled considerable evidence on the clinical benefits of antihypertensive therapy in hypertensive patients of all ages. The advantage of treatment has been observed in the first few years of treatment; even partial blood pressure reduction has been reported to reduce the risk of cardiovascular events (Taguchi and Freis, 1974). In younger patients, it is imperative to obtain adequate control of blood pressure in the hope of preventing a premature cardiovascular catastrophe. In older patients, alteration of lifelong life-style habits may be difficult. Yet most clinicians place a high priority in modification of life-style, rather than in medical therapy, for the treatment of hypertension in this age group. For this reason, it is appropriate to make an assessment of life-style, economic and psychosocial conditions before a therapeutic intervention is made in the elderly hypertensive patient.

The goals of therapy should be directed to careful and individualized treatment programs. Safety, convenience and simplicity are important characteristics of the therapeutic regimen. One must be certain that the patient understands and accepts the rationale of treatment.

Frequently, compliance with therapy is a major drawback to adequacy of control. Treatment compliance can be improved by psychosocial support from family, friends or visiting nurse. Aggressive and overzealous treatment is more harmful than beneficial. In some instances, it is better to accept improvement rather than normalization of blood pressure levels. Persons with otherwise limited life expectancy, or those gravely debilitated, are not candidates for antihypertensive treatment.

Non-pharmacologic management

Non-pharmacologic intervention is a well-accepted measure of reducing blood pressure and may even be used as the sole treatment of blood pressure control in patients with mild hypertension. Measures include weight reduction, lowering of dietary sodium intake, decreased alcohol consumption, exercise and behaviour modification.

Several studies have reported an association between obesity and hypertension, independent of the effect of age (Kannel *et al.*, 1967; Berchtold *et al.*, 1981). A recent Australian survey in 1550 male and female subjects aged 25–64 years showed that 30 per cent of hypertension could be attributed to obesity (MacMahon *et al.*, 1984). A low calorie diet is advisable for an overweight hypertensive patient. Reduction of body weight by 5–10 per cent may result in reduction of 5–10 mmHg in diastolic blood pressure (Reisin *et al.*, 1978; Stamler *et al.*, 1980). This decrease in blood pressure can be accomplished despite variations in salt intake and may be enough to restore normal blood pressure levels or decrease the requirements of antihypertensive medications (Tuck *et al.*, 1981).

Extreme caution should be exercised in prescribing hypocaloric diets to elderly obese patients. As discussed before, elderly patients have abnormal cardiovascular reflexes which makes them particularly sensitive to orthostatic hypotension. The use of hypocaloric diets results in natriuresis and attenuation of the sympathetic system which may enhance the propensity to orthostatic hypotension (Landsberg and Young, 1978).

Dietary sodium restriction has been advocated as an important component of the treatment of hypertension. In recent years the concept of sodium restriction has been challenged by those who believe that salt consumption is not the culprit of the hypertensive process and by those who place more importance on dietary chloride consumption than on sodium consumption (Whitescarve *et al.*, 1985). Whatever the case, it is well accepted that salt excess may negate the beneficial effects of antihypertensive medications and the surreptitious use of salt may bring harmful consequences in a subgroup of hypertensive patients. Reduction of dietary sodium chloride intake to 2 or 3 g/day produces a significant reduction in blood pressure of hypertensive patients (Parijs *et al.*, 1973).

It may be difficult for the elderly patient to tolerate a severely restricted salt intake, but a modest decrease, usually between 90 and 120 mmol/day, may prove beneficial. Notwithstanding, extracellular volume may be substantially affected by restriction of salt, making the elderly patient more vulnerable to orthostatic changes in blood pressure.

The extent of the influence of alcohol in elevating blood pressure has been emphasized by several studies (Klatsky *et al.*, 1977; Criqui *et al.*, 1981; Cooke *et al.*, 1982). In the Australian survey already referred to, 11 per cent of hypertension in males and 1 per cent in females could be attributable to alcohol (MacMahon *et al.*, 1984). The association of alcohol consumption and hypertension has a relation of cause and effect, since blood pressure is reduced by alcohol withdrawal and re-emerges when alcohol ingestion is resumed (Saunders, Beevers and Paton, 1982). A consumption of 1–4 drinks per day may raise blood pressure significantly. However, recent studies indicate that a small amount of alcohol intake, less than 2oz (57g) per day, may decrease the risk of cardiovascular complications (Hennekens *et al.*, 1979; Willet *et al.*, 1980). There is no doubt that beneficial effects can be derived from a restrained intake of alcohol in younger people. However, elderly individuals are better off abstaining from alcohol, since it can produce other adverse effects which are potentially disastrous.

The role of exercise as a therapeutic modality to lower blood pressure has been argued for many years. Large-scale controlled trials have been difficult to design. Generally, two primary forms of exercise are known. Dynamic (isotonic or aerobic) exercise occurs when skeletal muscles contract, resulting in a change of the length of the muscle without changes in tension within the muscle. Paradigms of dynamic exercise are walking, jogging, swimming, bicycling and dancing. By contrast, static or isometric exercise occurs when skeletal muscle contracts resulting in a change of tension without changes in length of the muscle. Static exercise includes lifting or pushing heavy objects.

The recommended exercise for young and older individuals is the dynamic exercise since it has a salutary effect on cardiovascular haemodynamics by decreasing blood pressure and peripheral vascular resistance. Elderly patients, specially those with poor cardiac reserve, should be advised against performing static exercise.

The beneficial cardiovascular effects of dynamic exercise and conditioning in the elderly hypertensive patient has been extensively reviewed (Gavras and Gavras, 1983). Regular controlled exercise can improve cardiopulmonary function and psychological wellbeing. As a precautionary measure, older patients should avoid strenuous physical activities and exposure to extremely high or low temperatures or high humidity. Finally, behavioural modification by biofeedback, yoga or transcendental meditation has also been used to decrease blood pressure (Patel and North, 1975; Benson *et al.,* 1974). Although their benefits in lowering blood pressure are questionable, they can help to improve psychologic stress.

Pharmacologic management

The Joint National Committee on Detection, Evaluation and Treatment of High Blood Pressure (1984) has provided guidelines for the use of pharmacotherapy in hypertensive patients. These guidelines may be beneficial to a large number of patients including the elderly population (*Tables 5.3* and *5.4*). For example, elderly patients with blood pressure levels of 170/95 mmHg levels are considered hypertensive in other age groups, but are normally not treated. However, if these levels of blood pressure are observed in a patient with evidence of congestive heart failure, cerebral haemorrhage or unstable angina, a beneficial effect may be derived from lowering blood pressure.

Table 5.3 Relative contraindications for drug treatment in elderly hypertensives

Systolic blood pressure	≦160 mmHg
Diastolic blood pressure	≦ 80 mmHg
No end-organ disease	
Significant side effects to therapy	

Table 5.4 Absolute indications for drug treatment in elderly hypertensives

Systolic blood pressure	≧180 mmHg
Diastolic blood pressure	≧ 95 mmHg
Presence of unstable angina or aortic aneurysm	
Prior complications of hypertension:	
cerebral haemorrhage	
congestive heart failure	
renal insufficiency	

After non-pharmacologic management has failed to control blood pressure, the next decision is to select the appropriate drugs for treatment. It is imperative that pharmacologic treatment should be judiciously instituted. Certain factors may alter our approach to the selection of drugs. Among these are (1) the level of blood pressure, (2) whether blood pressure elevation is purely systolic or a combination of systolic and diastolic, (3) the presence of complications or other diseases, (4) interaction with other drugs, and (5) the psychosocial and economic aspects of the patient and his environment. A conscientious, broad analysis of the patient must be made before embarking on any specific therapy.

Advanced age leads to alterations in the pharmacokinetics and pharmacodynamics of drugs. These alterations may lead to an enhanced or diminished drug effect.

Absorption, distribution, metabolism and excretion are pharmacokinetic processes which determine the final plasma concentration of drugs. In elderly patients the rate of absorption is lowered, mostly as a result of a generalized decrease in gastric acidity, intestinal blood flow and gastrointestinal motility. The distribution of the drug is affected by body mass, volume of distribution, the binding to plasma proteins and red cells, regional blood flow and tissue permeability (Croaks, Malley and Stevenson, 1976). The body mass of elderly patients is smaller than that of younger subjects, whereas body fat increases from 18 to 36 per cent. Total body fluid, extracellular fluid volume and plasma volume show significant decrements. A fall in albumin and a rise in gamma globulin may occur. These changes disrupt the proportion of protein-bound and free drug. As a consequence, there is a higher than normal plasma concentration. In addition, binding to red cells may be diminished; this also affects the volume of distribution. Furthermore, regional flow may be decreased due to a low cardiac output, and tissue permeability may be affected by changes in connective tissue structures.

Table 5.5 Pharmacology of commonly used diuretics

Drug	*Action*	*Dose range** (mg/day)	*Adverse effects*
Thiazides and related:	Initial natriuresis with		
Hydrochlorothiazide	decreased ECF volume	25–50	Hypokalaemia
Chlorthalidone	and cardiac output.	25–50	Hypernatraemia
Metolazone	Late: restoration of	2.5–5.0	Hypovolaemia
Indapamide	volume and cardiac	0.5–2.0	Hyperglycaemia
	output; decrease in		Hypercalcaemia
	peripheral resistance		Hyperuricaemia
			Hypercholesterolaemia
			Azotaemia
Loop:			
Furosemide		20–80	Same as thiazides, etc.,
Bumetanide		0.5–2.0	except that hypocalcaemia
Ethacrynic acid		50–100	(instead of hypercalcaemia)
			may occur with all loop
			diuretics
Potassium-sparing:			
Spironolactone	Aldosterone antagonist at distal tubular site	25–75	Hyperkalaemia
Triamterene	Inhibit Na–K exchange	100–200	
Amiloride	at distal tubular site	2.5–5.0	

*Doses recommended in elderly patients.

The metabolism of drugs is also affected in the elderly (see Chapter 9). Most drugs are metabolized in the liver through enzymatic microsomal processes. As senescence occurs, there is a decrease in the oxidation and reducing capacity of hepatic microsomal enzymes. In addition, hepatic blood flow tends to decrease. The final result of these changes is a prolongation of the plasma half-life of the drug.

Except for a few drugs which are excreted in the bile, renal excretion is the usual route of elimination of most drugs. As mentioned earlier, renal blood flow and glomerular filtration rate are diminished with age. Accordingly, a prolongation of half-life is observed for those drugs eliminated by the kidney. Dosage and/or interval adjustments are therefore necessary to reduce the risk of toxic effects.

Antihypertensive drugs

In view of the difficulties of elderly patients with the handling of drugs, it is practical and safe to start antihypertensive treatment with low dosages, carefully titrating while on the watch for side effects. The stepped-care approach has been used widely and effectively since it is simple and, to a certain extent, rational. Its major drawback

Table 5.6 Pharmacology of sympatholytic diuretics

Drug	*Action and characteristics*	*Dose range** (mg/day)	*Adverse effects*
β-adrenergic blockers	Unknown action		
Cardioselective:			
Metoprololol	Lipid soluble	25–100	Heart block
Atenololol	Water soluble	25–100	Bronchospasm
Acebutolol	Water soluble, ISA, MSA		Impair hypoglycaemic response
			Aggravate claudications
Non-selective:			Decompensate latent
Timolol	Lipid soluble	5–30	Heart failure
Pindolol	Lipid soluble, ISA	2.5–100	CNS symptoms
Propranolol	Lipid soluble, MSA	10–240	
Nadolol	Water soluble	40–160	
Alpha-1-antagonist:			
Prazosin	Peripheral alpha-adrenergic blocker	1–10	Orthostatic hypotension diarrhoea
Alpha-2-antagonists:			
Methyldopa	↓CNS sympathetic outflow	250–1500	Sedation, fatigue, hepatitis, fever, Coombs' positive
Clonidine		0.05–0.6	Sedation, dry mouth, withdrawal syndrome
Guanabenz			
Central and peripheral depletors:			
Reserpine	↓Norepinephrine at central and peripheral nerve endings	0.1–0.25	Sedation, depression, confusion, nasal stuffiness
Peripheral depletors:			
Guanethidine	↓Norepinephrine stores at peripheral nerve endings	10–25	Orthostatic hypotension and diarrhoea
Guanadrel			
Pargyline			

ISA, intrinsic sympathomimetic activity; MSA, membrane stabilizing activity.
*Doses recommended for elderly patients.

is that it does not consider pathophysiological processes and accompanying diseases or complications affecting cardiovascular integrity. In older individuals who may be plagued with other diseases and complications, it is more practical to select the most appropriate and favourable antihypertensive drugs.

Table 5.7 Pharmacology of vasodilators

Drug	*Action*	*Dose range** (mg/day)	*Adverse effects*
Hydralazine	Arteriolar	10–200	Heachache, tachycardia, aggravates angina nausea, tremors
Minoxidil	Arteriolar	2.5–20	As above, severe sodium retention, hirsutism, pericardial effusion, reversible ECG changes
For emergencies:			
Diazoxide	Arteriolar	30–200 mg bolus	Reflex tachycardia, hyperglycaemia, sodium retention
Nitroprusside	Arteriolar and venous	Infusion, needs monitoring	Nausea, vomiting, muscle tremors
Nitroglycerin	Arteriolar and venous	Infusion, needs monitoring	Headaches, tachycardia

*Dose suggested for elderly patients

Antihypertensive drugs are classified into five broad categories: diuretics, sympathetic inhibitors, vasodilators, angiotensin-converting enzyme inhibitors, and calcium channel blockers. The actions, dosage and side effects of the most commonly employed antihypertensive drugs are given in *Tables 5.5–5.7*.

Diuretics

The efficacy, safety, tolerance and low cost of diuretics as well as the longer experience with their use have influenced clinicians to select them as the best initial drug in the treatment of hypertension. In fact, most controlled clinical trials which demonstrate a decline in cardiovascular morbidity and mortality used diuretics as initial treatment. Diuretics can be divided into three groups, according to their site of action: (1) thiazides and chemically related compounds chorthalidone, metozalone and indapamide; (2) loop diuretics, such as furosemide, bumetanide and ethacrynic acid; (3) potassium-sparing diuretics such as spironolactone, triamterene and amiloride.

The initial antihypertensive action of thiazides is exerted through a diuretic and natriuretic effect on the distal convoluted tubule. As a consequence there is a decrease in extracellular and plasma volume, cardiac output and peripheral resistance. During long-term treatment, however, extracellular volume and cardiac output are restored and the main antihypertensive action of thiazides is mediated by a decreased peripheral vascular resistance. The exact mechanism by which these changes occur remains unknown. At any rate, it is well accepted that the mechanism involved in long-term use of thiazide is not mediated through a decrease in extracellular and plasma volume.

The major adverse effects of thiazides are summarized in *Table 5.5*. Hypokalaemia, hyponatraemia, metabolic alkalosis, hypercalcaemia, hyperuricaemia, azotaemia, hypercholesterolaemia and hyperglycaemia can develop with the use of thiazides. Of these complications, hypokalaemia (<2.5 mEq/l) is of particular importance since it may give rise to severe arrhythmias, especially in those patients receiving digitalis preparations. It is therefore important to measure serum potassium and other biochemical factors at regular intervals in patients receiving thiazides.

In elderly patients thiazide therapy can begin with single daily dose in the morning (see doses in *Table 5.5*). If the response is not adequate after 2 weeks of therapy, the dose can be increased to the maximum for that particular preparation. Further increases in dose are not justifiable since they do not improve the effectiveness of the drug. Moreover, the tendency to dehydration, postural hypotension and hypokalaemia is increased.

Other thiazide-related diuretics such as chlorthalidone, metolazone and indapamide share a similar mode of action and, with a few exceptions, similar side effects. Nevertheless, in patients with renal insufficiency, thiazides lose their effectiveness. In this setting, metolazone and indapamide retain effectiveness even when renal failure is severe.

Loop diuretics are unsuitable for the long-term treatment of patients with essential hypertension. These agents have a short duration of action, requiring at least 3 doses daily to maintain their effectiveness. Furosemide, ethacrynic acid and bumetanide are the loop diuretics at present available. Their main use is in hypertensive patients with an already compromised renal function; they are particularly useful in the prevention of sodium retention in patients with renal insufficiency and receiving sympatholytic or vasodilator therapy.

Potassium-sparing diuretics include spironolactone, triamterene and amiloride. They are weak diuretics and antihypertensive agents when compared to the thiazides and loop diuretics. Their main use is in combination with other diuretics to prevent excessive potassium loss.

Spironolactone is a competitive antagonist of aldosterone that inhibits sodium and potassium exchange in the distal tubule. Triamterene and amiloride inhibit sodium potassium exchange independent of aldosterone. The main problem with potassium-sparing diuretics is the development of a potentially dangerous hyperkalaemia. The elderly and diabetics who have a tendency to hypoaldosteronism are particularly prone to develop hyperkalaemia. Potassium plasma levels must be carefully monitored when elderly patients receive these agents.

Sympathetic inhibitors

The sympathetic inhibitors may be classified, according to their site of action, into (1) drugs blocking adrenergic receptors, (2) drugs which stimulate the alpha-adrenergic receptors, (3) drugs acting by depletion of catecholamines at the prejunctional site, and (4) drugs blocking peripheral adrenergic neurons. The commonly used sympathetic inhibitors are listed in *Table 5.6*.

Beta receptor blockers have been used as first-line treatment, particularly in Europe. Some clinicians prefer to use them in the young hypertensive population. These agents are usually indicated in those hypertensive patients with arrhythmias, coronary heart disease, unstable angina, recent myocardial infarction, migraine and diuretic-induced complications. With proper patient selection, beta-blockers are safe and efficacious. Patients with frank congestive heart failure, cardiac conduction defects, bradyarrhythmias, asthma, chronic obstructive pulmonary disease, peripheral vascular disease and insulin-dependent diabetes mellitus should not be treated with beta-blockers (Kotler, Berman and Rubenstein, 1966).

The various beta-adrenoreceptor antagonists differ in receptor selectivity and sympathomimetic, membrane stabilizing and solubility properties. Their exact mechanism of action remains poorly understood. A decrease in cardiac output, suppression of plasma renin and central vasomotor action have been the major mechanisms considered. Not all beta-blockers have these effects and may share a similar antihypertensive effect despite the fact they may lack one or the other of these actions.

Beta-blockers are clearly indicated in the subgroup of elderly patients with hyperkinetic circulation and in the subgroup, recently described by Topol, Traill and Fortuin (1985), who exhibit concentric hypertrophy, congestive heart failure but higher ejection fraction than other hypertensives. However, in the large majority of elderly patients *beta-blockers should be used with extreme caution.* As already mentioned, the haemodynamic response to exercise may be rather poor in the elderly and beta-blockers may further impair the response. For patients with mild to moderate hypertension it is preferred to use water-soluble agents that do not penetrate the blood–brain barrier and do not produce central nervous system symptoms that may simulate those due to senility. Elderly patients may suffer from conditions such as chronic obstructive pulmonary disease, sick sinus syndrome, peripheral vascular insufficiency, congestive heart failure and conduction defects which may contraindicate the use of beta-blockers.

Prazosin, an alpha-l-adrenoreceptor blocking agent, reduces peripheral resistance without inducing reflex tachycardia. Its major drawback is that it may produce syncopal attacks after the first dose (Rosendorff, 1976). Patients should be advised to start with the smallest dose, remain in bed for several hours after taking the first dose and be extremely cautious when arising from bed. Prazosin has been used as monotherapy, but it causes sodium and fluid retention and usually requires the concomitant administration of a diuretic.

Alphamethyldopa, clonidinine and *guanabenz* reduce sympathetic outflow through the stimulation of alpha-2 receptors in the central nervous system. Common side effects from these drugs are sedation, drowsiness, lethargy, dry mouth and impotence. Allergic or idiosyncratic side effects are observed with the use of alphamethyldopa. Drug fever, positive Coombs' test, leucopenia and thrombocytopenia have also been reported. In general, elderly patients are more susceptible than younger patients to the side effects of alphamethyldopa. It is therefore recommended, in elderly patients, to initiate therapy with a lower dose (i.e. 125 mg twice a day) and gradually increase the dose not to exceed 1–2 g/day. Alphamethyldopa causes sodium and water retention, and concomitant diuretic treatment is necessary. Postural hypotension is one of the most dangerous complications in elderly patients; thus, care should be taken to warn and instruct them of that possibility.

Clonidine or [(2,6-dichlorobenzylidene)amino]guanidine (Guanabenz) may be good alternative therapy in those patients who have contraindications to the use of beta-blockers. As with alphamethyldopa, therapy should begin with low doses and diuretic therapy will be required to avoid fluid and sodium retention. Postural or exercise hypotension is not seen as frequent as with alphamethyldopa; when it occurs it is usually observed in extremely hypertensive patients. Abrupt withdrawal of clonidine and Guanabenz leads to increases in blood pressure greater than those pre-existing levels. This phenomenon is due to a sudden release of catecholamines and can be controlled by an alpha-adrenoreceptor antagonist such as prazosin or phentolamine. Clearly, these drugs can become dangerous in patients with poor compliance or those who have poor supervision.

Reserpine depletes catecholamines from peripheral adrenergic nerve endings and in central adrenergic neurons. Its main advantage is low cost and a long duration of action. However, it may caused drowsiness, confusion, forgetfulness and mental depression. Thus, its use is not recommended in elderly patients who, in fact, have a great propensity to many of these symptoms with senility.

Guanethidine, pargyline and *trimetaphan* act by inhibiting the release of norepinephrine from the adrenergic nerves endings. In doing this, they inhibit cardiovascular reflexes, decrease venous return and cardiac output. These changes are accompanied by severe orthostatic hypotension which may be a serious problem to the elderly individual. We restrict the use of these drugs to the elderly with uncontrolled hypertension who have failed to respond to other medication. Otherwise, we do not use them at all in the elderly.

Vasodilators

Vasodilators (*Table 5.7*) have a direct relaxation effect on the vascular smooth muscle without participation of the autonomic nervous system. Some, such as hydralazine, minoxidil and diazoxide, have purely arteriolar effects. Others, such as sodium nitroprusside and nitrates, exhibit both arteriolar and venous dilatory actions. Arteriolar vasodilators tend to induce reflex tachycardia, increase venous return and increase cardiac output. The result is a hyperkinetic circulatory effect. This condition can be brought under control by a beta-blocker. By contrast, arteriolar and venous dilators do not produce reflex tachycardia or alterations in myocardial contractility. All vasodilators, however, tend to cause water and sodium retention and should always be combined with diuretic therapy.

Hydralazine has been used in the treatment of hypertension in the elderly. Its main problems are tachycardia, headaches, anginal attacks and fluid retention. In rare instances, a lupus-like syndrome, which is indistinguishable from chronic arthritis, may be observed with prolonged administration of hydralazine in doses greater than 300 mg/day (Perry, 1973). Discontinuation of the drug is associated with regression of the syndrome.

Minoxidil is the most potent oral vasodilator available (Gottlieb, Thomas and Chidsey, 1972). It is reserved as one of the last alternatives in subjects in whom blood pressure control is difficult or in those with renal insufficiency. Concomitant therapy with beta-blocker to avoid severe reflex tachycardia and with a potent diuretic to counteract fluid retention is necessary (Gilmore, Weil and Chidsey, 1970). Its major side effects are hirsutism, pericardial effusion and bizarre electrocardiographic changes.

Diazoxide, nitroprusside and *nitroglycerin* are powerful vasodilators that must be given intravenously in hypertensive emergencies or crisis. Diazoxide is administered by bolus injections (150–300 mg). In the geriatric patient, the unpredictable results of such procedure may lead to dangerous episodes of hypotension. Mini-bolus injections (50 mg) are more reliable and safe. The drug must be administered rapidly to prevent binding to protein and a potent diuretic should be administered concomitantly to avoid fluid retention (Finnerty, 1974). It is not recommended in patients with cerebrovascular and coronary insufficiency, or those suspected of having aortic dissection.

Sodium nitroprusside is the treatment of choice of hypertensive emergencies in all age groups. It is administered as a continuous infusion and permits strict control of blood pressure. Nevertheless, constant monitoring and adjustment of the rate of infusion is needed. Its effect is transient and, if stopped suddenly, blood pressure may increase to pretreatment levels in less than 15 min. At the initiation of treatment, other antihypertensive agents should be started by the oral route. Nitroprusside reduces preload and afterload and is therefore the drug of choice in hypertensive patients with congestive heart failure. It also decreases left ventricular work in patients without hypertension and pump failure. Nitroprusside is metabolized in the liver to thiocyanate, which is then excreted by the kidneys. This creates a potential risk of cyanide toxicity in patients with liver disease and of thiocyanate toxicity in those patients with renal disease. When prolonged infusions are administered for 2–3 days, thiocyanate levels should be measured to maintain levels below 10 mg/dl.

Another alternative when severe hypertension is present is the use of nitroglycerin by intravenous route. Close monitoring of the rate of infusion and blood response is mandatory. Toxic effects of nitrates may be observed in patients with significant hepatic or renal disease.

Angiotensin-converting enzyme inhibitors

Angiotensin-converting enzyme (ACE) inhibitors are effective agents in the treatment of hypertensive disorders. Angiotensin-converting enzyme catalyses the formation of angiotensin II from angiotensin I and, in addition, it transforms bradykinin into inactive products. Inhibition of the enzyme results in a vasodilatory effect without sodium retention; in fact, there is a tendency to a small natriuretic action (Gavras, Brunner and Gavras, 1981). The antihypertensive action of ACE inhibitors is not entirely understood, but it is attributed mostly to the suppression of the vasoconstrictor effect of angiotensin II. Blockade of the action of catecholamines and the degradation of bradykinin may be contributing factors.

Captopril was the first ACE inhibitor available. Some physicians now use it in the treatment of mild hypertension. It is a very useful drug in the therapy of congestive heart failure. The haemodynamic actions of captopril include a reduction in the peripheral vascular resistance (afterload), a decline in right atrial pressure and pulmonary artery resistance (preload), and increase in cardiac output in patients with heart failure (Levine, Olivari and Cohn, 1984). As a result, an increase in renal blood flow and glomerular filtration rate occurs, provided renal artery stenosis is absent (Hollenberg, 1984). Postural changes, tolerance and sodium retention have not been reported with captopril. It has been used as monotherapy in hypertensive patients. The recommended starting dose is 6.25–12.5 mg/day, and if necessary, the dose can be gradually increased to a maximum of 150 mg/day. Hypersensitivity reactions, proteinuria and leucopenia with agranulocytosis are rare complications that have been reported with doses over 150 mg/day (Jenkins *et al.*, 1985). Leucopenia is most likely to occur in immunocompromised patients and proteinuria in severely hypertensive patients. These effects are usually transient and reversible with discontinuation of therapy. *Enalapril* is now under extensive evaluation, and in general has similar effects to captopril.

Calcium channel blockers

Calcium channel blockers are a novel group of drugs which prevent vascular smooth muscle cell contraction by reducing calcium influx to cells through the slow inward channels. This action results in a generalized vasodilatation and lowers cardiac preload and afterload (Lehmann *et al.*, 1983). Verapamil, nifedipine and diltiazem are at present available for use in angina pectoris, Prinzmetal angina and supraventricular tachycardia (Antman *et al.*, 1980; Stone *et al.*, 1980). Their use in hypertension has not been approved by the Food and Drug Administration, but the experience accumulated thus far indicates that verapamil and nifedipine are effective for the treatment of the hypertensive patient. Elderly subjects have an antihypertensive response greater than individuals younger than 40 years of age (Buhler, 1984).

Verapamil has anti-arrhythmic action and is useful in the treatment of refractory supraventricular arrhythmias. Hypotensive effects are observed at doses of 120–240 mg/day. In contrast to nifedipine, it does not produce reflex tachycardia or salt and fluid retention (Bartorelli *et al.*, 1980). The main side effect of verapamil is constipation (Doyle, 1983). Verapamil has a negative inotropic action which could predispose to heart failure. Therefore, it should be carefully used in geriatric patients.

Nifedipine is another therapeutic option for the hypertensive patient. Its use includes hypertensive emergencies or crises, where it is administered by the sublingual route in a dose of 10–20 mg (Raemsch and Sommer, 1983). Its efficacy has also been documented in the long-term management of hypertension in doses of 60–120 mg. Its effectiveness is increased when combined with diuretics and beta-blockers. The main side effects of nifedipine are leg oedema, facial flushing and reflex tachycardia. Nifedipine has been used as monotherapy in geriatric patients. Long-acting preparations are available and useful.

Rationale of therapy

Non-pharmacologic measures have limited success in the geriatric individual, since major changes in life-style are difficult to accomplish in this group. Sodium restriction, weight reduction, regular exercise and relaxation techniques may be beneficial. If an adequate trial of these non-pharmacological measures does not control blood pressure, drug therapy should be considered.

The great majority of geriatric patients with a sustained diastolic blood pressure >95 mmHg or isolated systolic blood pressure >180 mmHg should be treated with antihypertensive drugs. The stepped-care approach completely ignores important factors in the life-style and clinical condition of the patient. Thus, treatment must be individualized and should be tailored to the needs of the patient, without producing notable effects on the patient's life-style and associated medical conditions. *Table 5.8* shows some medical problems in the elderly which may require alterations of the therapeutic approach.

Absence of complications or other important disease processes permits initiation of treatment with small doses of a diuretic, preferably a long-acting thiazide. One-half of the usual dose with modest restriction of sodium intake to 4 g/day reduces the degree of volume contraction and its complications. Loop diuretics should be reserved for those hypertensive patients with heart failure and renal insufficiency. Therapeutic failure with diuretics alone should lead to the use of other agents such as

Table 5.8 Use of drugs in elderly patients with hypertension and associated medical conditions

Condition	*Advantageous drug*	*Drug to avoid or use with caution*
Congestive heart failure	Diuretic, vasodilator, ACEI, CCB	Beta-blocker
Coronary artery disease	Beta-blocker, CCB	Clonidine on withdrawal
Diabetes mellitus	Vasodilators (prazosin)	Diuretics
Peripheral vascular disease	Vasodilator	Beta-blocker
Renal insufficiency	Loop diuretics, vasodilators	Thiazides, beta-blockers, ACEI
Pulmonary disease	Prazosin, CCB, beta-blockers with ISA	Beta-blockers
Orthostatic hypertension	Non-selective beta-blockers, ACEI	Alphamethyldopa, guanethidine
Depression	Diuretics	Reserpine
Aortic dissection	Trimethaphan (emergent control)	Diazoxide, hydralazine

ACEI, angiotensin-converting enzyme inhibitor; CCB, calcium channel blocker

beta-blockers, alphamethyldopa or clonidine. As mentioned earlier, beta-blockers should be avoided in patients with left ventricular dysfunction, bronchospasm or diabetes (Grinblatt and Koch-Weser, 1974; Beumer, 1974). If patients fail to achieve control of blood pressure with a diuretic and sympatholytic agents, a vasodilator is then indicated. In this regard, hydralazine or prazosin can be used. Minoxidil should be reserved for those patients with refractory hypertension. Another alternative in elderly patients is the use of ACE inhibitors as third or fourth step drugs. At present, their safety in this age group has not been established. However, recent data suggests that side effects are minimal if given at low doses (Jenkins *et al.*, 1985), and in the future they may be particularly suitable as the first step of drug therapy.

Elderly patients with congestive heart failure and hypertension benefit from the use of vasodilators that reduce afterload. Hydralazine, prazosin, captopril and calcium channel blockers can accomplish this; they can potentiate the use of diuretics and digitalis.

Beta-blockers reduce myocardial oxygen consumption through their negative chronotropic and inotropic effect. Therefore, they are extremely useful in patients with coronary insufficiency. In patients with bradycardia at rest, the use of beta-blockers with intrinsic sympathomimetic action may be desirable (Wahl, Turlpaty and Singh, 1985). Calcium channel blockers may be used alone or in combination with beta-blockers to treat patients with hypertension and symptomatic coronary heart disease. Verapamil should be used cautiously in the uncontrolled hypertensive, since it may precipitate heart failure (Singh and Roche, 1977). Nifedipine is very useful in the hypertensive patient with uncontrolled angina.

Patients with hypertension and peripheral vascular disease may greatly benefit from vasodilators, calcium channel blockers and ACE inhibitors. Many beta-blockers aggravate symptoms of peripheral vascular disease because of their tendency to raise peripheral vascular resistance. On the other hand, beta-blockers with intrinsic sympathomimetic activity such as pindolol or acebutolol do not increase peripheral resistance and are indicated for the treatment of hypertensive patients with peripheral vascular disease (Wallam *et al.*, 1979).

Renal insufficiency may be aggravated by the aging process and/or blood pressure elevation. Hypertension contributes to progressive renal deterioration;

conversely, hypertension may arise from advancing renal failure. Renal function must be protected by adequately lowering blood pressure and by the use of antihypertensive drugs which do not alter renal functional integrity.

Loop diuretics, metolazone and indapamide are more effective diuretics than thiazides in the presence of moderate to severe renal insufficiency. In this setting, as mentioned elsewhere, potassium-sparing diuretics are contraindicated because of the danger of hyperkalaemia. Antihypertensive agents which do not impair renal blood flow and glomerular filtration rate should be used in patients with moderate to severe renal insufficiency. In this group, sympatholytic agents such as alpha-methyldopa, clonidine and guanabenz, vasodilators such as hydralazine, prazosin and minoxidil, the calcium channel blockers, and ACE inhibitors can be used. Agents that are excreted by the kidney should have appropriate dosage adjustments.

Hypertension may be encountered in 80 per cent of patients with advanced renal disease. In 90 per cent of these patients hypertension arises because of fluid and sodium retention (sodium dependent), whereas in 10 per cent of patients increased levels of plasma renin are associated with elevation of blood pressure (renin dependent) (Vertes *et al.*, 1969). When hypertension is sodium dependent, removal of fluid by dialysis may control blood pressure (Cangiano *et al.*, 1976). This is not the case in patients with renin-dependent hypertension. Instead, potent antihypertensive agents such as ACE inhibitors or minoxidil must be used for blood pressure control.

Hypertensive patients with chronic obstructive pulmonary disease are at risk of developing complications with the use of sympathomimetic amines, since these agents have a tendency to raise blood pressure. Beta-blockers are also contra-indicated. If the clinical situation warrants the use of a beta-blocker, cardioselective agents or beta antagonists with intrinsic sympathomimetic activity are the best choice. It should be remembered that cardioselectivity is only relative and increasing the dose of the beta-blocker may provoke a pulmonary reaction. Reserpine and alphamethyldopa may precipitate or aggravate an asthmatic condition. Most patients with chronic obstructive pulmonary disease will benefit from the use of the alpha-adrenergic antagonist prazosin, or from calcium channel blockers because they produce bronchodilatation (Altounyan, 1967; Rowlands, Stollard and Littler, 1984; Tinkelman, 1985).

Orthostatic hypotension occurs in less than 5 per cent of healthy elderly patients. However, hypovolaemia, aggressive diuretic therapy, sympatholytic and vaso-dilator agents may produce substantial orthostatic hypotension and disabling symptoms. In addition, orthostatic hypotension associated to recumbent hypertension is a difficult problem to treat. Sympatholytic agents except clonidine and reserpine aggravate the condition and are not indicated for control of recumbent hypertension. Beta-blockers may be beneficial because they raise peripheral resistance, an effect which may dissipate with time. The patients should be instructed to wear tightly fitting support stockings to avoid blood pooling in lower extremities and elevate the head of bed with 6 in. (150 mm) of blocks for better control of blood pressure. In some cases this phenomenon may be observed after eating a meal (Lipit *et al.*, 1983). Thus, patients must be cautioned of orthostatic symptoms after meals.

Depression is commonly observed in geriatric patients. The most important consideration in a hypertensive patient is that some antihypertensive drugs may induce depression. Drugs like reserpine, alphamethyldopa, clonidine, beta-blockers and thiazides are known to produce depressive reactions. The recognition of drug-induced depression is important since it can be reversed by discontinuation of treatment.

Treatment of renovascular hypertension

The development of *de novo* hypertension or the aggravation of a pre-existing hypertension in patients over the age of 60 should alert the physician to the presence of renovascular hypertension. The most common cause of renovascular disease in this age group is arteriosclerosis. The lesions are usually bilateral, progressive and may ultimately lead to renal impairment. Even if blood pressure is controlled the lesion may lead to progressive obstruction with significant loss of renal function. Refractoriness to treatment is common. Moreover, side effects are rather frequent and may induce poor compliance. On the other hand, surgery may present the following disadvantages: significant morbidity and mortality, increased relapse rates, failure of cure or no improvement, increased cost and prolonged hospitalization.

The development of percutaneous transluminal angioplasty (PTA) by Gruntzig *et al.* (1978) has been a major advance in the treatment of renovascular hypertension. A soft, flexible double lumen catheter with an inflatable balloon may stretch vessel walls and enlarge the vessel lumen. This procedure has been successfully used in elderly patients and in patients with bilateral stenotic lesions and post-transplant renovascular hypertension. In contrast to surgery, it is a simple procedure with a low cost and short period of hospitalization. The potential risks of PTA include rupture of the vascular wall, peripheral embolization, segmental renal infarcts and acute renal failure after injection of radiocontrast material. Finally, it may be successful in the recurrent cases of renal artery stenosis, and at present it is the treatment of choice in elderly, uncontrolled hypertensives with a high risk for surgery.

References

ALPERT, N.R., GALE, H.H. and TAYLOR, N. (1967). The effect of age on contractile protein ATPase activity and the velocity of shortening. In *Factors Influencing Myocardial Contractility,* edited by K. Kwalen, R.D. Tang and J. Robert, pp. 1154–1162. New York; Academic Press

ALTOUNYAN, R.E.C. (1967). Inhibition of experimental asthma by a new compound—disodium cromoglycate. *Acta Allergy,* **22,** 487

ANTMAN, E.M., STONE, P.H., MULLER, J.E. and BRAUNWALD, E. (1980). Calcium channel blocking agents in the treatment of cardiovascular disorders. Part I: Basic and clinical electrophysiologic effects. *Annals of Internal Medicine,* **93,** 875–885

AUSTRALIAN NATIONAL BLOOD PRESSURE STUDY MANAGEMENT COMMITTEE (1979). Initial results of the Australian therapeutic trial in mild hypertension. *Clinical Science,* **57,** 449s–454s

AUSTRALIAN NATIONAL BLOOD PRESSURE STUDY MANAGEMENT COMMITTEE (1980). The Australian therapeutic trial in mild hypertension. *Lancet,* **1,** 1261

BARTORELLI, C., MAGRINI, F., MORUZZI, P., OLIVARI, M.T., POLESE, A., FIORENTINI, C. and GUAZZI, M. (1980). Hemodynamic effects of a calcium ion antagonist (nifedipine) in hypertension. Therapeutic implications. *Clinical Science,* **55,** Suppl., 291S–292S

BENSON, H., ROSNER, R.A., MARZETTA, B.R. and KLEMCHUK, H.P. (1974). Decreased blood pressure in borderline hypertensive subjects who practise meditation. *Journal of Chronic Diseases,* **27,** 163–169

BERCHTOLD, P., JORGENS, V., FINKE, C. and BERGER, M. (1981). Epidemiology of obesity and hypertension. *International Journal of Obesity,* **5,** Suppl. 1, 1–7

BEUMER, H.M. (1974). Adverse effects of beta-adrenergic receptor blocking drugs on respiratory function. *Drugs,* **7,** 130

BRANDFRONBRENER, M., LANDOWNE, M. and SHOCK, M.W. (1955). Changes in cardiac output with age. *Circulation*, **12**, 557–576

BRAVO, E.L., TARAZI, R.C., FOUAD, F.M., VIDT, D.G. and GIFFORD, R.W., Jr. (1981). Clonidine suppression test: a useful aid in the diagnosis of pheochromocytoma. *New England Journal of Medicine*, **305**, 12

BUHLER, F. (1984). Calcium metabolism and calcium channel blockers for understanding and treating hypertension. *American Journal of Medicine*, **77**(6B), 15

CANGIANO, J.L., RAMIREZ MUXO, O., RAMIREZ-GONZALEZ, R., TREVINO, A. and CAMPOS, J.A. (1976). Normal renin uremic hypertension. A study of cardiac hemodynamics, plasma volume, extracellular fluid volume and renin angiotensin system. *Archives of Internal Medicine*, **136**, 17–23

CHRISTENSEN, N.J. (1973). Plasma noradrenaline and adrenaline in patients with thyrotoxicosis and myxoedema. *Clinical Science and Molecular Medicine*, **45**, 163

COLANDREA, M.A., FRIEDMAN, G.D., NICHAMAN, M.Z. and LYND, C.N. (1970). Systolic hypertension in the elderly. *Circulation*, **41**, 239–245

COLE, R.M. and YATES, P.O. (1967). The occurrence and significance of intracerebral microaneurysms. *Journal of Pathology and Bacteriology*, **93**, 393–411

CONN, J.W. (1977). Primary aldosteronism. In *Hypertension*, edited by J. Genest, E. Koiw and O. Kuchel, pp. 768–780. New York; McGraw-Hill

COOKE, K.M., FROST, G.W., THORWELL, I.R. and STOKES, G.S. (1982). Alcohol consumption and blood pressure. Survey of the relationship at a health screening clinic. *Medical Journal of Australia*, **1**, 65–69

CRANE, M.G. and HARRIS, J.J. (1976). Effect of aging on renin activity and aldosterone excretion. *Journal of Laboratory and Clinical Medicine*, **87**, 947–959

CRIQUI, M.H., WALLACE, R.B., MISHKEL, M., BARNETT-CORNER, E. and HEISS, G. (1981). Alcohol consumption and blood pressure. The Lipid Research Clinics Prevalence Study. *Hypertension*, **3**, 557–565

CROAKS, J., MALLEY, K. and STEVENSON, H. (1976). Pharmacokinetics in the elderly. *Clinical Journal of Pharmacokinetics*, **1**, 280–296

DARMADY, E.M., OFFER, J. and WOODHOUSE, M.A. (1973). The parameters of the aging kidney. *Journal of Pathology*, **109**, 195–207

DEPARTMENT OF HEALTH (1966). Hypertensive heart diseases in adults, United States 1960–62. *National Center for Health Statistics*, Series II, no. 13

DOYLE, A.E. (1983). Comparison of beta-adrenoreceptor blockers and calcium antagonists in hypertension. *Hypertension*, **5**(II), 103–108

DUNILL, M.S. and HALLEY, W. (1973). Some observations on the quantitative anatomy of the kidney. *Postgraduate Medical Journal*, **110**, 113–121

ESLER, M., SKEWS, H., LEONARD, P., JACKMAN, G., BOBIK, A. and KORNER, P. (1981). Age-dependence of noradrenaline kinetics in normal subjects. *Clinical Science*, **60**, 217–219

FINNERTY, F.A. (1974). Diazoxide. *American Heart Journal*, **88**, 265–268

FRENCH, J.E., JENNINGS, M.P., POOLE, J.C.F. *et al.* (1963). Intimal changes in the arteries of the aging swine. *Proceeding of Royal Society of Biology*, **158**, 24

GANGULY, A., DOWDY, A.J., LAETSCHER, J.A. and MELADA, G.A. (1973). Anomalous postural response of plasma aldosterone concentration in patients with aldosterone producing adrenal adenoma. *Journal of Clinical Endocrinology and Metabolism*, **36**, 401–402

GAVRAS, H., BRUNNER, H.R. and GAVRAS, I. (1981). Captopril in the treatment of hypertension. *Annals of Internal Medicine*, **95**, 505–506

GAVRAS, H. and GAVRAS, I. (1983). *Hypertension in the Elderly*, pp. 99–117. Boston; Wright

GERRITY, R.G. and CLIFF, W.J. (1981). The aortic tunica intima in young and aging. *Hypertension*, **3**, 148–153

GERSTENBLITH, G., FREDERIKSEN, J., YIN, F.C., FORTIUN, N.J., LAKATTA, E.G. and WEISFELDT, M.L. (1977). Echocardiographic assessment of a normal adult aging population. *Circulation*, **56**, 273–277

GILMORE, E., WEIL, J. and CHIDSEY, C.A. (1970). Treatment of essential hypertension with a new vasodilator in combination with beta-adrenergic blockade. *New England Journal of Medicine*, **282**, 521–527

GOTTLIEB, T.B., THOMAS, R.C. and CHIDSEY, C.A. (1972). Pharmacokinetic studies of minoxidil. *Clinical Pharmacology and Therapeutics*, **13**, 346

GRIBBIN, B., PICKERING, T., SLEIGHT, P. and PETO, R. (1971). Effect of age and high blood pressure on baroreflex sensitivity in man. *Circulation Research*, **29**, 424–431

GRINBLATT, D.J. and KOCH-WESER, J. (1974). Adverse reaction to receptor blocking drugs. A report from the Boston Collaborative Drug Surveillance Programme. *Drugs*, **7**, 118

GRUNTZIG, A., KUHLMANN, U., VETTER, W., LUTOLF, U., MEIER, B. and SIEGENTHALER, W. (1978). Treatment of renovascular hypertension with percutaneous transluminal dilatation of a renal artery stenosis. *Lancet,* **1,** 801–802

GUBNER, R.S. (1962). Systolic hypertension: a pathogenetic entity. *American Journal of Cardiology,* **9,** 773–776

HAUDENSCHILD, C.C., PRESCOTT, M.F. and CHOBANIAN, A.V. (1981). Aortic endothelial and subendothelial cells in experimental hypertension and aging. *Hypertension,* **3,** 148–153

HENNEKENS, C.A., WILLET, W., ROSNER, B., COLE, D.S. and MAYRENT, S.L. (1979). Effects of beer, wine and liquor in coronary deaths. *Journal of American Medical Association,* **242,** 1973–1974

HOLLENBERG, N.K. (1984). Renal hemodynamics in essential and renovascular hypertension. Influence of Captopril. *American Journal of Medicine,* **76**(5B), 22–27

HUNT, J.C. and STRONG, C.G. (1973). Renovascular hypertension. Mechanisms, natural history and treatment. *American Journal of Cardiology,* **32,** 562–566

HYPERTENSION DETECTION AND FOLLOW-UP PROGRAM COOPERATIVE GROUP (1979a). Five year findings of the Hypertension Detection and Follow-up Program I. Reduction in mortality of persons with high blood pressure, including mild hypertension. *Journal of American Medical Association,* **242,** 2562–2571

HYPERTENSION DETECTION AND FOLLOW-UP PROGRAM COOPERATIVE GROUP (1979b). Five year findings of the Hypertension Detection and Follow-up Program II. Mortality by race, sex and age. *Journal of American Medical Association,* **242,** 2572–2577

HYPERTENSION DETECTION AND FOLLOW-UP PROGRAM COOPERATIVE GROUP (1985). Five years findings of the Hypertension Detection and Follow-up Programs. Prevention and reversal of left ventricular hypertrophy with antihypertensive drug therapy. *Hypertension,* **7,** 105–112

IBRAHIM, M.M., TARAZI, R.C., DUSTAN, H.P., BRAVO, E.L. and GIFFORD, R.W. Jr. (1975). Hyperkinetic heart in severe hypertension, a separate clinical hemodynamic entity. *American Journal of Cardiology,* **35,** 667–674

JENKINS, A.C., DRESLINSKI, G.R., TADROS, S.S., GROEL, J.J., FOND, R. and HERCZEG, S.A. (1985). Captopril in hypertension. Seven years later. *Journal of Cardiovascular Pharmacology,* **7**(S1), S96–S100

JOINT NATIONAL COMMITTEE ON DETECTION, EVALUATION AND TREATMENT OF HIGH BLOOD PRESSURE (1984). 1984 report. *Archives of Internal Medicine,* **144,** 1045–1057

JULIUS, S., AMERY, A., WHITLOCK, L.S. and CONWAY, J. (1967). Influence of age on the hemodynamic response to exercise. *Circulation,* **36,** 222–230

KANNEL, W.B. and BRAND, F.N. (1985). Cardiovascular risks factors in the elderly. In *Principles of Geriatric Medicine,* edited by R. Andres, F.L. Bierman and W.R. Hazzard, p. 116. New York; McGraw-Hill

KANNEL, W.B., BRAND, N., SKINNER, J.T., DOWBER, T.R. and McNAMARA, P.M. (1967). The relation of adiposity to blood pressure and development of hypertension. *Annals of Internal Medicine,* **67,** 48–59

KANNEL, W.B., DAWBER, T.R., SORLIE, P. and WOLF, P.A. (1976). Components of blood pressure and risk of atherothrombotic brain infarction. The Framingham Study. *Stroke,* **7,** 327–331

KIMBERLY, R.P., BOWDEN, R.E., KEISER, H.R. and PLATZ, P.H. (1978). Reduction of renal function by newer nonsteroidal antiinflammatory drugs. *American Journal of Medicine,* **64,** 804–807

KLATSKY, A., FRIEDMAN, G.D., SIEGELAUF, M.S. and GERARD, M.J. (1977). Alcohol consumption and blood pressure. *New England Journal of Medicine,* **296,** 1194–1200

KOTLER, M.N., BERMAN, L. and RUBENSTEIN, A.H. (1966). Hypoglycemia precipitated by propranolol. *Lancet,* **2,** 1389–1390

LAKATTA, E.G., GERSTENBLITH, G., ANGELL, C.S., SCHOCK, N.W. and WEISFELDT, M.L. (1975). Prolonged contraction duration in aged myocardium. *Journal of Clinical Investigation,* **55,** 61–68

LANDSBERG, L. and YOUNG, J.B. (1978). Fasting, feeding and regulation of the sympathetic nervous system. *New England Journal of Medicine,* **298,** 1295–1301

LEHMANN, H.U., HOCHREIN, H., WITT, E. and MIES, H.W. (1983). Hemodynamic effects of calcium antagonists. *Hypertension,* **5**(II), 67–73

LEVINE, T.B., OLIVARI, M.T. and COHN, J.N. (1984). Hemodynamic and regional blood flow response to captopril in congestive heart failure. *American Journal of Medicine,* **76**(5B), 38–42

LIPITZ, L.A., NYQUIST, P. Jr, WEI, J.W. and ROWE, J.W. (1983). Postprandial reduction in blood pressure in the elderly. *New England Journal of Medicine,* **309,** 81–83

LOPEZ-OVEJERO, J.A., WEBER, M.A., DRAYER, J.M., SEALEY, J.E., and LARAGH, J.H. (1978). Effect of indomethacin alone and during diuretic or beta adrenoreceptor blockade therapy on blood pressure and the renin system in essential hypertension. *Clinical Science of Biology and Medicine,* **55,** 203s–205s

MACMAHON, S.W., BLAKET, R.B., MACDONALD, G.J. and HALL, W. (1984). Obesity, alcohol consumption and blood pressure in Australian men and women. The National Heart Foundation of Australia Risk Factor Prevalence Study. *Journal of Hypertension,* **2,** 85–91

MANGER, W.M. and GIFFORD, R.W. (1977). In *Pheochromocytoma,* edited by W.M. Manger and R.W. Gifford, p. 45. Berlin; Springer

MANNIX, H., PYORTEK, L.J., CROMBIE, H.D. and CANALIS, E. (1980). Hyperparathyroidism in the elderly. *American Journal of Surgery,* **139,** 581–585

MASTER, A.M. and OPPENHEIMER, E.T. (1929). A simple exercise tolerance test for circulating efficiency with standard tables for normal individuals. *American Journal of Medical Sciences,* **177,** 223–243

MESSERLI, F.H., SUNDGAARD-RIIS, D., VENTURA, H.O., DUNN, F.G., GLADE, L.B. and FROHLICH, E.D. (1983). Essential hypertension in the elderly: hemodynamics, intravascular volume, plasma renin activity and circulating catecholamine levels. *Lancet,* **2,** 983–986

MESSERLI, F.H., VENTURA, H.D. and ANRODEO, C. (1985). Osler's maneuver and pseudohypertension. *New England Journal of Medicine,* **312,** 1548–1550

MILLER, J.A., McDONALD, R.K. and SHOCK, N.W. (1951). The renal extraction of p-amino-hippurate in the aged individual. *Journal of Gerontology,* **6–9,** 213

MILLER, J.H., McDONALD, R.H. and SHOCK, N.W. (1952). Age changes in the maximal rate of renal tubular reabsorption of glucose. *Journal of Gerontology,* **7,** 196–199

MINAKER, K.L., ROWE, J.W. and SPARROW, D. (1980). Impaired cardiovascular adaptation to vasodilation in the elderly. *Gerontologist,* **25,** 162

MORGAN, T., ADAM, W., GILLIES, A., MORGAN, G., ARLSON, M. and CARNEY, S. (1978). Hypertension treated by salt reduction. *Lancet,* **1,** 227–230

NIARCHOS, A.P. and LARAGH, J.H. (1980). Hypertension in the elderly. *Modern Concepts of Cardiovascular Diseases,* **49,** 43

OSTFELD, A.M., SHEKELLE, R.B., KLAWANS, H. and TUFO, H.M. (1974). Epidemiology of stroke in an elderly welfare population. *American Journal of Public Health,* **64,** 450–458

PARIJS, J., JOOSENS, J.V., LINDEN, L.V.D., VERSTREKEN, G. and AMERY, A. (1973). Moderate sodium restriction and diuretics in the treatment of hypertension. *American Heart Journal,* **85,** 22–34

PATEL, C. and NORTH, W.R.S. (1975). Randomized controlled trials of yoga and biofeedback in management of hypertension. *Lancet,* **2,** 93

PERRY, H.M. (1973). Late toxicity to hydralazine resembling lupus erythematosus or rheumatoid arthritis. *American Journal of Medicine,* **54,** 58–72

PFEFFER, R.I. (1978). Estrogen use, hypertension and stroke in postmenopausal women. *Journal of Chronic Diseases,* **31,** 389–398

PORT, S., COBB, F.R., COLEMAN, R.E. and JONES, R.H. (1980). Effect of age on the response of the left ventricular ejection fraction to exercise. *New England Journal of Medicine,* **303,** 1133–1137

PROPER, R. and WALL, F. (1972). Left ventricular stroke volume measurements not affected by chronologic aging. *American Heart Journal,* **83,** 843–845

RAEMSCH, K.D. and SOMMER, J. (1983). Pharmacokinetics and metabolism of nifedipine. *Hypertension,* **5,** 1118–1124

REISIN, E., ABEL, R., MODAN, M., SILVERBERG, D.S., ELIAHOU, H.E. and MODAN, B. (1978). Effect of weight loss without salt restriction on the reduction of blood pressure in overweight hypertensive patients. *New England Journal of Medicine,* **298,** 1–6

RODEHEFFER, R.J., GERSTENBLITH, G., BECKER, L.C., FLEG, J.L., WEISFELDT, M. and LAKATTA, E.G. (1980). Exercise cardiac output is maintained with advancing age in healthy human subjects: cardiac dilation and measured stroke volume compensate for diminished heart rate. *Circulation,* **69,** 203

ROSENDORFF, C. (1976). Prazosin. Severe side effects are dose dependent. *British Medical Journal,* **2,** 508

ROSS RUSSELL, R.W. (1963). Observations on intracerebral aneurysms. *Brain,* **86,** 425–442

ROWE, J.W. and TROEN, B.R. (1980). Sympathetic nervous system and aging in man. *Endocrinology Review,* **1,** 167

ROWLANDS, B.D, STOLLARD, T.J. and LITTLER, W.A. (1984). Continuous ambulatory monitoring of blood pressure and assessment of cardiovascular reflexes in the elderly hypertensive. *Journal of Hypertension,* **2,** 615–622

SAUNDERS, J.B., BEEVERS, D.G. and PATON, A. (1982). Alcohol induced hypertension. *Lancet,* **2,** 653–656

SCHOKEN, D. and ROTH, G. (1977). Reduced beta adrenergic receptor concentrations in aging man. *Nature,* **267,** 856–858

SHIMADA, K., KITAZUMI, T., SADAKANE, N., HISAKOZA, O. and OZAWA, T. (1985). Age-related changes of baroreflex function, plasma norepinephrine and blood pressure. *Hypertension,* **7,** 113–117

SINGH, B.N. and ROCHE, A. (1977). Effects of intravenous verapamil on hemodynamics in patients with heart disease. *American Heart Journal,* **94,** 593–599

STAMLER, J., FARINARO, E., MOJONNIER, L.M., HALL, Y., MASS, D. and STAMLER, R. (1980). Prevention and control of hypertension by nutritional hygienic means: long-term experience of the Chicago Coronary Prevention Evaluation Program. *Journal of the American Heart Association,* **243,** 1819–1823

STERN, M.P., BROWN, B.W., HASKELL, W.L., FARQUHAR, H.W., WEHRLE, C. and WOOD, P.D.S. (1976). Cardiovascular risk and use of estrogens or estrogen–progestogen combination. Stanford Three-community Study. *Journal of the American Heart Association,* **235,** 811–815

STEWART, B.H., BRAVO, E.L., HAAGA, J., MEANEY, T.F. and TARAZI, R. (1978). Localization of pheochromocytoma by computed tomography. *New England Journal of Medicine,* **299,** 460–461

STONE, P.A, ANTMAN, E.M., MULLER, F.E. and BRAUNWALD, E. (1980). Calcium channel blocking agents in the treatment of cardiovascular disorder. Part II. Hemodynamic effects and clinical application. *Annals of Internal Medicine,* **93,** 886–904

STRANDELL, T. (1964). Heart rate, arterial lactate concentration and oxygen intake during exercise in old men compared with young men. *Acta Physiologica Scandinavica,* **60,** 197–216

STRANDELL, T. (1976). Cardiac output in old age. In *Cardiology in Old Age,* edited by F.I. Caird, J.L.C. Dall and R.O. Kennedy, pp. 81–100. New York; Plenum Press

TAGUCHI, J. and FREIS, E.D. (1974). Partial reduction of blood pressure and prevention of complication in hypertension. *New England Journal of Medicine,* **291,** 329–331

TAKAZAKURA, E., SAWABU, N., HANDA, A., TAKADA, A., SHINODA, A. and TAKEUCHI, J. (1974). Intrarenal vascular changes with age and disease. *Kidney International,* **2,** 224

TARAZI, R.C. and LEVY, M.N. (1982). Cardiac responses to increased afterload. *Hypertension,* **4,** Suppl. II, 8–18

TARAZI, R. (1984). Hypertension in the elderly. In *Nephrology,* vol. II, edited by R. Robinson, pp. 1154–1162. New York; Springer

TINKELMAN, D.G. (1985). Calcium channel blocking agents in the prophylaxis of asthma. *American Journal of Medicine,* **78**(2B), 35–38

TOPOL, E.J., TRAILL, T.A. and FORTUIN, N.J. (1985). Hypertensive hypertrophic cardiomyopathy of the elderly. *New England Journal of Medicine,* **312,** 277–283

TUCK, M.L., SOWERS, J., DORNFELD, L., KLEDZIK, G. and MAXWELL, M. (1981). The effect of weight reduction on blood pressure, plasma renin activity and plasma levels in obese patients. *New England Journal of Medicine,* **304,** 930–933

UNITED STATES PUBLIC HEALTH HOSPITAL COOPERATIVE STUDY GROUP (1972). Morbidity and mortality in mild essential hypertension. *Circulation Research,* **30/31,** Suppl., 110

VANTOSH, A., LAKATTA, E.G., FLEG, J.L., WEISS, J., KALLMAN, C., WEISFELDT, M. and GERSTENBLITH, G. (1980). Ventricular dimension changes during submaximal exercise: effect of aging in normal men. *Circulation,* **62,** 111–129

VERTES, V., CANGIANO, J.L., BERMAN, L.B. and GOULD, A.B. (1969). Hypertension in end stage renal disease. *New England Journal of Medicine,* **280,** 978–981

VESTAL, R.E., WOOD, A.J.J. and SHAND, D.G. (1979). Reduced beta adrenoreceptor sensitivity in the elderly. *Clinical Pharmacology and Therapeutics,* **26,** 181–186

VETERANS ADMINISTRATION COOPERATIVE STUDY GROUP (1967). Effects of morbidity in hypertension I. Results in patients with diastolic blood pressure averaging 115 through 129 mmHg. *Journal of the American Medical Association,* **202,** 1028

VETERANS ADMINISTRATION COOPERATIVE STUDY GROUP (1970). Effects of morbidity in hypertension II. Results in patients with diastolic blood pressure average 90 through 114 mmHg. *Journal of American Medical Association,* **213,** 1143–1152

WAHL, J., TURLAPATY, P. and SINGH, B.N. (1985). Comparison of acebutolol and propranolol in essential hypertension. *American Heart Journal,* **109,** 313–321

WALLAM, G.L., CODY, R.J., TARAZI, R.C. and BRAVO, E.L. (1979). Acute hemodynamic effects and cardioselectivity of acebutolol, practolol and propranolol. *Clinical Pharmacology and Therapeutics,* **25,** 813–820

WEIDMANN, P., DE-MYTTENAERE-BURSZTEIN, S., MAXWELL, M.H. and DE LIMA, J. (1975). Effect of aging on plasma renin and aldosterone in normal man. *Kidney International,* **8,** 325–333

WEISFELDT, M.L. (1980). Aging of the cardiovascular system. *New England Journal of Medicine,* **303,** 1172

WHITE, E.A., SCHAMBELAN, M., ROST, C.R., BIGLIERI, E.G., MOSS, A.A. and KOROBKIN, M. (1980). Use of computed tomography in diagnosing the cause of primary aldosteronism. *New England Journal of Medicine,* **303,** 1503–1507

WHITESCARVE, S.A., OTT, C.E., JACKSON, B., GUTHRIE, H.G.P. and KOTCHEN, T.A. (1985). Hypertension and sodium salts. *Science,* **228,** 352

WILLET, W., HENNEKENS, C.H., SIEGEL, A.J., ADNER, M.M. and CASTELLI, W.P. (1980). Alcohol consumption and high-density lipoprotein cholesterol in marathon runners. *New England Journal of Medicine,* **303,** 1159–1161

WOLF, R.C., GHERMAN, C.F., SAUER, J.D, FISK, H.L. and LEVERLY, B.R. (1973). A new urinary assay for separate normetanephrine and metanephrine with application to the diagnosis of pheochromocytoma. *Clinical Science Molecular Medicine,* **45,** 2635

ZIEGLER, M.G., LAKE, C. and KOPIN, J. (1976). Plasma noradrenaline increases with age. *Nature,* **261,** 333–334

Chapter 6

The aging kidney and calcium-regulating hormones: vitamin D metabolites, parathyroid hormone and calcitonin

David Galinsky, Yitzhak Meller and Shraga Shany

Introduction

During the past fifteen years, great progress has taken place in the understanding of the role of vitamin D, its metabolites, and related hormones and minerals in humans. It was previously thought that either a lack of food intake or non-exposure to sunshine constituted the sole causes of rickets in childhood and osteomalacia in adulthood. This concept changed when it was determined that active vitamin D is not absorbed by the gut or produced by the skin, but rather the more sophisticated metabolites (hormones) produced by the kidney (DeLuca, 1975).

Aging is a physiological process affecting the total body, and specifically every cell, organ and system (Comfort, 1979; Fries, 1980). For instance, renal function declines with age (Davies and Shock, 1950; Macias Nuñez, 1983), and renal impairment is a well-recognized cause of calcium malabsorption and bone disease due to impaired production of the renal metabolites of vitamin D (1,25-dihydroxyvitamin D and 24,25-dihydroxyvitamin D). This process is also accompanied by changes in parathyroid hormone (PTH), calcitonin (CT) and oestrogens, and mainly affects the bone.

The clinical implications should be considered within the context of geriatric medicine. Here, the association of impaired social status in terms of nutritional deficiency, the effects of biological decline, multiple pathology, and the loss of functional ability with immobilization and lack of sun exposure all interact, demanding a comprehensive approach.

This chapter reviews the physiological basis by which the calcium-regulating hormones are affected by the aging process; it also deals with the common medical implications related to those hormones, and with the most advisable therapeutic management of these conditions.

Renal calcium and phosphate homeostasis

The human body loses calcium via three organs: the skin, the gastrointestinal tract (GIT) and the kidney. Undoubtedly the kidney plays the most important role in calcium excretion.

The daily urinary excretion of calcium varies considerably among young adults. The oral intake of calcium and its intestinal absorption have only a slight effect on daily urinary excretion. The kidney has but a limited ability to conserve calcium and thus there is always an essential calcium loss even in the presence of severe hypocalcaemia (Popovtzer and Knochel, 1980; Ardaillou, 1982). The upper normal range of calcium excretion per day in young adults is about 300 mg.

Renal excretion of ions can be described as a two-component system comprising glomerular filtration and tubular reabsorption. In young adults, 90 per cent of filtered calcium is reabsorbed in the proximal nephron — 60–70 per cent in the pars convoluta and 10–20 per cent in the pars recta. Only 5–10 per cent of the filtered load of calcium is reabsorbed along the distal convoluted tubule (Popovtzer and Knochel, 1980). The tubules reabsorb ionized calcium more easily than calcium bound to citrate, sulphate, phosphate and gluconate. The urinary excretion of calcium depends very much on the accompanying anion and on urine pH (Popovtzer and Knochel, 1980; Ardaillou, 1982).

The urinary excretion of calcium and that of sodium are intimately related. Factors that affect the renal excretion of sodium such as extracellular fluid (ECF) expanders, diuretic agents and steroids alter the renal excretion of calcium in various ways (e.g. steroids cause hypercalciuria). PTH and thiazides reduce urinary calcium excretion but induce a natriuresis (Ardaillou, 1982). Nevertheless, these two ions do not share the same mechanisms of transport along the nephron.

Changes in the filtered load of calcium may also affect its excretion. Thus, hypocalcaemia, regardless of its cause, is associated with hypocalciuria. The renal capacity to excrete calcium is severely compromised by a reduction in glomerular filtration rate (GFR), usually in chronic renal failure. Two factors contribute to this observation: secondary hyperparathyroidism and resistance to vitamin D (Popovtzer and Knochel, 1980; Ardaillou, 1982; Heckel and Hofeldt, 1982).

Calcium and phosphate movements are closely related and coupled in ECF, bone, gut and kidney. Acute and chronic phosphate loads decrease the urinary excretion of calcium, while phosphate depletion leads to hypercalciuria (Popovtzer and Knochel, 1980). Phosphate depletion enhances renal synthesis of 1,25-dihydroxyvitamin D ($1,25(OH)_2D$) which stimulates intestinal calcium absorption (Birge *et al.*, 1981; Ardaillou, 1982).

About 80 per cent of serum phosphate is filtered and the ratio of different phosphorus anions in the urine depends on its pH. Phosphate is the major urinary buffer accounting for most of the titrable acidity. Seventy to ninety per cent of phosphate is reabsorbed in the proximal nephron and none in the loop of Henle (Popovtzer and Knochel, 1980). There is a nephronal heterogeneity regarding phosphate handling: deep nephrons save phosphate, while superficial ones lose it.

Urinary excretion of phosphate depends to a great extent on oral intake. Increased dietary phosphate is associated with hyperphosphaturia depending on the state of parathyroid activity. High levels of PTH increase the phosphaturic response to phosphate load (Aurbach, Marx and Spiegel, 1981; Birge *et al.*, 1981).

Since the solubility product of calcium and phosphate in the urine is normally exceeded, several modifying factors are necessary to prevent the formation of calcium phosphate stones. Many observations show the dependence of renal handling of phosphate on serum levels of calcium, which are regulated by PTH and vitamin D metabolites. Increased levels of serum calcium, which are the result of higher calcium intake depending on dose and site of entry (oral or intravenous), usually decrease the urinary excretion of phosphate. These interrelationships are variable and complex because of the accompanying changes in serum PTH levels (Popovtzer and Knochel, 1980; Ardaillou, 1982).

Changes in renal handling of calcium and phosphate with age

It is assumed that age-related changes of the kidney occur in healthy people without any primary or secondary diseases that affect the kidney such as hypertension, diabetes or atherosclerosis. These changes have already been described in previous chapters of this book and in other texts (Shapiro, Porush and Kahn, 1978; Feinstein and Friedman, 1979; Goldman, 1979; Bichet and Schrier, 1982; Frocht and Fillit, 1984).

The serum levels of the electrolytes including calcium and phosphate remain relatively stable throughout a person's life. However, the efficiency of the homeostatic mechanisms that maintain electrolyte and acid-base balance is somewhat diminished. This means that the aging kidney has a reduced capacity to deal with drastic changes in serum levels of different electrolytes (Bichet and Schrier, 1982; Frocht and Fillit, 1984). For example, in the elderly, the reaction to immobilization, particularly when due to paralysis or a fracture, is exaggerated and may rapidly produce urinary calcium excretion in excess of 500 mg/24 h and lead to calcium stone formation.

It is customary to find relatively lower normal serum levels of calcium and higher serum levels of phosphate in the elderly as compared to young adults. In the aged, hypocalciuria and hyperphosphaturia are often found to be the results of functional renal impairment which characterizes the aging kidney. The latter is also characterized by reduced phosphate T_m. In addition, it should be noted that the elderly suffer more than young people from a variety of primary and secondary renal diseases which profoundly influence the renal handling of calcium and phosphate: Paget's disease, hyperthyroidism, malignancies, vitamin D deficiency, hyperparathyroidism and diabetes mellitus (Gregerman and Bierman, 1981; Heckel and Hofeldt, 1982). Yet one-third of patients aged 65 or older have glomerular and tubular function no different from that seen in younger people. In the majority of healthy elderly people, the loss of renal mass and function due to aging causes neither signs nor symptoms (Shapiro, Porush and Kahn, 1978).

Normal physiology of the calcium-regulating hormones

Parathyroid hormone

Parathyroid hormone (PTH) is a single-chain polypeptide molecule composed of 84 amino acids. The amino acid sequences of bovine, porcine and human PTH are now well known (Aurbach, Marx and Spiegel, 1981).

The intact biologically active PTH molecule is the major secretory product of the gland. It has a circulating half-life measured in minutes and is cleaved into amino- and carboxy-terminal fragments (at site 34 in the chain) in the kidney and liver. Only a small amount of the intact hormone is filtered and degraded by the kidney. The amino-terminal fragments, which are biologically active, have a very short circulating half-life (minutes) and are taken up by specific receptors in the kidney and bone and, to a lesser extent, are filtered and degraded by the kidney. Carboxy-terminal fragments are biologically inactive and have a circulating half-life measured in hours. They are eliminated from the circulation solely by glomerular filtration and degradation. Thus PTH in the serum is heterogeneous, but is mainly composed of carboxy-terminal fragments (Ardaillou, 1982; Broadus, 1982).

The effects of PTH on bone and kidney involve activation of adenyl-cyclase and increased formation of cyclic AMP which serves as the main mediator of this peptide hormone (Aurbach, Marx and Spiegel, 1981). PTH-responsive adenylate cyclase activity has been located in the terminal segments of the distal convoluted tubule and the first part of the collecting duct.

There is no evidence that a trophic factor influences PTH secretion or that innervation of the glands is important in the control of secretion. The major regulator of both PTH synthesis and secretion is the concentration of ionized calcium in the ECF. Serum calcium concentration is maintained within a very narrow range, primarily due to a feedback mechanism in which minimal hypocalcaemia increases the synthetic and secretory rate of PTH which then restores it to normocalcaemia by its action on bone and kidney (Broadus, 1982). Serum levels of phosphate are not feedback regulated, and they therefore vary over a relatively wide range. There also exists a calcium independent or non-suppressible portion of PTH secretion, which represents about 15 per cent of the normal secretion rate.

A variety of other ionic and hormonal factors influence the rate of PTH secretion including serum magnesium levels, catecholamines, calcitonin, gastrointestinal hormones and vitamin D metabolites (Birge *et al.*, 1981; Broadus, 1982). It is not yet clear whether these factors have a direct effect on the parathyroid cells or an indirect one, mediated by the associated systemic hypocalcaemia (except for vitamin D metabolites, which have direct effects on and specific receptors in the gland). Some of the catecholamines may act through a release of the stored hormone, while only hypocalcaemia stimulates both synthesis and secretion.

PTH is primarily responsible for the regulation of calcium metabolism in humans. The hormone recruits calcium from available sources in order to combat hypocalcaemia. This control is a result of (1) a direct effect on calcium and phosphate transport in the kidney, (2) a direct effect on calcium mobilization from the skeleton, and (3) stimulation of the active vitamin D metabolite synthesis in the kidney, with consequent indirect control of the intestinal absorption of calcium and phosphate (Broadus, 1982).

PTH has two principal effects on renal ion transport: (a) it decreases proximal tubular phosphate reabsorption causing marked phosphaturia; (b) it increases calcium reabsorption in the distal nephron causing a decrease in urinary calcium excretion (Ardaillou, 1982; Broadus, 1982).

Calcitonin

Calcitonin (CT) is a peptide hormone produced by the C cells of the thyroid gland. It is a 32 amino acid polypeptide. The amino acid sequences of CT molecules from five species (human, bovine, porcine, ovine and salmon) reveal close homologies for only parts of the residues of the 32 amino acids, so most radioimmunoassays developed for CT are relatively species-specific (Barlet, 1982).

The entire 32 amino acid sequence of CT is required for biological activity. CT molecules from different species and synthetic analogues have different hypocalcaemic potencies. For example, in humans, salmon CT is 10 times more potent than human CT on a weight basis (Barlet, 1982).

The details of CT synthesis, storage and secretion are less well understood than those of PTH. The primary stimulus for CT production and release is an increase in serum levels of ionized calcium.

The effects of CT on bone, kidney and gut are mostly mediated by cyclic AMP (Broadus, 1982).

The half-life for human CT is approximately 5 min. The principal organs responsible for the clearance and destruction of CT are the kidney, liver and possibly bone. It is cleared and metabolized by the kidney, rather than simply being filtered into the urine (Austin and Heath, 1981; Calmettes and Moukhtar, 1982).

There exists an as yet unexplained discrepancy between the pharmacological actions of CT as shown in experimental and some clinical situations, and the understanding of the physiological role and significance of CT for the human being. Metabolic consequences of clinical CT deficiency or excess are unknown in man. Studies on CT physiology in other species show that besides the known effects of CT as a serum calcium-lowering and phosphate-lowering factor and PTH antagonist, it also has a role in gastrointestinal function (Ziegler, Deutschle and Raue, 1984). According to this latter concept, CT acts to conserve ingested calcium and thus to preserve the skeleton, especially in calcium-consuming processes such as growth, pregnancy and lactation, and fracture healing.

CT inhibits directly, rapidly and profoundly both osteoclastic bone resorption and periosteocytic osteolysis. Its net influence on serum calcium depends on the rate of pre-existing bone resorption. The greatest effects of the hormone are seen under circumstances in which bone resorption is increased, as in (1) young growing animals, (2) bone which has been pre-stimulated by PTH or vitamin D, or (3) disease states associated with an increase in bone resorption and bone turnover such as Paget's disease and primary hyperparathyroidism (MacIntyre, 1983). The reduction in serum phosphate produced by CT appears to result both from an inhibition of phosphate mobilization derived from bone resorption and a direct stimulation of phosphate uptake into bone (MacIntyre, 1983).

The role of CT in the stimulation of osteoblastic bone formation is still controversial. Some investigators have found that pharmacological doses of CT have no effect on bone formation, while others have found it stimulatory (Aurbach, Marx and Spiegel, 1981; Broadus, 1982).

When a calcium-rich diet is consumed, the gastrointestinal hormones increase in the blood and stimulate CT secretion. In the case of fast calcium absorption and the start of hypercalcaemia, there may be an intensified CT release. The hormone then inhibits the secretory processes of digestion (gastric secretion) causing changes in intraluminal pH, and thus delaying calcium absorption and preventing hypercalcaemia. It seems that CT is an antihypercalcaemic hormone rather than a hypocalcaemic one (Cooper *et al.*, 1978; Ziegler, Deutschle and Raue, 1984).

The literature regarding the renal action of CT is confusing and filled with conflicting results depending especially on the different hormonal doses used in various experiments in different species. High doses of CT lead directly to transient increases in the excretion of calcium and phosphate in urine, while low doses tend to do the opposite (Borlé, 1983). These effects are due to the direct influence of the hormone on proximal tubular ion transport. In contrast to the long-lasting effects of CT on bone, all the renal tubular effects are transient and limited in time to the actual period of hormonal stimulation. No direct effect of CT on vitamin D metabolism in the kidney has been demonstrated. In fact, there is little evidence to suggest that the renal effects of CT are of physiological or even pathophysiological relevance (Ardaillou, 1982; Borlé, 1983; Ziegler, Deutschle and Raue, 1984).

There is a progressive decrease of CT secretion in both sexes with age, which indicates the importance of CT in age-related bone loss. Because women are CT deficient relative to men, their accelerated loss of bone mass, especially after menopause, may be related to decreased CT levels. The factors responsible for these age- and gender-related events have not been defined, but oestrogens have been implicated through a stimulatory effect on CT secretion (Stevenson, 1982; Taggart *et al.*, 1982; Deftos, 1984).

Vitamin D

Vitamin D and its metabolites play an important role in calcium and phosphate homeostasis. The consequences of vitamin D deficiency are rickets in children or osteomalacia in adults. Studies in recent years have contributed significantly to our understanding of the metabolism and the mode of action of vitamin D.

Vitamin D is supplied to the body by both endogenous production and diet. Sunlight promotes vitamin D_3 cholecalciferol synthesis in the skin by the ultraviolet photolysis of 7-dehydrocholesterol. The rate of synthesis is related to the amount of ultraviolet radiation and to the duration of exposure to this light. Seasonal variations in ultraviolet radiation are associated with variations in endogenous vitamin D_3 production and account for the seasonal fluctuations in the serum levels of vitamin D metabolites in normal young adults (Juttman *et al.*, 1981). Such a seasonal variation was also recorded in the elderly (Morris *et al.*, 1984). Although the natural diet of man is poor in vitamin D, egg yolk, fatty fish and milk fat are relatively rich in vitamin D_3. Vitamin D_2 (ergocalciferol) is the synthetic form of vitamin D obtained by ultraviolet irradiation of ergosterol from fungi and yeasts. Some foods, such as margarine and oils, are fortified with vitamin D_2 in the USA, Israel and some other countries. Both vitamin D_3 and vitamin D_2 have identical metabolic pathways and the same nutritional value in man.

Vitamin D, like other fat-soluble nutrients, requires micelle formation in the intestinal lumen for its absorption. It is absorbed primarily from the duodenum and jejunum into the lymph (Maislos, Silver and Fainaru, 1981). Vitamin D itself does not show any biological activity. This compound must be further hydroxylated to more polar compounds before it can manifest its activity. Vitamin D and its metabolites are transported in blood bound to a specific carrier protein (Haddad and Walgate, 1976). This vitamin D binding protein, which is produced by the liver, has an α-globulin electrophoretic mobility and a molecular weight of $52–59 \times 10^3$ (Imawari, Kida and De Goodman, 1976).

The first step in vitamin D metabolism takes place in the liver (*Figure 6.1*). As a result of the action of vitamin D 25-hydroxylase, the vitamin is hydroxylated in the C-25 position to yield 25-hydroxyvitamin D (25-OH-D). The rate of 25-OH-D production is not influenced by variations in the circulating concentrations of either calcium or phosphate, or by product formation (Bhattacharya and DeLuca, 1973). In fact, most of the available vitamin D is hydroxylated in the liver to 25-OH-D. Consequently 25-OH-D is the major vitamin D compound in the circulation (Mawer *et al.*, 1973) and its serum levels reflect the vitamin D status of the body.

The 25-OH-D is further hydroxylated at the C_1 position to produce the active form of vitamin D, namely $1,25(OH)_2D$ (*Figure 6.1*). The kidney is the major site of $1,25(OH)_2D$ synthesis (Fraser and Kodicek, 1970). The renal production of $1,25(OH)_2D$, which is carried out by the enzyme 25-OH-D-1α-hydroxylase, is closely controlled. High PTH and low serum levels of calcium and phosphate enhance its production (DeLuca, 1975; Fraser, 1980) and a number of hormones such as oestrogen and prolactin have been found to have a similar effect (Spanos,

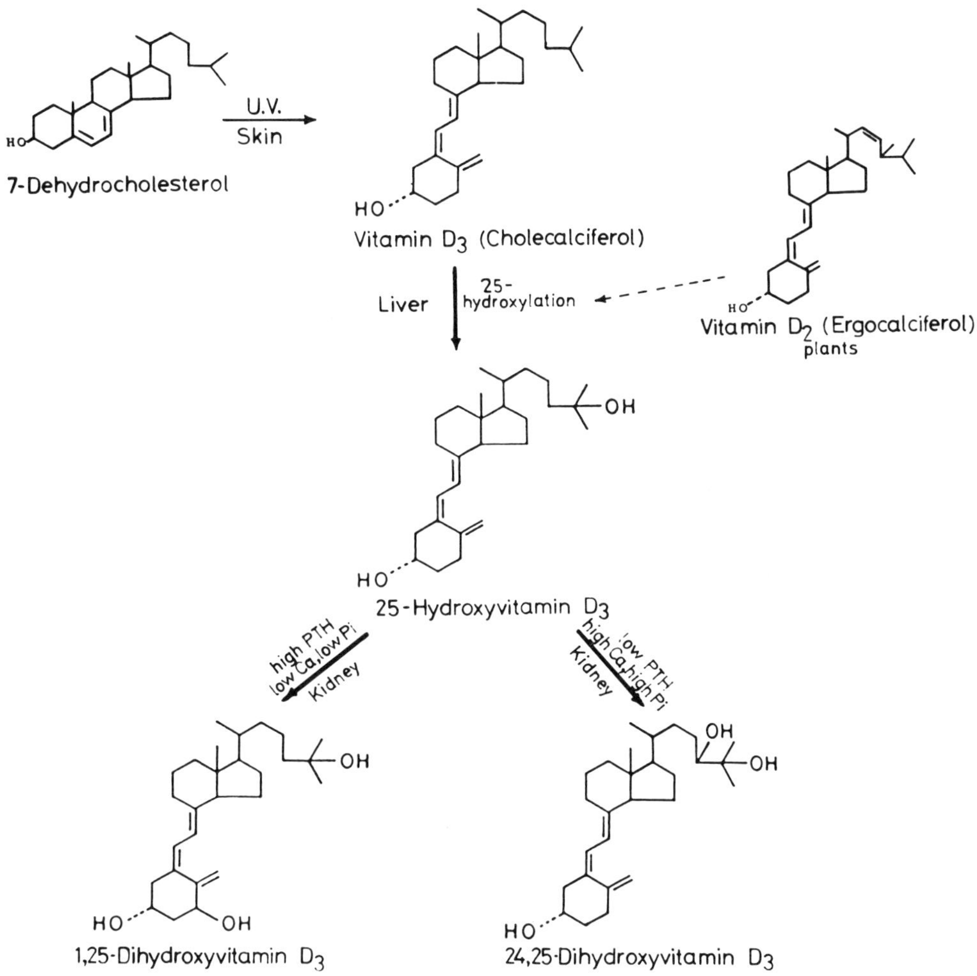

Figure 6.1 The metabolism of vitamin D

Pike and Haussler, 1976; Castillo, Tanaka and DeLuca, 1977). The main activity of $1,25(OH)_2D$ is the enhancement of calcium absorption in the gut. The mechanism of action includes a direct effect of $1,25(OH)_2D$ on the mucosal luminal membrane, resulting in changes in membrane lipid structure. These changes lead to an increase in membrane fluidity and thereby to an increase in calcium absorption (Rasmussen *et al.*, 1982).

On the other hand, $1,25(OH)_2D$ is responsible also for a sequence of events which leads to the production of calcium binding protein (CaBP) in the mucosal cells (Wasserman and Taylor, 1968). In this regard, $1,25(OH)_2D$ may be considered a hormone. It is produced in the kidney; the intestine is its target tissue, and it is responsible for the production of new proteins. Its mode of action is similar to that of the steroid hormones. $1,25(OH)_2D$ enters the mucosal cell and binds to a specific high affinity cytosolic receptor which transports it to the nucleus. There it promotes the production of mRNA to CaBP. This mRNA is translated on the ribosomes to give the CaBP (Haussler and McCain, 1977). The latter has a key role in calcium transport in the mucosal cell and in the rate of calcium efflux from the cell across its basolateral membrane (Rasmussen *et al.*, 1982). $1,25(OH)_2D$ also stimulates the active transport of phosphate in the gut (Walling and Kimberg, 1975).

The bone is also a target tissue for $1,25(OH)_2D_3$. Specific cytosolic receptors for this active metabolite of vitamin D have been identified in bone cells (Edelstein, 1974). In bone, $1,25(OH)_2D$, together with PTH, stimulates bone resorption (Rasmussen and Bordier, 1974). The ability of $1,25(OH)_2D$ to cause calcium mobilization from bone enables the skeleton reservoir to be utilized in cases of low calcium intake, or in cases of high calcium requirement. In the kidney, $1,25(OH)_2D$ increases calcium reabsorption.

It may be concluded that $1,25(OH)_2D$ is responsible for the known calcaemic effect of vitamin D by increasing intestinal calcium uptake, by decreasing renal calcium loss and by releasing calcium from bone.

Another dihydroxyvitamin D metabolite produced by the kidney is 24,25-dihydroxyvitamin D ($24,25(OH)_2D$) (*Figure 6.1*). The renal 25-OH-D-24-hydroxylase is responsible for the hydroxylation of the 25-OH-D in the C-24 position. The rate of production of $24,25(OH)_2D$ is well controlled. In fact, whereas high PTH and low serum levels of calcium and phosphate are required for $1,25(OH)_2D$ synthesis, the opposite physiological conditions enhance $24,25(OH)_2D$ production (DeLuca, 1975). Moreover, high $1,25(OH)_2D$ levels stimulate the renal 24-hydroxylase to produce $24,25(OH)_2D$ (Zerwekh *et al.*, 1983).

The serum $24,25(OH)_2D$ concentrations in normal healthy adults range from 1.6 to 4.4 ng/ml (Shany *et al.*, 1984). These levels are in the order of 100-fold higher than the normal serum concentrations of $1,25(OH)_2D$. Although the physiological role of $24,25(OH)_2D$ is still controversial, evidence has recently been presented which suggests that it may play a significant role in bone mineralization (Bordier *et al.*, 1978; Hodsman *et al.*, 1983). The exact biological role of $24,25(OH)_2D$ as well as other newly recognized vitamin D metabolites needs further investigation.

The aging kidney and PTH, CT and vitamin D metabolites

The endocrine changes caused by aging are well known: glandular atrophy and fibrosis are common; the serum levels of hormones tend to remain normal or altered; there is a decreased synthetic, secretory and degradative rate of hormones; target tissues and cells become less sensitive (more resistant) to the hormonal actions and there is a reduced ability of the glands to cope with sudden increased demands (Heckel and Hofeldt, 1982).

Parathyroid hormone

The interrelationship between the aging kidney and the aging parathyroid gland is unique because the latter is an independent one not regulated by other trophic (brain) endocrine factors, and its direct major target organ is the kidney itself.

There is no evidence to indicate that primary age-related changes in the parathyroid gland *per se* cause the increased serum levels of PTH usually observed in the elderly (Gregerman and Bierman, 1981). It is clear that many age-related alterations occurring in other organs (kidney, gut, bone, female genital system) indirectly influence the activity of the parathyroid gland (Johnston and Epstein, 1982).

It should be stressed that what is called the 'normal elderly' is a highly heterogeneous population including subjects suffering from: simple senile osteoporosis, sex-hormone-related postmenopausal osteoporosis, different incidences and kinds of hip and other fractures, different degrees of renal failure, varying levels of physical activity and related factors (exposure to sunshine, calcium and vitamin content in the diet). There are many differences between old women and old men, between the younger age group (65–73 years old) and very old people (>80 years old), between races and geographic areas of living. This heterogeneity provides a simple explanation for the controversial and even conflicting data concerning PTH levels in the aged (Berlyne *et al.*, 1975; Gregerman and Bierman, 1981; Johnston and Epstein, 1982; Deftos, 1984).

While reviewing the literature about age-related changes in serum PTH levels and in renal functions, two key questions should be asked: (1) do the increased recorded PTH levels represent an accumulation of inactive fragments of the hormone as a result of age-related deterioration of renal functions (i.e. a blockage in the degradation and excretion of the hormone), or (2) do active peptides indicate the development of real secondary hyperparathyroidism, which signifies genuine increased production and secretion of the hormone in response to other age-related changes in calcium metabolism?

The peripheral and intraglandular metabolism of PTH results in the production of peptide fragments of the molecule. Thus, serum contains a mixture of PTH molecules, including the intact molecule (bioactive) and fragments from various regions of the molecule, but especially the C-terminal peptide (inactive) and the NH_2-terminal peptide (active). The reports concerning serum PTH levels in the elderly used all kinds of methods to measure different PTH fragments (Roof *et al.*, 1976; Wiske *et al.*, 1979; Knorring *et al.*, 1982; Lips *et al.*, 1983). Thus, it is not surprising that the differences in concentration of the hormone found in this population may relate to those fragments of PTH detected by the particular assay used. On the other hand, this wide range of values for serum PTH may also reflect the underlying heterogeneity of this population as mentioned above.

From a practical point of view, most studies show high serum PTH concentrations in the elderly. A variety of pathogenic mechanisms closely related to each other (a multifactorial approach to aetiology) are proposed to be the reasons for this age-related secondary hyperparathyroidism which undoubtedly contributes to age-related bone loss and osteoporosis (Gallagher, Riggs and DeLuca, 1980).

It is impossible to ignore the similarity between the state of calcium and phosphate metabolism and calcium-regulating hormones in the elderly and in acute or chronic renal failure. Indeed, apart from the age-related changes in glomerular and tubular functions which cause a delay in PTH catabolism, impaired synthesis of $1,25(OH)_2D$ contributes to secondary hyperparathyroidism. This is due to age-related diminished activity of the 1-hydroxylase enzyme, which consequently leads to diminished intestinal Ca absorption and the lack of its direct inhibitory effect on the parathyroid gland (Goldman, 1979; Gregerman and Bierman, 1981; Heckel and Hofeldt, 1982).

Two other major factors contribute to this phenomenon: (1) increased skeletal and renal resistance to PTH due to age-related changes in target cells (maybe due to a reduction in number and quality of receptors) and the relative uraemia (Gregerman and Bierman, 1981; Heckel and Hofeldt, 1982; Deftos, 1984; Francis,

Peacock and Barkworth, 1984); (2) the relative state of vitamin D deficiency in the aged, not related to renal impairment *per se* (Johnston and Epstein, 1982; Deftos, 1984).

Calcitonin

CT secretion is regulated by a variety of factors. These include age and sex, calcium and related ions, gastrointestinal hormones, neuroendocrine factors and species. Different CT secretion rates, according to age and sex, have been found in various species including cattle, rats, dogs, salmon and humans (Deftos *et al.*, 1980; Birge *et al.*, 1981; Deftos, 1981; Barlet, 1982; Meller *et al.*, 1984b).

There is some controversy in the literature concerning age-related changes of serum CT levels in humans. Most studies show a decline in serum CT concentrations with aging (Deftos *et al.*, 1980; Shamonki *et al.*, 1980; Austin and Heath, 1981; Birge *et al.*, 1981; Deftos, 1981; Taggart *et al.*, 1982; MacIntyre, 1983), while others fail to demonstrate it (Body and Heath, 1983; Meller *et al.*, 1985). Nevertheless, there is now consensus that in both sexes CT secretion progressively declines with age (Deftos, 1984). Evidence has accumulated in clinical studies to implicate CT in the pathogenesis of age-related osteopenia. The principal skeletal effect of CT is to inhibit bone resorption: a main skeletal defect in osteoporosis is increased bone resorption (Johnston and Epstein, 1982). Therefore, it is not surprising to discover that studies of CT treatment indicate the role played by this hormone in osteoporosis (Jowsey *et al.*, 1978; MacIntyre, 1983).

The majority of reports in humans show that women of any age, but especially the elderly (postmenopausal), have lower serum CT levels than do men (Deftos, 1981; MacIntyre, 1983; Meller *et al.*, 1984b, 1985). Calcium-stimulation studies of CT secretion in women with osteoporosis suggest a deficient CT response in comparison to normal women (Taggart *et al.*, 1982). Calcitonin and gonadal steroids may be linked in the pathogenesis of postmenopausal osteopenia. Since oestrogen receptors are not present in bone cells, oestrogens must exert their skeletal effects indirectly, by stimulating CT secretion. Pregnancy and oestrogen therapy have been reported to increase serum CT levels, and higher CT concentrations have been found in the middle of the menstrual cycle (Stevenson, 1982; Taggart *et al.*, 1982; MacIntyre, 1983; Deftos, 1984).

Many effects of CT on renal physiology have been demonstrated in the past (Borlé, 1983). The significance of age- and sex-related changes in serum CT levels in renal handling of calcium and phosphate homeostasis is still unknown (Ardaillou, 1982; Heckel and Hofeldt, 1982; Borlé, 1983).

Vitamin D metabolites

Various degrees of vitamin D deficiency are common among elderly people. In many studies concerning healthy elderly people, significantly low serum levels of 25-OH-D were determined in comparison to normal healthy young adults (Hodkinson *et al.*, 1979; Lawson *et al.*, 1979; Galinsky *et al.*, 1982). This decline in serum 25-OH-D levels in the elderly is explained by disturbances in mobility which lead to reduced exposure to sunshine, by inadequate general nutrition and by low content of vitamin D in diets.

In addition to these reasons, a vitamin D intestinal malabsorption has been recorded in elderly people (Barragry *et al.*, 1978). Hepatic disorders, such as bile duct obstruction due to carcinoma or stones, decrease the intraluminal bile salts required for normal vitamin D absorption (Wills and Savory, 1984). Other factors, such as intestinal mucosal disease (Meredith and Rosenberg, 1980) or pancreatic exocrine deficiency (Hahn *et al.*, 1979), may contribute to this malabsorption. The existence of an enterohepatic cycle of vitamin D and its metabolites (Wiesner *et al.*, 1980) might lead to a loss of some endogenous vitamin D metabolites, as well as exogenous ones, in malabsorption disorders. Cholestyramine therapy may induce malabsorption of vitamin D since this drug diminishes the luminal bile salts (Parfitt *et al.*, 1982). Depression or loss of hepatic 25-hydroxylase in some hepatic disorders, such as alcoholic liver disease and chronic active liver disease, could be a contributory factor to the low serum 25-OH-D levels in the elderly. The pharmacological use of anticonvulsant drugs such as phenobarbital and diphenylhydantoin also reduces serum 25-OH-D levels (Parfitt and Kleerekoper, 1980). Low serum 25-OH-D concentrations in nephrotic syndrome can result from urinary excretion of 25-OH-D (Barragry *et al.*, 1977). Such a loss of 25-OH-D was reported recently in uraemic patients treated with continuous ambulatory peritoneal dialysis (Aloni, Shany and Chaimovitz, 1983).

Low concentrations of serum 1,25$(OH)_2$D in the elderly have also been recorded (Gallagher *et al.*, 1979). There is no doubt that the reduction in renal function is part of the aging process. Whether the decreased renal 1α-hydroxylation is an isolated process or part of the general aging process of the kidney occurring in elderly people should be further investigated. These low serum concentrations of 1,25$(OH)_2$D are accompanied by increased levels of serum PTH. The decreased 1,25$(OH)_2$D levels result in a decrease in intestinal calcium absorption, which in turn causes increased PTH secretion (Tsai *et al.*, 1984). A poor response of the renal 1α-hydroxylase, which was found to be negatively correlated with age, was obtained following PTH infusion (Tsai *et al.*, 1984). This phenomenon is related to decreased renal function due to aging.

In postmenopausal women the lack of oestrogen may contribute to the reduced levels of 1,25$(OH)_2$D. Oestrogen enhances renal 1,25$(OH)_2$D production (Castillo, Tanaka and DeLuca, 1977). Recently, an induction of 1,25$(OH)_2$D cytosolic receptor production by oestrogen was described in the rat uterus (Levy *et al.*, 1984). Due to these findings, the lack of oestrogen in postmenopausal women may cause an alteration in the target tissue, in addition to reduced renal 1α-hydroxylation.

Recently, interest has been shown in the biological role of 24,25$(OH)_2$D. Evidence has been presented which suggests that this metabolite plays a significant role in bone mineralization (Bordier *et al.*, 1978; Hodsman *et al.*, 1983). Serum levels of 24,25$(OH)_2$D were found to be increased together with CT levels during fracture healing in young human adults (Meller *et al.*, 1984a). These findings indicate a possible role of 24,25$(OH)_2$D in bone healing. Serum levels of 24,25$(OH)_2$D in elderly people were found to be low (Weisman *et al.*, 1981; Galinsky *et al.*, 1982). This reduction in serum 24,25$(OH)_2$D is greater than the general reduction in vitamin D levels in the elderly. Galinsky *et al.* (1982) have shown a rise in serum 25-OH-D following vitamin D administration in a group of elderly people. At the same time, serum 24,25$(OH)_2$D concentrations were not affected by the treatment. These results represent a significant failure of an essential function of the aging kidney.

The above findings are in accordance with the observation that serum 24,25$(OH)_2D$ levels did not increase in elderly patients during fracture healing (Meller *et al.*, 1985). This is of course in contrast to the findings observed in young adults (Meller *et al.*, 1984a). This fact may be at least partially responsible for the slow healing of fractures in geriatric patients.

Clinical implications

The most common diseases affecting the calcium-regulating hormones in the elderly are discussed in this section. There is a high incidence of renal disease among the elderly (Samiy, 1983; Frocht and Fillit, 1984), not only as an isolated disease, but associated with other pathology, such as arteriosclerosis, diabetes, malignancies, or combined with other conditions such as multiple drug therapy, or water and electrolyte impairment. Since the kidney is the main producer of 1,25$(OH)_2D$, parenchymal damage in chronic renal disease impairs the production of this active hormone. This vitamin D-resistant uraemia has therapeutic implications, as is discussed below (Brickman, Coburn and Norman, 1972). Also, the same condition can diminish or antagonize the 1α-hydroxylase by phosphate retention and acidosis, in spite of elevated blood levels of PTH (Mason *et al.*, 1980).

The two main determinants of effective calcium absorption are the amount of calcium in the diet and the efficiency of its absorption. The daily recommendation for calcium intake in the USA is 800 mg (National Research Council, 1980); in the UK, 500 mg (Department of Health and Social Security, 1969). Actually, one-fourth of USA females of all ages are found to ingest less than 300 mg/day (Heaney *et al.*, 1982). Other studies conducted with the same purpose conclude that low calcium intake is a common condition among the elderly (Nordin, 1960). Moreover, the intestinal calcium absorption efficiency decreases after middle age (Avioli, McDonald and Lee, 1965; Bullamore *et al.*, 1970).

Preliminary observations (S. Shany, personal communication, 1984) in vitamin D metabolite feeding experiments in old people show that the polar compounds (25-OH-D and 1α-OH-D) are well absorbed, but that the native vitamin D_2 is very poorly absorbed.

Since vitamin D is a fat-soluble compound, its absorption is mainly into the lymph tract (Maislos, Silver and Fainaru, 1981) and requires the participation of bile salts. On the other hand, the polar vitamin D metabolites are absorbed mainly into the portal blood. Probably a decrease in bile salts in the elderly contributes to this difference. In any case, vitamin D levels are commonly low among the geriatric population. In many European countries, and especially in the UK, serum 25-OH-D is lower than in the younger population (Parfitt *et al.*, 1982). Mean values are frequently under 5 ng/ml. The main reasons are deficient diet and lack of exposure to sunlight. In the USA, because the addition of vitamin D to milk and to other nutrients is very common, the deficiency is related much more to pathological conditions such as malabsorption as a result of different gastrointestinal ailments, or loss of 25-OH-D in the urine, as in the nephrotic syndrome.

As a consequence of the high incidence of neurological and musculoskeletal disease among the elderly, loss of mobility, homebound confinement and lack of sun exposure are the expected outcome. This dreadful sequence of events exacerbates the negative calcium balance, producing a daily loss of 200–300 mg of calcium in addition to the deficient intake mentioned above. This phenomenon has already been addressed by various investigators (Donaldson *et al.*, 1970; Preece *et al.*, 1975).

Since serum calcium became a routine determination, more cases of hyperparathyroidism have been discovered (Pearson, 1984). Among the elderly, females are much more affected than males. Indeed, the incidence of hyperparathyroidism in females over 60 years of age was 188.5 per 100 000 population, 7 times the incidence found before the introduction of the screening of calcium. The most common symptoms were weakness, mental slowdown and decreased mobility. Since high levels of PTH are common within the elderly, hypercalcaemia is of paramount importance in the diagnosis of this disease.

It is well known that multiple pathology is the rule for the elderly. The number of diseases suffered is in the range of three to six and the amount of involvement of different organs and systems is quite extensive (Williamson, 1967). However, there is a long list of pathological conditions within the elderly which specifically affect the hormones and minerals discussed here. For example in diabetes, a significant decrease in serum $1,25(OH)_2D$ and an increase in $24,25(OH)_2D$ is the pattern. Those patients also have reduced vitamin D-dependent CaBP in the kidney (Raisz and Kream, 1983).

In hyperthyroidism, increased bone resorption may be responsible for an increase in serum calcium concentration, a decrease in serum PTH and $1,25(OH)_2D$, and a decrease in intestinal absorption of calcium (Haldiman *et al.*, 1980).

Metabolic acidosis produces a negative calcium balance probably due to increased dissolution and impaired formation of minerals and deficient activation of vitamin D (Reddy *et al.*, 1982). The association between chronic liver disease, chronic alcoholism and osteoporosis has also been reported already (Paterson and Losowsky, 1967).

In the last few years, different studies have been devoted to the fall of oestrogen levels in postmenopausal osteoporosis and related hormones (Gallagher, Riggs and DeLuca, 1980; Lund *et al.*, 1982). From these studies it transpired that there is a correlated decrease in CT and $1,25(OH)_2D$, with a subsequent decrease in calcium absorption. Parathyroid hormone can be either normal or decreased in Type I osteoporosis (postmenopausal, age 55–70) or elevated in Type II osteoporosis (senile, age 70–85) (Riggs and Melton, 1983). The greatest medical importance of the fall in oestrogen levels is that it creates a tendency to fractures, especially of the hip, vertebrae and distal forearm. It has been estimated that about 70 per cent of fractures in persons aged 45 and older are attributable to osteoporosis (Iskrant and Smith, 1969). The cost of osteoporosis in the USA in 1983 was estimated to be 3.8 billion dollars (Kelsey, 1984).

Osteomalacia is a very common disease among the elderly (Exton Smith, 1973). Basically, a lack of vitamin D is the cause. Other contributory factors include malnutrition, long confinement indoors, malabsorption, gastrectomy, liver and biliary tract diseases. The incidence is about 4 per cent among women admitted to geriatric departments (Anderson *et al.*, 1966). In a careful study, Aaron *et al.* (1974) showed that the incidence of osteomalacia among 102 females with fractures was about 20–30 per cent; for men, 40 per cent.

In the elderly, multiple diseases necessitate the use of several drugs simultaneously (Klein, German and Levine, 1981). There is a group of drugs which have in common the enhancement of the negative calcium balance with the consequent increase in bone loss. Among these drugs, mention should be made of glucocorticoids, furosemide, aluminium, isoniazide and tetracycline. This clinical observation is probably based on interference with the metabolism of vitamin D or the increase in the urinary excretion of calcium and phosphate (Hahn, Boisseau and Avioli, 1974; Spencer, Kramer and Osis, 1982).

Special attention should be given to the combined use of drugs inducing calcium depletion, such as corticosteroids, isoniazid and aluminium hydroxide in patients with tuberculosis; or, in chronic alcoholism, the intake of aluminium/antacids for gastritis and hyponutrition. Drugs originating alteration of the hydroxylation of vitamin D in the liver, such as barbiturates and diphenylhydantoin, should also be considered in this context (Bouillon *et al.*, 1975).

Another clinical implication of bone loss — osteoporosis and fractures — is that over a period of 10 years, 75 per cent of patients lose 10 cm in height. Height loss and kyphosis are the major permanent sequelae (Scott, 1984).

Therapeutic management

Some of the diseases discussed in this chapter affect the kidney, and as a consequence the calcium-regulating hormone system is impaired. Since this malfunction causes bone disorders, the bone should be considered as the target tissue for therapeutic management. In any case in which altered vitamin D metabolism is secondary to diseases such as diabetes, hyperthyroidism or acidosis, adequate treatment of the latter should be a priority.

The vitamin D metabolites are already low in normal aging people (Slovik *et al.*, 1981; Galinsky *et al.*, 1982). For several reasons, the vitamin D requirement increases with age, and a total supply of 15–20 μg/day (600–800 iu) from all sources, is recommended (Parfitt *et al.*, 1982). Special attention should be paid to persons most likely to need supplementation, such as the housebound, persons with malabsorption, and persons with interruption of the enterohepatic circulation. Osteomalacia is less common in the USA than in Europe, but subclinical vitamin D deficiency may contribute to the pathogenesis of hip fractures, both through increased liability to fall and through PTH-mediated bone loss. It is worth mentioning that the use of native vitamin D has limitations. For example, the use of 40 000 u (1 mg) of vitamin D causes no change in serum calcium and phosphate, and has negligible effects on calcium absorption in a group of patients with chronic renal failure (Gotloib *et al.*, 1978).

In the section dealing with clinical implications, it was reported that a preliminary study (S. Shany, personal communication, 1984) suggested that polar compounds are better absorbed than the native vitamin D. In this study, done on a group of 9 residents in a home for the aged, who were not taking any drugs and who did not suffer from liver or kidney diseases or malabsorption, 3000 u/day of vitamin D in arachis oil was administered for 5 months; no rise occurred in the serum level of 25-OH-D, $1,25(OH)_2D$ or $24,25(OH)_2D$. On the other hand, the administration of 25 μg/day of 25-OH-D for 7 days produced a significant increase in all the metabolites. This finding probably provides clues about the future use of this metabolite as a way of overcoming the decreased absorption of vitamin D in the intestinal tract in the elderly.

The limitations in the therapeutic use of native vitamin D increase the interest in its metabolites. Brickman, Coburn and Norman (1972) showed, in a group of patients with advanced renal failure, that significant responses were obtained from daily treatment with only 0.25 to 2 μg of $1,25(OH)_2D$ for 6–10 days; serum calcium and phosphate rose, intestinal calcium absorption increased by 30 per cent to 220 per cent. Gallagher *et al.* (1982) found that $1,25(OH)_2D$ given in a daily dose of 0.5–0.75 μg significantly reduced the vertebral fracture rate in patients with postmenopausal osteoporosis.

$1,25(OH)_2D$ is also useful in the treatment of osteomalacia (Exton Smith, 1973). It has been shown that in doses of 0.025–0.125 mg (1000–5000 iu) daily during a period of 1–3 months, there is a striking symptomatic improvement, with the disappearance of muscular weakness and bone pains. It is customary to administer oral calcium supplements (1 g daily).

The oral administration of 1–2 μg daily of 1α-hydroxyvitamin D (1α-OH-D), a potent synthetic analogue of vitamin D, is known to reverse many of the clinical symptoms of bone disease associated with chronic renal failure (Gotloib *et al.*, 1978). 1α-hydroxyvitamin D_3 (1α-OH-D_3) was also demonstrated to be an important agent in the treatment of osteoporosis. Lund *et al.* (1975) treated a group of patients with synthetic 1α-OH-D_3 for 3–4 months. The compound was given at a daily oral dose of 2 μg together with an oral supplement of 1 g of calcium. Clinically there was a striking improvement in the patients' physical fitness. Increased bone formation and mineralization were seen on iliac crest bone biopsy, and this was supported by increased osteoblastic activity demonstrated by measurement of alkaline phosphatase activity. Bone histology furthermore showed a reduced bone resorption, which was supported by a reduced urinary excretion of total hydroxyproline. Photon absorptiometry of the forearm showed significant increased bone density in all patients. The serum concentrations of 25-OH-D and PTH were not significantly affected by the treatment. This observation was also supported later on by Nordin *et al.* (1980). On the other hand, controversial studies done with the same purpose with vitamin D and 1α-OH-D_3 reached the conclusion that treatment with these agents had no preventive effect on postmenopausal calcium loss (Christiansen *et al.*, 1980, 1981).

Although the function of $24,25(OH)_2D$ is still unclear, it appears that this metabolite may ultimately prove beneficial to patients with chronic renal disease and dialysis osteomalacia, who do not respond to $1,25(OH)_2D$ treatment (Hodsman *et al.*, 1983).

It should also be emphasized that excessive intake of vitamin D or of its metabolites may result in hypercalcaemia and extra-osseous calcification, particularly in arterial walls and in the kidney, leading to chronic renal failure (Parfitt *et al.*, 1982). The dose of vitamin D that causes significant hypercalcaemia is highly variable between individuals, but is rarely less than 1000 μg/day. Higher doses can cause hypercalciuria, nephrolithiasis and possibly impaired renal function. Vitamin D administration may increase plasma cholesterol, but there is no convincing evidence that the risk of myocardial infarction is increased. The recommended total supply for the elderly of 20 μg/day is most unlikely to be harmful, except in patients with sarcoidosis or renal calculi.

Although the problem of osteoporosis is beyond the scope of this chapter, it is worth mentioning a few highlights on this issue. Among the elderly there is a high risk group permanently threatened by falls and fractures. The combination of biological, social and pathological factors (Raisz, 1984) is the reason for the high risk. This group should be identified in the community by adequate preventive programmes in order to avoid further deterioration (Lowther, McLeod and Williamson, 1970; Galinsky, Schneiderman and Lowenthal, 1983).

Physical activity should be considered among the basic measures in the treatment of osteoporosis. The weight of evidence favours the concept that exercise can prevent involutional changes in body composition (Aloia, 1981).

The role played by calcium is also of paramount importance in the treatment of osteoporosis. Different reasons for loss of calcium were investigated in the aged (Spencer, Kramer and Osis, 1982). As a consequence of those reasons, the calcium intake in the diet requires special consideration. It is suggested that the mean requirement in perimenopausal women should be approximately 1.0 g calcium daily and in the oestrogen-deprived postmenopausal, approximately 1.5 g calcium daily (Heany, 1984). This is also the recommendation of the Consensus Development Conference on Osteoporosis from the National Institute of Health (1984).

The fall of oestrogen levels during menopause and its relationship to osteoporosis has already been proved (Shamonki *et al.*, 1980; Christiansen, Christensen and Transbol, 1981). The administration of oestrogens increased $1,25(OH)_2D$, increased calcium absorption from the intestine (Lund *et al.*, 1982), increased bone mineral content (BMC) (Jensen, Christiansen and Transbol, 1982) and reduced the fracture rate (Riggs *et al.*, 1982). The best results were obtained by a combination of oestrogen, calcium and fluoride (Riggs *et al.*, 1982). It is worth mentioning that in their very thorough study, Gambrell, Maier and Sanders (1983) reached the conclusion that oestrogen therapy for postmenopausal women does not increase the risk of breast cancer and may afford some protection. Progestogen added to postmenopausal oestrogen therapy significantly decreases the risk of this malignancy.

The doses recommended by the Consensus Development Conference on Osteoporosis are 0.625 mg conjugated equine oestrogen, or 25 μg of mestronal and 2 mg of oestradiol valcrate daily (National Institute of Health, 1984).

Another agent that should be considered in osteoporosis is fluoride therapy (Riggs, 1984a, 1984b). A retrospective study showed that this significantly decreases the occurrence of vertebral fractures (Riggs *et al.*, 1982). It is agreed that the optimal dosage is 50–70 mg of sodium fluoride daily combined with 1000–1500 mg of supplementary elemental calcium.

There are studies which suggest a possible beneficial effect of calcitonin in osteoporosis (Pecile, 1981). In a controlled study carried out on a group of osteoporotic patients (from 76 to 89 years old) (Jimenez Herrero, 1983) receiving 100 iu of synthetic salmon calcitonin on an intermittent schedule for a period of 3 years, a functional improvement was obtained: lower prescription of analgesics and skeletal X-rays revealed a lower frequency of new vertebral compression or collapse in patients receiving this treatment compared to other groups.

With regard to the management of hyperparathyroidism among the elderly, it is important to report the experience of Hodkinson, Peacock and Nordin (1971). They no longer recommended surgery on asymptomatic patients with primary hyperparathyroidism unless the serum calcium is above 11.5 mg/l. In addition, the problem of confusion or dementia should be considered. The papers surveyed provide no real basis for expecting an improvement in dementia in those affected patients in whom primary hyperparathyroidism is found once the effect of competing pathologies has been ruled out. If for any reason it was felt that hypercalcaemia might be relevant to the dementia, then perhaps the effect of dichloromethylene diphosphonate (Shane, Baquirau and Bilezikian, 1981) could be tried as, even if calcium were only lowered for 16–18 weeks, this should be adequate to see if there were any improvement.

Acknowledgement

The authors wish to express their gratitude to Mrs M Duman for her excellent and devoted secretarial help.

References

AARON, J.E., GALLAGHER, J.C., ANDERSON, J., STASIAK, L., LONGTON, E.B., NORDIN, B.E.C. *et al.* (1974). Frequency of osteomalacia and osteoporosis in fractures of the proximal femur. *The Lancet*, **I**, 229–233

ALOIA, J.F. (1981). Exercise and skeletal health. *Journal of the American Geriatrics Society*, **29**(3), 104–107

ALONI, Y., SHANY, S. and CHAIMOVITZ, C. (1983). Losses of 25-hydroxyvitamin D in peritoneal fluid: possible mechanism for bone disease in uremic patients treated with chronic ambulatory peritoneal dialysis. *Mineral and Electrolyte Metabolism*, **9**, 82–86

ANDERSON, I., CAMPBELL, A.E.R., DUNN, A. and RUNCIMAN, J.B.M. (1966). Osteomalacia in elderly women. *Scottish Medical Journal*, **2**, 429–436

ARDAILLOU, R. (1982). The endocrinology of renal calcium and phosphate homeostasis. In *Endocrinology of Calcium Metabolism*, edited by J.A. Parsons, pp. 41–54. New York; Raven Press

AURBACH, G.D., MARX, S.J. and SPIEGEL, A.M. (1981). Parathyroid hormone, calcitonin and the calciferoles. In *Textbook of Endocrinology*, edited by R.W. Williams, pp. 922–1031. Philadelphia; Saunders

AUSTIN, L.A. and HEATH, H. (1981). Calcitonin, physiology and pathophysiology. *New England Journal of Medicine*, **304**, 269–278

AVIOLI, L.V., McDONALD, J.E. and LEE, S.W. (1965). The influence of age on the intestinal absorption of 47Ca absorption in postmenopausal osteoporosis. *Journal of Clinical Investigation*, **44**, 1960–1967

BARLET, J.P. (1982). Comparative physiology of calcitonin. In *Endocrinology of Calcium Metabolism*, edited by J.A. Parsons, pp. 235–270. New York; Raven Press

BARRAGRY, J.M., FRANCE, M.W., CARTER, N.D. *et al.* (1977). Vitamin D metabolism in nephrotic syndrome. *The Lancet*, **II**, 629–632

BARRAGRY, J.M., FRANCE, M.W., CORLESS, D., GUPTA, S.P., SWITALA, S., BOUCHER, B.J. and COHEN, R.D. (1978). Intestinal cholecalciferol absorption in the elderly and in younger adults. *Clinical Science and Molecular Medicine*, **55**, 213–220

BERLYNE, G.M., BEN-ARI, J., KUSHELEVSKY, A., IDELMAN, A., GALINSKY, D., HIRSCH, M. *et al.* (1975). The etiology of senile osteoporosis: secondary hyperparathyroidism due to renal failure. *Quarterly Journal of Medicine*, **175**, 505–521

BHATTACHARYA, M.H. and DELUCA, H.F. (1973). The regulation of rat liver calciferol-25-hydroxylase. *Journal of Biological Chemistry*, **248**, 2969–2973

BICHET, D.G. and SCHRIER, R.W. (1982). Renal function and diseases in the aged. In *Clinical Internal Medicine in the Aged*, edited by R.W. Schrier, pp. 211–221. Philadelphia; Saunders

BIRGE, S.J., HAHN, T.J., WHYTE, M.P. and AVIOLI, L.V. (1981). Hormonal regulation of mineral metabolism. *International Reviews of Physiology*, **24**, 201–241

BODY, J.J. and HEATH, H. (1983). Effects of age, sex, calcium and total thyroidectomy on circulating monomeric calcitonin (CT) concentrations (abstract). *Calcified Tissue International Supplement*, **35**, 171

BORDIER, P., RASMUSSEN, H., MARIE, P., MIRAVET, L., GUERIS, J. and RYCKWAERT, A. (1978). Vitamin D metabolites and bone mineralization. *Journal of Clinical Endocrinology and Metabolism*, **46**, 284–294

BORLÉ, A.B. (1983). Calcitonin and the regulation of calcium transport and of cellular calcium metabolism. *Triangle*, **22**(2/3), 75–80

BOUILLON, R., REYNAERT, J., CLAES, J.H., LISSEUS, W. and DE MOOR, P. (1975). The effect of anticonvulsant therapy on serum levels of 25-hydroxyvitamin D, calcium, and parathyroid hormone. *Journal of Clinical Endocrinology and Metabolism*, **41**(6), 1.130–1.135

BRICKMAN, A.S., COBURN, J.W. and NORMAN, A.W. (1972). Action of 1,25-dihydroxycholecalciferol, a potent, kidney-produced metabolite of vitamin D_3, in uremic man. *New England Journal of Medicine*, **287**, 891–895

BROADUS, A.E. (1982). Mineral metabolism. In *Endocrinology and Metabolism,* edited by P. Felig, J.D. Baxter, A.E. Broadus and L.A. Frohman, pp. 967–988. New York; McGraw-Hill.

BULLAMORE, J.R., GALLAGHER, J.C., WILKINSON, R., NORDIN, B.E.C. and MARSHALL, D.H. (1970). Effect of age on calcium absorption. *The Lancet,* **II,** 535–537

CALMETTES, C. and MOUKHTAR, M.S. (1982). Immunoassay of human calcitonin in health and disease. In *Endocrinology of Human Metabolism,* edited by J.A. Parsons, pp. 211–234. New York; Raven Press

CASTILLO, L., TANAKA, Y. and DELUCA, H.F. (1977). The stimulation of 25-hydroxyvitamin D_3-1-hydroxylase by estrogen. *Archives of Biochemistry and Biophysics,* **179,** 211–217

CHRISTIANSEN, C., CHRISTENSEN, M.S., McNAIR, P., HAGEN, G., STOCKLUND, T.E. and TRANSBOL, I. (1980). Prevention of early postmenopausal bone loss: controlled 2 year study in 315 normal females. *European Journal of Clinical Investigation,* **10,** 273–279

CHRISTIANSEN, C., CHRISTENSEN, M.S., RODBRO, P., HAGEN, G. and TRANSBOL, I. (1981). Effect of 1,25 dihydroxyvitamin D_3 in itself or combined with hormone treatment in preventing postmenopausal osteoporosis. *European Journal of Clinical Investigation,* **11,** 305–309

CHRISTIANSEN, C., CHRISTENSEN, M.S. and TRANSBOL, I. (1981). Bone mass in postmenopausal women after withdrawal of oestrogen/gestagen replacement therapy. *The Lancet,* **II,** 459–461

COMFORT, A. (1979). *The Biology of Senescence,* 3rd edn, pp. 81–86. New York; Elsevier

COOPER, C.W., BOLMAN, R.M., LINEHON, W.M. and WELLS, S.A. (1978). Interrelationship between calcium, calcemic hormones and gastrointestinal hormones. *Recent Progress in Hormone Research,* **34,** 259–290

DAVIES, D.F. and SHOCK, N.W. (1950). Age changes in glomerular filtration rate, effective renal plasma flow and tubular excretory capacity in adult males. *Journal of Clinical Investigation,* **29,** 496–507

DEFTOS, L.J. (1981). Regulation of calcitonin secretion: effects of species, age and sex. In *Proceedings of the Seventh International Conference on Calcium Regulating Hormones,* edited by D.V. Chohen, pp. 266–270. International Congress Series 511. Amsterdam; Excerpta Medica

DEFTOS, L.J. (1984). Calcitonin and parathyroid hormone in osteoporosis. In *Osteoporosis, National Institute of Health Consensus Development Conference,* edited by L.E. Shulman, pp. 66–69. Bethesda, Maryland; National Institute of Health

DEFTOS, L.J., WEISMAN, M.H., WILLIAMS, G.W., KARPF, D.B., FRUMAR, A.M., DAVIDSON, B.J. *et al.* (1980). Influence of age and sex on plasma calcitonin in human beings. *New England Journal of Medicine,* **302,** 1351–1353

DELUCA, H.F. (1975). The kidney as an endocrine organ involved in the function of vitamin D. *American Journal of Medicine,* **58,** 39–47

DEPARTMENT OF HEALTH AND SOCIAL SECURITY (1969). Recommended intakes of nutrients for the United Kingdom, No. 120. London; HMSO

DONALDSON, C.L., HULLEY, S.B., VOGEL, J.M., HATTNER, R.S., BAYYERS, J.H. and McMILLAN, D.E. (1970). Effect of prolonged bed rest on bone mineral. *Metabolism,* **19,** 1074–1084

EDELSTEIN, S. (1974). Vitamin D binding proteins. In *The Metabolism and Function of Vitamin D,* edited by D.R. Fraser, Special Publication No. 3, p. 43. London; Biochemical Society

EXTON SMITH, A.N. (1973). Musculo skeletal system. Bone aging and metabolic bone disease. In *Textbook of Geriatric Medicine and Gerontology,* edited by J.C. Brocklehurst, pp. 476–491. Edinburgh; Churchill Livingstone

FEINSTEIN, E.I. and FRIEDMAN, E.A. (1979). Renal disease in the elderly. In *Clinical Geriatrics,* edited by I. Rossman, pp. 224–238. Philadelphia; Lippincott

FRANCIS, R.M., PEACOCK, M. and BARKWORTH, S.A. (1984). Renal impairment and its effects on calcium metabolism in elderly women. *Age and Ageing,* **13,** 14–20

FRASER, D.R. (1980). Regulation of the metabolism of vitamin D. *Physiological Reviews,* **60,** 551–613

FRASER, D.R. and KODICEK, E. (1970). Unique biosynthesis by kidney of a biologically active vitamin D metabolite. *Nature,* **228,** 764–770

FRIES, J.F. (1980). Aging, natural death, and the compression of morbidity. *New England Journal of Medicine,* **303,** 130–135

FROCHT, A. and FILLIT, H. (1984). Renal disease in the geriatric patient. *Journal of the American Geriatrics Society,* **32**(1), 28–43

GALINSKY, D., OREN, A., ZUILI, I., YANKOWITZ, N., LOWENTHAL, M. and SHANY, S. (1982). Disturbance of 24,25-dihydroxyvitamin D in healthy elderly. In *Osteoporosis,* edited by J. Menczel, G. Robin and M. Makin, pp. 55–60. Chichester, UK; Wiley

GALINSKY, D., SCHNEIDERMAN, K. and LOWENTHAL, M.N. (1983). A homecare unit: geriatrically oriented and hospital based with the active involvement of the family physician. *Israel Journal of Medical Sciences,* **19,** 841–844

GALLAGHER, J.C., JERPBACK, C.M., JEE, W.S.S., JOHNSON, K.A., DELUCA, H.F. and RIGGS, B.L. (1982). 1,25 dihydroxyvitamin D_3: short and long term effects on bone and calcium metabolism in patients with postmenopausal osteoporosis. *Proceedings of the National Academy of Sciences of the United States of America,* **79,** 3325–3329

GALLAGHER, J.C., RIGGS, B.L. and DELUCA, H.F. (1980). Effect of estrogen on calcium absorption and serum vitamin D metabolites in postmenopausal osteoporosis. *Journal of Clinical Endocrinology and Metabolism,* **51**(6), 1359–1364

GALLAGHER, J.C., RIGGS, B.L., EISMAN, J., HAMSTRA, A., ARNAUD, S.B. and DELUCA, H.F. (1979). Intestinal calcium absorption and serum vitamin D metabolites in normal subjects and osteoporotic patients: effects of age and dietary calcium. *Journal of Clinical Investigation,* **64,** 729–736

GALLAGHER, J.C., RIGGS, B.L., JERPBACK, C.M. and ARNAUD, C.D. (1980). The effect of age on serum immunoreactive parathyroid hormone in normal and osteoporotic women. *Journal of Laboratory and Clinical Medicine,* **95,** 373–385

GAMBRELL, R.D., MAIER, R.C. and SANDERS, B.E. (1983). Decreased incidence of breast cancer in postmenopausal estrogen/progestogen users. *Obstetrics and Gynecology,* **62,** 435–443

GOLDMAN, R. (1979). Decline in organ function with aging. In *Clinical Geriatrics,* edited by I. Rossman, pp. 23–59. Philadelphia; Lippincott

GOTLOIB, L., MINES, M., MAZUR, Y., SKLAN, D., GARMIZO, A.L., JANCU, J. *et al.* (1978). 1 hydroxycholecalciferol: a promising therapeutic approach for renal osteodystrophy. *Israel Journal of Medical Sciences,* **14,** 731–735

GREGERMAN, R.I. and BIERMAN, E.L. (1981). Aging and hormones. In *Textbook of Endocrinology,* edited by R.W. Williams, pp. 1192–1212. Philadelphia; Saunders

HADDAD, J.G. and WALGATE, J. (1976). 25-hydroxyvitamin D transport in human plasma. *Journal of Biological Chemistry,* **251,** 4803–4809

HAHN, T.J., BOISSEAU, V.C. and AVIOLI, L.V. (1974). Effect of chronic corticosteroid administration on diaphyseal and metaphyseal bone mass. *Journal of Clinical Endocrinology and Metabolism,* **39,** 274–282

HAHN, T.J., SQUIRES, A.E., HALSTEAD, L.R. and STROMINGER, D.B. (1979). Reduced serum 25-hydroxyvitamin D concentration and disordered mineral metabolism in patients with cystic fibrosis. *Journal of Pediatrics,* **94,** 39–42

HALDIMAN, B., KAPTEIN, E.M., SINGER, F.R., NIOLOFF, J.T. and MASSRY, S.G. (1980). Intestinal calcium absorption in patients with hyperthyroidism. *Journal of Clinical Endocrinology and Metabolism,* **51,** 995–997

HAUSSLER, M.R. and McCAIN, T.A. (1977). Basic and clinical concepts related to vitamin D metabolism and action. *New England Journal of Medicine,* **297,** 1041–1050

HEANEY, R.P. (1984). Role of calcium in pathogenesis, prophylaxis and treatment of osteoporosis. In *Osteoporosis, National Institute of Health Consensus Development Conference,* edited by L.E. Shulman, pp. 46–48. Bethesda, Maryland; National Institute of Health

HEANEY, R.P., GALLAGHER, J.C., JOHNSTON, C.C., NEER, P., PARFITT, A.M. and WHEDON, G.D. (1982). Calcium nutrition and bone health in the elderly. *American Journal of Clinical Nutrition,* **36,** 986–1013

HECKEL, R.H. and HOFELDT, F.D. (1982). Endocrinology and metabolism in the elderly. In *Clinical Internal Medicine in the Aged,* edited by R.W. Schrier, pp. 222–255. Philadelphia; Saunders

HODKINSON, A., PEACOCK, M. and NORDIN, B.E.C. (1971). Asymptomic hyperparathyroidism. *The Lancet,* **II,** 49

HODKINSON, H.M., BRYSON, E., KLENERMAN, L., CLARKE, M.B. and WOOTON, R. (1979). Sex, sunlight, season, diet and the vitamin D status of elderly patients. *Journal of Clinical and Experimental Gerontology,* **1,** 13

HODSMAN, A.B., WONG, E.G.C., SHERRARD, D.J., BRICKMAN, A.S., LEE, D.B.N., SINGER, F.R. *et al.* (1983). Preliminary trials with 24,25 dihydroxyvitamin D_3 in dialysis osteomalacia. *American Journal of Medicine,* **74,** 407–414

IMAWARI, M., KIDA, K. and DE GOODMAN, W.S. (1976). The transport of vitamin D and its 25-hydroxy metabolite in human plasma. Isolation and partial characterization of vitamin D and 25-hydroxyvitamin D binding protein. *Journal of Clinical Investigation,* **58,** 514–523

ISKRANT, A.P. and SMITH, R.W. Jr. (1969). Osteoporosis in women 45 years and over related to subsequent fractures. *Public Health Reports,* **84,** 33–38

JENSEN, G.F., CHRISTIANSEN, C. and TRANSBOL, I. (1982). Treatment of postmenopausal osteoporosis. A controlled therapeutic trial comparing oestrogen/gestagen, 1,25-dihydroxyvitamin D_3 and calcium. *Clinical Endocrinology (Oxford),* **16**(5), 515–524

JIMENEZ HERRERO, F. (1983). Calcitonin in senile osteoporosis: clinical effects. In *Proceedings of the Tenth European Congress of Clinical Gerontology* (Budapest, Hungary), p. 79

JOHNSTON, C.C. and EPSTEIN, S. (1982). The endocrinology of osteoporosis. In *Endocrinology of Calcium Metabolism,* edited by J.A. Parsons, pp. 467–484. New York; Raven Press

JOWSEY, J., RIGGS, B.L., KELLY, P.J. and HOFFMAN, D.L. (1978). Calcium and salmon calcitonin in treatment of osteoporosis. *Journal of Clinical Endocrinology and Metabolism,* **47,** 633–639

JUTTMAN, J.R., VISSER, T.J., BUURMAN, C., DEKAM, E. and BERKENHAGER, J.C. (1981). Seasonal fluctuations in serum concentrations of vitamin D metabolites in normal subjects. *British Medical Journal,* **282,** 1349–1352

KELSEY, S.L. (1984). Osteoporosis: prevalence and incidence. In *Osteoporosis, National Institute of Health Consensus Development Conference,* edited by L.E. Shulman, pp. 25–28. Bethesda, Maryland; National Institute of Health

KLEIN, L.E., GERMAN, P.S. and LEVINE, D.M. (1981). Adverse drug reactions among the elderly: a reassessment. *Journal of the American Geriatrics Society,* **29**(11), 525–529

KNORRING, J.V., SLATIS, P., WEBER, T.H. and HELENIUS, T. (1982). Serum levels of 25-hydroxyvitamin D, 24,25-dihydroxyvitamin D and parathyroid hormone in patients with femoral neck fractures in southern Finland. *Clinical Endocrinology,* **17,** 189–194

LAWSON, D.E.M., PAUL, A.A., BLACK, A.E., COLE, T.J., MANDELL, A.R. and DAVIE, M. (1979). Relative contributions of diet and sunlight to vitamin D state in the elderly. *British Medical Journal,* **2,** 303–305

LEVY, J., ZUILI, I., YANKOWITZ, N. and SHANY, S. (1984). Induction of cytosolic receptors for 1,25-dihydroxyvitamin D_3 in the immature rat uterus by oestradiol. *Journal of Endocrinology,* **100,** 265–269

LIPS, P., HACKENG, W.H.L., JONGEN, M.J.M., VAN GINKEL, F.C. and NETELENBOS, J.C. (1983). Seasonal variations in serum concentrations of parathyroid hormone in elderly people. *Journal of Clinical Endocrinology and Metabolism,* **57,** 204–206

LOWTHER, C.P., McLEOD, R.D.M. and WILLIAMSON, J. (1970). Evaluation of early diagnostic services for the elderly. *British Medical Journal,* **1,** 275–277

LUND, B., HJORTH, L., KJAER, J., REIMANN, J., FRIIS, T., ANDERSEN, R.B. *et al.* (1975). Treatment of osteoporosis of aging with 1α-hydroxycholecalciferol. *The Lancet,* **II,** 1168–1171

LUND, B., SORENSON, O.H., LUND, B. and AGNER, E. (1982). Serum 1,25-dihydroxyvitamin D in normal subjects and in patients with postmenopausal osteopenia. Influence of age, renal function and oestrogen therapy. *Hormone and Metabolic Research,* **14**(5), 271–274

MACIAS NUÑEZ, J.F. (1983). Aspectos morfologicos, funcionales y patologicos del rinon del viejo. *Nefrologia,* **3**(1), 1–7

MACINTYRE, I. (1983). The physiological actions of calcitonin. *Triangle,* **22,** 69–74

MAISLOS, M., SILVER, J. and FAINARU, M. (1981). Intestinal absorption of vitamin D steroids: differential absorption into lymph and portal blood in the rat. *Gastroenterology,* **80,** 1528–1534

MASON, R.S., LISSNER, D., WILKINSON, M. and POSEN, S. (1980). Vitamin D metabolites and their relationship to azotaemic osteodystrophy. *Clinical Endocrinology,* **13,** 375–385

MAWER, E.B., BACKHOUSE, J., TAYLOR, C.M., LUMB, G.A. and STONBURY, S.W. (1973). Failure of formation of 1,25-dihydroxycholecalciferol in chronic renal failure. *The Lancet,* **I,** 626–631

MELLER, Y., KESTENBAUM, R.S., SHANY, S., GALINSKY, D., ZUILI, I., YANKOWITZ, N. *et al.* (1985). Parathormone, calcitonin and vitamin D metabolites during normal fracture healing in geriatric patients. *Clinical Orthopaedics and Related Research* (in press)

MELLER, Y., KESTENBAUM, R.S., SHANY, S., ZUILI, I., YANKOWITZ, N., GIAT, J. *et al.* (1984a). Parathyroid hormone, calcitonin, and vitamin D metabolites during normal fracture healing in humans. *Clinical Orthopaedics and Related Research,* **183,** 238–245

MELLER, Y., KESTENBAUM, R.S., YAGIL, R. and SHANY, S. (1984b). The influence of age and sex on blood levels of calcium-regulating hormones in dogs. *Clinical Orthopaedics and Related Research,* **187,** 296–299

MEREDITH, S.C. and ROSENBERG, I.H. (1980). Gastrointestinal-hepatic disorders and osteomalacia. *Clinical Endocrinology and Metabolism,* **9,** 131–150

MORRIS, H.A., MORRISON, G.W., BURR, M., THOMAS, D.W. and NORDIN, B.E.C. (1984). Vitamin D and femoral neck fractures in elderly South Australian women. *Medical Journal of Australia,* **140,** 519–521

NATIONAL INSTITUTE OF HEALTH (1984). *Osteoporosis. Consensus Development Conference Statement,* Vol. 5, No. 3. Bethesda, Maryland; National Institute of Health

NATIONAL RESEARCH COUNCIL (1980). Recommended dietary allowances, 9th edn. Food and Nutrition Board. Washington D.C.; National Academy of Sciences, NAS/NRC

NORDIN, B.E.C. (1960). Osteoporosis and calcium deficiency. In *Bone as a Tissue,* edited by K. Rodahl, J.T. Nicholson and E.M. Brown Jr., pp. 44–66. New York; McGraw-Hill

NORDIN, B.E.C., HORSMAN, A., CRILLY, R.G., MARSHALL, D.H. and SIMPSON, M. (1980). Treatment of spinal osteoporosis in postmenopausal women. *British Medical Journal,* **280,** 451–454

PARFITT, A.M., GALLAGHER, J.C., HEANEY, R.P., JOHNSTON, C.C., NEER, R. and WHEDON, G.D. (1982). Vitamin D and bone health in the elderly. *American Journal of Clinical Nutrition,* **36,** 1014–1031

PARFITT, A.M. and KLEEREKOPER, M. (1980). The divalent ion homeostasis system: physiology and metabolism of calcium, phosphorus, magnesium and bone. In *Clinical Disorders of Fluid and Electrolyte Metabolism,* edited by M. Maxwell and C.R. Kleeman, pp. 269–398. New York; McGraw-Hill

PATERSON, C.R. and LOSOWSKY, M.S. (1967). The bone in chronic liver disease. *Scandinavian Journal of Gastroenterology,* **2,** 293–300

PEARSON, M.W. (1984). Asymptomatic primary hyperparathyroidism in the elderly. *Age and Ageing,* **13,** 1–5

PECILE, A. (1981). *Calcitonin: Chemistry, Physiology, Pharmacology and Clinical Aspects,* p. 396. Amsterdam; Excerpta Medica

POPOVTZER, M.M. and KNOCHEL, J.P. (1980). Disorders of calcium, phosphorus, vitamin D and parathyroid hormone activity. In *Renal and Electrolyte Disorders,* 2nd edn, edited by R.W. Schrier, pp. 223–297. Boston; Little, Brown

PREECE, M.A., TOMLINSON, S., RIBOT, C.A., PIETREK, J., KORN, H.T., DAVIES, D.M. *et al.* (1975). Studies of vitamin D deficiency in man. *Quarterly Journal of Medicine* (New Series), **44,** 575–589

RAISZ, L.G. (1984). Management of osteoporosis: endocrinological perspective. In *Osteoporosis, National Institute of Health. Consensus Development Conference,* edited by L.E. Shulman, pp. 85–87. Bethesda, Maryland; National Institute of Health

RAISZ, L.G. and KREAM, B.E. (1983). Regulation of bone formation (second of two parts). *New England Journal of Medicine,* **309**(2), 83–89

RASMUSSEN, H. and BORDIER, P. (1974). *The Physiological and Cellular Basis of Metabolic Bone Disease.* Baltimore; Williams and Wilkins

RASMUSSEN, H., MATSUMATO, T., FONTAINE, O. and GOODMAN, D.P.B. (1982). Role of changes in membrane lipid structure in the action of 1,25-dihydroxyvitamin D_3. *Federation Proceedings,* **41**(1), 72–77

REDDY, G.S., JONES, G., KOOH, S.W. and FRASER, D. (1982). Inhibition of 25 hydroxyvitamin D_3-1-hydroxylase by chronic metabolic acidosis. *American Journal of Physiology,* **243**(L), 265–271

RIGGS, B.L. (1984a). Treatment of osteoporosis with sodium fluoride: an appraisal. In *Bone and Mineral Research Annal 2,* edited by W.A. Peck, pp. 366–393. New York; Elsevier

RIGGS, B.L. (1984b). Treatment of osteoporosis with sodium fluoride and by other regimens that increase bone mass. In *Osteoporosis, National Institute of Health Consensus Development Conference,* edited by L.E. Shulman, pp. 55–58. Bethesda, Maryland; National Institute of Health

RIGGS, B.L. and MELTON, J.L. (1983). Evidence for two distinct syndromes of involutional osteoporosis. *American Journal of Medicine,* **75,** 899–901

RIGGS, B.L., SEEMAN, E., HODGSON, S.F., TAVES, D.R. and O'FALLON, W.M. (1982). Effect of the fluoride/calcium regimen on vertebral fracture occurrence in postmenopausal osteoporosis. *New England Journal of Medicine,* **306,** 446–450

ROOF, B.S, PIEL, C.F., HANSEN, J. and FUDENBERG, H.H. (1976). Serum parathyroid hormone levels and serum calcium levels from birth to senescence. *Mechanism of Ageing and Development,* **5,** 289–304

SAMIY, A.H. (1983). Renal disease in the elderly. *Medical Clinics of North America,* **67**(2), 463–480

SCOTT, W.W. Jr. (1984). Osteoporosis — related fractures syndromes. In *Osteoporosis, National Institute of Health Consensus Development Conference,* edited by L.E. Shulman, pp. 20–24. Bethesda, Maryland; National Institute of Health

SHAMONKI, I.M., FRUMAR, A.M., TATARYN, I.V., MELDRUN, D.R., DAVIDSON, B.H., PARTHEMORE, J.G. *et al.* (1980). Age related changes of calcitonin secretion in females. *Journal of Clinical Endocrinology and Metabolism,* **50**(3), 437–439

SHANE, E., BAQUIRAU, D.C. and BILEZIKIAN, J.P. (1981). Effects of dichloromethylene diphosphonate on serum and urinary calcium in primary hyperparathyroidism. *Annals of Internal Medicine,* **95,** 23–27

SHANY, S., RAPOPORT, J., GOLIGORSKY, M., YANKOWITZ, N., ZUILI, I. and CHAIMOVITZ, C. (1984). Losses of 1,25- and 24,25-dihydroxycholecalciferol in the peritoneal fluid of patients treated with continuous ambulatory peritoneal dialysis. *Nephron,* **36,** 111–113

SHAPIRO, W.B., PORUSH, J.G. and KAHN, A.I. (1978). Medical renal diseases in the aged. In *Clinical Aspects of Aging,* edited by W. Reichel, pp. 199–211. Baltimore; Williams and Wilkins

SLOVIK, D.M., ADAMS, J.S., NEER, R.M., HOLICK, M.F. and POTTS, J.T. (1981). Deficient production of 1,25 dihydroxyvitamin D in the elderly osteoporotic patients. *New England Journal of Medicine,* **305**(7), 372–374

SPANOS, E., PIKE, J.W. and HAUSSLER, M.R. (1976). Circulating 1-alpha,25-dihydroxyvitamin D in the chicken: enhancement by injection of prolactin and during egg laying. *Life Sciences,* **19,** 1751–1756

SPENCER, H., KRAMER, L. and OSIS, D. (1982). Factors contributing to calcium loss in aging. *American Journal of Clinical Nutrition,* **36,** 776–787

STEVENSON, J.C. (1982). Regulation of calcitonin and parathyroid hormone secretion by estrogens. *Maturitas,* **4,** 1–7

TAGGART, H.M., CHESNUT, C.H., IVEY, J.L., BAYLINK, D.J., SISOM, K., HUBER, M.B. *et al.* (1982). Deficient calcitonin response to calcium stimulation in postmenopausal osteoporosis. *The Lancet,* **I,** 475–477

TSAI, K.S., HEATH, H., KUMAR, R. and RIGGS, B.L. (1984). Impaired vitamin D metabolism with aging in women. *Journal of Clinical Investigation,* **73,** 1668–1672

WALLING, M.W. and KIMBERG, D.V. (1975). Effects of 1α,25-dihydroxyvitamin D_3 and solanum glaucophyllum on intestinal calcium and phosphate transport and on plasma calcium, magnesium and phosphate levels in the rat. *Endocrinology,* **97,** 1567–1576

WASSERMAN, R.H. and TAYLOR, A.M. (1968). Vitamin D dependent calcium-binding protein. *Journal of Biological Chemistry,* **243,** 3987–3993

WEISMAN, Y., SCHEN, R.J., EISENBERG, Z., EDELSTEIN, S. and HARELL, A. (1981). Inadequate status and impaired metabolism of vitamin D in the elderly. *Israel Journal of Medical Science,* **17,** 19–21

WIESNER, R.H., KUMAR, R., SEEMAN, E. and GO, V.L.W. (1980). Enterohepatic physiology of 1.25-dihydroxyvitamin D_3 metabolites in normal man. *Journal of Laboratory and Clinical Medicine,* **96,** 1094–1100

WILLIAMSON, J. (1967). Detecting disease in clinical geriatrics. *Gerontologia Clinica,* **9,** 236–242

WILLS, M.R. and SAVORY, J. (1984). Vitamin D metabolism and chronic liver disease. *Annals of Clinical and Laboratory Science,* **14**(3), 189–197

WISKE, P.S., EPSTEIN, S., BELL, N.H., QUEENER, S.T., EDMONDSON, J. and JOHNSTON, C.C. (1979). Increase in immunoreactive parathyroid hormone with age. *New England Journal of Medicine,* **300,** 1419–1421

ZERWEKH, J.E., McPHAUL, J.J., PARKER, T.F. and PAK, C.Y. (1983). Extra-renal production of 24.25-dihydroxyvitamin D in chronic renal failure during 25-hydroxyvitamin D_3 therapy. *Kidney International,* **23,** 401–406

ZIEGLER, R., DEUTSCHLE, U. and RAUE, F. (1984). Calcitonin in human pathophysiology. *Hormone Research,* **20,** 65–73

Chapter 7

Proximal tubular function and renal acidification in the aged

Jose M. Tabernero Romo

Introduction

As a consequence of the increase in life expectancy in the general population, the number of elderly persons continues to rise. This has meant that more attention must be paid to the possible existence of specific characteristics in this sector of the population when its members become ill. The kidney of elderly persons presents a series of characteristic modifications consecutive to organic or functional disturbances of the structures which constitute the organ. One such structure is the renal tubule whose physiology and pathology are dealt with in this chapter.

The proximal tubule

The proximal tubule reabsorbs a large fraction (two-thirds) of the glomerular filtrate. Sodium, several other solutes and water are reabsorbed at a high rate. Active sodium reabsorption and hydrogen ion secretion are the essential processes to which transport of chloride, several organic solutes and water are coupled by a variety of mechanisms. Fluid transport is isosmotic, so that concentration gradients of solute across the wall are small. Functionally, the proximal tubule can be divided into three segments:

(1) Initial portion of the convoluted segment. Sodium metabolism in this portion occurs through cells and intercellular spaces. Entry of sodium across luminal membranes is passive and occurs (a) by diffusion, (b) coupled to the transport of other solutes (e.g. glucose, amino acids and phosphate), and (c) in exchange with H^+ secreted from cell to lumen. Sodium extrusion from cells into the intercellular spaces and across the basalateral membrane is an active process. Preferential reabsorption of bicarbonate resulting from H^+ secretion occurs in this segment, with bicarbonate concentration falling and chloride concentration increasing as the fluid progresses along this segment of the tubule. The reabsorption of glucose and amino acid is active, is coupled to sodium transport and is essentially complete in this segment.

(2) Distal part of the convoluted segment. The luminal fluid of this segment is characterized by a low concentration of bicarbonate and by the absence of glucose and amino acid. The high concentration of chloride in the lumen favours

its diffusion to the cell. Sodium reabsorption in this segment occurs by active transport and passive flow.

(3) Straight segment. This segment is the main site of secretion of organic acids (penicillin, uric acid, etc.). Its rate of sodium and fluid transport is slower.

Physiology of urinary acidification

The human body produces hydrogen ions as a consequence of daily metabolism (Lennon and Leman, 1966). Plasma bicarbonate is consumed upon combining with the endogenously produced protons. One of the most important roles of the kidney lies in regulating acid-base balance; it does this by maintaining plasma bicarbonate within normal ranges and by excreting H^+ generated by the body's metabolism. The kidney performs these processes by reabsorbing through the tubules the bicarbonate filtered by the glomerulus and then by regenerating the consumed bicarbonate, at the same time excreting H^+. We shall look at these processes step by step.

Theoretically there should be three general sources of endogenous fixed acid during the metabolism of neutral foodstuffs (Relman, 1964):

(1) The oxidation of sulphur to sulphate. In this sense the sulphur-containing amino acids methionine and cystine act as donors of hydrogen ions.
(2) During the course of metabolism of neutral carbohydrates, fats and nucleoproteins a great variety of moderately strong organic acids are formed: lactic acid, citric acid, keto acids and uric acid.
(3) The hydrolysis of phosphoesters. In this way the phosphate-containing components of the diet act as a source of hydrogen ions.

The production of hydrogen ions is greater in children than in adults due to bone formation. It is known that for every 10 mmol of calcium retained for the formation of hydroxyapatite, 8–9 mmol of H^+ are released. Accordingly, the greater or lesser production of hydrogen ions depends on the positive balance of calcium produced during bone development.

Eighty-five per cent of the reabsorption of filtered bicarbonate (approximately 4500–5000 mEq/day) takes place in the proximal tubule (*Figure 7.1*). The other 15 per cent is reabsorbed in the distal convoluted tubule. The hydration of CO_2 catalysed by carbonic anhydrase (CA) in the proximal tubular cells produces HCO_3^- + H^+ ($CO_2 + H_2O \rightleftharpoons HCO_3^- + H^+$). The H^+ is exchanged with the tubular lumen sodium which arises from the reaction $NaHCO_3 \rightleftharpoons HCO_3^- + Na^+$. H^+ secretion is carried out actively and sodium enters the cell passively; from the cell, Na^+ passes into the peritubular fluid by an active mechanism and is followed passively by the bicarbonate ion in order to maintain electroneutrality. In the tubular lumen, the H^+ ions are combined with the HCO_3^- to give H_2CO_3. By the action of CA, which is also found in the brush border of the proximal tubular cells, this acid is transformed into $CO_2 + H^+$ and OH^- which is completely reabsorbed by the cell where it gives rise to $HCO_3^- + H^+$. In the light of all this, two points are of interest: for every mEq of HCO_3^- reabsorbed, 1 mEq of H^+ is secreted; each H^+ secreted is absorbed again in the form of H_2O. Hence, the 4500 hydrogen ions secreted to reabsorb the HCO_3^- do not pass into what constitutes the final urine.

This system of bicarbonate reabsorption and H^+ excretion should be considered as being of low gradient and of great efficiency, because 85 per cent of the

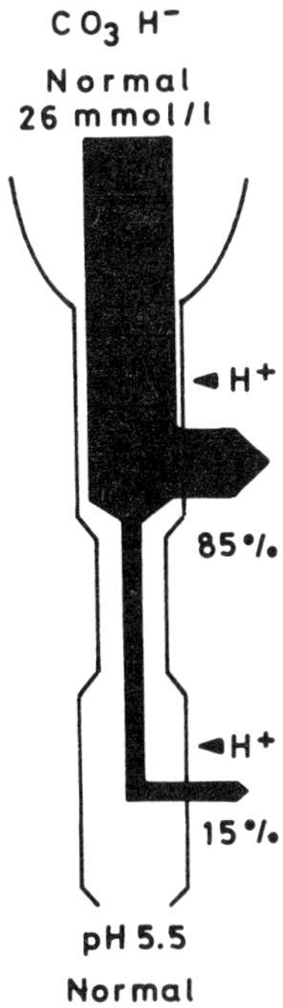

Figure 7.1 Normal renal bicarbonate reabsorption

bicarbonate filtered is reabsorbed. The reabsorption of HCO_3^- in the proximal convoluted tubule is influenced by the following:

(1) The concentration of potassium. Hypokalaemia stimulates bicarbonate reabsorption; hyperkalaemia depresses it (Relman, 1964).
(2) P_{CO_2} levels. The rise of P_{CO_2} in arterial blood is linked to an increase in bicarbonate reabsorption (Rector *et al.*, 1960; Malnic, Mello and Giebich, 1972).
(3) Extracellular volume. It has been shown that a decrease in extracellular space is related to an increase in bicarbonate. Conversely, its expansion is linked to a decrease in its reabsorption (Schwartz and Relman, 1967).
(4) Glomerular filtration. Bennet, Falkingburg and Springer (1975) have reported that by maintaining constant the three factors just considered, the reabsorption of $NaHCO_3$ is directly proportional to the glomerular filtration rate (GFR).
(5) Parathyroid hormone (PTH). This has been shown to inhibit bicarbonate reabsorption in the proximal tubule (Rodriguez-Soriano *et al.*, 1967).

In the distal tubule, the small part of the bicarbonate which escapes proximal reabsorption is reabsorbed. This is carried out in the same way as happens in the proximal tubule, except that at this level there is no CA in the tubular lumen and thus the dehydration of carbonic acid is slower.

Another essential role of the kidney is the regeneration of the consumed bicarbonate, which is accomplished by tubular secretion of H^+. For this process to occur, the presence of buffers in the urine is necessary (*Figure 7.2*). These buffers are mainly phosphate and ammonium, which upon binding to the hydrogen ions give

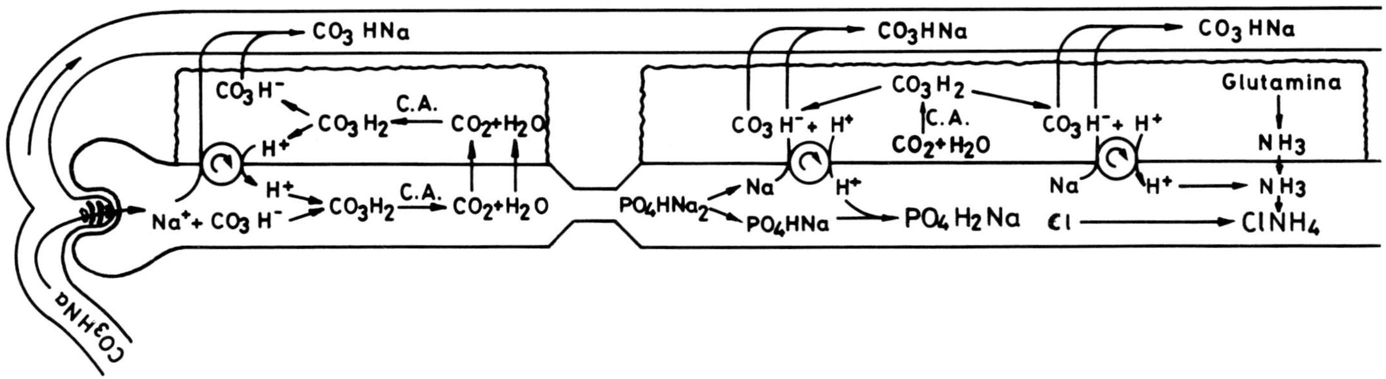

Figure 7.2 Normal renal bicarbonate reabsorption and acid excretion

rise to titratable acids and ammonium ions. It should be pointed out that although this was classically thought to take place at distal tubule level, the formation of titratable acid and NH_4 ions can already be observed at proximal level.

In contrast to the situation in the proximal tubule, H^+ regeneration in the distal tubule and collecting duct is a low capacity (only 15 per cent of the filtered bicarbonate is reabsorbed), high gradient system, since the pH of the distal tubular fluid is appreciably lower than that of the proximal tubule and therefore the difference in the H^+ concentration between the inside of the cells and the tubular lumen is greater (Morris, Sebastian and MacSherry, 1972). The difference in the concentration of hydrogen ions beyond which it is not possible to overcome the gradient is 1000 to 1, which implies a pH of 4.4 at a blood pH of 7.4 (Pitts, 1944; Relman, 1964). The possibility of overcoming such a high gradient makes the presence of CA in the distal tubule unnecessary and, in fact, absence has been demonstrated.

Titratable acid

Titratable acid (TA) is formed in the tubular lumen (*Figure 7.2*). Dibasic sodium phosphate (Na_2HPO_4) present in the urine releases a Na^+ ion which is exchanged for H^+ from the tubular cell (Pitts, 1944). The H^+ binds to the phosphate to give titratable acid in the form of monobasic sodium phosphate (NaH_2PO_4). The Na^+ ion enters the cell passively and from there it passes to the peritubular fluid where it binds to the HCO_3^- originating in the cell to give rise to sodium bicarbonate. The buffer : phosphate ratio in the urine depends on the phosphate present in the diet.

Excretion of ammonium

The second way of eliminating hydrogen ions (*Figure 7.2*) in exchange with Na^+ in the distal tubule is on the basis of NH_3, which upon combining with such hydrogen ions in the tubular lumen, is transformed into NH_4 which is then eliminated in the urine; NH_3 is synthesized in the tubular cells themselves, mainly from glutamine, alanine, glycolate, glutamic acid and other nitrogen compounds (Pitts, 1944). The diffusion of NH_3 towards the tubular lumen or towards the peritubular fluid is passive. Other factors which play a role in the synthesis and secretion of NH_3 are the intracellular serum potassium concentration, hyponatraemia, the plasma glutamic acid content and plasma aldosterone (Wrong, 1965; Goodman, Fuiz and Cahill, 1967).

The presence of buffers in the urine is essential for adeqúate H^+ excretion; without them, it would only be possible to excrete minimum amounts of H^+ ions which, since they would be free, would decrease the pH of the urine to very low values (4.0) which in turn would inhibit the secretion of new hydrogen ions (Narins, 1978).

The sum of titratable acid and ammonium ions excreted in the urine, less the bicarbonate excreted, is known as net acid excretion (NAE).

Exploratory methods for renal acidifying capacity

Together with the clinical data which can lead the physician to suspect the existence of some disturbance in renal acidification, it is also necessary to evaluate the acid-base equilibrium in blood, the urinary pH and NAE.

When a disturbance in tubular acidification exists, a hyperchloraemic metabolic acidosis in blood will become apparent. Under such circumstances, the urinary pH will show the following characteristics: it may be acid, with normal NAE values, as in the case of proximal bicarbonate wasting or type 2 renal tubular acidosis (RTA); it may be consistently higher than 6.2 with a lowered NAE, as in the case of type I or distal RTA, or it may be acid, with subnormal NAE values; this is characteristic of type 4 RTA (see below). In order to confirm diagnosis, overload tests must be carried out.

(a) Exploration of the renal capacity to secrete hydrogen ions

Before performing the test, it is necessary to eliminate the existence of urinary infection. This exploration is carried out by administration of an acute or chronic loading with ammonium chloride, calcium chloride or arginine chloride; the most commonly used substance is NH_4Cl (Wrong and Davies, 1959). The acid overload leads to metabolic acidosis and as plasma bicarbonate decreases, so does the pH of

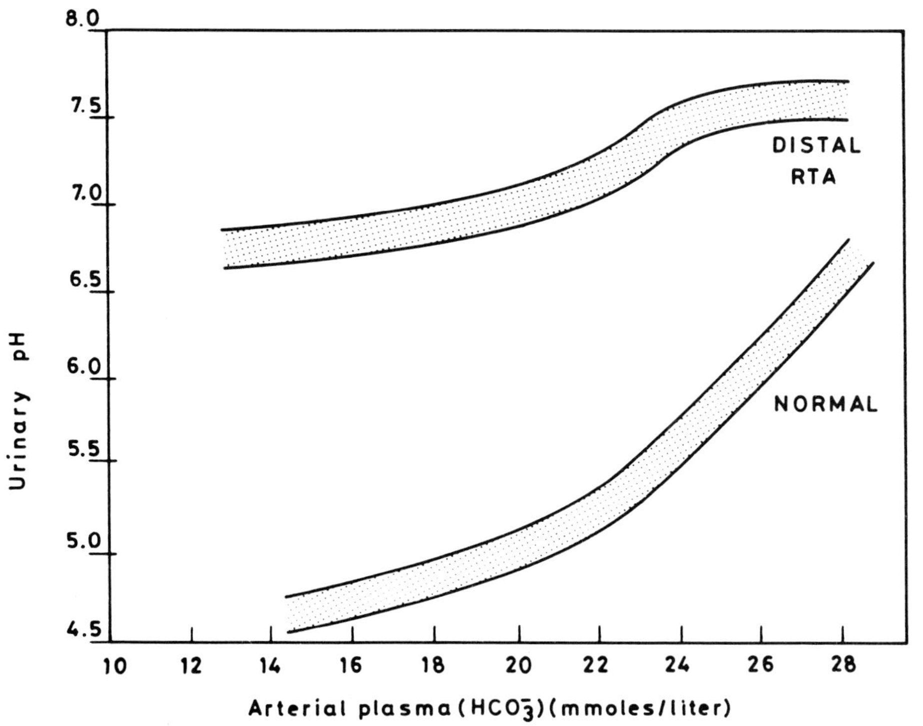

Figure 7.3 Relationship between urinary pH and plasma bicarbonate concentration in patients with distal type 1 RTA

the urine (*Figure 7.3*). In normal individuals, and according to the fall in plasma bicarbonate levels (approximately 4 mEq/l), the pH of the urine should fall below 5.2 and the levels of NH_4 and TA should reach values of 33–75 μEq/min and 24–51 μEq/min, respectively.

(b) Bicarbonate reabsorption capacity

The aim of this test is to determine the renal threshold for bicarbonate. After acidification of the internal environment by an acid load, 1M sodium bicarbonate is infused slowly, in order to avoid plasma volume expansion, and the levels of urinary bicarbonate are measured. Above a given level of plasma bicarbonate, part of the bicarbonate filtered is lost in the urine. At this level we say that the renal bicarbonate threshold has been reached. In children, under normal conditions, this point is reached at 22 mEq/l and in adults at 25–26 mEq/l of plasma bicarbonate.

Classification of types of tubular acidosis

According to physiopathological criteria, it has been traditionally admitted that two forms of RTA exist: the classical form or type 1, with tubular incapacity to excrete hydrogen ions, and the proximal form or type 2, with a defect in the proximal tubular reabsorption of bicarbonate. A third kind, type 3 or 'mixed', shows features of the two previous forms.

More recently, a fourth type (type 4) has been described in patients with CRF (Sebastian *et al.*, 1973; Perez, Oster and Vaamonde, 1974; Schambelan, Sebastian and Biglieri, 1980). This type has been interpreted as the expression of a defect in the secretion of H^+ and K^+ ions in the distal tubule and has been related to a deficit in aldosterone.

Wrong and Davies (1959) have described a kind of distal and incomplete tubular acidosis in which in basal conditions there is no metabolic acidosis and H^+ excretion is appreciably normal; but if the situation is stressed with NH_4Cl overload, the urinary pH does not fall in a similar way to normal conditions.

Distal or type 1 RTA

This process is characterized by a hyperchloraemic metabolic acidosis consecutive to the renal tubular incapacity to excrete the daily net load, with a deficit in TA and NH_4; thus the capacity to lower the urinary pH is impaired. It may have a primary, sporadic or inherited origin or may be secondary to other processes (Seldin and Wilson, 1966; Morris and Fundenberg, 1967; Buckalew *et al.*, 1974) such as (a) autoimmune diseases — of outstanding interest among these are Sjögren syndrome, SLE and primary biliary cirrhosis; (b) processes which cause nephrocalcinosis; (c) drugs — of these the most representative are amphotericin B and lithium; (d) certain other renal diseases, such as in patients receiving cadaveric kidney transplants, chronic hydronephrosis, etc., may have complete or incomplete renal tubular acidosis.

The primary defect is the tubular incapacity to establish an adequate gradient of hydrogen ions between the blood and the tubular fluid, in spite of the low levels of plasma bicarbonate.

The defect in urinary acidification is currently thought to arise as a consequence of the reduction of the distal H^+ secretory capacity. Such a reduction would be due to a renal defect in H^+ secretion or to a passive back-leak of hydrogen ions out of the tubular lumen to the cell (Halperin *et al.*, 1974; Sebastian and Morris, 1977a).

The positive balance of hydrogen ions is followed by physiopathological changes (Albright *et al.*, 1946; Pines and Mudge, 1955; Relman, 1964), such as hyperchloraemic metabolic acidosis, which induces the release of calcium from bone tissue; the excess of calcium released is eliminated by the kidney, leading to hypercalcuria, nephrolithiasis and nephrocalcinosis. The hypercalcuria is associated with elevated citrate levels in the urine. The lack of Na^+/H^+ exchange means that sodium is lost in the urine with the resulting contraction in extracellular space, which in turn leads to secondary hyperaldosteronism and hence to hypokalaemia, a classical manifestation of this process.

As a result of the urinary H^+ deficit, the urinary pH will be consistently greater than 6.0, with a low excretion of NH_4 and titratable acid and a bicarbonate excretion not greater than 3 per cent.

The clinical spectrum of distal RTA is manifested by a delay in growth (currently this can be avoided), accompanied by osteomalacia. In children, it is common to find hypercalcuria together with nephrolithiasis and nephrocalcinosis. Polyuria and hypokalaemia are frequent manifestations.

The diagnosis of distal RTA centres on the study of the urinary pH in conditions (metabolic acidosis) in which the acidification of urine should be maximum. The urinary pH is alkaline and remains thus without evident modifications after an acid overload (see *Figure 7.3*). The high pH, together with reduced plasma bicarbonate levels, leads to the diagnosis of distal RTA.

This process is controlled by continuous administration of alkaline products such as sodium bicarbonate or sodium or potassium citrate. Supplements of potassium are often necessary. The levels of urinary calcium are the most sensitive indicator for therapy and should be kept below 2 mg/kg/day.

Proximal (type 2) RTA

The disturbance in this process lies in a defect of the proximal tubule to reabsorb bicarbonate, when plasma bicarbonate levels are normal, which leads to hyperchloraemic hyperkalaemic metabolic acidosis (Rodriguez-Soriano *et al.*, 1967; Morris, 1968). This is not a very common state and although it may appear sporadically or for hereditary reasons, most cases are secondary to hereditary diseases affecting the proximal tubule (cystinosis, Wilson's syndrome, fructose intolerance, etc.) or to the use of drugs or toxic substances (outdated tetracyclines, streptozotocin, lead, etc.). These situations have also been described in states of both vitamin D_3 deficiency or dependency. Other diseases which affect the kidney, such as amyloidosis, multiple myeloma, renal transplant and medullary cystic disease can also lead to this kind of RTA (Narins, 1978).

The decrease in proximal tubular capacity to reabsorb bicarbonate means that when bicarbonate has exceeded the tubular reabsorption capacity it is lost through the urine. Up to the moment when this level of bicarbonate reabsorption is reached, all the HCO_3^- filtered is reabsorbed. Accordingly, in situations of established metabolic acidosis, NAE is normal and hence the urinary pH is acid. The diagnostic criteria for proximal or type 2 RTA involve the demonstration that urinary bicarbonate levels, after establishing normal plasma bicarbonate levels, are greater than 15 per cent of the bicarbonate filtered (Morris, 1968).

The loss of urinary bicarbonate leads to a contraction in extracellular volume, which gives rise to secondary hyperaldosteronism and the resulting hypokalaemia. The clinical symptomatology originating this process is scanty and when it occurs in children only growth retardation is observed.

The absence of manifestations such as hypercalcuria, nephrocalcinosis, renal lithiasis, bone lesions and all those disorders related to alterations in calcium metabolism, so characteristic of distal RTA in this process, is attributed to the capacity shown by the kidneys to excrete the endogenous load of acids.

Patients with proximal RTA need important amounts of alkaline substances, generally bicarbonate, to control the metabolic acidosis. Doses usually range between 3 and 5 mEq/day. The hydrochlorothiacids have been used with noteworthy success in the treatment of this process.

Mixed or type 3 RTA

There are mixed forms in which both proximal and distal defects are observed. Morris, Sebastian and MacSherry (1972) and Rodriguez-Soriano, Vallo and Garcia (1975) consider them to be not so much a different form of the previous groups, but rather variants of one of them.

Type 4 RTA

During the 1970s a new kind of renal tubular acidosis was described by Sebastian *et al.* (1973) and Perez, Oster and Vaamonde (1974), characterized by the presence of hyperchloraemic metabolic acidosis; however, this kind is associated with hyperkalaemia which is different from the other types of acidosis described. The process has mainly been described in situations of hypoaldosteronism and renal impairment (Schambelan, Sebastian and Hulter, 1978). The most frequent hypoaldosteronisms are those secondary to hyporeninism and these mainly appear in diabetic patients with a moderate to severe degree of renal impairment. They can also be present, although less commonly, in chronic renal failure, generally of interstitial origin (Perez, Siegel and Schreiner, 1972; Schambelan, Stockigt and Biglieri, 1972; Weidmann *et al.*, 1973; Brown *et al.*, 1973; Gossain *et al.*, 1973; Halperin *et al.*, 1974). This type of RTA is most frequently found in adults, and hence its interest.

Hyperkalaemia, a characteristic feature of this process, arises as a result of a deficit in aldosterone. Furthermore, diabetics have an insulin deficit which prevents the metabolism of glucose and the subsequent entry of potassium into the cell (Goldfarb *et al.*, 1976); hyperglucaemia *per se,* due to its osmotic effect, leads to the exit of potassium and water from inside the cell. In particular cases, associated with these factors there is a certain degree of renal tubular resistance to the action of mineralo-corticoid hormones (MCH) (Perez, Pelleya and Oster, 1982). Until a very pronounced degree is reached, renal impairment does not interfere with the genesis of hyperkalaemia.

The metabolic acidosis arises as a result of a tubular defect in H^+ excretion. The urinary characteristics of this process are the existence of a very low NAE, with an acid urinary pH; this is what differentiates it from the disturbance shown in type I or distal RTA. The mechanism which causes this disturbance is not due, as in the case of type I RTA, to a derangement of the secretion of hydrogen ions, nor to an incapacity to create a gradient between the cell and the tubular lumen. The process arises as a consequence of a decrease in urinary buffers, principally NH_3, which neutralize the H^+ secreted. This decrease in NH_3 is closely related to hypo-aldosteronism and the hyperkalaemia which it induces. Sebastian *et al.* (1977b) have described a close negative linear correlation between the NH_4 load in urine and serum potassium. The role of renal insufficiency in the pathogenesis of this disturbance in acidification is important. In most cases of hypoaldosteronism, renal impairment is necessary for the disturbance to become manifest (Perez, Oster and Vaamonde, 1976; Schambelan and Sebastian, 1979; Grande *et al.*, 1984). The conjunction of both processes is necessary since, separately, neither of them is able to induce the disturbance in acidification.

The origin of an acid urinary pH has not been fully elucidated. Because of the lack of sufficient urinary buffers, it is possible that small amounts of H^+ secreted could remain free and active in the urine, depressing the urinary pH considerably (Grande *et al.*, 1984). Only 0.1 mEq/l of free hydrogen ions in the urine are needed for the pH to fall to a value of 4. This could be the reason why the urinary pH is acid, in spite of the existence of metabolic acidosis.

Administration of endogenous MCH in patients with type 4 RTA ameliorates or corrects the metabolic acidosis (Sebastian *et al.*, 1977b; Schambelan and Sebastian, 1979). Furosemide, with fewer side effects, also improves the process (Sebastian, Schambelan and Sutton, 1984). Both drugs decrease the hyperkalaemia and augment urinary ammonium excretion.

Disturbances in renal tubular acidification in the elderly

Renal tubular acidification capacity, like many other renal functions, is currently being studied in the elderly. The findings reported up to the present are incomplete. Certain defects in the acidification of the urine have been described, although they have not been reported as leading to important changes in the homeostasis of the internal environment.

The first references to this problem are the reports by Shock and Yiengst (1948), who described that the pH and the CO_2 content in the blood of elderly individuals do not show any significant differences compared with a group of young controls. These data were later confirmed by all the different authors who have been involved in such research up to the present (Hilton, Goodbody and Kreusi, 1955; Adler *et al.*, 1968; Agarwal and Cabebe, 1980; Macias *et al.*, 1983).

There are, however, certain discrepancies regarding the behaviour of the aging kidney when challenged with an acid overload. In this sense, Shock and Yiengst (1948) and later Hilton, Goodbody and Kreusi (1955) described the decrease in pH and blood CO_2 content as being more intense and more prolonged in elderly subjects than in younger populations. None of these studies, however, examined the urinary acidification capacity of the kidney testing the urinary pH and NAE. Most authors (Adler *et al.*, 1968; Agarwal and Cabebe, 1980; Macias *et al.*, 1983) who later studied this particular aspect found that CO_2 levels descend in a similar way to that found in the young control groups with which the elderly subjects are compared; however, what is evident from some of these studies is that plasma bicarbonate decreases more in some groups than in others, although in an identical fashion to their control counterparts. Such differences indicate the degree of absorption of the acid, administered in an overload and generally in the form of ammonium chloride. According to a study carried out by Macias *et al.* (1983) on renal tubular bicarbonate reabsorption, elderly people reach the bicarbonate reabsorption threshold at plasma bicarbonate levels of 25.6 ± 1.6 mmol/l, similar to the young controls (25.9 ± 1.6 mmol/l).

Most authors, although not all, seem to accept that the kidney in the elderly has difficulty in getting rid of the acid overload. Adler *et al.* (1968) found that after 8 h the aging kidney excretes only 18 ± 5 per cent of the acid overload, whereas middle-aged persons excrete 30 ± 7 per cent and young persons 35 ± 6 per cent. Expressed as NAE, these data represent 100 μEq/min for young persons, compared with 39 μEq/min for the elderly. Agarwal and Cabebe (1980) described similar behaviour in persons of advanced age who showed a significantly reduced acid excretion compared with healthy young persons; one intermediate age group showed a significant decrease in NAE compared with the young persons, although it was higher, but without statistical significance, compared with the elderly group. The NAE values were: young group, 78.6 ± 3.5 μmol/min; middle-aged group, 54.5 ± 10.5 μmol/min; elderly group, 47.3 ± 7.26 μmol/min. The decrease observed in NAE is related to a lower NH_4 excretion, the excretion of titratable acid being similar to that of young persons.

The urinary pH after an acid overload in both studies showed that the urine becomes acid; however, whereas Agarwal and Cabebe (1980) observed that the difference in the fall in pH was significant (4.5 ± 0.1 for the young individuals versus 4.93 ± 0.07 for the elderly), Adler *et al.* (1968) reported that in the elderly the fall was more intense: young individuals, 4.96 ± 0.52 versus 4.85 ± 0.23 for the elderly. Although there are differences between the studies carried out, there is one common aspect and this is the apparent discordance between an acid urinary pH and a depressed NAE due to a lower NH_4 urinary excretion rate.

Similar findings to those which we have just looked at have also been described, although indirectly, by Henneman, Wallach and Dempsey (1962) when studying the effect of the acid pH of the urine as a factor which favours the formation of uric acid renal stones. These authors found that their series of patients with recurrent uric acid renal stones presented an acid urinary pH with a low NH_4 excretion rate and normal titratable acid. A NH_4Cl acid overload was seen to induce a characteristic decrease of the urinary pH, but the NH_4 excretion rate increased less intensely and more slowly than what was observed in control individuals and was disproportionately low for the urinary pH exhibited. A characteristic feature, common to all these patients, was their age — all were over 60.

The decrease in urinary NH_4 has been interpreted in different ways by different authors. According to Adler *et al.* (1968), the lower excretion of NH_4 would be the result of the decrease in glomerular filtration rate, i.e. consequent upon the decrease in functioning nephrons. In favour of such a hypothesis is the important rise taking place in NH_4 excretion when this is calculated by relating it to 100 ml of GFR. These data are in agreement with what has been reported by Wrong and Davies (1959) and Relman (1964), who showed that the decrease in NH_4 secretion in different types of renal disease was directly related to the decrease in the GFR. Simpson (1971) and Cogan and Rector (1986) have described that as functional renal mass is reduced by disease, there is an adaptative increase in ammonia production by individual nephrons in the residual parenchyma, although an important decrease in renal mass results in an absolute decrease in ammonia production.

For Agarwal and Cabebe (1980), the defect in NH_4 excretion is the result of an intrinsic tubular defect, inherent to the aging process. They arrive at this conclusion from the fact that, in their series of elderly patients, they found a significant reduction in NH_4 excretion, which was unaccompanied by a significant decrease in GFR. They also observed that when the urinary NH_4 levels are expressed relative to 100 ml of GFR, this latter parameter remained lower than that observed in young individuals. They therefore conclude that the defect in acidification is independent of GFR. The fact that this defect in acidification can already be observed in the middle-aged group of individuals suggests to them that the defect is progressive as age advances. These authors have postulated that the disturbance in acidification could be the result of a lesion of the collecting tubule, which in turn would be responsible for the defect in concentration shown by the elderly. Such a notion, however, cannot be justified since it has not been shown that the defect in concentration is consecutive to a lesion in the collecting tubule, but rather to a reduced formation of free water as Macias *et al.* (1978) have shown.

Regardless of whether this is a problem of aging which affects the tubule in its capacity to acidify the urine, or whether it is a problem related to the decrease in GFR which may appear with age, the fact is that in persons of advanced age the urinary pH falls adequately with disproportionately low NH_4 levels when the kidneys are challenged with an acid overload. The lack of H^+ excretion as NH_4 is not compensated by a higher excretion of titratable acid (Agarwal and Cabebe, 1980; Macias *et al.*, 1983). This behaviour is different from what has been reported by Pitts (1948), Milne, Stanbury and Thomson (1952) and Bricker and Fine (1981) when studying disturbances in urinary acidification. These authors have described an inverse linear correlation between the urinary pH and NH_4 excretion values; this correlation has not been observed in the elderly.

Certain factors such as plasma sodium or potassium levels, and also the nutritional status of the individuals studied, can affect the secretion of NH_3 to form NH_4 (Macias *et al.*, 1983). Hyponatraemia and deficient nutritional states have often been described in the elderly, so these factors should be taken into account when evaluating the renal tubular acidification capacity. In any case, these factors cannot be very important, since in the studies described such anomalies are not reported (Adler *et al.*, 1968; Agarwal and Cabebe, 1980; Macias *et al.*, 1983).

Aldosterone deficiency is one factor which may indeed be of importance in attempting to account for the decrease in renal NH_4 excretion in the elderly. Aldosterone deficiency can lead to a disturbance in renal tubular acidification through the following mechanisms:

(1) A decrease in the tubular reabsorption of sodium is accompanied by a decrease in the electronegativity of the tubular lumen which hinders the secretion of H^+ apart from decreasing the conductance of active protons in the distal nephron.
(2) Aldosterone deficiency has a direct effect on renal ammonia synthesis and excretion (Crabe and Nichols, 1960; Perez, Oster and Vaamonde, 1976; Hulter *et al.*, 1977; Sebastian *et al.*, 1977b; Al-Awqati, 1978; Arruda and Kurtzman, 1980).
(3) Indirectly, the decrease in extracellular volume, brought about by hypoaldosteronism, can lead through a reduction in renal blood flow and in GFR to a deficit in glutamine uptake by the tubular cell and hence to a decrease in the synthesis and secretion of NH_3 (Wrong and Davies, 1959; Schambelan, Sebastian and Biglieri, 1980).
(4) Another mechanism is through a disturbance in sodium and potassium exchange in the distal and collecting tubules. The transport of sodium in the distal nephron is the result of distal delivery of sodium on one hand, and the presence of aldosterone on the other. The hydrosaline depletion which occurs in hypoaldosteronism exacerbates sodium transport in the proximal tubule, such that the distal sodium load is low, in turn creating a decrease in the exchange of sodium for potassium and hydrogen ions. Accordingly, when adrenalectomized animals are challenged with a saline overload, favouring the exchange of sodium

for potassium and hydrogen ions, hyponatraemia decreases and the secretion of NH_4 increases to levels similar to those observed in normal animals (Hulter *et al.*, 1977; Ditella *et al.*, 1978).

(5) Hyperkalaemia, secondary to aldosterone deficiency, has also been postulated to be the responsible factor in the inhibition of NH_3 production. Tannen (1977), Sebastian *et al.* (1977b) and Schambelan and Sebastian (1979) have described an inverse linear correlation between the levels of serum potassium and renal NH_4 excretion in patients with hypoaldosteronism treated with 9α-fluorohydrocortisone. This correlation has also been described by Szylman *et al.* (1976).

In recent years the disturbance in renal acidification shown by patients suffering from hypoaldosteronism has been described (Sebastian *et al.*, 1973; Perez, Oster and Vaamonde, 1974; Kurtzman, 1983). This corresponds to a type 4 RTA which is characterized by an acid urinary pH with a poor NAE owing to a decrease in NH_4 excretion. This process is generally accompanied by a moderate degree of renal impairment. As shown by several different works dealing with renal tubular acidification in individuals of advanced age, the exact circumstances are found in this kind of patient for such a disturbance in renal acidification to arise. Accordingly, the workers who have studied the renin–angiotensin–aldosterone axis in elderly patients (Noth *et al.*, 1977; see also Chapter 4) have reported that, as age advances, aldosterone and PRA levels decrease to a level which in elderly patients is quite significant compared with young populations. The studies which have examined renal tubular acidification (Adler *et al.*, 1968; Agarwal and Cabebe, 1980; Macias *et al.*, 1983) have shown that the urinary pH in elderly patients, following an acid overload, is strongly acid, although with a reduced NAE owing to a reduced renal excretion of NH_4. Furthermore, in persons older than 40, it has been shown that the GFR decreases; this may become significant in the elderly, and in some of them may even lead to moderate renal impairment (Davies and Shock, 1950; Macias *et al.*, 1981).

The fact that in the elderly there is no repercussion on the internal environment, in spite of there being urinary data in favour of a possible defect in renal tubular acidification owing to a deficit in aldosterone, could be related to the intensity of the process. As has been pointed out, for aldosterone deficiency to become manifest as renal tubular acidosis, with metabolic acidosis, the conjunction of hypoaldosteronism and CRF is necessary. In the patients studied by the authors mentioned above, the age ranges were wide, which could mean that the degree of hypoaldosteronism was not homogeneous. Although these patients have a significant reduction in GFR with respect to the young population, they mostly present acceptable GFR levels and only a few of them show a GFR as decreased as that observed in patients diagnosed with type 4 RTA (Grande *et al.*, 1984).

Another factor which could influence the lack of clinical expression in this process is the absence of potassium retention in the elderly. It is a generally accepted (although unexplained) fact that elderly people exhibit a decrease in total body potassium (Lye, 1981) with a low plasma potassium level. As has been pointed out above, the rise in serum potassium is one of the most important factors through which aldosterone deficiency inhibits ammonia production and secretion. The incidence of these three factors would mean that under basal conditions the elderly would not show any overt manifestation in their acid-base balance and that the deficit in H^+ excretion would only become apparent after an acid overload. This clinical situation could be called an incomplete form of type 4 RTA.

Although persons of advanced age have the necessary capacity to present these disturbances, it is pertinent to evaluate together all the factors which may intervene, before accepting or discarding such a hypothesis.

Renal handling of glucose

The glucose freely filtered in the glomerulus is almost entirely reabsorbed in the proximal convoluted tubule. Of the 180 g of glucose filtered each day, less than 180 mg will be found in the urine. The reabsorption of glucose takes place in the S1 segment of the proximal convoluted tubule, and this is closely related to the reabsorption of sodium; such that if the tubular fluid did not contain Na^+, only a small part of the glucose would be reabsorbed and vice versa.

The fact that glucose is reabsorbed against a concentration gradient suggests that it is governed by an active transport mechanism; in fact, it is linked to the transport of sodium and has thus been called secondary active transport. The dependence of the reabsorption of glucose and of other solutes on the presence of sodium can be seen in

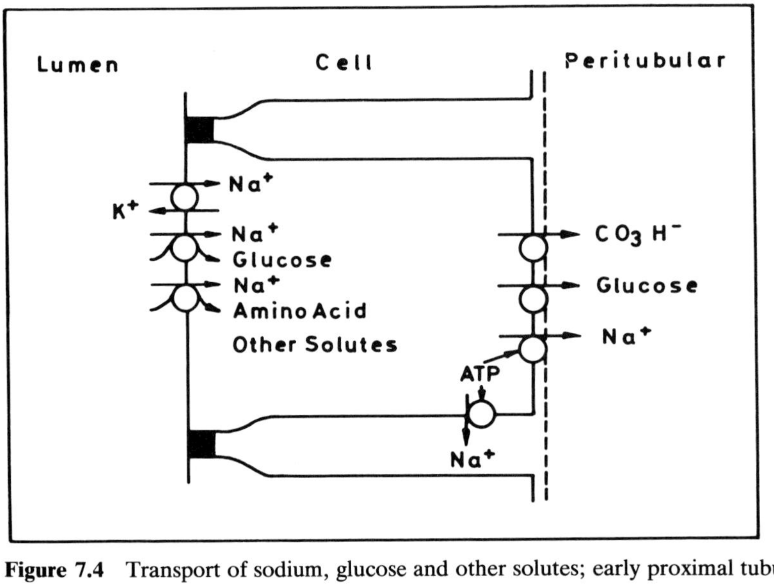

Figure 7.4 Transport of sodium, glucose and other solutes; early proximal tubular

Figure 7.4. Sodium transport occurs in two steps, located respectively in peritubular and intercellular and in the cell lumen membranes. At peritubular and intercellular level, a 'sodium pump' or Na^+–K^+ATPase-dependent pump actively transports sodium from the inside of the cell to the peritubular fluid. The primary step in sodium transport lowers the concentration of cell sodium, thus providing a sodium concentration difference from lumen to cell. At the same time, the exit of cell sodium also causes the voltage to be negative. The difference in concentration and voltage produced are the driving forces which favour the passive transport of sodium from the tubular lumen to the interior of the cell.

Such passive reabsorption of sodium is linked to the reabsorption of glucose. It is accepted that the same carriers which transport glucose into the cell are used by sodium. These carriers, situated on the luminal cell membrane, have binding sites for glucose and sodium. When such binding sites are facing the lumen, they capture both elements. Translocation of the carriers such that they face the inside of the cell leads to the entrance of sodium and glucose. The secondary active transport of glucose means that its intracellular concentration is high. The high intracellular concentration drives the passive exit of these substances from the cell at the peritubular border. Permeability to these solutes is high at the peritubular border, facilitating this step. The high permeability to glucose at the peritubular membrane is provided by a carrier that is not dependent on sodium (Silverman, 1976).

Other solutes such as amino acids use similar mechanisms for their tubular reabsorption, although the carriers are different. All the carriers can at some point become completely saturated by an excess of substrate to be transported. At this point, the tubular cell has reached the maximum transport capacity (T_m) for that particular product and all of it which cannot be reabsorbed is lost in the urine. Each substrate has its own T_m.

The mechanism of glucose reabsorption reaches saturation when plasma glucose levels rise to values above 150–180 mg/dl, which represents a filtered load of 300–375 mg/min of glucose. However, before saturation of glucose transport is reached, the sugar begins to appear in the urine. The level of filtered glucose at which it begins to appear in the urine is said to be the glucose renal tubular threshold; from this moment onwards, the loss of glucose in urine is progressive and total saturation of the transport mechanism is reached (T_mG). Above this level all the glucose filtered is lost in the urine.

Most of the nephrons are saturated over a relatively narrow glucose concentration range. This means that maximum glucose transport is fairly constant in normal subjects. However, T_mG varies with the changes in Na^+ reabsorption taking place in the proximal tubule. T_mG varies directly with the glomerular filtration rate; a saline overload depresses the T_m of glucose, whereas contraction of the extracellular volume stimulates it. All this indicates that there is no absolutely constant value for the T_mG, but rather that it depends on the prevailing clinical situation.

Glucosuria can occur in any situation which involves a rise in plasma glucose concentrations and which implies a saturation of the tubular mechanisms of glucose transport. The appearance of glucose in the urine arises when glycaemia is higher than the T_mG. Diabetes mellitus is a characteristic example of glucosuria due to saturation.

Glucosuria can also arise secondary to a disturbance in glucose transport, which may either be congenital or acquired. This abnormality is known as renal glucosuria.

Modifications in renal handling of glucose with age

Few authors have devoted much attention to the renal handling of glucose in elderly people. In a study carried out by Macias *et al.* (1979) it was observed that the glucose reabsorption threshold was normal in 10 patients with an age range of 65–75 years. Only the work by Miller, McDonald and Shock (1952) is outstanding, in which the maximum glucose transport in persons of different ages with a range of 20–90 years was studied. From their work, it can be seen that a decrease takes place in T_mG parallel to the increase in age, varying from a mean value of 358.7 mg/min/litre/1.73 m^2 in the third decade of life to 219 mg/min/litre/1.73 m^2 in the ninth decade, with an inverse linear correlation between age and the T_mG; the percentage annual decrease was about 0.68 per cent. Upon comparing the decrease in T_mG with the drop in glomerular filtrate, it may be seen that the regression of both is very similar with respect to age. Furthermore, the GFR : T_mG ratio of glucose remains constant throughout the individual's lifespan.

All these data show that the progressive decrease in tubular reabsorption of glucose is related to the progressive loss of other renal functions, and mainly to the GFR. The fact that the GFR : T_mG ratio remains normal means that the functioning nephrons are working at normal capacity, and that the problem lies in the fact that their number decreases with age. These findings are in agreement with what was reported by Bricker, Morrin and Kime (1960) as the 'intact nephron hypothesis', according to which parallel to the decrease in renal function, whatever its cause, some nephrons undergo a serious degree of morphological and functional deterioration, whereas others which remain 'intact' undergo morphological and functional adaptations with normal or even increased functional capacity.

Although from a pathophysiological point of view this disturbance is not of very great importance, it can be of considerable interest from the point of view of everyday clinical practice. It should be taken into account that in situations of a discrete rise in glycaemia, elderly persons show a greater tendency to glucosuria than their younger counterparts at equivalent blood glucose concentrations, owing to the decrease in their T_mG. This does not mean that the person in question is diabetic, and hence in the elderly individual with glucosuria, plasma glucose levels should be monitored before starting treatment with oral hypoglucaemiant agents or with insulin. Even in the case of diabetics, this disturbance in tubular glucose reabsorption should be born in mind. Elderly patients whose diabetes is acceptably under control may have glucosuria. All this points to the notion that in all cases of diabetic or non-diabetic glucosuria, the plasma glucose levels should be evaluated.

References

ADLER, S., LINDEMAN, R.D., YIENGST, M.J., BEARD, E. and SHOCK, N.W. (1968). Effect of acute acid loading on urinary acid excretion by the aging human kidney. *Journal of Laboratory and Clinical Medicine,* **72,** 278–289

AGARWAL, B.N. and CABEBE, F.G. (1980). Renal acidification in elderly subjects. *Nephron,* **26,** 291–295

AL-AWQATI, Q. (1978). H^+ transport in urinary epithelia. *American Journal of Physiology,* **235,** F77–F78

AL-AWQATI, Q., NORBY, L.H., MUELLER, A. and STEINMETZ, P.R. (1976). Characteristics of stimulation of H^+ transport by aldosterone in turtle urinary bladder. *Journal of Clinical Investigation,* **58,** 351–358

ALBRIGHT, F., BURNETT, C.H., PARSON, W., REIFENSTEIN, E.C. Jr. and ROSS, A. (1946). Osteomalacia and late rickets: the various etiologies met in the United States with emphasis on that resulting from a specific form of renal acidosis, the therapeutic indication for each etiological subgroup, and the relationship between osteomalacia and Milkman's syndrome. *Medicine,* **25,** 339–479

ARRUDA, J.A.L., BALLE, D.E., SEHY, J.T., ROSEMAN, N.K., BORONOWSKI, R.L. and KURTZMAN, N.A. (1981). Hyperkalemia and renal insufficiency: role of selective aldosterone deficiency and tubular unresponsiveness to aldosterone. *American Journal of Nephrology,* **1,** 160–167

ARRUDA, J.A.L. and KURTZMAN, N.A. (1980). Mechanism and classification of deranged distal urinary acidification. *American Journal of Physiology,* **239,** 515–523

BENNET, C., FALKINGBURG, N. and SPRINGER, P. (1975). Glomerulo-tubular balance for bicarbonate in man. *Nephron,* **14,** 237–241

BRICKER, N.S. and FINE, L.G. (1981). The renal response to progressive nephron loss. In *The Kidney,* 2nd edn, edited by B. Brenner and F. Rector Jr., 1084 pp. Philadelphia; Saunders

BRICKER, N.S., MORRIN, P.A.F. and KIME, S.W. Jr. (1960). The pathologic physiology of chronic Bright's disease. An exposition of the 'intact nephron hypothesis'. *American Journal of Medicine,* **28,** 77–98

BROWN, J.J., CHINN, R.H., FRASER, R., LEVER, A.F., MORTON, J.J., ROBERTSON, J.J. *et al.* (1973). Recurrent hyperkalaemia due to selective aldosterone deficiency: correction by angiotensin infusion. *British Medical Journal,* **1,** 650–655

BUCKALEW, V.M., PURVIS, M.L., SHULMAN, M.G., HERNDON, C.N. and RUDMAN, D. (1974). Hereditary renal tubular acidosis. *Medicine (Baltimore),* **53,** 229–234

COGAN, M.G. and RECTOR, F.G. (1986). Acid-base disorders. In *The Kidney,* 3rd edn, edited by B. Brenner and F.G. Rector, pp. 457–518. Philadelphia; Saunders

CRABBE, J. and NICHOLS, G. (1960). Effect of adrenalectomy, aldosterone and dehydration on electrolyte metabolism of rat cortex slices. *American Journal of Physiology,* **199,** 871–875

DAVIES, D.F. and SHOCK, N.W. (1950). Age changes in glomerular filtration rate, effective renal plasma flow, and tubular excretory capacity in adult males. *Journal of Clinical Investigation,* **29,** 496–507

DITELLA, P.G., SODHI, B., McCREARY, J., ARRUDA, J.A.L. and KURTZMAN, N.A. (1978). Mechanism of metabolic acidosis of selective mineralocorticoid deficiency. *Kidney International,* **14,** 466–477

GOLDFARB, S., COX, M., SINGER, I. and GOLDBERG, M. (1976). Acute hyperkalemia induced by hyperglycemia: hormonal mechanisms. *Annals of Internal Medicine,* **84,** 426–432

GOODMAN, A.E., FUIZ, R.E. and CAHILL, G.F. (1967). Renal gluconeogenesis in acidosis, alkalosis and potassium deficiency; its possible role in regulation of renal ammonium production in dog and rat. *American Journal of Physiology,* **213,** 969–975

GOSSAIN, N.V., FERRARA, E.V., WERKE, E., SRIVASTAVA, L., PRIVIRETA, P.J. and HANENSON, I. (1973). Impaired renin responsiveness with secondary hypoaldosteronism. *Archives of Internal Medicine,* **132,** 885–890

GRANDE, J., MACIAS, J.F., MIRALLES, J.M. and TABERNERO, J.M. (1984). Plasma renin activity, plasma aldosterone and distal urinary acidification in diabetics with chronic renal failure. In *Proceedings of the European Dialysis and Transplant Association — European Renal Association* (Florence 1984), edited by A.M. Davison and P.J. Guillou, vol. 21, pp. 801–807. London; Pitman

HALPERIN, M.L., GOLDSTEIN, M.B., HAIG, A., JOHNSON, M.D. and STINEBAUG, H. (1974). Studies on the pathogenesis of type I (distal) renal tubular acidosis as revealed by urinary PCO_2 tension. *Journal of Clinical Investigation,* **53,** 669–677

HENNEM, P.H., WALLACH, S. and DEMPSEY, E. (1962). The metabolic defect responsible for uric acid stone formation. *Journal of Clinical Investigation,* **41,** 537–542

HILTON, G.F., GOODBODY, M.F. and KREUSI, O.R. (1955). The effect of prolonged administration of ammonium chloride on the blood acid-base equilibrium of geriatric subjects. *Journal of the American Geriatrics Society,* **3,** 697–703

HULTER, H.N., ILMICKI, L.P., HARBOTTLE, J.A. and SEBASTIAN, A. (1977). Impaired renal H^+ secretion and NH_3 production in mineralocorticoid-deficient glucocorticoid-replete dogs. *American Journal of Physiology,* **232,** F136–F146

KURTZMAN, N.A. (1983). Acquired distal renal tubular acidosis. *Kidney International,* **24,** 807–819

LENNON, E.J. and LEMAN, J. JR. (1966). Defense of hydrogen ion concentration in chronic metabolic acidosis. *Annals of Internal Medicine,* **65,** 265–271

LYE, M. (1981). Distribution of body potassium in healthy elderly subjects. *Gerontology,* **27,** 286–292

MACIAS, J.F., GARCIA, C., BONDIA, A., RODRIGUEZ, J.L., CORBACHO, L., TABERNERO, J.M. *et al.* (1978). Renal handling of sodium in old people: a functional study. *Age and Ageing,* **7,** 178–181

MACIAS, J.F., GARCIA, C., TABERNERO, J.M., BONDIA, A., RODRIGUEZ, J.L., CORBACHO, L. *et al.* (1981). Estudio del filtrado glomerular en viejos sanos. *Revista Española de Geriatria y Gerontologia,* **16,** 113–117

MACIAS, J.F., GARCIA, C., TABERNERO, J.M., BONDIA, A., RODRIGUEZ, J.L., CORBACHO, L. *et al.* (1983). Comportamiento del riñon del viejo en la sobrecarga de acidos. *Nefrologia,* **3,** 11–16

MACIAS, J.F., GARCIA, C., TABERNERO, J.M., RODRIGUEZ, J.L., CORBACHO, L., BONDIA, A. *et al.* (1979). Estudio de la reabsorcion de glucosa en el viejo. En *Proceedings de X Congreso Espanol de Geriatria.* Santiago de Compostela, 1979, 585 pp. Barcelona; Graficas Poutica

MALNIC, G., MELLO, G. and GIEBICH, G. (1972). Micropuncture study of renal tubular hydrogen ion transport in the rat. *American Journal of Physiology,* **222,** 147–153

MILLER, J.H., McDONALD, R.K. and SHOCK, N.W. (1952). Age changes in the maximal rate of renal tubular reabsorption of glucose. *Journal of Gerontology,* **7,** 196–200

MILNE, M.D., STANBURY, S.W. and THOMSON, A.E. (1952). Observations on the Fanconi syndrome and renal hyperchloraemic acidosis in adults. *Quarterly Journal of Medicine,* **21,** 61–68

MORRIS, R.C. Jr. (1968). An experimental renal acidification defect in patients with hereditary fructose intolerance. II Its distinction from classic renal tubular acidosis: its resemblance to the renal acidification defect associated with the Fanconi Syndrome of children with cystinosis. *Journal of Clinical Investigation,* **47,** 1648–1663

MORRIS, R.C. Jr. and FUNDENBERG, H.H. (1967). Impaired renal acidification in patients with hypergamma globulinemia. *Medicine (Baltimore),* **46,** 57–79

MORRIS, R.C., SEBASTIAN, A. and MacSHERRY, E. (1972). Renal acidosis. *Kidney International,* **1,** 322–340

NARINS, R.G. (1978). The renal acidosis. In *Acid-base and Potassium Homeostasis,* edited by B. Brenner and J.H. Stein, *Contemporary Issues in Nephrology,* Vol. 2, pp. 30–64. New York; Churchill Livingstone

NOTH, R.H., LASSMAN, M.N., TAN, S.Y., FERNANDEZ CRUZ, A. Jr. and MULROW, P.J. (1977). Age and renin aldosterone system. *Archives of Internal Medicine,* **137,** 1414–1417

PEREZ, G.O., OSTER, J.R. and VAAMONDE, C.A. (1974). Renal acidosis in renal potassium handling in selective hypoaldosteronism. *American Journal of Medicine,* **57,** 809–816

PEREZ, G.O., OSTER, J.R. and VAAMONDE, C.A. (1976). Renal acidification in patients with mineralocorticoid deficiency. *Nephron,* **17,** 461–473

PEREZ, G.O., PELLEYA, R. and OSTER, J.R. (1982). Renal tubular hyperkalemia. *American Journal of Nephrology,* **2,** 109–114

PEREZ, G., SIEGEL, L. and SCHREINER, G.E. (1972). Selective hypoaldosteronism with hyperkalemia. *Annals of Internal Medicine,* **76,** 757–763

PINES, K. and MUDGE, G.H. (1955). Renal tubular acidosis with osteomalacia: report of three cases. *American Journal of Medicine,* **11,** 302–311

PITTS, R. (1944). *Physiology of the Kidney and Body Fluids,* 3rd edn. Chicago; Year Book

PITTS, R. (1948). The renal excretion of acid. *Federation Proceedings,* **7,** 418–423

RECTOR, F.C., SELDIN, D.W., ROBERTS, A.D. and SMITH, J.S. (1960). The role of plasma CO_2 tension and carbonic-anhydrase activity in the renal absorption of bicarbonate. *Journal of Clinical Investigation,* **39,** 1706–1712

RELMAN, A.S. (1964). Renal acidosis and renal excretion of acid in health and disease. *Archives of Internal Medicine,* **12,** 295–347

RODRIGUEZ-SORIANO, J., BIOCHES, H., STARK, H. and EDLEMAN, C.M. Jr. (1967). Proximal renal tubular acidosis: a defect in bicarbonate reabsorption with normal urinary acidification. *Pediatric Research,* **1,** 81–98

RODRIGUEZ-SORIANO, J., VALLO, A. and GARCIA FUENTES, M. (1975). Distal renal tubular acidosis in infancy: a bicarbonate wasting state. *Journal of Pediatrics,* **86,** 528–534

SCHAMBELAN, M., STOCKIGT, J.R. and BIGLIERI, E.G. (1972). Isolated hypoaldosteronism in adults. A renin-deficiency syndrome. *New England Journal of Medicine,* **287,** 573–578

SCHAMBELAN, M. and SEBASTIAN, A. (1979). Hyporeninemic hypoaldosteronism. *Archives of Internal Medicine,* **24,** 385–405

SCHAMBELAN, M., SEBASTIAN, A. and BIGLIERI, E.G. (1980). Prevalence, pathogenesis and functional significance of aldosterone deficiency in hyperkalemic patients with chronic renal insufficiency. *Kidney International,* **7,** 89–101

SCHAMBELAN, M., SEBASTIAN, A. and HULTER, H.N. (1978). Mineralocorticoid excess and deficiency syndromes. In *Acid-base and Potassium Homeostasis,* edited by B. Brenner and J.H. Stein, *Contemporary Issues in Nephrology,* Vol. 2, pp. 232–268. New York: Churchill Livingstone

SCHWARTZ, W.B. and RELMAN, A.S. (1967). Effect of electrolyte disorders on renal structure and function. *New England Journal of Medicine,* **276,** 452–457

SEBASTIAN, A. and MORRIS, R.C. Jr. (1977a). Renal tubular acidosis. *Clinical Nephrology,* **7,** 216–230

SEBASTIAN, A., McSHERRY, E., SCHAMBELAN, M., BIGLIERI, E. and MORRIS, R.C. (1973). Renal tubular acidosis (RTA) in patients with hypoaldosteronism caused by renin deficiency. *Clinical Research,* **21,** 706–714

SEBASTIAN, A., SCHAMBELAN, M., LIDENFELD, S. and MORRIS, R.C. Jr. (1977b). Amelioration of metabolic acidosis with fluorocortisone therapy in hyporeninemic hypoaldosteronism. *New England Journal of Medicine,* **297,** 576–583

SEBASTIAN, A., SCHAMBELAN, N. and SUTTON, J.M. (1984). Amelioration of hyperchloremic acidosis with furosemide therapy in patients with chronic renal insufficiency and type 4 renal tubular acidosis. *American Journal of Medicine,* **4,** 287–300

SELDIN, D. and WILSON, J.D. (1966). Renal tubular acidosis. In *The Metabolic Basis of Inherited Disease,* edited by J.B. Stanbury, S.B. Wyngaarden and D.S. Frederickson, pp. 1230–1246. New York; McGraw-Hill

SHOCK, N.W. and YIENGST, M.J. (1948). Experimental displacement of the acid-base equilibrium of the blood in aged males. *Federation Proceedings,* **7,** 114–119

SILVERMAN, M. (1976). Glucose transport in the kidney. *Biochemica et Biophysica Acta,* **457,** 303–308

SIMPSON, D.P. (1971). Control of hydrogen ion homeostasis and renal acidosis. *Medicine (Baltimore),* **50,** 503–542

SZYLMAN, P., BETTER, O.S., CHAIMOWITZ, C. and ROSLER, A. (1976). Role of hyperkalemia in the metabolic acidosis of isolated hypoaldosteronism. *New England Journal of Medicine,* **294,** 361–365

TANNEN, R.L. (1977). Relationship of renal ammonia production and potassium homeostasis. *Kidney International,* **11,** 453–456

WEIDMANN, P.P., REINHART, R., MAXWELL, M.H., ROWE, P., COBURN, J.W. and MASSRY, S.G. (1973). Syndrome of hyporeninemic hypoaldosteronism and hyperkalemia in renal disease. *Journal of Clinical Endocrinology and Metabolism,* **36,** 965–977

WRONG, O. (1965). Urinary hydrogen ion excretion. *Journal of Clinical Pathology,* **18,** 520–527

WRONG, O. and DAVIES, H.E. (1959). The excretion of acid in renal disease. *Quarterly Journal of Medicine,* **28,** 259–313

Chapter 8

Changes in renal function and morphology in aging laboratory animals

José M. López Novoa and Inmaculada Montañes

Introduction

During the last century the average life expectancy has shown an upward trend in developing countries, and the elderly constitute a growing proportion of the population in these countries (see the Preface, pp. xi–v). Among the diseases responsible for the morbidity and mortality in this sector of the population, renal diseases occupy an important place. The literature contains a number of clinical studies dealing with the impairment of renal function in aging patients. However, the studies dealing with age-related changes in the structure and function of laboratory animals are scarce and scattered, and only a few topics from among the functional alterations such as proteinuria or impairment of the concentrating ability have been adequately studied. The purpose of this chapter is thus to review these studies in an attempt to give a unifying version of the phenomena described.

Studies of the spontaneous modification in structure and function of the kidney with aging in laboratory animals are important, not only because they serve as models of aging, leading to a more precise knowledge of the biochemical and molecular mechanism which induces such an alteration, together with a better control of the experimental procedures than in human studies, but also because in long-term studies on laboratory animals, the investigator must know what changes are due to the factor under study and what must be attributed to the natural senescence of the animal.

Most of the studies on this topic have been performed on albino laboratory rats, probably because of their relatively low cost, easy maintenance, adequate body size, well-established 'normal' renal function and short lifespan. It must be remembered, however, that the rat kidney differs from its human counterpart in many important respects, especially those involving medullary function.

Spontaneous kidney disease in aging rats, first reported early in this century (McCoy, 1908), has been subsequently described for all the most used strains: Sprague–Dawley (Ashworth, Erdmann and Arnold, 1960; Gray, 1963; Foley, Jones and Osborn, 1964; Berg, 1965; Bolton, Benton, Maclay *et al.*, 1976), Wistar (Arataki, 1926; Andrew and Pruett, 1957; Pollard and Kajima, 1970; Elema, Koudstaal and Arends, 1971), Fisher 344 (Bolton, Benton and Maclay, 1976; Coleman *et al.*, 1977), Lewis (Bell *et al.*, 1984) and other less used strains of this species.

The most evident effects of this spontaneous nephropathy is proteinuria, which begins at maturity and increases continuously with age. There is also a reduction in the glomerular filtration rate and renal blood flow and impairment in the urinary concentrating mechanisms, although the animal generally dies of non-renal problems.

Microscopically, the changes are consistent in the strains studied. In brief, the lesion is focal and segmental, affecting both glomeruli and tubules. The glomerular disease is characterized by a thickening of the capillary basement membrane and Bowman's capsule, an increase in mesangial matrix, segmental sclerosis of isolated capillary loops and, later, segments of tufts; finally, hyalinization and sclerosis of the glomeruli are observed. Adhesion between tufts and Bowman's capsule, glomerular crescents and protein precipitates into Bowman's space are also common findings. Tubular lesions are characterized by epithelial atrophy and secondary hyperplasia, cast formation and tubule obstruction, with massive dilatation and, finally, fibrotic degeneration. The interstitium is infiltrated with mononuclear cells and also becomes fibrotic. All these changes will be detailed later in this chapter.

There is no marked heterogeneity in the severity and the time course of the lesions among the different strains of laboratory rats. Thus, the inbred Lewis strain was seen to develop little proteinuria and few morphological changes with age, whereas in the Fisher 344 strain these alterations appear at an accelerated rate; the Sprague–Dawley and Wistar strains show an intermediate behaviour.

The renal lesions associated with age are also sex- and diet-dependent. Male animals are much more likely to develop the disease than females, an aspect first described by Blatherwick and Medlar (1937), and subsequently confirmed by several workers (Sellers *et al.*, 1950; Linkswiler, Reynolds and Baumann, 1952). When male rats are castrated before puberty, protein excretion is similar to that recorded in females. However, when castrated as adults, protein excretion falls, although it remains abnormal (Linkswiler, Reynolds and Baumann, 1952). Androgen therapy increases protein excretion in both castrated males and normal females, whereas adrenalectomy decreases spontaneous proteinuria in males, but not in females, and blocks renin-induced proteinuria (Addis *et al.*, 1950).

Another factor that plays a major role in the development of spontaneous renal lesions with age is the diet, especially with respect to protein intake. In 1928, Newburg and Curtis observed that a diet enriched with beef liver produced several renal lesions in their laboratory rats. Blatherwick and Medlar (1937) and Medlar and Blatherwick (1937) extended these observations and also noted spontaneous, although less severe, lesions in their control rats given a standard diet. Saxton and Kimball (1941) focused their attention on the association between aging and nephrosis in the rat, confirming the effect of a high protein diet in accelerating the process.

Since these early reports, numerous studies have focused on the effect of diet on the spontaneous nephrosis associated with age, confirming that rats fed a high protein diet develop nephropathy at an earlier age and with greater severity than rats allowed a standard diet and that food (protein)-restricted rats were partially protected from such renal damage (Rumsfeld, 1956; Kennedy, 1957; Simms and Berg, 1957; Berg and Simms, 1960; Wachtel, Cole and Rosen, 1966; Lalich, Faith and Harding, 1970; Lalich and Allen, 1971; Elema and Arends, 1975; Tucker, Mason and Beauchene, 1976).

The influence of diet in this 'disease' of aging is much more evident in males than in females (Sellers *et al.*, 1950; Linkwiler, Reynolds and Baumann, 1952; Elema and Arends, 1975). Unilateral nephrectomy accelerates the appearance of the lesion in both sexes in all the rat strains studied, although this acceleration is seen to

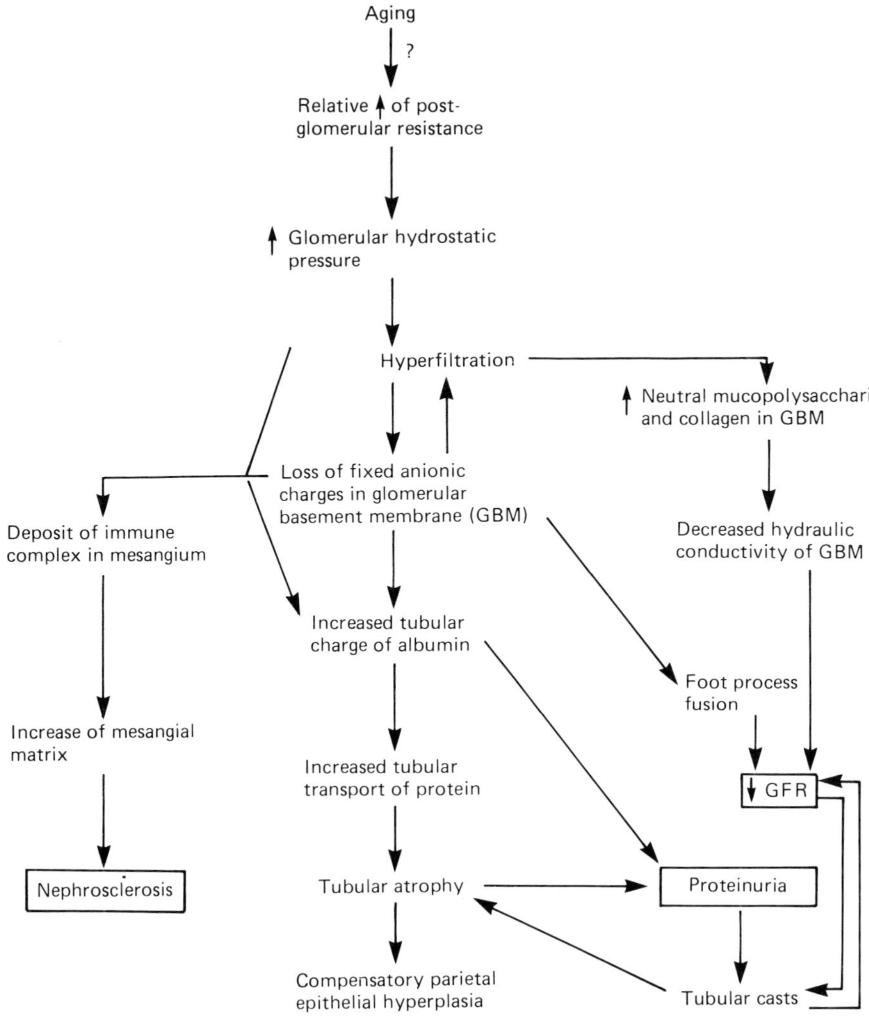

Figure 8.1 Hypothetical physiopathological mechanism of nephrosclerosis and proteinuria in aging rats

be greater in young than in old animals (Moore and Hellman, 1930; Kennedy, 1957; Wachtel, Cole and Rosen, 1966; Lalich and Allen, 1971; Striker *et al.*, 1969).

Radiation also enhances the development of renal lesions, especially in the uninephrectomized animal (Wachtel, Cole and Rosen, 1966); this has also been observed in the Chinese hamster (Guttman and Kohn, 1960).

In the following pages we shall review the changes produced in laboratory animals by the aging process, together with the physiopathology of such alterations. *Figure 8.1* schematically represents the relationship between the functional and morphological changes described in the text.

Histological changes

Among the studies reviewed there is complete agreement that in laboratory rats over 1 year of age (about one-half of the lifespan in this species) the kidney shows a great number of structural changes. This observation had already been reported early in this century (McCoy, 1908). These changes have been described in both Sprague–Dawley and Wistar strains, as well as in other less common strains such as Fisher 344 or WAG I Rij rats. However, the precise age of the appearance of structure abnormalities in the laboratory rat has not been fully elucidated and may be obscured by the differences between sexes and the animal strains studied.

It is of considerable significance that, according to several authors, abnormalities in the renal corpuscle and tubule of male rats have been noted as early as 3 months of age (young adult animals) (Hirokawa, 1975; Bolton *et al.*, 1976), whereas others (Haley and Bulger, 1983) are not of this opinion. However, pathological changes are much more common by 12 months of age (Berg, 1965; Gray, Weaver and Purmalis, 1974; Kraus and Cain, 1974; Couser and Stilmant, 1975; Bolton *et al.*, 1976).

Glomerulus

Most of the histological studies of the aging rat have reported simplification or *fusion of the foot processes of the podocytes* (Gray, Weaver and Purmalis, 1974; Kraus and Cain, 1974; Causer and Stilmant, 1975; Hirokawa, 1975). However, Haley and Bulger (1983) reported that in 12-month-old male Sprague–Dawley rats, podocytic cell bodies, pedicels and even foot processes were essentially normal in size, shape and space.

The observation of the fusion of foot processes in aging rats is not surprising in view of the fact that proteinuria is commonly found in rats from the fifth month of life and increases with age (Neuhaus and Flory, 1978) and foot process fusion has been observed in many forms of kidney diseases associated with proteinuria (Brenner, Hostetter and Humes, 1978). This process, also termed 'effacement', occurs when the complex relationship between individual foot processes of the visceral epithelial cells are replaced by a continuous band of cytoplasm adjacent to the lamina rara externa of the basal membrane; the mechanism of this structural alteration is not completely understood. However, Seiler, Venkatachalam and Cotran (1975) have recently demonstrated in the rat kidney that intra-arterial infusion of polycationic substances such as protamine sulphate, which interacts with membrane-associated anionic sites, causes structural alterations of the visceral epithelial cells very similar to foot process fusion. It should also be noted that regions without the normal structure of alternating foot processes along short segments of the basement membrane, especially near the mesangial region between adjacent capillary loops, have been observed in normal glomeruli (Jörgensen, 1966).

Although proteinuria will be dealt with specifically in another part of this chapter, it should be mentioned here that in the paper of Haley and Bulger (1983) in which foot process fusion was not observed in 12-month-old rats, the proteinuria reported was markedly lower than in other reports with rats of the same age (Neuhaus and Flory, 1978). In addition, Haley and Bulger (1983), using scanning electron microscopy, reported that many areas which in young rats are occupied by pedicels and trabeculae, appeared to be replaced with an amorphous veil of cytoplasm in old animals. Transmission electron microscopy reveals that the thin cytoplasmic extensions observed by scanning microscopy originate from both cell bodies and primary processes and overlay podocytic cell bodies and pedicels. The space enclosed by these cytoplasmic expansions was clearly extracellular. Similar structures have been described by Elias *et al.* (1964) and later by Yoshinary and Fujita (1982) in the rabbit. In the original description of Elias *et al.* (1964) these structures were termed 'podocytic membranes' since they appeared as attenuated portions of the podocytic cell body; under each membrane was observed a 'subpodocytic lacuna', the floor of which was formed by pedicels. The authors suggested that the membrane could form a second filtration barrier. However, in later studies, Yoshinary and Fujita (1982) disagreed with this suggestion, reporting that podocytic membranes appeared as flattened extensions of primary processes which formed broad cytoplasmic bands over the pedicels and provided no impediment to the filtration.

In the rat, structures similar to the podocytic membranes, but unrelated to aging, have been described by Kondo, Takizawa and Akikusa (1981) in Sprague–Dawley rats undergoing chronic nephrotoxic nephritis. These animals showed a kind of cyst formed by dome-like extensions of primary podocyte processes.

Parietal epithelium

The *epithelium lining the inside of Bowman's capsule* has frequently been reported to be modified in aging male Sprague–Dawley rats, adopting the form of the cells lining the proximal tubule; this phenomenon has been described as 'tubularization' (Foley *et al.*, 1964; Gray, Weaver and Purmalis, 1974; Bolton *et al.*, 1976; Haley and Bulger, 1983). In the normal rat glomerulus, the parietal epithelial cells are simple, squamous in character. At the urinary pole, where the initial segment of the proximal tubule has its origin, there is usually an abrupt transition from the parietal epithelial cells to the taller columnar cells typical of the proximal tubules (Tisher, 1981). In the tubularization phenomenon, the normally squamous parietal layer of Bowman's capsule is progressively transformed into a columnar epithelium that is continuous with the proximal tubule cells, and extends from the urinary pole of the capsule to variable distances, in some cases involving the whole of Bowman's capsule. The ultrastructure of this cell was almost identical to that of the epithelial cell of the first portion of the proximal tubule, with a well-defined brush border, apical vesicles and extensive basolateral cellular interdigitations. According to Haley and Bulger (1983) the percentage of glomeruli affected by this tubularization process and its severity increase with age. These authors also observed that there were no differences between superficial and juxtamedullary nephrons in the severity or percentage of affectation of their glomeruli.

Hypertrophy of the parietal epithelium is also frequent in the aged male mouse (Crabtree, 1940; Pfeiffer, Emmel and Gardner, 1940; Dietert, 1967; Melis, Palermo and Motta, 1974), whereas it is a very uncommon finding in female mice, unless injected with androgens (Selye, 1939). Furthermore, mature castrated males did not show parietal hypertrophy, unless injected with testosterone (Crabtree, 1941). All these data suggest that the parietal epithelium in this species is highly sensitive to androgens. Hypertrophy of the parietal epithelium has also been described in man (Eisen, 1946; MacPherson, 1963; Reidbord, 1968) and in several other mammals (Von Mollendorf, 1930; Helmholtz, 1935). There are other factors unrelated to age which have also been reported to cause hypertrophy of the parietal epithelium. These factors include a reduction of functional renal mass (Lalich and

Allen, 1971; Andrews, 1981), overnutrition (Kennedy, 1957; Lalich and Allen, 1971) and hypertension (Haensly *et al.*, 1982).

The process of tubularization seems to occur by transformation of the original squamous epithelial cells into tubular-like ones by proximal tubule cells. The two main arguments for this suggestion of Haley and Bulger (1983) were the absence of mitosis and the appearance of some zones containing cells with an increased complexity which seems to be intermediate between parietal and tubular cells. It should be pointed out that the parietal, visceral and proximal tubule epithelia originate from the same group of cells in the metanephric blastema (Potter, 1972).

The functional significance of this phenomenon of tubularization in the aged male rat is not difficult to understand. As will be detailed below, the proximal tubules of aged rats undergo a series of modifications, mainly tubular atrophy, loss of brush border, impairment of cellular function and cell necrosis, which leads to an impairment of the reabsorption capacity of this segment of the nephron. This causes a limitation in the reabsorptive capacity of the kidney and, speculatively, causes some unknown alteration in body fluid homeostasis which induces metaplasia among the cell types related to the proximal tubule epithelium in order to improve the reabsorptive capacity, thus expanding morphologically and functionally the proximal tubule along the Bowman's capsule. This theory, suggested by Haley and Bulger (1983), could also account for the increase of proximal tubule-like epithelium into the Bowman's capsule after reduction of the functional renal mass.

Basement membrane

The other important alteration consistently found in the glomeruli of aged rats is a *thickening of the basement membrane.* Thus, whereas in the adult Sprague–Dawley rat (>3 months old), the basement membrane has an average width of 0.12 μm, in the old rat (ca 12 months old) the width of the membrane is almost twice as large (Haley and Burger, 1983). In the aged Lewis rat, the thickness of the basement membrane is about 50 per cent greater than that of adult male rat (Bell *et al.*, 1984). However, in spite of this thickening of the basal membrane, its permeability to protein increases, as reflected in the albuminuria consistently found in the aged rat (Blatherwick and Medlar, 1937; Berg, 1965; Kraus and Cain, 1974; Couser and Stilmant, 1975; Bolton *et al.*, 1976; Neuhaus and Flory, 1978). The fact that the basement membrane may become more permeable to proteins is explained by diminished histochemical staining of acid mucopolysaccharide groups (Ashworth, Erdmann and Arnold, 1960; Rosenquist and Bernick, 1971; Couser and Stilmant, 1975; Bolton *et al.*, 1976). In the normal rat, these anionic sites are constituents of the lamina rara interna and lamina rara externa and other components of the glomerular capillary wall and so contribute to the creation of a charge barrier which hinders the filtration of anionic plasma proteins such as albumin (Caulfield and Farquhar, 1976; Kawar and Farquhar, 1979). The loss of these charges would, in turn, allow the passage through the glomerular barrier of increased amounts of albumin, and subsequently, once the reabsorptive capacity of the tubular cells has been exceeded, proteinuria will become apparent. These mechanisms will be studied in greater depth in the section devoted to the physiopathology of proteinuria.

Furthermore, the increased staining by neutral mucopolysaccharides and collagen, as described in the aged rat by Ashworth, Erdmann and Arnold (1960) and Rosenquist and Bernick (1971), together with the increased width of the basal membrane, would diminish the hydraulic conductivity of the filtration barrier and, subsequently, the glomerular filtration rate, as will be detailed later in this chapter.

Mesangial cells

Changes in *mesangial cells* with aging in the experimental animal have also received some attention. The accumulation of IgM in the glomerular mesangium has been reported in old Sprague–Dawley, Lewis and Fisher rats (Hirokawa, 1975; Couser and Stilmant, 1975, 1976; Bolton *et al.*, 1976). In addition, the area of the mesangial cells increases with age in the Lewis rat (Bell *et al.*, 1984), but these phenomena have not been associated with any inflammatory response. These IgM deposits do not fix complement either *in vivo* or *in vitro*, and can be eluted with acid or potassium thiocyanate, but not with PBS or saline (Couser and Stilmant, 1975, 1976; Bolton *et al.*, 1976). Occasionally, they are associated with deposits of fibrin IgG, C_3 and rarely, IgE or IgA; generally, however, only IgM is present. Furthermore, the failure to find other serum proteins with the same distribution as IgM argues against non-specific protein trapping by the mesangium (Bolton *et al.*, 1976). These authors also found that the amount of IgM in the mesangium of aged Sprague–Dawley rats did not bear any close relationship with the degree of proteinuria. They also observed IgM deposits in several different strains of rats, some of which developed proteinuria and glomerular sclerosis, while others did not (Bolton *et al.*, 1976).

However, Couser and Stilmant (1975), who described a pattern of IgM distribution very similar to that of Bolton *et al.* (1976), reported a good correlation between the amount of IgM deposited in the mesangium and the proteinuria observed in Sprague–Dawley rats. Moreover, Elema and Arends (1975) described a different pattern of immunofluorescence images. Working with aged Wistar rats, these authors found a spontaneous glomerular hyalinosis and sclerosis which resembled focal glomerular sclerosis in man. Deposits of immunoglobulins and complement were found only in a pattern suggestive of insudated material and not in the mesangial cells. Thus, at the present time there is some evidence that the IgM represents an elutable immune complex being processed by the mesangium, although its role in the pathogenesis of glomerular sclerosis in aging rats is not evident. Similar findings have been reported by Markham, Sutherland and Mardiney (1973) in mice and by Proskitt *et al.* (1974) in monkeys.

The aging process has been associated with changes in immune function (Yunis, Fernándes and Stutman, 1971; MacKay, 1972; Walford, 1974) and an auto-immune phenomenon has been postulated to be important in the pathogenesis of spontaneous renal lesions in rats (Couser and Stilmant, 1976) and mice (Guttman, Wuepper and Fudenberg, 1967; Peter, 1973). Thus, although the mesangial IgM appears to be an incidental finding and the humoral immune system does not seem to be involved in the pathogenesis of the lesion (Couser and Stilmant, 1975; Bolton *et al.*, 1976), it is possible that the cellular immune system could be related with the lesion. Evidence for its participation comes from the observation that neonatal thymectomy and irradiation accelerate the damage (Guttman and Kohn, 1960; Wachtel, Cole and Rosen, 1966), whereas the addition of thyroid supplements may exacerbate the development of the disease (Addis *et al.*, 1950).

Starvation significantly protects rats against glomerular lesions (Saxton and Kimball, 1941; Simms and Berg, 1957; Berg and Simms, 1960; Wachtel, Cole and Rosen, 1966). Starvation is related to the cellular immune system because it produces involution of the lymphoid organs and lymphopenia, with a reduction in

IgM and, especially, IgG antibody production (Yunis, Fernandes and Stutman, 1971; Chandra, 1975). Although these observations (protection of the lesion with depressed capacity after neonatal thymectomy) seem to be antagonistic, they can be reconciled by the demonstration by Folch and Waksman (1974) of the existence of a 'splenic suppressor cell' of thymic origin which is present in large numbers at birth, but declines with age. In addition, there appear to be decreasing amounts of thymic hormone with increasing age (Bach, Dardenne and Bach, 1973). Thus, there is some indirect evidence which implicates the cell-mediated immune system as an aetiologic factor in glomerular sclerosis of the aging rat. However, the precise participation of the immune system in the renal aging process is yet to be completely defined.

Tubule

Changes in tubular cells in aged laboratory animals have received less attention than glomerular changes. Haley and Bulger (1983) reported that the proximal tubule of the 12-month-old Sprague–Dawley rat showed several degenerative changes; these were more evident in the proximal tubule. The pars convoluta exhibited focal cellular necrosis, focal brush border loss, regions with low cell height, bulbous projections and irregular profiles. The cells of these areas frequently showed increased numbers of apical vesicles, heterophagic vacuoles and protein absorption droplets. Mitochondria were few in number and irregular in shape and were seen to have lost their characteristic orientation perpendicular to the plasma of the basal lamina. Some proximal tubules were found to be completely atrophic.

The pars recta was generally less damaged than proximal portions of the pars convoluta. However, proximal portions of the par recta and outer stripe of the medulla were frequently collapsed and contained large intercellular spaces. Cells of these regions also contained protein absorption droplets and large number of apical vesicles and heterophagic vacuoles, organelles rarely found in these cells in the younger rat. Otherwise, the cells of this region were normal in appearance. No noteworthy modifications were observed in most distal segments of the nephron, although occasionally hyaline casts were seen in the thick ascending limbs and collecting ducts. At ultrastructural level, the epithelia of both segments contained protein absorption droplets, heterophagic vacuoles and abundant cytoplasmic vesicles, features that are unusual in the young rat.

The papillary epithelium, which in the young rat is a monolayer of simple cuboidal cells (Kül and Setekleiv, 1973), was observed in the aged rat to suffer varying degrees of hyperplasia, ranging from a few layers of cuboidal epithelium to areas of heavily stratified, columnar epithelium (Haley and Bulger, 1983).

The causes of the tubular alterations with age is uncertain. However, most reports support the concept that glomerular disease precedes tubular alterations (Lalich, Faith and Harding, 1970; Gray, Weaver and Purmalis, 1974; Hirokawa, 1975; Bolton *et al.*, 1976; Bell *et al.*, 1984). In this sense, Bolton *et al.* (1976) found a good correlation between glomerular damage in both proteinuric and non-proteinuric rats of several strains (Sprague–Dawley, Fisher 344 and Lewis), whereas the tubular histologic grade only paralleled proteinuria increasing with age. Furthermore, Bell *et al.* (1984) observed that glomerular changes correlated closely with the presence of dilated protein-filled tubules and that the animals with protein casts had significantly a thicker glomerular basement membrane and more mesangium than animals without protein casts. These facts strongly suggest that glomerular damage precedes tubular lesions and that these latter are closely related with proteinuria. Accordingly, it is possible that the initiating pathogenetic event is an excessive leakage of plasma protein through an abnormally permeable glomerular basement membrane, as described previously in this chapter. This would oblige the tubular cells, starting with the most proximal areas, to strongly develop the protein reabsorptive mechanisms. This is accomplished in the renal tubule by a process of pinocytosis (Carone *et al.*, 1979) and its excessive development in the aging rat can be reflected by the presence along the whole nephron of abnormal amounts of protein absorption droplets, heterophagic vacuoles and cytoplasmic vesicles — features only rarely seen in young rats.

The presence of protein droplets (the so-called hyalin droplets) in the proximal convoluted tubule and sometimes in epithelial cells of the glomerular tuft is a common finding in conditions accompanied by proteinuria (Heptinstal, 1966). The droplets have also been observed in rats and mice injected with large amounts of protein (Oliver, McDowell and Lee, 1954; Shuster and Callaghan, 1961); in these animals heterophagic vacuoles and lysosomes are also abundant (Anderson and Recant, 1962). Such intracellular modifications are often accompanied by atrophy and a flattening of the epithelium (Heptinstal, 1966), similar to those reported for the aging rat.

Excessive protein reabsorption could induce changes in the intracellular metabolism and become toxic for the epithelial cell, in a way similar to that reported for the nephrotoxicity induced by light chains (Preuss *et al.,* 1974; Martínez-Maldonado, Benabe and López-Novoa, 1983). Although the acute addition of proteins isolated from the urine of subjects with nephrotic syndrome had no toxic effects on kidney slices *in vitro,* whereas light chains from the urine of myeloma patients did induce some metabolic changes (Preuss *et al.,* 1974), it is possible that chronic exposure to urinary proteins could become toxic for the epithelial cells. This mechanism also accounts for the fact that the most affected cells are proximal ones, which are subject to the maximal protein overload and are hence responsible for the reabsorption of the small amounts of protein present in the urine under normal conditions (Maack, 1975).

Increased filtration of plasma proteins therefore seems to be at least one major pathogenetic event responsible for the alterations in the tubular epithelium in the aging experimental animals.

Interstitium

Changes in the renal interstitium of aging experimental animals have not been extensively studied, in spite of the importance of the interstitium in physiological processes such as urine concentration and the dilution or conservation of urea. It has been reported that cortical interstitium in aging rats showed infiltration of macrophages and mononuclear and polymorphonuclear cells, particularly in relation to blood vessels (Bolton *et al.*, 1976; Haley and Bulger, 1983); this results in variable degrees of interstitial fibrosis (Bell *et al.,* 1984).

Histological studies on the rat have not found any pathological alterations in blood vessels in relation to age (Blatherwick and Medlar, 1937; Saxton and Kimball, 1941; Andrew and Pruett, 1957; Pollard and Kajima, 1970; Elema, Koudstaad and Lambert, 1971; Gray, Weaver and Purmalis, 1974; Couser and Stilmant, 1975; Elema and Arends, 1975; Bell *et al.,* 1984), whereas the predominant changes in man are vascular and ischaemic in nature (see Chapter 1).

Functional changes

Proteinuria

We have already mentioned that proteinuria is the most consistent change in renal function observed in the aging rat. The urinary excretion of protein, increasing with age, has generally been ascribed to a spontaneous development of renal lesion or glomerulosclerosis. We have also discussed the main factors that control the severity of the renal lesion: diet, strain, sex and the functional renal mass. In the present section we will thus review the characteristics of age-related proteinuria and the mechanism determining protein excretion and its modifications.

Age-dependent changes in the excretion of protein in the urine of male rats were first described by Addis (1931) and Blatherwick and Medlar (1937). Sellers *et al.* (1950) first pointed to the clear difference in protein excretion between males and females of the same strain. These authors and Perry (1965) demonstrated that prostatic and testicular secretion were not responsible for this difference, thus documenting the renal origin of the protein. Proteinuria has been reported to correlate with the severity of glomerular lesions (Blatherwick and Medlar, 1937; Berg, 1967). However, Elema and Arends (1975) described manifest proteinuria in male rats before overt morphological changes could be evidenced.

With respect to the time course of the proteinuria, Bolton *et al.* (1976) reported that, up to 2 months of age, Sprague–Dawley rats did not show detectable protein in urine using a dipstick test. By 3 months, evident proteinuria ($>$10 mg/day) was observed in 25 per cent of the male rats, and this proportion increased with age. In contrast, female rats did not show proteinuria until at least 18 months of age, and the percentage of females with proteinuria was consistently lower than that of males of the same age. Neuhaus and Flory (1978), using a more precise assay for proteins in males of the same strain, reported an average excretion of 10.6 mg/day in 1-month-old rats, increasing up to 50 mg/day in 2-month-old animals.

Examination of the composition of urinary proteins in young males revealed the essential absence of albumin, an abundance of α-globulin being the most characteristic feature of the proteinuria. Bolton *et al.* (1976) suggested that this α-globulin was of tubular origin, and Neuhaus and Flory (1978) identified most of it as a specific sex-dependent protein called $\alpha_{2\mu}$-globulin. In the young male rat this globulin represents 25–30 per cent of the total urinary protein (Neuhaus and Flory, 1975); $\alpha_{2\mu}$-globulin is produced by males at puberty (Roy, Neuhaus and Hermison, 1966). It is of hepatic origin (Roy and Neuhaus, 1966) and its synthesis is reported to be under the control of androgens and glucocorticoids (Roy and Neuhaus, 1967; Irwin, Lane and Neuhaus, 1971). Its presence in urine is due to its low molecular weight (18–20 000 D), which allows it to pass freely through the normal glomerular barrier.

As the rat ages, albumin begins to appear in the urine, constituting the major component of urinary protein in the middle-aged proteinuric rat (Bolton *et al.*, 1976; Neuhaus and Flory, 1978). The beginning of the albuminuric phase coincides with the appearance of the histological lesion in the kidney, suggesting that an increased leakage of plasma albumin stems from the development of renal lesions (Neuhaus and Flory, 1978).

Old proteinuric animals excreted protein in urine in a profile similar to normal rat serum. This evolution of selective (albumin) to non-selective proteinuria, described by Perry (1965) and Couser and Stilmant (1975), demonstrates a progressive loss of glomerular barrier selectivity.

The age-related changes in glomerular barrier have been already described in detail in this chapter. We shall now revise the relationship between such changes and the permeability of the glomerulus to protein, as well as the mechanism that would lead to such abnormalities; we shall use as an example another model of spontaneous proteinuria which has been extensively studied: severe reduction of renal mass.

Considerable evidence is now available to indicate that, in addition to molecular size and haemodynamic parameters, other factors influence the normal glomerular filtration of macromolecules (Brenner, Ichikawa and Deen, 1981). Differences in the fractional clearance of macromolecules with similar sizes but with different charges have been reported, and such differences cannot be accounted for by differences in tubular reabsorption (Myers, Deen and Brenner, 1975). This suggests that besides a size selectivity, the glomerular capillary wall also has charge selectivity. Albumin at least is restricted to a much greater extent than would be predicted from considering its size alone. Chang *et al.* (1975) demonstrated that the passage of polyanions through the capillary wall is restricted. Albumin is a polyanion at the pH of plasma, and the anomalous low filtration rate of this protein may largely be the consequence of the charge-selective properties of the capillary wall.

A likely explanation for this selective restriction to filtration of circulating polycations is electrostatic hindrance resulting from some fixed, negatively charged component of the glomerular capillary wall, as demonstrated by Rennke and Venkatachalam (1977, 1978), who used clearance of molecules with different charges. In addition, the existence of highly anionic structural elements in the normal capillary wall has been deduced from the pronounced histochemical affinity of all component layers of the glomerular capillary wall for cationic stains such as ruthenium red, alcian blue, lysozyme or colloidal iron (Latta, Johnston and Stanley, 1975; Kanwar and Farquhar, 1979). The glomerular epithelial cell and its foot processes are covered with a surface coat of acidic glycoproteins, so-called sialoproteins or glomerular polyanions, that are highly negatively charged. Furthermore, the epithelial slit diaphragm, a thin membrane lying between the channels formed by the interdigitating foot process, partly consist of sialoproteins (Spiro, 1967). The glomerular basement membrane and the endothelial cell coat have also been shown to contain these substances (Spiro, 1967). The most important functional electrostatic barriers to circulating polyanions seem to be the structures closest to the capillary lumen, i.e. the endothelium and the innermost layer of the glomerular basement membrane, the lamina rara interna (Latta and Johnston, 1976; Rennke and Venkatachalam, 1977).

In the aged rat a diminished histochemical staining of the acid mucopolysaccharide groups present in the glomerular capillary wall has been described (Ashworth, Erdmann and Arnold, 1960; Rosenquist and Bernick, 1971; Couser and Stilmant, 1975). This could explain the high rates of albumin present in the urine of these animals. However, Bolton *et al.* (1976) concluded that alterations in the sialoprotein barrier to filtered protein appear to have no role in this process, although most of the authors conclude that alterations in charge selectivity of the glomerular barrier is a key event in the development of proteinuria (Haley and Bulger, 1983). In addition, these and other histological changes often observed in the aged rat, such as foot process fusion, are also characteristic of pathological states accompanied by proteinuria (Brenner, Hostetter and Humes, 1978).

In the knowledge of the mechanism that leads to such alterations of great interest are the observations of Michael, Blau and Vernier (1970) that in the experimental nephrotic syndrome induced by aminonucleoside in the rat, the decrease in glomerular sialoprotein appears to coincide in time not only with the onset of proteinuria, but also with the morphological appearance of foot process fusion. Since negatively charged surface coats can influence the stability of plasma membranes, and polycations can influence several morphological alterations in many types of cells, Seiler *et al.* (1977) were prompted to study the effect of perfusing rat kidneys with highly cationic polymers such as protamine sulphate or poly-L-lysine. These authors reported that these manoeuvres induced foot process fusion and a loss of the fixed negative charges of the glomeruli, alterations very similar to those seen in proteinuric states and as the experimental nephrotic syndrome induced by puromycin aminonucleoside or in the aging kidney in rats.

The similarity of the polycation-induced lesion at ultrastructural levels to those seen in the aging kidney and in human or experimental nephrotic syndrome raises the question of a common denominator in the course of the morphological changes as well as of the proteinuric characteristics of such situations. In this sense, the common event to all these pathological states would be loss of glomerular fixed negative charges, which leads not only to diminished staining with cationic stains, but also to an increased polyanion filtration fraction and hence to albuminuria. Another consequence of the reduced negative fixed charges could be foot process fusion, as suggested by Seiler *et al.* (1977). These authors proposed that the normal crossed finger-like appearance of foot processes is due to mutual electrostatic repulsion of the highly charged cationic coat covering each individual process. When disease, age or polycation treatment reduces the sialoprotein coat, the electrostatic repulsive forces disappear, leading to the appearance of fused foot processes. This hypothesis was supported by the observation that foot processes fused by polycation treatment can be rapidly sent apart by treatment with the strongly polyanion heparin (Seiler *et al.*, 1977).

Such findings strongly point to another question. What is the cause of the loss of anionic charges in the glomeruli of the aged rat? To our knowledge no study has been designed to answer this question in the aging rat. However, there is another well-studied model of spontaneous and progressive glomerulosclerosis, i.e. that resulting from severe reduction of renal mass, which has important similarities with the aging kidney and may shed some light on its pathogenetic mechanisms (see Chapter 3).

As described in detail by Shimamura and Morrison (1975), adult rats subjected to surgical resection of approximately 80 per cent of their total renal mass showed an increase in the mass and function of their remaining kidney tissue within the first 3 months after nephrectomy. This hypertrophy was accompanied by ultrastructural alterations, including vacuolization of glomerular epithelial cells, deposition of osmophilic droplets within the cells and fusion of foot processes. Later, more severe abnormalities appeared, such as expansion of the mesangial matrix and denudation of cells from areas of the glomerular basement membrane. These structural alterations lead to progressive glomerular hyalinization and, ultimately, to glomerular sclerosis. All these changes, very similar to those found in the kidneys of aged rats, have also been observed in other models of severe reduction of renal mass (Purkerson, Hoffsten and Klahr, 1976; Olson *et al.*, 1982); the similarities, however, are not only histological. The severe reduction of functional renal mass induces massive proteinuria in spite of the marked reduction in glomerular filtration rate (Chanutin and Ferris, 1932). The severity and the time course of this functional lesion is partially prevented by dietary protein restriction (Meyer *et al.*, 1983;

Hostetter, 1984) as occurs in aged rats (Elema and Arends, 1975; Tucker, Mason and Beauchene, 1976).

There is enough evidence to demonstrate that proteinuria in the rat with severely reduced kidney mass is due to the loss of the size and charge selectivity of the glomerular filtration barrier (Robson *et al.*, 1979; Olson *et al.*, 1982). There is also evidence to support the notion that the early morphological derangements observed in subtotally nephrectomized rats are caused by an increase in glomerular pressure and flow by a mechanism similar to that proposed for arterial hypertension (Hostetter, 1984). However, it appears unlikely that systemic hypertension *per se* could account completely for the functional and structural alterations reported. For example, rats subjected to partial infarction of one kidney develop acute severe hypertension, but they did not develop histological renal lesions in a short-term follow-up (Purkerson, Hoffsten and Klahr, 1976). Conversely, when the arterial pressure of rats with severe reduction of renal mass was maintained between normal limits with antihypertensive drugs, renal lesions still became apparent, although the degree of damage was reduced (Purkerson, Hoffsten and Klahr, 1976). In aged animals, glomerular sclerosis also occurs in the animals which did not develop arterial hypertension. It therefore appears reasonable to conclude that the changes in glomerular dynamics and structure observed in rats with a severe reduction of renal mass and in senescent animals are not simply a consequence of systemic arterial hypertension, but rather that they depend on the modification of intrarenal resistance.

It has been reported that the pre/postglomerular resistance ratio, one of the major determinants of glomerular filtration (Brenner, Ichikawa and Deen, 1981), is reduced in the older Wistar rat, with the presence of a 10–15 per cent increase in total renovascular resistance (Göthberg and Folkow, 1983). These data suggest a structural narrowing of mainly the postglomerular vessel, a phenomenon that involves an increase in capillary pressure and the filtration fraction. Hence, the haemodynamic changes described above will lead to an increase of ultrafiltrate movement across the capillary wall and, subsequently, to an increased transcapillary movement of macromolecules due to convective forces. As substances exist in plasma which are polycations at physiological pH, the increased traffic of such molecules through the capillary wall would have an injurious effect on its charge barrier in a way similar to that described for polycation infusion (Seiler *et al.*, 1977) inducing foot process fusion and favouring the passage of albumin across the wall.

Finally, there is a growing body of evidence to suggest that the loss of glomerular fixed negative charges and the subsequently increased transglomerular traffic of albumin may facilitate the accumulation of macromolecules within the glomerular mesangium (Farquhar and Palade, 1961; Hoyer, Elema and Vernier, 1976), thereby influencing the site and magnitude of immune complex and non-immune circulating aggregate deposition within the glomerular wall and mesangium (Couser *et al.*, 1978). The presence within the mesangium of such aggregates could be a continuous stimulus to mesangial matrix production, the ultimate result of which might be glomerular sclerosis, as suggested by several workers (Hoyer, Elema and Vernier, 1976; Velosa *et al.*, 1977; Olson *et al.*, 1982). Although these studies have been performed on models of proteinuria and glomerulosclerosis by aminonucleoside or severe renal mass reduction, it is likely that the physiopathology of the lesions observed in the aged rat is very similar.

It must be noted that, as detailed earlier in this chapter, a consistent finding in the kidney of aged rats is an increase in the area of mesangial cells (Bell *et al.*, 1984) and accumulation of IgM and IgG in the glomerular mesangium (Couser and Stilmant, 1975; Hirokawa, 1975; Bolton *et al.*, 1976). These alterations, as suggested for other models of proteinuria, would result in glomerular sclerosis, the main histological manifestation observed in the kidney of senescent rats.

Glomerular filtration rate

Reports devoted to the study of glomerular filtration rate (GFR) in aged laboratory animals are scarce and controversial. Working with 2-year-old male Fisher 344 rats, an age which can be considered as senescence in this strain, Bengele, Mathias and Alexander (1981) observed that aged rats showed a higher GFR than young ones, although this difference became non-significant when GFR was factored by kidney weight. This finding was also confirmed by the same group in a later study (Bengele *et al.*, 1981). These authors also reported that saline infusion induced a slight but significant decrease in GFR in aged rats, whereas no significant differences were found in the young animals (Bengele, Mathias and Alexander, 1981). In addition, a high potassium diet induced a decrease in GFR in aged but not in young rats (Bengele *et al.*, 1983).

By way of contrast, Haley and Bulger (1983), working with male Sprague–Dawley rats, reported that 12-month-old animals showed a 60 per cent reduction in GFR as compared with 5- and 3-month-old rats. Booker and Williams (1981) observed in 12-month-old rats of the same strain a 15 per cent decrease in GFR which was accompanied by a 50 per cent decrease in superficial single-nephron GFR. These authors suggested that this decrease in SNGFR is mostly the result of a marked increase in afferent arteriolar resistance, with no change in GFR or Kf. However, Gothberg and Folkow (1983), in experiments with isolated perfused kidneys, have reported that in the aged Wistar rat the ratio of pre-glomerular to post-glomerular resistances is reduced, a result which does not support the hypothesis of Booker and Williams. Again this important difference between the several studies must be attributed to the difference in behaviour between rat strains and to the differences in the design of the study, taking into account also that in the studies of Bengele *et al.* (1981, 1983) most of the manoeuvres performed induced decreases in GFR, a fact suggestive of the lability of GFR in aged animals.

Electrolyte handling

Bengele, Mathias and Alexander (1981) have studied the hydroelectrolyte balance and the renal response to volume expansion in aged (24 months) male Fisher 344 rats, in comparison with young animals. They found that, in basal conditions, no significant differences could be noted between young and old rats. However, after an isotonic saline infusion (7 per cent of body weight) the old animals excreted a lower proportion of the sodium infused than young ones. This agrees with a decrease in GFR and blood pressure observed in aged but not in young rats. A similar difference was observed when the expansion was made with blood, with the exception that under these conditions GFR did not change in either group. The authors concluded that the aged rats are significantly less efficient in the excretion of a sodium load than the young animals, although the mechanisms of these differences could not be deduced from their data.

The same group (Bengele *et al.*, 1983) has also studied the ability of aged rats of the same strain to adapt themselves to a chronic potassium load. Although when on a normal potassium diet or after an acute potassium injection, potassium excretion was similar in both young and aged animals, after 5 weeks on a high potassium diet, urinary potassium excretion increased in both groups, although the increment was markedly smaller in aged rats. Plasma potassium concentration and urine volume increased similarly in both groups, while GFR was lower in the aged rats. A major difference between young and aged animals on a normal potassium diet was the decreased activity of the enzyme Na–K–ATPase in the renal medulla of the aged rats. In contrast, no differences in Na^+–K^+–ATPase activity were observed in renal cortex and colon. The chronic administration of a high K^+ diet significantly increased ATPase activity in the kidney and colon of young rats, but such an increment was not observed in the renal cortex of aged rats. In these animals, ATPase activity in colon and renal medulla increased at a ratio similar to that noted in the young animals and thus the absolute activity of the enzyme in the renal medulla after chronic potassium administration remains significantly lower in old than in young rats.

The authors explained the failure of aged rats to exhibit renal adaptation to potassium on the basis of the reduced amount of the enzyme detected in the renal medulla of the aged rats. Other data exist to the effect that Na–K–ATPase activity was reduced in total kidney homogenates (Beauchene, Fanestil and Barrows, 1965) and in kidney cortex (Gambert, Ingbar and Hagen, 1981) of aged rats. A delayed or diminished ability of enzyme adaptation is a recognized general characteristic of aging individuals (Sartin *et al.*, 1980). It has also been reported that the decrease of Na–K–ATPase in the kidney of aged rats is dependent on thyroid hormone, and that the response of renal Na^+–K^+–ATPase to thyroid hormone decreases with age (Gambert, Ingbar and Hagen, 1981). A decrease in activity with age in the rat has also been reported for other renal membrane-bound enzymes such as maltose and alkaline phosphatase, this decrease in activity being due to a decrease in the number of units rather than to changes in the function of the enzymes (O'Bryan and Lowenstein, 1974). This deficiency in transport units could therefore be responsible for the failure of renal adaptation to chronic potassium administration in aged rats. The capacity of these animals adequately to handle acute potassium loads can be explained by the fact that acute changes in potassium transport are not related to renal Na^+–K^+–ATPase activity (Katz and Lindheimer, 1975).

Urinary concentration

In 1956, Friedman, Hinke and Friedman observed that the injection of hypertonic sodium into the common carotid artery of non-anaesthetized, hydrated rats produced a smaller antidiuretic effect in senescent than in younger animals. They attributed the decrease in antidiuretic effect in aged rats to a failure of the neurohypophysis to react to the stimulation of hypertonic saline solutions. The same authors also observed an impairment of the concentrating ability in their senescent animals (Friedman and Friedman, 1957).

Later studies by Dicker and Nunn (1958) concluded that in the rat there is no evidence of a decline with age in neurohypophyseal response to hypertonic stimulation and that the smaller antidiuretic effect observed after intracarotid injection of hypertonic saline in aged rats appears to be based on a lack of kidney response to vasopressin. This contention is further supported by the fact that there is little evidence for impairment of neurohypophyseal function in aged rats (Rodeck, Lederis and Heller, 1960; Dunhue, 1965).

Recently, Bengele *et al.* (1980), using clearance techniques, performed a study of the renal concentrating and diluting ability of 1-year-old male Fisher 344 rats, whose average lifespan is 30 months (Masoro, 1980). They observed that under basal conditions aged rats exhibited polydipsia and polyuria. In addition, when subjected to water deprivation, they observed a markedly impaired concentrating ability. They concluded therefore that the decreased concentrating ability in their aged rats was due to an alteration in renal response to antidiuretic hormone rather than to a decrease in vasopressin release from the pituitary. Furthermore, the decreased concentrating ability in aged rats could not be explained by a possible change in sodium transport in the distal nephron, and neither could any decrease be detected in the interstitial tonicity of the papilla. These authors (Bengele *et al.*, 1982) postulated that there might be an impairment of the ability of vasopressin to affect water permeability in the collecting duct epithelium. This problem was further studied by Beck and Yu (1982) in the same strain of rats, who focused their research on the cellular mechanism that mediates renal response to vasopressin.

The hydro-osmotic effect of vasopressin is believed to be mediated through cAMP generation in the collecting duct cells (Grantham and Orloff, 1961; Orloff and Handler, 1967). Beck and Yu therefore compared vasopressin-dependent cAMP generation between animals of different ages. They observed that basal cAMP production was decreased in aged rats when compared with young animals. In addition, the cAMP increase induced by exogenous vasopressin observed in young rats was abolished in aged rats, which showed normal phosphodiesterase (the enzyme that catabolizes cAMP) activity, suggesting that the decrease of cAMP in aged rats was at least in part due to a decrease in adenylate cyclase activity. Taking all the available data together, it is possible to conclude that old rats show an impaired ability to concentrate urine; this would at least be partly due to a decrease in vasopressin-dependent cAMP generation which occurs during or prior to the step of vasopressin-dependent adenylate cyclase activation in the kidney.

However, the mechanism of this lack of activation on other possible pathogenic mechanisms involved in the impairment of renal concentration related with senescence in the rat is not known. Additionally, as far as we know, no studies on this phenomenon in other laboratory animals have been published.

Hormones with renal action

It is generally accepted that plasma renin activity (PRA) decreases progressively in non-hypertensive men over the age of 60 (Weidmann *et al.*, 1975, 1978). However, the changes in PRA in the laboratory rat were dependent on the strain studied. Thus, in Kyoto–Wistar rats, the basal plasma renin activity and renin content of the kidney are not different in young and 12-month-old rats (Sen, Smeby and Bumpus, 1972; Aoi and Weinberger, 1976). In the same strain, the responsiveness of PRA to various stimuli decreases progressively with aging (Forman and Murlow, 1974).

In contrast, Hayashi *et al.* (1981) have reported that 13–18-month-old Wistar male rats showed lower values of PRA than 3–6-month-old animals. They also observed that the content of renin in both superficial and juxtamedullary nephrons was decreased in the aged animals, concluding that the decreased PRA in these animals was a consequence of the decreased number of functioning nephrons.

With respect to aldosterone, to our knowledge there is only one paper in the literature which has examined the concentrations of this hormone in aged rats. In this study, Bengele *et al.* (1983) found similar plasma aldosterone levels in young and 24-month-old Fisher 344 rats. We do not know of any study dealing with other hormones related to renal function in laboratory animals.

In conclusion, studies dealing with this topic are scarce and sometimes contradictory, and the precise changes in the kidney-related hormones in aged animals should be the object of further research.

References

ADDIS, T. (1931). Proteinuria and cylinduria. *Proceedings of the California Academy of Medicine,* **38,** 52

ADDIS, T., MARMORSTON, J., GOODMAN, H.C., SELLERS, A.L. and SMITH, M. (1950). Effect of adrenalectomy on spontaneous and induced proteinuria in the rat. *Proceedings of the Society for Experimental Biology and Medicine,* **74,** 43–46

ANDERSON, M.S. and RECANT, L. (1962). Five structural alterations in the rat kidney following intraperitoneal bovine albumin. *American Journal of Pathology,* **40,** 555–570

ANDREW, W. and PRUETT, D. (1957). Senile changes in the kidneys of Wistar Institute rats. *American Journal of Anatomy,* **100,** 51–69

ANDREWS, P.M. (1981). The presence of proximal tubule-like cells in the kidney parietal epithelium in response to unilateral nephrectomy. *Anatomical Records,* **200,** 61–65

AOI, W. and WEINBERGER, M.H. (1976). The effect of age and norepinephrine on renin release by rat kidney slices *in vitro. Proceedings of the Society for Experimental Biology and Medicine,* **151,** 47–52

ARATAKI, M. (1926). On the postnatal growth of the kidney with special reference to the number and size of the glomeruli (albino rat). *American Journal of Pathology,* **36,** 399–436

ASHWORTH, C.T., ERDMANN, R.R. and ARNOLD, N.J. (1960). Age changes in the renal basement membrane in rats. *American Journal of Pathology,* **36,** 165–180

BACH, J.F., DARDENNE, M. and BACH, M. (1973). Demonstration of a circulating thymic hormone in mouse and man. *Transplantation Proceedings,* **5,** 99–104

BEAUCHENE, R.E., FANESTIL, D.D., and BARROWS, C.H. Jr. (1965). The effect of age on active transport and sodium–potassium activated ATPase activity in renal tissue of rats. *Journal of Gerontology,* **20,** 306–310

BECK, N. and YU, B.P. (1982). Effect of aging on urinary concentrating mechanism and vasopressin-dependent cAMP in rats. *American Journal of Physiology,* **204,** F121–F125

BELL, R.H. Jr., BÖRJESSON, B.A., WOLF, P.L., FERNÁNDEZ-CRUZ, L., BRIMM, J.E., LEE, S. *et al.* (1984). Quantitative morphological studies of aging changes in the kidney of the Lewis rat. *Renal Physiology,* **7,** 176–184

BENGELE, H.H., MATHIAS, R.S. and ALEXANDER, E.A. (1981). Impaired natriuresis after volume expansion in the aged rat. *Renal Physiology,* **4,** 22–29

BENGELE, H.H., MATHIAS, R.S., PERKINS, J.H. and ALEXANDER, E.A. (1981). Urinary concentrating defect in the aged rat. *American Journal of Physiology,* **240,** F147–F150

BENGELE, H.H., MATHIAS, R.S., PERKINS, J.H., McNAMARA, E.R. and ALEXANDER, E.A. (1983). Impaired renal and extrarenal potassium adaptation in old rats. *Kidney International,* **23,** 684–690

BERG, B.N. (1965). Spontaneous nephrosis with proteinuria, hyperglobulinemia and hypercholesterolemia in the rat. *Proceedings of the Society for Experimental Biology and Medicine,* **119,** 416–420

BERG, B.N. (1967). Longevity studies in rats. II. Pathology of aging rats. In *Pathology of Laboratory Rats and Mice,* edited by Cotchin and Roe, pp. 749–786. Oxford; Blackwell

BERG, B.N. and SIMMS, H.S. (1960). Nutrition and longevity in the rat. II. Longevity and onset of disease with different levels of food intake. *Journal of Nutrition,* **71,** 255–263

BLATHERWICK, N.R. and MEDLAR, E.M. (1937). Chronic nephritis in rats fed high protein diets. *Archives of Internal Medicine,* **59,** 572–596

BOLTON, W.K., BENTON, F.R., MACLAY, J.G. and STURGILL, B.C. (1976). Spontaneous glomerular sclerosis in aging Sprague–Dawley rats. *American Journal of Pathology,* **85,** 277–300

BOOKER, B. and WILLIAMS, R. (1981). Glomerular hemodynamics in aged rats. *Kidney International,* **19,** 195

BRENNER, B.M. HOSTETTER, T.H. and HUMES, H.D. (1978). Molecular basis of proteinuria of glomerular origin. *New England Journal of Medicine,* **298,** 826–833

BRENNER, B.M., ICHIKAWA, I. and DEEN, W.M. (1981). Glomerular filtration. In *The Kidney*, 2nd edn, edited by B.M. Brenner and F.C. Rector, pp. 289–327. Philadelphia; Saunders

CARONE, F.A., PETERSON, D.R., OPARIL, S. and PULLMAN, T.N. (1979). Renal tubular transport and catabolism of proteins and peptides. *Kidney International*, **16**, 271–278

CAULFIELD, J.P. and FARQUHAR, M.G. (1976). Distribution of anionic sites in glomerular basement membranes. Their possible role in filtration and attachment. *Proceedings of the National Academy of Sciences of the USA*, **73**, 1646–1649

CHANDRA, R.R. (1975). Antibody formation in first and second generation offspring of nutritionally deprived rats. *Science*, **190**, 289–290

CHANG, R.L.S., DEEN, W.M., ROBERTSON, C.R. and BRENNER, B.M. (1975). Permselectivity of the glomerular capillary wall. III Restricted transport of polyanions. *Kidney International*, **8**, 212–218

CHANUTIN, A. and FERRIS, E. (1932). Experimental renal insufficiency produced by partial nephrectomy. *Archives of Internal Medicine*, **49**, 767–787

COLEMAN, G.L., BARTHOLD, S.W., OSBALISTON, C.W., FOSTER, S.S. and JONAS, A.M. (1977). Pathological changes during aging in barrier-reared Fischer 344 male rats. *Journal of Gerontology*, **32**, 258–278

COUSER, W.G., HOYER, J.R., STILTMAN, M.M., JERMANOWICH, N.B. and BELOK, S. (1978). Effect of amino nucleocide nephrosis on immune complex localization in autologous immune complex nephritis in the rat. *Journal of Clinical Investigation*, **61**, 561–572

COUSER, W.G. and STILMANT, M.M. (1975). Mesangial lesions and focal glomerular sclerosis in the aging rat. *Laboratory Investigation*, **33**, 491–501

COUSER, W.G. and STILMANT, M.M. (1976). The immunopathology of the aging rat. *Journal of Gerontology*, **31**, 13–22

CRABTREE, C. (1940). Sex differences in the structure of Bowman's capsule in the mouse. *Science*, **91**, 299

CRABTREE, C. (1941). Structure of Bowman's capsule in castrated and testosterone-treated male mice as an index of hormonal effects on renal cortex. *Endocrinology*, **29**, 197–203

DAVIES, D.F. and SHOCK, N.W. (1950). Age changes in glomerular filtration rate, effective renal plasma flow and tubular excretory capacity in adult males. *Journal of Clinical Investigation*, **29**, 496–507

DICKER, S.E. and NUNN, J. (1958). Antidiuresis in adult and old rats. *Journal of Physiology*, **141**, 332–336

DIETERT, S.E. (1967). The columnar cells occurring in the parietal layer of Bowman's capsule. *Journal of Cell Biology*, **35**, 435–444

DUNIHUE, F.W. (1965). Reduced cell granularity, pituitary neurosecretory material and width of the zona glomerulosa in aging rats. *Endocrinology*, **77**, 948–951

EISEN, H.N. (1946). Adenonatoid transformation of the glomerular capsulous epithelium. *American Journal of Pathology*, **22**, 597–600

ELEMA, J.D. and ARENDS, A. (1975). Focal and segmental glomerular hyalinosis and sclerosis in the rat. *Laboratory Investigation*, **33**, 491–501

ELEMA, J.D., KOUDSTAAL, J., LAMBERTS, H.B. and ARENDS, A. (1971). Spontaneous glomerulosclerosis in the rat. *Archives of Pathology*, **91**, 418–425

ELIAS, H., ALLARA, E., ELIAS, P.M. and KRISHNA MURTHY, A.S. (1964). The podocytes, reexamined. *Journal Microskopische Anatomische Forschung*, **72**, 344–365

FARQUHAR, M.G. and PALADE, G.E. (1961). Glomerular permeability. II. Ferritin transfer across the glomerular capillary wall in nephrotic rats. *Journal of Experimental Medicine*, **114**, 699–716

FOLCH, H. and WAKSMAN, B.H. (1974). The splenic suppressor cell. I. Activity of thymus-dependent adherent cells: changes with age and stress. *Journal of Immunology*, **133**, 127–139

FOLEY, W.A., JONES, D.C.L., OSBORN, G.K. and KIMELDORF, W.H. (1964). A renal lesion associated with diuresis in the aging Sprague–Dawley rat. *Laboratory Investigation*, **13**, 439–450

FORMAN, B.H. and MURLOW, P.J. (1974). Effect of plasma renal activity in the spontaneously hypertensive rat. *Circulation Research*, **35**, 215–221

FRIEDMAN, S.M. and FRIEDMAN, C.L. (1957). Salt and water balance in aging rats. *Gerontologia*, **1**, 107–121

FRIEDMAN, S.M., HINKE, J.A.M. and FRIEDMAN, C.L. (1956). Neurohypophyseal responsiveness in the normal and senescent rat. *Journal of Gerontology*, **2**, 286–291

GAMBERT, S.R., INGBAR, S.H. and HAGEN, T.C. (1981). Interaction of age and thyroid hormone status or Na^+, K^+, ATPase in rat renal cortex and liver. *Endocrinology*, **108**, 27–30

GRANTHAM, J.J. and ORLOFF, J. (1968). Effect of prostaglandin E_2 on the permeability response of the isolated collecting tubule to vasopressin adenosine 3′5′ monophosphate and theophylline. *Journal of Clinical Investigation*, **47**, 1154–1158

GÖTHBERG, G. and FOLKOW, B. (1983). Age-dependent alterations in the structurally determined vascular resistance, pre- to postglomerular resistance ratio and glomerular filtration capacity in kidneys, as studied in aging normotensive rats and spontaneously hypertensive rats. *Acta Physiologica Scandinavica*, **117**, 547–555

GRAY, J.E. (1963). Naturally occurring and sulfonamide-induced lesions in rats during a 1-year toxicity study. *American Journal of Veterinary Research*, **24**, 1044–1059

GRAY, J.E., WEAVER, R.N. and PURMALIS, A. (1974). Ultrastructural observations of chronic progressive nephrosis in the Sprague–Dawley rat. *Veterinary Pathology*, **11**, 153–164

GUTTMAN, P.H. and KOHN, H.I. (1960). Progressive intercapillary glomerulosclerosis in the mouse, rat and Chinese hamster associated with aging and x-ray exposure. *American Journal of Pathology*, **37**, 293–304

GUTTMAN, P.H., WUEPPER, K.D. and FUDENBERG, H.H. (1967). On the presence of γG and ß1C globulins in renal glomeruli of aging and neonatally x-irradiated mice. *Vox Sanguinis*, **12**, 329–339

HAENSLY, W.E., GRANGER, H.J., MORRIS, A.C. and CIOFFE, C. (1982). Proximal tubule-like epithelium in Bowman's capsule in spontaneously hypertensive rats. Changes with age. *American Journal of Pathology*, **107**, 92–97

HALEY, D.P. and BULGER, R.E. (1983). The aging male rat: structure and function of the kidney. *The American Journal of Anatomy*, **167**, 1–13

HAYASHI, M., SARUTA, T., NAKAMURA, R., KITAJIMA, W. and KOTO, E. (1981). Effect of aging on single nephron renin content in rats. *Renal Physiology*, **4**, 17–21

HELMHOLTZ, H.F. (1935). The presence of tubular epithelium within the glomerular capsule in mammals. *Proceedings of the Staff Meetings of the Mayo Clinic*, **10**, 110–112

HEPTINSTALL, R.H. (1966). *Pathology of the Kidney*, 2nd edn, p. 1047. Boston; Little, Brown

HIROKAWA, K. (1975). Characterization of age-associated kidney disease in Wistar rats. *Mechanisms of Aging and Development*, **4**, 301–316

HOSTETTER, T.H. (1984). The hyperfiltering glomerulus. *Medical Clinics of North America*, **68**, 387–398

HOYER, J.R., ELEMA, J. and VERNIER, R.L. (1976). Unilateral renal disease in the rat II. Glomerular mesangial uptake of coloidal carbon in unilateral aminonucleotide nephrosis and nephrotoxic serum nephritis. *Laboratory Investigation*, **34**, 250–253

IRWIN, J.F., LANE, S.E. and NEUHAUS, O.W. (1971). Synergistic effect of glucocorticoids and androgens on the biosynthesis of a sex-dependent protein in the male rat. *Biochimica Biophysica Acta*, **252**, 328–334

JÖRGENSEN, F. (1966). *The Ultrastructure of the Normal Human Glomerulus*. Copenhagen; Ejnar Munksgaard

KANWAR, Y.S. and FARQUHAR, M.G. (1979). Anionic sites in the glomerular basement membrane. *In vivo* and *in vitro* localization of the laminae rarae by cationic probes. *Journal of Cell Biology*, **81**, 137–140

KATZ, A.I. and LINDHEIMER, M.D. (1975). Relation of Na-K-ATPase to acute changes in renal tubular sodium and potassium transport. *Journal of General Physiology*, **66**, 209–222

KENNEDY, G.C. (1957). Effects of old age and over-nutrition on the kidney. *British Medical Bulletin*, **13**, 67–70

KÜL, F. and SETEKLEIV, J. (1973). Physiology of ureter and renal pelvis. In *Handbook of Physiology*, Section 8, Renal Physiology, edited by J. Orloff and R.W. Berliner. Washington; American Physiological Society

KONDO, Y., TAKIZAWA, J. and AKIKUSA, B. (1981). Cystic alterations of glomerular epithelial cells in experimental chronic nephritis in the rat. *Biomedical Research*, **2** (Supplement): Scanning Microscopy in Biology and Medicine, 311–316

KRAUS, B. and CAIN, H. (1974). Uber eine spontane Nephropathie bei Wistarratten. Die Licht- und Elektronenmicroskopischen Glomerulumveränderungen. *Virchows Archiv* (Pathology and Anatomy), **363**, 343–358

LALICH, J.J. and ALLEN, J.R. (1971). Protein overload nephropathy in rats with unilateral nephrectomy. II. Ultrastructural study. *Archives of Pathology*, **91**, 372–382

LALICH, J.J., FAITH, G.C. and HARDING, G.E. (1970). Protein overload nephropathy. *Archives of Pathology*, **89**, 548–559

LATTA, H. and JOHNSTON, W.H. (1976). The glycoprotein membrane as a filtration barrier. *Journal of Ultrastructural Research*, **57**, 65–72

LATTA, H., JOHNSTON, W.H. and STANLEY, T.M. (1975). Sialoglycoproteins and filtration barriers in the glomerular capillary wall. *Journal of Ultrastructural Research*, **51**, 354–359

LINKSWILER, H., REYNOLDS, M.S. and BAUMANN, C.A. (1952). Factors affecting proteinuria in the rat. *American Journal of Physiology*, **168**, 504–508

MAAK, T. (1975). Renal handling of low molecular weight proteins. *American Journal of Medicine*, **58**, 57–64

McCOY, G.W. (1908). Pathological conditions found in rats: observations based upon examination of 50,000 rats in the laboratory of the Public Health and Marine Hospital Service, San Francisco, *California Public Health Reports*, **23**, 1363–1383

MacKAY, I. (1972). Aging and immunological function in man. *Gerontology*, **18**, 285–304

MacPHERSON, D.J. (1963). Metaplasia of renal glomerular capsular epithelium. *Journal of Clinical Pathology*, **16**, 220–222

MARKHAM, R.V., SUTHERLAND, J.C. and MARDINEY, M.R. Jr. (1973). The ubiquitous occurrence of immune complex localization in the renal glomeruli of normal mice. *Laboratory Investigation*, **29**, 111–120

MARTÍNEZ-MALDONADO, M., BENABE, J.E. and LÓPEZ-NOVOA, J.M. (1983). Acute renal failure associated with tubulo-interstitial diseases, including papillary necrosis. In *Acute Renal Failure*, edited by B.M. Brenner and J.M. Lazarus, p. 452. Philadelphia; Saunders

MASRO, E.J. (1980). Mortality and growth characteristics of rat strains commonly used in aging research. *Experimental Aging Research*, **6**, 219–233

MEDLAR, E.M. and BLATHERWICK, N.R. (1937). The pathogenesis of dietary nephritis in the rat. *American Journal of Pathology*, **13**, 881–896

MELIS, M.F., PALERMO, C.D. and MOTTAR, P. (1974). Scanning and transmission electron microscopy′ observations and the columnar cells of the parietal layer of the Bowman's capsule in normal mice. *Journal of Microscopy*, **19**, 247–257

MEYER, T.W., HOSTETTER, T.H., RENNKE, H.G., NODDIN, J.L. and BRENNER, D.M. (1983). Preservation of renal structure and function by long term protein restriction in rats with reduced nephron mass. *Kidney International*, **23**, 218 (Abstract)

MICHAEL, A.F., BLAU, E. and VERNIER, R.L. (1970). Glomerular polyanion alteration in aminonucleoside nephrosis. *Laboratory Investigation*, **23**, 619–624

MOORE, R.A. and HELLMAN, L.M. (1930). The effect of unilateral nephrectomy on the senile atrophy of the kidney in the white rat. *Journal of Experimental Medicine*, **51**, 51–57

MYERS, B.D., DEEN, W.M. and BRENNER, B.M. (1975). Effects of norepinephrine and angiotensin II on the determinants of glomerular ultrafiltration and proximal tubule fluid reabsorption in the rat. *Circulation Research*, **37**, 101–109

NEUHAUS, O.W. and FLORY, W. (1975). The effect of dietary protein on the excretion of $\alpha 2\mu$, the sex-dependent protein of the adult male rat. *Biochimica Biophysica Acta*, **411**, 74–86

NEUHAUS, O.W. and FLORY, W. (1978). Age-dependent changes in the excretion of urinary proteins by the rat. *Nephron*, **22**, 570–576

NEWBURG, L.H. and CURTIS, A.C. (1928). Production of renal injury in the white rat by the protein of the diet. *Archives of Internal Medicine*, **42**, 801–821

O'BRYAN, D. and LOWENSTEIN, L.M. (1974). Effect of aging on renal membrane bound enzyme activities. *Biochimica Biophysica Acta*, **339**, 1–9

OLIVER, J., McDOWELL, M. and LEE, Y.C. (1954). Cellular mechanism of protein metabolism in the nephron. 1. The structural aspects of proteinuria. Tubule absorption, droplet formation and the disposal of proteins. *Journal of Experimental Medicine*, **99**, 589

OLSON, J.L., HOSTETTER, T.H., RENNKE, H.G., BRENNER, B.M. and VENKATACHALAM, M.A. (1982). Altered change and size selective properties of the glomerular wall. A response to reduced renal mass. *Kidney International*, **22**, 112–126

ORLOFF, J. and HANDLER, J.S. (1967). The role of adenosine 3′,5′-phosphate in the action of antidiuretic hormone. *American Journal of Medicine*, **42**, 757–768

PERRY, S.W. (1965). Proteinuria in the Wistar rat. *Journal of Pathology and Bacteriology*, **89**, 729–733

PETER, G.P. (1973). Possible immune origin of age-related pathological changes in long-lived mice. *Journal of Gerontology*, **28**, 265–275

PFEIFFER, C.A., EMMEL, V.M. and GARDNER, W.U. (1940). Renal hypertrophy in mice receiving estrogens and androgens. *Yale Journal of Biology and Medicine*, **12**, 493–501

POLLARD, M. and KAJIMA, M. (1970). Lesions in aged germ-free Wistar rats. *American Journal of Pathology,* **61,** 25–31

POTTER, E.L. (1972). *Normal and Abnormal Development of the Kidney,* pp. 3–71. Chicago; Year Book

PREUSS, H.G., WEISS, F.R., IANMARINO, R.M., HAMMACK, W.J. and MURDAUGH, H.V. Jr. (1974). Effects on rat kidney slice function *in vitro* of proteins from the urines of patients with myelomatosis and nephrosis. *Clinical Science and Molecular Medicine,* **46,** 283–294

POSKITT, T.R., FORTWENGLER, H.P. Jr., BOBROW, J.G. and ROTH, J.G. (1974). Naturally occurring immune complex glomerulonephritis in monkeys (*Macaca inus*). I. Light immunofluorescence and electron microscopic studies. *American Journal of Pathology,* **76,** 145–159

PURKERSON, M.L., HOFFSTEN, P.E. and KLAHR, S. (1976). Pathogenesis of glomerulopathy associated with renal infarction in rats. *Kidney International,* **9,** 407–417

REIDBORD, H.G. (1968). Metaplasia of the parietal layer of Bowman's capsule. *American Journal of Clinical Pathology,* **50,** 240–242

RENNKE, H.G. and VENKATACHALAM, M.A. (1977). Glomerular permeability: *in vitro* tracer studies with polyanionic and polycationic ferritins. *Kidney International,* **11,** 44–53

ROBSON, A.M., MOR, J., ROOT, E.R., JAGER, B.V., SHANKEL, S.W., INGELFINGER, J.R., KIENSTRA, R.A. and BRICKER, N.S. (1979). Mechanism of proteinuria in nonglomerular disease. *Kidney International,* **16,** 416–429

RODECK, H., LEDERIS, K. and HELLER, H. (1960). The hypothalamus–neurohypophyseal system in old rats. *Journal of Endocrinology,* **21,** 225–228

ROSENQUIST, T.M. and BERNICK, S. (1971). Histochemistry of renal basal lamenae: adolescent compared with senescent rats. *Journal of Gerontology,* **26,** 176–185

ROY, A.K. and NEUHAUS, O.W. (1966). Proof of the hepatic synthesis of a sex-dependent protein in the rat. *Biochimica Biophysica Acta,* **127,** 82–87

ROY, A.K. and NEUHAUS, O.W. (1967). Androgenic control of a sex-dependent protein in the rat. *Nature,* **214,** 618–620

ROY, A.K., NEUHAUS, O.W. and HARMISON, C.R. (1966). Preparation and characterization of a sex-dependent rat urinary protein. *Biochimica Biophysica Acta,* **127,** 72–81

RUMSFELD, H.W. Jr. (1956). Role of dietary protein in normal rat proteinuria. *American Journal of Physiology,* **184,** 473–478

SARTIN, J., CHANDHURI, M., OBENRADER, M. and ADELMAN, R.C. (1980). The role of hormones in changing adaptative mechanisms during aging. *Federation Proceedings,* **39,** 3163–3167

SAXTON, J.A. and KIMBALL, G.C. (1941). Relation of nephrosis and other diseases of albino rats to age and to modification of diet. *Archives of Pathology,* **32,** 951–965

SEILER, M.W., RENNKE, H.G., VENKATACHALAM, M.A. and COTRAN, R.S. (1977). Pathogenesis of polycation-induced alterations ('fusion') of glomerular epithelium. *Laboratory Investigation,* **36,** 48–61

SEILER, M.W., VENKATACHALAM, M.A. and COTRAN, R.S. (1975). Glomerular epithelium: structural alterations induced by polycations. *Science,* **189,** 390–393

SELLERS, A.L., GOODMAN, H.G., MARMORSTON, J. and SMITH, M. (1950). Sex difference in proteinuria in the rat. *American Journal of Physiology,* **163,** 662–667

SELYE, H. (1939). The effect of testosterone on the kidney. *Journal of Urology,* **42,** 637–641

SEN, S., SMEBY, R.R. and BUMPUS, F.M. (1972). Renin in rats with spontaneous hypertension. *Circulation Research,* **31,** 876–880

SHIMAMURA, T. and MORRISON, A.B. (1975). A progressive glomerulosclerosis occurring in partial five-sixths nefrectomy. *American Journal of Pathology,* **79,** 95–101

SHUSTER, S. and CALLAGHAN, P. (1961). Protein excretion and droplet formation in the mammalian kidney. *British Journal of Experimental Pathology,* **42,** 1–6

SIMMS, H.S. and BERG, B.N. (1957). Longevity and the onset of lesions in male rats. *Journal of Gerontology,* **12,** 244–252

SPIRO, R.G. (1967). Studies on the renal glomerular basement membrane: preparation and chemical composition. *Journal of Biological Chemistry,* **242,** 1915–1932

STRIKER, G.E., NAGLE, R.B., KOHNER, P.W. and SINUCLER, E.A. (1969). Response to unilateral nephrectomy in old rats. *Archives of Pathology,* **87,** 439–442

TISHER, C.C. (1981). Anatomy of the kidney. In *The Kidney,* 2nd edn, edited by B.M. Brenner and F.C. Rector Jr, pp. 3-76. Philadelphia; Saunders

TUCKER, S.M., MASON, R.L. and BEAUCHENE, R.E. (1976). Influence of diet and feed restriction on kidney function of aging male rats. *Journal of Gerontology,* **31,** 264–270

VELOSA, J.A., GLASSER, R.J., NEVINS, T.E. and MICHAEL, A.F. (1977). Correlation with immunopathological changes, macromolecular kinetics and polyamino loss. *Laboratory Investigation,* **36,** 527–534

VENKATACHALAM, M.A. and RENNKE, H.G. (1978). The structural and molecular basis of glomerular filtration. *Circulation Research,* **43,** 337–347

VON MOLLENDORF, W. (1930). Der Exkretionsapparat. In *Handbuch der Microskopischen Anatomie des Menschen,* edited by W. von Mollendorf, Vol. VII (pt. 1), pp. 61–65. Berlin; Springer

WACHTEL, L.W., COLE, L.J. and ROSEN, V.J. (1966). X-ray induced glomerulosclerosis in rats: modification of lesion by food restriction, uninephrectomy and age. *Journal of Gerontology,* **21,** 442–448

WALFORD, R.L. (1974). Immunologic theory of aging. Current status. *Federation Proceedings,* **33,** 2020–2027

WEIDMANN, P., BERETTA-PICCOLI, C., ZIEGLER, W.H., KEUSH, G., GLÜCK, Z. and REUBI, F. (1978). Age versus urinary sodium for judging renin aldosterone and catecholamine levels. Studies in normal subjects and patients with essential hypertension. *Kidney International,* **14,** 619–628

WEIDMANN, P., DE MYTTENAERE-BURSZTEIN, S., MAXWELL, M.H. and DE LIMA, J. (1975). Effect of aging on plasma renin and aldosterone in normal man. *Kidney International,* **8,** 325–333

YOSHINARI, T. and FUJITA, T. (1982). Scanning electron microscope studies on rabbit renal glomerulus with special reference to 'podocytic membrane' of Elias and to pored domes on capillary epithelium. *Archives of Histology of Japan,* **45,** 49–109

YUNIS, E.J., FERNANDES, G. and STUTMAN, O. (1971). Susceptibility to involution of the thymus-dependent lymphoid system and autoimmunity. *American Journal of Clinical Pathology,* **56,** 280–292

Chapter 9

Pharmacokinetics in the aged

A. Domínguez-Gil, M.J. García and A.S. Navarro

Introduction

The aim of pharmacokinetics research is to characterize the processes of absorption, distribution, metabolism and excretion after the administration to the organism of substances with pharmacological activity. Whereas the first two processes determine the access of the drug to its site of action, metabolism and excretion contribute to the elimination of the drug from the organism. The dynamic equilibrium set up between these processes regulates the levels of drug in the organism and is frequently correlated with the intensity of the pharmacological effect. Absorption regulates the incorporation of the drug into the systemic circulation through the mechanisms of passive diffusion or active transport. Absorption is defined by the rate at which it takes place, by the absorption constant and by the fraction of drug absorbed. The absorption of a drug is governed by factors related to the chemical structure of the agent (molecular weight, lipophilia, degree of ionization, etc.), to the form of administration (solution, tablets, capsules, etc.) and by physiopathological factors (age, cardiac disease, etc.). The fraction of drug which reaches the systemic circulation in an unaltered state is defined by the drug's bioavailability, a parameter which should be characterized in the design of new dosing forms or for new drugs which are administered by an extravascular route.

When a drug is administered orally, it should be taken into account that it may undergo what is known as the 'first-pass effect'. This phenomenon leads to a decrease in the apparent absorption of the drug as a result of the fact that on passing through the gastrointestinal tissues and the liver the agent is transformed and only a part of the absorbed fraction reaches the systemic circulation unaltered; this in turn means that the bioavailability of certain drugs administered by this route can be considerably reduced, not because the drugs do not have good oral absorbance but because they have undergone this first-pass effect. Among the drugs which could be mentioned in this sense are the following: desipramine; hydralazine; isoproterenol; lidocaine; methylphenidate; morphine; nitroglycerin; pentazocine, propoxyphene; propranolol; salicylamide.

For practical purposes, the concept of bioavailability is employed to indicate the amount of dose which reaches the systemic circulation in an unaltered state without taking into account the causes which have led to modifications in this fraction. The estimation of this parameter is generally made on the basis of the values of the area under the plasma concentration–time curve obtained after intravenous and extravascular administration.

Distribution regulates the access of the drug to the different organs and tissues of the body. It is calculated through the apparent distribution volume, which expresses the volume of the organism into which a given dose of drug is distributed. Different factors, such as plasma protein binding and tissue binding, lead to non-physiological values for this parameter, which accounts for the concept of the apparent value. The distribution parameter furnishes information about the degree of distribution, but only rarely coincides with the true value; even in those cases in which the distribution volume calculated corresponds to a physiological value, it cannot be inferred that such a value reflects the true distribution volume. To calculate this parameter we use the relationship between the amount of drug present in the organism and its plasma concentration once distribution equilibrium has been reached. Generally, it can be said that the value of the distribution volume calculated in this way will be greater than the real value when the drug shows affinity for tissue proteins, and the opposite will be true when its affinity is greater for plasma proteins. The concentration reached by the drug thus depends on the dose absorbed and the volume into which it is distributed.

Metabolism includes the chemical transformations which the drug undergoes inside the organism. Generally, these take place in the liver, although some substances are metabolized in other organs (kidney, lung). Metabolism is usually quantified according to the fraction of drug excreted in an unaltered state through the kidney, or by the urinary excretion of metabolites. In recent years, attempts have been made to characterize the kinetic profile of metabolites as a complementary contribution to information concerning this process. The characterization of the kinetic profile of a given metabolite is of particular interest when a considerable fraction of the dose is transformed metabolically, when the elimination of that metabolite is the slowest process in the sequence of events taking place between absorption and elimination, and when clearance of the metabolite is less than that of the parent drug.

Although most metabolites are eliminated faster than the drug administered, they are often governed by the rate of their formation. Some biotransformation processes are dose-dependent, as in the case of diphenylhydantoin, such that the elimination rate depends on the amount of drug administered. In other cases, the biotransformation processes are time-dependent such as with carbamazepine, owing to an autoinduction phenomenon. The parameter most commonly used to express the elimination rate of drugs is the *plasma half-life* or the time necessary for the plasma concentration of the drug to be reduced by half. This parameter constitutes a characteristic of each drug and can range from 30 min for penicillin G to 130 h in the case of phenobarbital. The elimination rate can also be expressed by the *plasma clearance,* which is the volume of plasma cleared in 1 min. Clearance can be described in terms of the eliminating organ, e.g. hepatic clearance, renal clearance or pulmonary clearance. It can also be described by the difference between renal excretion and elimination by all other processes, e.g. renal clearance and extrarenal clearance. Total clearance is the sum of the clearances by each of the eliminating organs and is one of the most common terms used in pharmacokinetics.

Interindividual variability in the response to a pharmacological treatment is sufficiently well documented in clinical practice and particularly so in the case of geriatric therapeutics.

With advanced aged, the response to drugs is modified as a result of the changes taking place in the processes defining the disposition kinetics of drugs, of the changes in receptor sensitivity and of the influence of associated pathological states

(Cohen, 1986). This is generally reflected in a requirement of lower doses in the elderly, compared with adult patients, and it is convenient to carefully monitor drug levels in order to individualize the doses administered.

The intensity and duration of the pharmacological effect of a drug are frequently related to its pharmacokinetic profile and principally to the concentration of free drug at the site of action. The concentrations reached by drugs in the different body organs and tissues depend on the equilibrium established between the kinetic processes of absorption, distribution, metabolism and excretion. Absorption determines the amount of drug which reaches the systemic circulation and the speed at which the process takes place. A decrease in the fraction of drug absorbed is equivalent to a decrease in the dose administered, with obvious clinical consequences. A decrease in the absorption rate, within certain limits, does not usually affect the response to the treatment. It should here be pointed out that a drug can be completely absorbed but at the same time present poor bioavailability as a result, for example, of an important first-pass effect, as in the case of the tricyclic antidepressants. In this case, a decrease in the response to the drug administered orally is associated with a decrease in serum levels caused by a low bioavailability, even though the drug has good absorption.

Distribution determines the access of the drug to the body organs and tissues and in this sense certain groups of drugs such as antibiotics, drugs which act on the CNS, etc., are of special importance. There are numerous factors which affect the penetration of drugs into tissues: their chemical structure, the serum concentration, their binding to proteins, their degree of biotransformation, their elimination rate, etc., as well as the modifications which take place in the body composition of the elderly.

Of interest are the modifications taking place in distribution as a result of the decrease in the elimination rate; this is one of the most significant alterations observed in the drug kinetics of the elderly.

Metabolism and excretion are the processes which govern the disappearance of a drug from the organism and they are frequently associated with a decrease in the intensity of the pharmacological effect.

From a kinetic point of view, the decrease in the elimination rate in elderly patients leads to higher values in the serum and tissue concentrations, in turn responsible for a stronger pharmacological response; this makes it necessary to reduce the dose administered, especially in drugs with a low safety margin such as cardiotonics, aminoglycoside antibiotics, antiarrhythmics, bronchodilators, etc.

The extraordinary development undergone by analytical methodology in recent years has made it possible to follow correctly the evolution of drugs and their metabolites within the organism by characterizing the processes which define their disposition kinetics. The monitoring of serum levels in geriatric patients means that it is possible to programme their dosage regimens correctly and this ensures greater efficacy and safety in pharmacological treatment. However, it should be pointed out that at the time of making a therapeutic decision, the data relating to plasma levels should be considered in the clinical context of the patient, and should never substitute observation and criteria of the clinician, but should rather be a complement to these.

There is ample evidence of pharmacodynamic alterations in the elderly. Accordingly, those drugs which act on the CNS induce an increased response which is not associated with modifications in the drug's pharmacokinetics. However, in other systems the same type of response does not occur, as is the case of drugs acting on the cardiovascular system (Vestal, 1978). The decrease in the intensity of the response is attributed to a decrease in the number of receptors, in the activity of the enzymes necessary to act as mediators on the drug's effect, etc. (Richey and Bender, 1977).

In view of the results obtained by numerous authors in studies carried out on animals and in man, O'Malley, Judge and Crooks (1976) have suggested that in geriatric patients a generalized decrease takes place in the function mediated by beta-receptors. This is manifested, for example, by an increased resistance to the effects of propranolol in the elderly and suggests a need to increase the dose of drugs whose action is localized on those receptors.

The response to drugs in the elderly may be modified by the influence of other factors associated with the aging process. Among these, the following are of importance:

(1) *Polypharmacy*. This is frequent in elderly patients and often leads to interactions which are manifested by an increased frequency in the appearance of adverse effects and toxicity.
(2) *Errors in medication* and in compliance. This is very common in elderly patients subjected to chronic treatments, particularly on complicated dosing schedules. A recommendable practice here is to try to make the dosage regimen as simple as possible for this kind of patient. Determination of their serum levels permits the clinician to detect the degree of compliance to the schedule prescribed.
(3) *States of malnutrition* which develop in the elderly are also responsible for alterations in the response to drugs.

All these factors justify the growing interest in geriatric pharmacology and the need for a careful control in the dosage schedule which must be supported by complete knowledge of drug pharmacokinetics in these patients.

Absorption

The aging process is accompanied by a series of physiological changes in the gastrointestinal tract which may induce alterations in drug absorption kinetics (Bender, 1968). Among such degenerative changes, the following are of interest: a delay in the gastric emptying time, which can have variable effects on the rate and extent of the absorption process; a decrease in gastric secretion, leading to an increase in the gastric pH which affects the ionization and consequently the solubility of certain drugs; an important reduction from 40 to 50 per cent in intestinal blood flow, leading to a decrease in drug absorption; atrophy of the macro- and microvellosities with an increase in connective tissue, and a decrease in gastrointestinal motility.

The kinetic modifications caused by such physiological changes exhibit great interindividual differences, even though the patients are of similar age; this is different to the kinetic modifications observed in paediatric populations and means that the kinetic parameters defining the absorption process are difficult to estimate in aging patients.

From the information available it is admitted that the absorption of sugars, vitamins and minerals is decreased. Accordingly, a decrease has been observed in the absorption of 3-methyl glucose, thiamine, galactose, calcium and organic iron (Triggs and Nation, 1975). These substances are absorbed through active transport mechanisms whose functionality may be reduced in this kind of patient. However, most drugs are absorbed by simple diffusion, which does not seem to be significantly modified with age, at least for a large number of drugs. The following is a list of drugs in which no modifications have been observed in the absorption process, compared with the data obtained in the young adult population: acetaminophen; indomethacin; lorazepam; paracetamol; phenylbutazone; propranolol; propicillin; sulphamethazole.

Nevertheless, certain drugs, such as digoxin or phenobarbital, exhibit pH-dependent absorption (Iisalo, 1977; Wettrell and Anderson, 1977; Tognoni *et al.*, 1983), such that a decrease in the absorption rate would be expected. In fact, the bioavailability of digoxin is decreased in geriatric populations (Lamy, 1982). The following list includes some drugs in which modifications in absorption have been reported in elderly patients:

Increased absorption	*Decreased absorption*
Chlormethiazole	Chlorazepate
Cimetidine	Chlordiazepoxide
Tetracyclines	Diazepam
	Iron salts
	Quinidine

It should be pointed out that the available data is somewhat scanty and has frequently been derived from studies with inadequate methodologies, which are hence inconclusive. In this sense, it is difficult to appreciate differences between geriatric and young adult patients by simple comparison of the values of the area under the plasma level curves (AUC) or the values of the maximum plasma concentrations reached. This is because in elderly patients simultaneous modifications take place in other parameters which are reflected in the value of the plasma clearance (Cl_p). Thus an increase in the AUC of the plasma levels observed in elderly patients does not necessarily imply an increase in absorption, since it could be due to a decrease in elimination or to modifications in the distribution processes. Hence for a comparison between the two populations, the AUC × Cl_p product should be used. In this sense, the AUC value of nitrazepam is significantly increased in elderly patients, principally due to a decrease in plasma clearance (Hirtz, 1980). Likewise, an increase may be seen in the bioavailability of propranolol as a consequence of the decrease of the first-pass effect, without this being involved in the absorption process.

The frequent association of several different drugs in the elderly may be responsible for modifications in absorption. Here we could mention the associations of tricyclic antidepressants and anticholinergic agents, or the association of tetracyclines with certain anti-acids. Other factors, such as changes in dietary habits, in dentition or in salivary flow, may be responsible for modifications in the plasma levels reached by certain drugs.

At present, most authors agree that in geriatric patients there are no important modifications in the rate and extent of the absorption process sufficient to justify changes in the dosage protocol.

Distribution

Distribution is an important kinetic process which determines the access of drugs to the different body organs and tissues and which may affect the pharmacological activity of numerous compounds (drugs). The changes observed in the distribution of drugs in geriatric populations are a result of the physiological changes which take place during the aging process, among which the following are outstanding:

(1) Changes in cardiac output. These have been calculated to decrease by 1 per cent per year from 30 years onwards and are manifested as alterations in tissue perfusion, thereby decreasing hepatic and renal blood circulation (Roddie and Wallace, 1978). This also affects the clearance for several drugs.
(2) Alterations in body composition. These are mainly manifested in a decrease in lean body mass and an increase in adipose tissues, particularly in women; such differences in fat content lead to a more extensive distribution of fat-soluble drugs in women. In general, it should be admitted that the changes in distribution with age principally depend on the hydrosolubility or liposolubility properties of the drug in question. In this sense, certain agents such as antipyrine, acetaminophen and ethanol, which are relatively hydrosoluble, will have a descended distribution in the elderly (O'Malley *et al.*, 1971; Chan *et al.*, 1975), whereas other liposoluble drugs such as lidocaine or diazepam will be more extensively distributed in such populations. This can be of great importance, since it may lead to a prolongation in the response to those drugs which have greater affinity for fatty tissues, especially when the dose has been established on the basis of the body weight of the patient. The aging process also leads to a decrease in body water and in extracellular fluid of between 20 and 40 per cent, respectively, which also affects the distribution of certain drugs.
(3) Changes taking place in the permeability of the biomembranes can influence the accessibility of drugs to the different body structures. Hence, studies carried out on epidural blockade clearly show that the amount of anaesthetic needed to block a certain area decreases with age (Bromage, 1962); this is attributed to a greater penetration capacity into the nerve fibres as a result of the degeneration of connective tissue and a delay in the removal of the drug due to a thickening of the vascular walls (Bender, 1965).

Other changes such as those related with the extra or intracellular pH or with the tissue binding of drugs may also be of interest, although they have not been sufficiently studied for conclusive results to be obtained.

Of all the factors which may affect the distribution of drugs, of greatest interest is that related to changes taking place in binding to plasma proteins: these may affect several kinetic processes and, in particular, distribution.

Although the content in total plasma proteins is not modified with age, a decrease takes place in the concentration of albumin accompanied by an increase in the concentration of globulins (Woodford-Williams *et al.*, 1964). The albumin:globulin ratio in young individuals has a value of 1.3, whereas in individuals older than 50 it only has a value of 1.0. Because drugs are mainly bound to albumin, a decrease in the degree of binding may be expected with age when drug plasma concentrations approach saturation capacity at the binding sites. *Table 9.1* shows the results obtained in studies on the binding capacity of drugs to plasma proteins in the elderly.

The clinical importance of the modifications in binding to plasma proteins is even greater if we consider that only the free fraction of drug has the ability to diffuse outside the systemic circulation, to the sites of action where they exert their pharmacological action and undergo the processes of biotransformation and

Table 9.1 Protein binding of several drugs in the elderly

Drugs with protein binding decreased in the elderly		*Drugs with protein binding unaltered in the elderly*
Phenytoin	(2–20%)	Phenylbarbituric acid
Carbenoxolone	(10%)	Benzylpenicillin
Propranolol	(60–62%)	Diazepam
Meperidine	(67–68%)	Desmethyldiazepam
Phenylbutazone	N.D.	Sulphadiazine
Tolbutamide	N.D.	Penicillin G
Chlormethiazole	N.D.	Quinidine
		Chlordiazepoxide

excretion (Greenblatt, Sellers and Shader, 1982). According to these considerations, the following may be established:

$$C^{ss} = \frac{\text{Dose per interval of time}}{\text{Clearance } (Cl_p)} \tag{9.1}$$

$$C_f^{ss} = \frac{\text{Dose per interval of time}}{\text{Free clearance } (Cl_f)} \tag{9.2}$$

where C^{ss} and C_f^{ss} are the mean concentrations at steady state of the total and free drug in plasma, respectively. Cl_f is free clearance, sometimes known as intrinsic clearance, which refers to the capacity of the clearing organs to remove the free drug.

Although it is frequently assumed that an increase in the free fraction implies an increase in Cl_p and in the intensity of the pharmacological effect, this is not always so, since the value of C^{ss} does not only depend on the free fraction, but also on the free clearance. For a given administration rate and free clearance value, C^{ss} will fall when the free fraction increases, whereas C_f^{ss}, and hence the intensity of the pharmacological action, will remain stable. In such circumstances, it is logical to expect that the therapeutic and toxic ranges, expressed as a function of concentration, should decrease significantly (Greenblatt *et al.*, 1980; Greenblatt, Sellers and Shader, 1982; Lamy, 1982) and as a consequence that the therapeutic ranges established in adult populations cannot be applied to geriatric patients.

The $Cl_p : Cl_f$ ratio will remain proportional if the fraction of free drug is only slightly modified interindividually. However, a clinically important reduction in the Cl_f associated with age may not be paralleled by a similar reduction in the Cl_p if the free fraction increases simultaneously. Thus, the data relating to total drug clearance in geriatric patients should be interpreted with caution if no information is available concerning the free fraction (Greenblatt, Sellers and Shader, 1982). Accordingly, it may happen that although a decrease in protein binding can induce an increase in transference to extravascular compartments, it will not necessarily produce a decrease in total plasma levels, as has been shown for chlormethiazole (Hirtz, 1980). This is possibly due to a drop in tissue protein binding simultaneously with the decrease in plasma protein binding.

The consequences of an increase in the free drug fraction depend on whether the drug is cleared by the kidney or by the liver and whether metabolism depends on the degree of hepatic extraction or on hepatic blood flow. For drugs with high extraction coefficients the result may be a decrease in clearance, which may be associated with a potential increase in the pharmacological response; this may make it necessary to correct the dosage regimen (Schumacher, 1980). However, what usually happens is an increase in clearance, either renal or hepatic: this effect compensates the greater free fraction because a decrease occurs in total levels such that no significant modification appears in the absolute amount of free drug and no correction in the dosage regimen is necessary.

Regardless of the possible modifications in the pharmacokinetic parameters, an increase in the fraction of free drug can increase the frequency of adverse reactions, as has been reported in the case of treatment with meperidine in elderly patients (Triggs and Nation, 1975).

Metabolism

Most drugs are eliminated from the organism through biotransformation processes of varying complexity. Only in a few cases, such as that of lithium or the aminoglycoside antibiotics, does elimination take place almost exclusively through renal excretion (Amdisem, 1975; Neu, 1982).

Metabolism can exert variable effects on the activities of drugs. When the activity is due to the drug itself, metabolism causes a decrease in the intensity and duration of the drug's effects. However, in certain cases metabolism can give rise to one or several active metabolites and the pharmacological activity will then depend on there being optimal hepatic function. *Table 9.2* shows some drugs whose metabolites are pharmacologically active.

Metabolism studies carried out in experimental animals with different drugs have shown that with advancing age a decrease takes place in the metabolic activity of the microsomes, in the liver weight:body weight ratio and in the activity of cytochrome P450, together with a reduced response to the effect of enzymatic inducers (Kato,

Table 9.2 Representative therapeutically important metabolites

Compound administered	*Metabolite*
Acetohexamide	Hydroxyhexamide
Acetylsalicylic acid	Salicylic acid
Amitriptyline	Nortriptyline
Amoxapine	8-Hydroxyamoxapine
Chloral hydrate	Trichloroethanol
Chlordiazepoxide	Desmethylchlordiazepoxide
Codeine	Morphine
Diazepam	Desmethyldiazepam
Doxepin	Desmethyldoxepin
Fluazepam	Desethylfluazepam
Glutethimide	4-Hydroxyglutethimide
Imipramine	Desipramine
Lidocaine	Desethyllidocaine
Loxapin	Desmethylloxapin
Meperidine	Normeperidine
Phenacetin	Acetaminophen
Phenylbutazone	Oxiphenbutazone
Prednisone	Prednisolone
Primidone	Phenobarbital
Procainamide	*N*-Acetylprocainamide
Propranolol	4-Hydroxypropranolol

Chiesara and Frontino, 1962; Kato *et al.*, 1964; Kato and Takanata, 1968). Even though in man there are no data relating hepatic microsome activity with age, the evidence does point to a decrease in the metabolism of several drugs in elderly patients. *Table 9.3* shows the effect of advanced age on the metabolic clearance of commonly used drugs.

Table 9.3 Effect of age on metabolic clearance of several drugs

Drug (route)	*Young*	*Elderly*	*Age groups studied*
Antipyrine (p.o.)	2.4 litres/h	1.5 litres/h[3]	20–50; 70–100
Antipyrine (i.v.)	34.6 ml/kg/h	28.2 ml/kg/h[3]	18–39; 60–92
Warfarin (p.o.)	3.80 ml/kg/h	3.26 ml/kg/h	20–40; 65–94
Phenytoin (i.v.; p.o.)	26.0 ml/kg/h	42.0 ml/kg/h[3]	20–43; 67–95
Diazepam (i.v.)	25.0 ml/min	25.0 ml/min	15–82
Paracetamol (p.o.)	777 ml/min/1.73 m^2	379 ml/min/1.73 m^2	22–27; 73–91

In those drugs whose clearance decreases in elderly patients, an increase will take place in the elimination half-life, leading to a progressive increase in serum concentrations; the possibility even exists of intoxication by overdose.

The decrease in biotransformation capacity in the elderly seems to be due to different factors: hepatic cell mass, enzyme activity, hepatic blood flow, plasma protein binding, drug distribution, nutritional status and enzyme induction (Crooks, O'Malley and Stevenson, 1976).

The biotransformation processes which are most significantly altered with age are the oxidation reactions, in particular hydroxylation (nortriptyline, phenytoin, quinidine, propranolol, etc.) and N-demethylation (amitriptyline, chlordiazepoxide, clobazan, chlorimipramine, etc.). Non-oxidative metabolism (acetylation conjugation) does not seem to be significantly modified by age, although more information is necessary to confirm this (Crooks, O'Malley and Stevenson, 1976; Hirtz, 1980).

Hepatic blood flow constitutes the main determining factor in the metabolic clearance of a large number of drugs. In geriatric patients a decrease of 40–45 per cent occurs, compared with values obtained in adults, as a result mainly of a decrease in cardiac output. One would therefore expect to find a decrease in the clearance of flow-dependent drugs, although the available data are rather conflicting. In this sense, for drugs with a high degree of hepatic extraction, such as propranolol, lidocaine and meperidine, a decrease occurs in clearance. Another of the factors which condition hepatic clearance is the binding of the drug to different blood components, in particular, to the plasma proteins, because only the free fraction can be cleared by the liver (Wilkinson and Shand, 1975).

Hence, for drugs widely bound to plasma proteins and in those drugs where the degree of binding is modified in geriatric patients, a modification will appear in the plasma clearance of the drug in question.

Elderly patients seem to be more resistant to the effect of enzymatic inducers which are always present in the environment. These include atmospheric pollutants, foods and components of tobacco smoke.

Renal excretion

The kidney is an important elimination route of drugs which are unaltered in the organism and also of their biotransformation products. Although most drugs are metabolized in the organism, a decrease in renal excretion usually leads to an accumulation of metabolites which may compromise the safety of a given pharmacological regimen.

The effective renal plasma flow (ERPF), which can be measured through the clearance of aminohippuric acid (AHA) or of iodopyracet (Diodrast), is modified with age according to the following expression:

$$\text{ERPF (ml/min/1.73 m}^2) = Cl_{\text{Diodrast}} = 840 - 6.44 \times \text{Age}$$

From this expression it may be inferred that the ERPF value decreases by approximately 1 per cent per year. If we take into account that the clearance of those drugs which are eliminated in an unaltered state through the kidney is limited by the renal blood flow, a decrease can be expected in clearance with age (Lamy, 1982).

Compared with the adult population, elderly individuals exhibit a 50 per cent decrease in renal function (Schumacher, 1980), with a drop in glomerular function and in tubular secretion; this may be seen by the clearance of inulin (Cl_{In}) and in the maximum tubular glucose uptake capacity (TmG) (Miller, McDonald and Shock, 1952) (see Chapters 1 and 7).

Although the degree of renal function is usually established on the basis of the creatinine clearance value or of serum creatinine, certain circumstances present in the elderly should be taken into account. As a consequence of the decrease in muscular mass and of lean body mass with respect to total body weight with age (Forbes and Reina, 1970; Bruce *et al.*, 1980), serum creatinine is not a good indicator for evaluating the degree of renal function in geriatric populations. Indeed, owing to a descended creatinine production, serum levels are maintained at normal levels, even though clearance may be lower than 50 ml/min. The creatinine clearance based on the determination of urinary excretion over 24 h and on the serum concentration of creatinine constitutes a truer indicator of renal function in the elderly. When it is not possible to carry out a complete urine collection, creatinine clearance may be estimated through serum creatinine according to equations or nomograms which consider the changes occurring with age (Siersbaeck-Nielsen *et al.*, 1971; Cockcroft and Gault, 1976).

The effect of the decrease in renal function with age on drug elimination is governed by the degree of utilization of the kidney as an excretion route. The clinical significance of such a decrease depends on the therapeutic range of the drug. Accordingly, the decrease in the elimination of penicillin is of little importance, whereas decreases in the elimination of digoxin or of aminoglycoside antibiotics may lead to very severe consequences (Ewy *et al.*, 1969).

For those drugs which are metabolized, a decrease in urinary excretion is manifested by a decrease in the elimination rate of their metabolites, as for example occurs with lidocaine.

The following is a list of drugs which are preferentially excreted through the kidney and whose elimination is decreased in the elderly: benzylpenicillin; digoxin; ethambutol; gentamicin; kanamycin; lithium; penicillin G; phenobarbital; practolol; propicillin; quinidine; sulphamethizole; tetracycline; tobramycin.

In order to avoid the accumulation which may take place in this kind of patient, it is necessary to adjust the dose according to the patient's cratinine clearance and to the parameters defining the elimination profile of the drug. Moreover, it should be remembered that the elderly patient is particularly prone to developing renal impairment due to frequent states of dehydration, congestive heart failure, hypotension, urinary retention, etc., which can contribute to a marked decrease in the elimination rate.

Elimination

Elimination encompasses a series of processes (metabolism, renal excretion, etc.) which contribute to the disappearance of the drug from the organism. The rate of elimination therefore significantly governs the duration of the effects achieved in a pharmacological treatment. The changes which may take place with age in the elimination rate of drugs is of special interest in those drugs with a narrow safety range: these are the aminoglycoside antibiotics, cardiotonic agents, hypoglycaemic agents, etc.

The parameter normally used to express the elimination rate is the plasma half-life, although it is more correct to use the plasma clearance. An increase in the elimination half-life increases the time needed to reach steady state and reduces the fluctuation between the maximum and minimum concentrations in a multiple dosage regimen, although it does not necessarily affect the degree of accumulation in the organism. The plasma clearance does not depend only on the elimination constant and hence determines the degree of accumulation in the organism. Both parameters may be differently modified in elderly patients. In this sense, the plasma clearance of diazepam is not significantly modified with age, whereas the elimination half-life is greater in elderly patients than in young individuals (Klotz, Avant and Hoyumpa, 1975). By contrast, for propicillin, the elimination constant is unmodified by age, although the decrease in the apparent distribution volume in elderly patients leads to a drop in the plasma clearance values. *Table 9.4* lists the drugs in which possible changes in the plasma clearance and elimination half-life have been studied in elderly patients. Generally, this kind of patient exhibits a decrease in the elimination capacity of drugs and this is manifested by a decrease in the plasma clearance and an increase in the elimination half-life.

Table 9.4 Modifications of Cl_p and $t_{\frac{1}{2}}$ in the elderly

Drug	Cl_p		$t_{\frac{1}{2}}$
Digoxin	50%	decrease	increase
Quinidine	30%	decrease	increase
Propranolol		increase	
Lithium	30–40%	decrease	
Chlordiazepoxide	20–40%	decrease	increase (2 times)
Desmethyldiazepam	50–70%	decrease	increase (3 times)
Theophylline	20–30%	decrease	
Cimetidine	30–50%	decrease	increase
Kanamycin		decrease	increase (2–3 times)
Acetaminophen		decrease	increase
Gentamicin		decrease	increase
Penicillin		decrease	
Tetracycline		decrease	
Tobramycin		decrease	
Chlormethiazole		decrease	
Antipyrine		decrease	
Sulphamethizole		decrease	
Cycloserine		decrease	
Phenytoin	40–60%	increase	
Tolbutamide		increase	

Pharmacokinetic approach to drug dosage in the elderly

The use of conventional drug dosing regimens in elderly patients has potential risks as a result of the modifications in the disposition kinetics of drugs with age. As has been mentioned above, in elderly patients a decrease takes place in plasma clearance compared with the values found in young adult pupulations, which often means that a reduction in the dose is necessary (Schumacher, 1980). Nevertheless, the possibility should also be considered of an increased pharmacological response due to increased sensitivity in the receptors, although the available information regarding this is rather scanty.

The application of pharmacokinetic criteria is of fundamental importance for establishing the correct dose of drugs in the elderly patient. This correction in the dosage regimen is particularly indicated when a decrease occurs in plasma clearance of drugs with a low therapeutic index, thereby offering a high risk of intoxication by overdose. Among those drugs which are of special interest in this sense are digoxin, nitrofurantoin, aminoglycoside antibiotics, tricyclic antidepressants, etc. (Richens and Warrinton, 1979; Davison, 1981).

Plasma clearance is the parameter which mainly controls the degree of drug accumulation during the course of therapeutic treatment. Equation (9.3) shows the relationship between drug serum levels at steady state (C_{av}^{ss}), the administration rate (D/τ) and plasma clearance (Cl_p):

$$C_{av}^{ss} = (f/Cl_p) \times (D/\tau) \tag{9.3}$$

where f is the bioavailability of the dosage form used. In order to apply this equation, it is necessary to assume that:

(1) The C_{av}^{ss} value is directly proportional to the intensity of the response.
(2) The variability in the magnitude of the response will allow the clinician to establish a range of C_{av}^{ss} values associated with therapeutic effects.
(3) The dose or the interval may be controlled by the clinician in order to achieve a desired C_{av}^{ss} value and hence a therapeutic response.
(4) The establishment of the dose is considerably influenced by the patient-dependent variables for a given drug, such as the bioavailability, plasma clearance and the response, which, logically, cannot be controlled by the clinician.

During the aging process, the changes taking place in the patient-dependent variables lead to alterations in the values of C_{av}^{ss} and, consequently, in the response if the dose administered is not modified.

Due to the wide interindividual variation shown by the parameters defining drug disposition in elderly patients, in order to modify the dose it is convenient to have individualized knowledge of the serum levels reached for a given dosage regimen. In this way it is possible to establish the $C_{av}^{ss}/D/\tau$ ratio in each patient, which is conditioned by the patient-dependent variables (f/Cl_p). Thus, and wherever possible, the serum drug levels in elderly patients should be monitored, especially when there is a risk of intoxication. For example in certain drugs, such as digoxin, quinidine, propranolol and theophylline, widely used in this kind of patient, variations of up to a magnitude of 10-fold are seen in the serum levels of patients receiving the same dose. Although the serum levels do not constitute an exact prediction of the pharmacological effect obtained, they are usually a better indicator than the actual dose administered to the patient (Sloan and Luderer, 1981).

For the monitoring of drug serum levels it is necessary to take into account that the therapeutic range should be considered as an approximate guide, in particular because this range has been established in clinical studies carried out in the adult population.

Lamy (1982) has reported that in geriatric patients the monitoring of serum levels is recommendable in the following situations: (a) when the serum levels/effect relationship is known; (b) for drugs with a low therapeutic index, i.e. in those cases where there is a high risk of passing from inefficient therapeutic levels to intoxication by overdose; (c) when it is difficult to evaluate the pharmacological or clinical effects; (d) when the patient is suspected of non-compliance with the prescribed medication; (e) when infradosing or overdosing is suspected.

The application of pharmacokinetic principles to the programming of dosage regimens allows the prediction of the serum concentrations and the possibility of correcting the dosing to fit the serum concentrations within the therapeutic range (Pippenger, 1979). For these predictions, it is possible to use the pharmacokinetic parameters established in a large population (Sheiner, Rosenberg and Marathe, 1977), the drug levels established in each individual patient (Jashvant, Unadkat and Rowland, 1982) or a combination of both sources of information. The use of the first source, the pharmacokinetic parameters established in a large population, has the disadvantage of presenting considerable interindividual variations, especially in those drugs which undergo a large degree of biotransformation.

The determination of the parameters of each individual patient presents several drawbacks, such as the time needed to perform the experiment, the discomfort for the patient and the high cost when hospitalization is necessary.

Different procedures have therefore been described for programming dosage regimens and these are more accurate than the first method (large populations) and simpler than the second (individual patient) and provide good information with a reduced number of blood samples.

When the initial dose of a drug is administered (D), the serum concentration (C) may be established from the following general expression:

$$C = D(Z) \cdot e^{-\beta\tau} \tag{9.4}$$

where β represents the terminal elmination phase constant, t is the time after administration once the absorption and distribution processes have been completed and (Z) is a factor which depends on the kinetic model and the administration route employed.

From three values obtained during the elimination phase it is possible to determine the parameters defining elimination and these allow us to estimate the serum concentrations at steady state. The serum concentration at the end of the dosage interval once steady state has been reached may be expressed by

$$C^{ss}_{min} = D_m \cdot (Z)\left(\frac{1}{1 - e^{-\beta\tau}}\right) e^{-\beta\tau} \tag{9.5}$$

where D_m is the maintenance dose and τ is the dosage interval. From equation (9.5) it is possible to calculate the maintenance dose to reach a desired C^{ss}_{min}:

$$D_m = \frac{C^{ss}_{min}}{(Z)} (1 - e^{-\beta\tau})\, e^{\beta\tau} \tag{9.6}$$

This method allows us to establish the desired serum levels according to the minimum pharmacokinetic information obtained in each of the patients after the administration of the first dose.

The validity of this method is conditioned by the exactness of the determination of the values of β and (Z).

The 'single-point single-dose' method is based on a single determination of the serum concentration carried out at a previously fixed time after the administration of a first dose. This method was first used for drugs with relatively long elimination half-lives, from 10 to 50 h, although recently its validity has been reported for drugs with short elimination half-lives, such as theophylline and chloramphenicol (Slattery, Gibaldi and Jeffery, 1980).

The methods described above permit the prediction of dosage intervals at the start of treatment by using the data supplied by an initial dose. However, it is common to start monitoring of the serum levels in patients who have been receiving pharmacological treatment for some time, perhaps even some years, as in the case of epileptic patients who do not respond to treatment. In those cases in which pharmacological treatment has been started, it is necessary to know the time taken for steady state to be reached, where correlations have been established between the serum levels and the efficacy or toxicity of the drug. For drugs which follow linear kinetics, i.e. drugs which are not dependent on either the dose administered or on the serum concentrations reached, the time necessary to reach steady state depends exclusively on the elimination constant of the drug and for practical purposes this is about 5 times the half-life value.

It should be pointed out that when monitoring of the serum levels is used, an optimal sampling time is established, according to the elimination half-life value and the dosage interval employed. If the determination of the serum values is carried out at this time, a good estimation can be obtained of the C_{av}^{ss} value from a single sample. Accordingly, for phenobarbital, the concentration determined at the end of the interval will give a good estimation (± 10 per cent) of the C_{av}^{ss} value. For other drugs with a faster elimination rate, it may be convenient to take blood samples close to the mid-point of the dosing interval, as long as at that time the absorption and elimination processes have been completed. Thus, for salicylates, procainamide and quinidine, blood sampling should be carried out immediately before the administration of a new dose. For digoxin and lithium, blood withdrawal should be performed at 8 and 12 h, respectively, after the last administration. The correct choice of the sampling time minimizes the errors introduced by the analytical techniques as well as the variations which occur as a consequence of the changes in the distribution volume.

Having chosen a suitable sampling time for the drug whose serum levels are to be monitored, a good estimation of the C_{av}^{ss} value may be obtained, related to the dose according to the following equation:

$$C_{av}^{ss} = \frac{f \cdot D}{K_e \cdot V_d \cdot \tau} = \frac{f \cdot D_m}{Cl_p \cdot \tau} \tag{9.7}$$

If the patient is undergoing a particular dosage regimen (D_1, τ_1) and a serum concentration C_{av1}^{ss} is reached once steady state is obtained, it is possible to know the factor Cl_p/f which for a given drug and in a given patient should be maintained constant (Q):

$$\frac{Cl_p}{f} = Q = \frac{D_1}{C_{av1}^{ss} \cdot \tau_1} \tag{9.8}$$

If the serum levels obtained at a steady state for the proposed dosage regimen (D_1, τ_1) are outside the therapeutic margin established, the dosing must be corrected, using the following:

$$D_2/\tau_2 = Q \,.\, C^{ss}_{av} \text{ desired} \tag{9.9}$$

Once the new corrected dose has been administered and after a period of about 5 times the elimination half-life of the drug in that particular patient, a new determination is made of the serum concentration (C^{ss}_{av2}). In general, in this first approximation it is possible to obtain acceptable correlation coefficients between the observed and predicted concentrations.

In view of the results obtained in numerous experimental and clinical studies, it is possible to affirm that the pharmacokinetics of a large number of drugs are altered in geriatric patients. Unfortunately, such alterations can affect the different pharmacokinetics parameters in various ways such that at present no general rule has been put forward. However, it is to be expected that this situation will improve in the foreseeable future and that greater information will become available to the clinician, who should be aware of the help of pharmacokinetics in establishing dosage regimens in elderly patients.

Misuse of some important drugs in the elderly in relation to renal function and disease

Given the complex changes in drug handling with age outlined above, it is not surprising that on occasion drugs are prescribed inappropriately in aged subjects. However, it is distressing to see just how frequently drugs are misused in elderly subjects, well-known traps for the unwary prescriber being forgotten or ignored. In this section we highlight some of the common and more important points in prescribing with reference to renal function and renal disease in the elderly; general guides to the use of drugs in established renal failure itself are those of Anderson *et al.* (1981), Bennett *et al.* (1977) and Briggs *et al.* (1984), and there are many reviews of drug use in the elderly (Papper, 1973; Hayes, Langman and Short, 1975; Ingman *et al.*, 1975).

One of the commonest problems in clinical practice is the inappropriate use of *digoxin* in elderly patients. The small muscle mass of the elderly patient in relation to body weight results in increased fraction of free drug, which must then be eliminated through kidneys affected by the functional and structural decline discussed in the preceding chapters. Cardiotoxicity is often compounded by hypokalaemia induced by the concomitant use of *diuretics*. The significance of this very common problem is the subject of lively debate (Kaplan *et al.*, 1985), but the balance of the evidence favours the idea that hypokalaemia in diuretic-treated patients, especially the elderly, *does* have a significant morbidity (see Chapters 4, 5 and 12). The use of potassium-sparing diuretics may have some advantages, as well as oral potassium supplementation, but the dangers of these must in turn be remembered (see Chapters 4 and 5). Whether digoxin improves the output of the heart in normal rhythm still remains the subject of debate and many elderly patients are not only taking toxic quantities of digoxin, but probably do not need it in the first place. Dall (1970) was able to discontinue the drug without detriment in 78 per cent of 80 elderly patients who had been taking it in the long term.

Aminoglycosides are exclusively removed by renal elimination, and the problems of aminoglycoside toxicity are compounded by their well-known propensity to cause renal tubular damage and even a polyuric acute renal failure (Neu, 1982). Thus, excessive dosage leads to even higher and rising plasma levels, with (in the case of gentamicin) both ototoxicity and nephrotoxicity. The fact that the acute renal failure is rarely accompanied by oliguria usually results in delay in diagnosis, so that the patient may be severely damaged before the true picture becomes evident. Tobramycin has a rather better record with regard to nephrotoxicity, but netilmicin has almost no ototoxicity and only minor nephrotoxicity; perhaps it should be employed as the drug of choice in the elderly, whose vestibular apparatus and hearing are often compromised already. *Aminoglycosides can only be used with safety in the elderly if the plasma concentrations can be monitored,* but under no circumstances should a starting dose of more than 160 mg/24 h of gentamicin be used.

Lithium is a valuable drug, especially in manic states, but it is a nephrotoxic drug with a very narrow therapeutic range (plasma lithium 0.4–0.7 mmol/l, toxicity $>$ 1.5 mmol/l) exclusively eliminated through the kidney. Usually, as with the aminoglycosides, the first effect is impairment of urinary concentrating ability, and renal failure, if induced, is polyuric rather than oliguric, so that diagnosis of renal damage may be delayed, and in addition to the already impaired ability of the elderly to conserve salt and water (see Chapter 4) is made worse.

Wallin *et al.* (1982) showed also that ^{51}Cr EDTA GFR measurements were below age-related control measurements from 20 to 80 years of age in patients treated with lithium, even those who had never had any clinical episodes of toxicity, and Hansen *et al.* (1982) found interstitial fibrosis, again in patients who had not experienced toxicity. Thus, lithium must be used with caution in the elderly. Foster, Gershell and Goldfarb (1977) suggest beginning with a dose of only 50–65 mg (1 mg/kg body weight) in elderly patients, repeated 2 or 3 times within 24 h if no side effects appear. Again, *the drug cannot be used safely unless it is possible to measure the plasma levels* at regular intervals. The dangers of such a slowly eliminated drug, should renal function become impaired during stable treatment, are obvious and often forgotten. If an elderly patient suffers diarrhoea or vomiting, or renal function falls for any reason, lithium must be stopped and only restarted after checking the plasma level.

A very large number of the elderly now take *non-steroidal anti-inflammatory drugs (NSAIDs)* for musculoskeletal problems of varying severity, some relatively trivial. It has been estimated that over 30 million Americans may be taking these drugs (Clive and Stoff, 1984), some of which are now available, like the prototype aspirin, over the pharmacist's counter without prescription. Thus, it may not be evident to the physician that a patient in front of him is taking NSAIDs, with all their varied renal effects.

NSAIDs have little or no effect on renal function in normal well-hydrated individuals with good cardiac outputs, but in any state of renal hypoperfusion (such as cardiac failure or volume depletion) there may be a profound fall in both renal blood flow and GFR (*Figure 9.1*). This arises at least in part from blockage by the drugs of compensatory mechanisms which increase cortical perfusion and the GFR, which depend upon the renal synthesis of vasodilator prostaglandins (principally PGI_2, prostacyclin, in man) (Ciabattoni *et al.*, 1984). One of the most dangerous features of patients taking NSAIDs in that conventional tests of renal function are normal — it is the *reserves* of renal function during hypovolaemic or hypotensive stress that are impaired. In addition, there may be retention of salt and water, leading

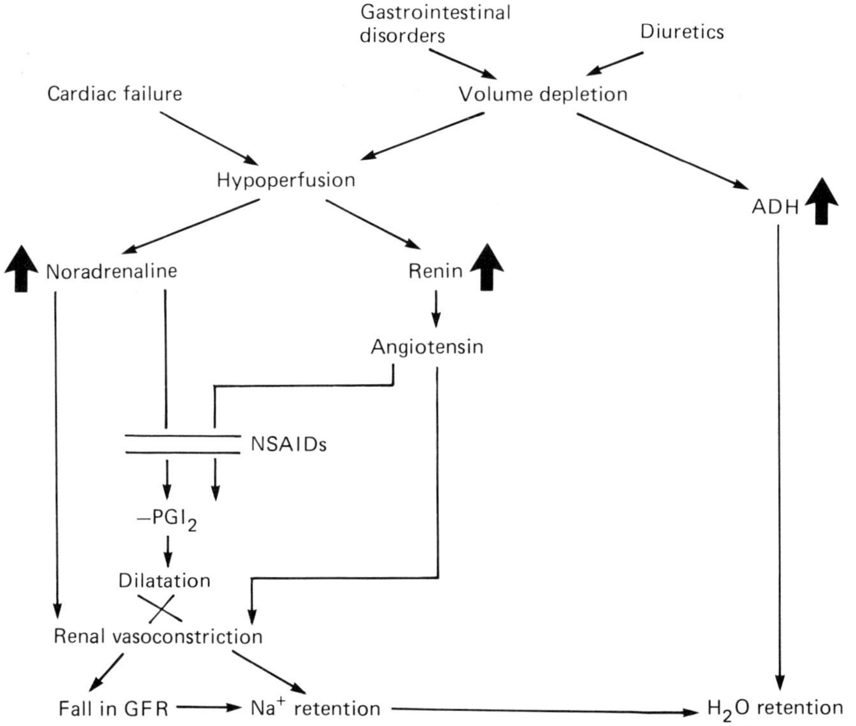

Figure 9.1 Some of the events during administration of non-steroidal anti-inflammatory agents. During renal hypoperfusion from any cause, noradrenaline and angiotensin secretion promote and perpetuate the hypoperfusion (left). Normally, this mechanism is balanced by the fact that both noradrenaline and angiotensin release lead to synthesis of prostacyclin (PGI_2) from arachidnoic acid in lipid plasma membranes via the enzyme cyclo-oxygenase. This PGI_2 induces renal vasodilatation, and helps preserve both renal blood flow and glomerular filtration rates in situations where renal perfusion is compromised, such as those shown at the top of the diagram. Administration of agents which block the production of prostaglandins block the production of the vasodilatory PGI_2, placing the kidney at risk from further vasoconstriction and a fall in perfusion and GFR. In normally hydrated and perfused individuals, however, no effect is evident. Because of simultaneous release of non-osmotically generated ADH (right), water is also retained as well as Na^+, and oedema may form. NSAIDs also block the production of renin and angiotensin (not shown in the diagram) and thus may precipitate hyperkalaemia

to either oedema or hypertension, and hyperkalaemia may be a problem. Interaction with concomitantly administered diuretics is an obvious danger (Taha *et al.*, 1985). Aspirin and diflusinal, ibuprofen, ketoprofen and fenoprofen, naproxen, indomethacin and zomepirac, the mefanamates, alclofenac and prioxicam, are all capable of this action, but other agents such as paracetamol, propoxyphene and azapropazone, not being prostaglandin synthetase inhibitors, do not. Some of these agents can induce an inflammatory interstitial nephritis, particularly fenoprofen, often accompanied by a nephrotic syndrome and sometimes acute renal failure. Occasionally, vasculitis may be seen (*Table 9.5*). The immunologic basis for these is not known, but oliguria may be prolonged and occasionally irreversible. Fenoprofen should, probably, not be used given the alternatives available. The considerable problems attending the use of these common drugs has led to several recent reviews of their effects on the kidney (Clive and Stoff, 1984; Garella and Matarese, 1984; Carmichael and Shankel, 1985).

Table 9.5 Renal syndromes caused by NSAIDs*
(From the literature review of Carmichael and Shankel, 1985)

Nephrotic syndrome	34
Acute interstitial nephritis	51
Acute tubular necrosis	29
Papillary necrosis	53
'Poor renal perfusion'	40
Glomerulonephritis/vasculitis	13
Other non-specified	102
	322

*In 274 patients, some of whom had more than one lesion.

Many antibiotics other than the aminoglycosides are excreted entirely or in part by the kidney, such as the *penicillins.* Usually these do not present problems, but if given in quantities far in excess of 20 g/24 h, they may accumulate and lead to a bleeding diathesis dependent upon platelet inhibition, or lead to an encephalopathy. Richet *et al.* (1970) found that neurological syndromes in patients with renal failure were most often due to abuse of drugs acting on the nervous system (at that time mostly barbiturates), but that the second commonest group at fault were antibiotics. First-generation cephalosporins and metronidazole may also give rise to encephalopathy.

The problems of inappropriately administered *hypotensive agents* in the elderly have been discussed in Chapters 5 and 12. Diabetes is common in the elderly subject, and may require treatment with oral hypoglycaemic agents. *Chlorpropamide* is excreted renally, has a very long half-life, and should never be used in the treatment of diabetes in the elderly (Stowers and Borthwick, 1977), since other safer hypoglycaemics such as tolbutamide and glibenclamide are available. Finally, *antidepressants* may inhibit bladder function, particularly imipramine but also tricyclic and tetracyclic agents, and may precipitate acute retention of urine in elderly males with subcritical bladder neck obstruction, usually the result of benign hypertrophy of the prostate. Before giving these drugs to the elderly, it is worth assessing prostatic size manually or by ultrasound, which will also reveal an enlarged, thickened bladder, or residual urine after micturition if not evident on palpation (see Chapter 19).

References

AMDISEM, A. (1975). Monitoring of lithium treatment through determination of lithium concentration. *Danish Medical Bulletin,* **22,** 277–291

ANDERSON, R.J., BENNETT, W.M., GAMBERTOGLIO, J.G. and SCHRIER, R.W. (1981). Fate of drugs in renal failure. In *The Kidney,* 2nd edn, edited by B.M. Brenner and F.C. Rector, pp. 2.659–2.700. Philadelphia; Saunders

BENDER, A.D. (1965). The effect of increasing age on the distribution of peripheral blood flow in man. *Journal of the American Geriatrics Society,* **13,** 192–198

BENDER, A.D. (1968). Effect of age on intestinal absorption: implications for drug absorption in the elderly. *Journal of the American Geriatrics Society,* **16**(1), 331–339

BENNETT, W.M., SINGER, I., GOLPER, T., FEIG, P. and COGGINS, C.J. (1977). Guidelines for drug therapy in renal failure. *Annals of Internal Medicine,* **86,** 754–783

BRIGGS, W.A., McDONALD, F.D., SILLIX, D.M. and McDOUGAL, M.L. (1984). Use of drugs in uremia and dialysis. In *Therapy of Renal Diseases and Related Disorders,* edited by W. Suki and S. Massry, pp. 567–586. Amsterdam; Nijhoff

BROMAGE, P.R. (1962). Exaggerated spread of epidural analgesia in arterosclerotic patients. *British Medical Journal,* **2,** 1.634–1.638

BRUCE, A., ANDERSON, M., ARVIDSSON, B. and ISAKSSON, B. (1980). Body composition. Prediction of normal body potassium, body water and body fat in adults on the basis of body height, body weight and age. *Scandinavian Journal of Clinical Laboratory Investigation,* **40,** 461–473

CARMICHAEL, T. and SHANKEL, S.W. (1985). Effects of non-steroidal anti-inflammatory drugs on prostaglandins and renal function. *American Journal of Medicine,* **78,** 992–1000

CHAN, K., KENDALL, M.J., MITCHARD, M., WELLS, W.D.E. and VICKERS, M.D. (1975). The effect of aging on plasma phetidine concentration. *British Journal of Clinical Pharmacology,* **2,** 297–302

CIABATTONI, G., CINOTTI, G.A., PIERUCCI, A., SIMPNETTI, B.M., MONZI, M., PUGLIESE, F. *et al.* (1984). Effects of sulindac and ibuprofen in patients with chronic glomerular disease. *New England Journal of Medicine,* **310,** 279–283

CLIVE, D.M. and STOFF, J.S. (1984). Renal syndromes associated with non-steroidal anti-inflammatory drugs. *New England Journal of Medicine,* **310,** 563–572

COCKCROFT, D.W. and GAULT, M.H. (1976). Prediction of creatinine clearance from serum creatinine. *Nephron,* **16,** 31–34

COHEN, J.L. (1986). Pharmacokinetic changes in aging. *American Journal of Medicine,* **80** (suppl. 5A), 31–38

CROOKS, J., O'MALLEY, K. and STEVENSON, I.H. (1976). Pharmacokinetics in the elderly. *Clinical Pharmacokinetics,* **1,** 280–296

DALL, J.L. (1970). Maintenance digoxin in elderly patients. *British Medical Journal,* **IV,** 69–72

DAVISON, W. (1981). Prescribing for the elderly. *The Practitioner,* **225,** 1.727–1.735

EWY, G.A., KAPADIA, G.G., YAO, L., LULLIN, M. and MARCUS, F.I. (1969). Digoxin metabolism in the elderly. *Circulation,* **39,** 449–453

FORBES, G.B. and REINA, J.C. (1970). Adult lean body mass declines with age; some longitudinal observations. *Metabolism,* **19,** 653–663

FOSTER, J.R., GERSHELL, W.J. and GOLDFARB, A.I. (1977). A lithium treatment in treatment in the elderly. *Journal of Gerontology,* **32,** 299–304

GARELLA, S. and MATARESE, R.A. (1984). Renal effects of prostaglandins and clinical adverse effects of non-steroidal anti-inflammatory agents. *Medicine (Baltimore),* **63,** 165–181

GREENBLATT, D.J., ALLEN, M.D., HARMATZ, J.S. and SHADER, R.I. (1980). Diazepam disposition determinants. *Clinical Pharmacology and Therapeutics,* **27,** 301–312

GREENBLATT, D.J., SELLERS, E.M. and SHADER, R.I. (1982). Drug disposition in old age. *New England Journal of Medicine,* **306,** 1.081–1.086

HANSEN, H.E., HESTBECH, J., SORENSEN, J.L., NORGAARD, K., HEISLSKOV, J. and AMDISEN, A. (1982). Chronic interstitial nephropathy on long-term lithium treatment. *Quarterly Journal of Medicine,* **48,** 577–591

HAYES, M.J., LANGMAN, M.J.S. and SHORT, A.H. (1975). Changes in drug metabolism with increasing age. II. Phenytoin clearance and protein binding. *British Journal of Clinical Pharmacology,* **2,** 73–78

HIRTZ, J. (1980). La pharmacocinetique du sujet âge. *Pharmaceutica Acta Helvetiae,* **55,** 72–78

IISALO, E. (1977). Clinical pharmacokinetics of digoxin. *Clinical Pharmacokinetics,* **2,** 1–16

INGMAN, S.R.I., LAWSON, E., PIERPAOLI, P.G. and BLAKE, P. (1975). A survey of the prescribing and administration of drugs in a long-term care institution for the elderly. *Journal of the American Geriatric Society,* **23,** 309–316

JASHVANT, D., UNADKAT, J.D. and ROWLAND, M. (1982). Further considerations of the 'single-point single-dose' method to estimate individual maintenance dosage requirements. *Therapeutic Drug Monitoring,* **4,** 201–208

KAPLAN, N.M., CARNEGIE, A., RASKIN, P., HILLER, J.A. and SIMMONS, M. (1985). Potassium supplementation in hypertensive patients with diuretic-induced hyperkalaemia. *New England Journal of Medicine,* **312,** 746–749

KATO, R., CHIESARA, E. and FRONTINO, G. (1962). Influence of sex difference on the pharmacological action and metabolism of some drugs. *Biochemical Pharmacology,* **11,** 221–227

KATO, R. and TAKANATA, A. (1968). Effect of phenobarbital on electron transport system, oxidation and reduction of drugs in liver microsomes of rats of different age. *Journal of Biochemistry,* **63,** 406–408

KATO, R., VASSANELLI, P., FRONTINO, G. and CHIESARA, E. (1964). Variation in the activity of liver microsomal drug-metabolising enzymes in rats in relation to age. *Biochemical Pharmacology,* **13,** 1.037–1.051

KLOTZ, U., AVANT, G.R. and HOYUMPA, A. (1975). The effects of age and liver disease in the disposition and elimination in adult man. *Journal of Clinical Investigation,* **55,** 347–359

LAMY, P.P. (1982). Comparative pharmacokinetic changes and drug therapy in an older population. *Journal of the American Geriatrics Society,* **30,** Suppl. No. 11, 11–19

MILLER, J.H., McDONALD, R.K. and SHOCK, N.W. (1952). Age changes in the maximal rate of renal tubular reabsorption of glucose. *Journal of Gerontology,* **7,** 196–200

NEU, H.C. (1982). Pharmacology of aminoglycosides. In *The Aminoglycosides,* edited by A. Whelton and H. Neu, pp. 125–142. New York; Marcel Dekker

O'MALLEY, K., CROOKS, J., DUKE, E. and STEVENSON, I.H. (1971). Effects of age and sex on human drug metabolism. *British Medical Journal,* **3,** 607–609

O'MALLEY, K., JUDGE, T.G. and CROOKS, J. (1976). Geriatric clinical pharmacology and therapeutics. In *Drug Treatment,* edited by G.S. Avery. Sydney; ADIS Press

PAPPER, S. (1973). The effects of age in reducing renal function. *Geriatrics,* **28,** 83–89

PIPPENGER, C.E. (1979). Therapeutic drug monitoring: an overview. *Therapeutic Drug Monitoring,* **1,** 3–9

RICHENS, A. and WARRINGTON, S. (1979). When should plasma drug levels be monitored? *Drugs,* **17,** 483–500

RICHET, G., DE NOVALIS, E.L. and VERROUST, P. (1970). Drug intoxication and neurological episodes in chronic renal failure. *British Medical Journal,* **2,** 394–399

RICHEY, D.P. and BENDER, A.D. (1977). Pharmacokinetic consequences of aging. *Annual Revision of Pharmacology and Toxicology,* **17,** 49–65

RODDIE, I.C. and WALLACE, W.K.M. (1978). Sistema cardiovascular. In *Fisiologia Patológica,* pp. 87–97. Barcelona; Salvat, S.A.

SCHUMACHER, G.E. (1980). Using pharmacokinetics in drug therapy VII: pharmacokinetic factors influencing drug therapy in the aged. *American Journal of Hospital Pharmacy,* **37,** 559–562

SHEINER, L.B., ROSENBERG, B. and MARATHE, V.V. (1977). Estimation of population characteristics of pharmacokinetic parameters from routine clinical data. *Journal of Pharmacokinetics and Biopharmaceutics,* **5,** 445–579

SIERSBAECK-NIELSEN, K., HANSEN, J.M., KAMPMANN, J. and KRISTENSEN, M. (1971). Rapid evaluation of creatinine clearance. *Lancet,* **1,** 1.123–1.134

SLATTERY, J.T., GIBALDI, M. and JEFFERY, R.K. (1980). Prediction of maintenance dose required to attain a desired drug concentration at steady-state from a single determination of concentration after an initial dose. *Clinical Pharmacokinetics,* **5,** 377–385

SLOAN, R.W. and LUDERER, J.R. (1981). Rational use of drugs levels. *American Family Physician,* **23,** 122

STOWERS, J.M. and BORTHWICK, L.J. (1977). Oral hyperglycaemic drugs: clinical pharmacologic and therapeutic use. *Drugs,* **14,** 14–56

TAHA, A., LENTON, R.J., MURDOCH, P.S. and PEDEN, N.R. (1985). Non-oliguric renal failure during treatment with mefanamic acid in elderly patients: a continuing problem. *British Medical Journal,* **291,** 661–662

TOGNONI, L., BELLANTUANO, M., BONATI, M., D'INCALCI, M., GERNA, M., LATINI, R. *et al.* (1983). Clinical relevance of pharmacokinetics. In *Handbook of Clinical Pharmacokinetics,* edited by M. Gibaldi and L.F. Prescott, pp. 1–34. Hong Kong; ADIS Health Science Press

TRIGGS, E.J. and NATION, R.L. (1975). Pharmacokinetics in the aged: a review. *Journal of Pharmacokinetics and Biopharmaceutics,* **3,** 387–418

VESTAL, R.E. (1978). Drug use in the elderly: a review of problems and special considerations. *Drugs,* **16,** 358–382

WALLIN, L., ALLING, L. and AURELL, M. (1982). Impairment of renal function in patients on long-term lithium treatment. *Clinical Nephrology,* **18,** 23–28

WETTRELL, G. and ANDERSSON, K.E. (1977). Clinical pharmacokinetics of digoxin in infants. *Clinical Pharmacokinetics,* **2,** 17–31

WILKINSON, G.R. and SHAND, D.G. (1975). A physiological approach to hepatic drug clearance. *Clinical Pharmacology and Therapeutics,* **18,** 377–390

WOODFORD-WILLIAMS, E., ALVARES, A.S., WEBSTER, D., LANDLESS, B. and DIXON, M.P. (1964). Serum protein patterns in 'normal' and pathological ageing. *Gerontology,* **10,** 86–99

Chapter 10

Summing up: what does decreased renal function in the aged mean?

S. de Castro del Pozo

Introduction

Reflections on this topic are not only of theoretical interest, but also imply certain ideas for clinical and preventative medicine which must be borne in mind by all those physicians caring for elderly persons, both ill and healthy, and which are elaborated upon in preceding chapters of this book.

(1) It is necessary to set down standards of normality and abnormality for functional exploration, *within the age range into which it has been agreed that 'elderly persons' fall.* One is aware that it is difficult to find groups of 'normal' elderly persons, but somehow this difficulty must be overcome. We shall then have at our disposal creditable references to judge the results of such assays in medical practice.

(2) It is important to bear in mind an aspect which is well established; given the reduced capacity of the kidney in the aged to eliminate exogenous substances, and drugs are examples of such substances (see Chapter 9), it is necessary to adjust the dosage to the patient's capacity, to avoid the consequences of excessive drug administration.

(3) The kidney of an elderly person is perfectly able to maintain the homeostasis of the internal milieu in *basal* conditions, i.e. following a normal life, but not in *exceptional* or *stressful* situations which demand maximum exercise of regulatory capacity. In this sense, it must be understood that the pathophysiological and clinical consequences of such situations are qualitatively identical to those observed in younger individuals, although in the elderly they can be more intense and are therefore more likely to reach the status of 'disease'; this is often more serious owing to the inability of these patients to adapt to maximum functional output. An example of this general idea (and of particular interest from the clinical point of view) is that, due to the relative incapacity of the aged kidney to conserve sodium and water and, to a lesser extent, to eliminate excesses of these substances, the *physician* may be obligated to ensure that intake is suitable and above all sufficient. Because this goal is linked to the conditions in which the elderly live, which are in turn dependent on their social situation, the possibility of achieving such a state fundamentally depends on improving the latter. Similarly, it should always be remembered that the elderly are particularly prone to sodium and water depletion, and this must be considered in any disease situation or circumstances which stress homeostasis. Some of these deviations may lead to circulatory insufficiency which needs prompt treatment to remedy them immediately, before renal function is fully compromised.

Is renal function decreased in the elderly?

At first it would appear that the answer to this question must be 'yes', since it is certain that the glomerular filtration rate is decreased (Shock, 1976; Macias Nuñez *et al.*, 1981) (see Chapter 2) and it is universally agreed that this parameter is an overall marker of renal function. However, it is not only the glomerular filtration rate (GFR) that is reduced, but also some functions of the tubulo-interstitial system, and the elimination of exogenous substances, such as iodopyracet (Diodrast) and para-aminohippuric acid (Davies and Shock, 1950; Dontas, Marketos and Papanayiotou, 1972), the reabsorption of sodium in the ascending limb of Henle's loop and in the distal segments of the nephron (Epstein and Hollenberg, 1976; Macias Nuñez *et al.*, 1978), and in the capacity to concentrate and dilute urine (Rowe, Shock and de Fronzo, 1976; Macias Nuñez *et al.*, 1978; Philips *et al.*, 1984).

The data available concerning the handling of glucose, amino acids, etc., in the proximal tubule are insufficient to draw conclusions, although it does appear that the glucose T_m is reduced in the aged, even though threshold values may be normal (Lindeman, 1975) (see Chapter 7). Data for plasma renin are inconclusive; whereas some workers (Weidmann *et al.*, 1975; North, Lassman and Tan, 1977) have reported diminished levels with a poor response to the stimuli of the upright position or to restricted saline intake, in contrast Crane and Harris (1976) have described normal basal values and a poor response, and Tuck, Williams and Cain (1973) did not detect any differences between values obtained in elderly patients and those in a young adult population. Some other findings point, albeit indirectly, to the notion that renin secretion is insufficient; for instance, hypertension in the elderly is of the low renin type, and accelerated hypertension is practically unknown in persons older than 70 (Parsons, 1977).

It is also possible that the capacity to hydroxylate 25-hydroxycholecalciferol is reduced (Gallagher *et al.*, 1979), although the low serum levels of vitamin D metabolites might rather be due to a deficit in the vitamin itself, a common finding in countries of northerly latitudes where there is little sun in winter.

Other functions, however, remain unaltered in some groups of elderly patients, such as the capacity to reabsorb bicarbonate. Regarding other aspects of renal function in the elderly, such as the handling of potassium which is not diminished when total potassium urinary output is considered (see Chapter 4), and the secretion of erythropoietin, the available information is very scanty, although there is no evidence of a decrease.

Accordingly, it is not correct to simply state that 'renal function is decreased in the aged', since it must be specified that only *some renal* functions are compromised.

When we consider those functions which *have* been shown to be diminished, we must of course take into account the procedure employed to establish the assumed 'reduction' and establish the concept of 'normality' and 'abnormality' in both the biological and medical sense. The truly 'normal' can only be established by a study conducted on a group of elderly 'patients', also healthy, and the results compared statistically: the concept of normality–abnormality is also statistically valid. When we say that renal function — or rather some renal functions — are reduced in the aged, what we mean is that they exhibit lower figures compared with younger adults. However, merely to say that they are 'reduced', which implies that they are abnormal, is superficial and inexact.

From another point of view, let us consider how paediatricians operate: they would never compare the functional yields of their young patients with those corresponding to older populations. Rather, they establish normal behaviour patterns for each age group according to the observations taken from that group. If we call renal functions 'abnormal' in the aged, then we should say the same about the neonatal kidney, since the inulin clearance is 39 ml/min/1.73 m^2 between days 2 and 8, while at 1–6 months it rises to 77 ml/min/1.73 m^2 (Goldsmith, 1978). If physicians who deal with the biologic–medical problems in the early stages of life act 'independently', so to speak, would it not be logical to behave similarly to the problems of the elderly?

Personally, I believe that this is the correct approach and thus when defining what is 'normal' and what is 'abnormal' in the aged we should free ourselves from the constraints of what has been established in young adult populations and attempt to establish absolute criteria for the special circumstances involved. Geriatrics is a speciality which has been (and indeed still is in many countries) in the hands of physicians who usually deal with younger adult populations, so that the professionals involved consider 'normal' only what they have observed in the majority of their patients (young adults).

In this way, having escaped from a relativistic outlook which has no justification, we arrive at the conclusion that the function of the kidney in the aged is *not* reduced, although it would be true to say that some of its functions do not exhibit the degree of competence or range of flexibility normally seen in healthy young adults, whereas others remain completely efficient.

In some ways it would be logical to terminate this contribution right here, since if the kidney in the elderly is not dysfunctional, but rather simply *different,* there is no point in attempting to investigate something which does not exist. However, let us now examine why the kidneys of the aged may differ from those of young adults.

Meaning of the behaviour of the aging kidney

Bearing in mind the similar behaviour of the remaining organs and tissues, we can state that the decrease in functional capacity with age compared to young adults is at least partially a logical event; since the kidney functions in unison with the rest ofthe body's activities, it would be unreasonable to suppose that it would conserve its full functional capacity with the passage of time if other organs do not.

It is not difficult to provide a teleological explanation for this phenomenon in the case of the relative reduction in excretory capacity, which seems to be the most affected, in terms of a logical adaptation to a lower calorie consumption and the decrease in lean body mass and parenchymal tissues, with fewer metabolic end products to eliminate. However, it is more difficult to explain in the same way the relative limitation in the *regulatory* functions of homeostasis. This is still possible, however, since it *can* be argued that the elderly are 'programmed' for a 'peaceful' life, and hence are less likely to confront adverse environmental situations which would demand maximum flexibility of such functions. This is not necessarily a true description of what really happens to the elderly, since it would imply that in some way the community 'protects' the elderly from stress, whereas it is common knowledge that this is often not the case: unfortunately, many old people have to live in a hostile environment owing to lack of family support, financial problems, etc.

The preceding chapters have pointed to considerable gaps in our knowledge of the function of the aging kidney. When we have more information regarding the individual behaviour of each and every aspect, then that will be the moment to study why some are more affected than others. However, if we attempt to assess the meaning of all these varied changes in renal function in the elderly, we would leave the framework of data and have to move into the field of pure speculation.

References

CRANE, M.G. and HARRIS, J.J. (1976). Effect of aging on renin activity and aldosterone excretion. *Journal of Laboratory and Clinical Medicine,* **87,** 947–959

DAVIES, D.F. and SHOCK, N.W. (1950) Age changes in glomerular filtration rate, effective renal plasma flow and tubular capacity in adult males. *Journal of Clinical Investigation,* **29,** 496–499

DONTAS, A.S., MARKETOS, S.G. and PAPANAYIOTOU, P. (1972). Mechanism of renal tubular defects in old age. *Postgraduate Medical Journal,* **48,** 295–303

EPSTEIN, M. and HOLLENBERG, N.K. (1976). Age as determinant of renal sodium conservation in normal man. *Journal of Laboratory and Clinical Medicine,* **82,** 411–417

GALLAGHER, J.C., RIGGS, B.L., EISMAN, J., HAMSTRA, A., ARNAUD, S.B. and DE LUCA, H.F. (1979). Intestinal calcium absorption and serum vitamin D metabolites in normal subjects and osteoporotic patients. *Journal of Clinical Investigation,* **64,** 729–736

GOLDSMITH, D.I. (1978). Clinical and laboratory evaluation of renal function. In *Pediatric Kidney Disease,* edited by C.M. Edelman, pp. 213–224. Boston; Little, Brown

LINDEMAN, R.D. (1975). Age changes in renal function. In *The Physiology and Pathology of Human Ageing,* edited by R. Goldman and M. Rochstein, pp. 19–38. New York; Academic Press

MACIAS NUÑEZ, J.F., GARCIA IGLESIAS, C., TABERNERO ROMO, J.M., BONDIA, A., RODRIGUEZ COMMES, J.L. and CORBACHO BECERRA, L. (1981). Estudio del filtrado glomerular en viejos sanos. *Revista Española de Geriatria y Gerontologia,* **16,** 113–124

MACIAS NUÑEZ, J.F., GARCIA IGLESIAS, C., TABERNERO ROMO, J.M., RODRIGUEZ COMMES, J.L. and CORBACHO BECERRA, L. (1978). Renal handling of sodium in old people: a functional study. *Age and Ageing,* **7,** 178–181

NORTH, R.H., LASSMAN, N. and TAN, S.Y. (1977). Age and the renin-aldosterone system. *Archives of Internal Medicine,* **137,** 1414–1417

PARSONS, V. (1977). What decreasing renal function means to aging patients. *Geriatrics,* **32,** 93–99

PHILIPS, P.A., ROLLS, B.J., LEDINGHAM, J.G., FORSLING, M.L., MORTON, J.J., CROWE, M.J. *et al.* (1984). Reduced thirst after water deprivation in healthy elderly man. *New England Journal of Medicine,* **311,** 753–759

ROWE, J.W., SHOCK, N.W. and DE FRONZO, R.A. (1976). The influence of age on the renal response to water deprivation in man. *Nephron,* **17,** 270–278

SHOCK, N.W. (1976). The effect of age on creatinine clearance in man: a cross-sectional and longitudinal study. *Journal of Gerontology,* **31,** 155–163

TUCK, M.L., WILLIAMS, G.H. and CAIN, J.P. (1973). Relation of age, diastolic pressure and known duration and presence of low renin essential hypertension. *American Journal of Cardiology,* **32,** 637–642

WEIDMANN, P., DE MYTTENAERE-BURZSTEIN, S., MAXWELL, M.H. and DE LIMA, J. (1975). Effect of aging on plasma renin and aldosterone in normal man. *Kidney International,* **8,** 325–333

Chapter 11

Incidence of renal diseases in a geriatric unit

F. Guillén Llera and P. Gil Gregorio

Introduction

As most of the diseases mentioned in this chapter have already been discussed in depth by other authors, a true understanding of its purpose will not be complete without first considering a number of introductory aspects. We will thus discuss the concept of the geriatric unit (GU) in order to define the type of patients it admits, then continue on to consider its status within the structure of a general hospital and its relationship with the other specializations which also treat elderly patients and, finally, the type of diseases, first general and then specifically renal, presented by the geriatric patients admitted.

Aging of populations; hospital geriatrics; general information

Aging of populations

The progressive aging of the population, especially in developed countries, has given rise to a constant increase in the percentage of people aged over 65 with respect to the total population. According to United Nations (1981) data, in 1980 this percentage had already reached 18 per cent in many European countries. In Switzerland, for example, life expectancy at birth is 72.7 years for men and 79.8 for women. Also, the progressively increasing proportion of the old and very old (in Europe, 2.8 per cent of women are over 80 years of age) is notable, as is also the case with life expectancy after 60 which, in the USA, is 18.8 years (see Preface).

Hospital geriatrics

This inexorable trend towards an aging population has rendered necessary implementation of new, specific systems of care which cover the needs of geriatric patients. The WHO (1974) has repeatedly recommended that steps be taken to plan and organize geriatric services and, very recently, the World Assembly on Ageing held in Vienna in 1982 has again emphasized these aspects (United Nations, 1982). The development of geriatrics is an unquestionable fact in many industrialized countries; in some cases it is recognized as a specialization in its own right (e.g. the UK, Denmark, Spain, Eire, Holland, Finland, Poland), but in any case always with special attention from within the departments of medicine (e.g. France, West Germany, Switzerland).

The availability of specialized hospital care for the elderly is thus indispensable; it is estimated that 10 beds are required per 1000 inhabitants over 65 to cover the short-, medium- and long-term hospitalization needs of this population group (British Medical Association, 1976).

Geriatric unit (Guillén Llera, 1981) means 'the level of care that, within a geriatric department integrated in a general hospital, gives specialized inpatient care to elderly patients who meet the criteria of "geriatric patient"'.

A hospitalized *geriatric patient* is that patient, usually over 65 years of age, who presents with an acute disease or an acute development of a chronic disease, especially if it tends towards disablement, if it is accompanied by other diseases (multiple pathology) or if its evolution is conditioned by psychological and/or social factors. The overall goal of the different levels of geriatric care (inpatient units, day hospital and home care) is to return the elderly patient to the community in a state of self-sufficiency; outpatient care and the community social services should ensure the maintenance of the high levels attained in the hospital.

General statistical information

This information is composed of the data obtained from the acute GU (32 beds) of the Geriatrics Department of the Central Red Cross Hospital in Madrid.

Table 11.1 contains the general data corresponding to 1984 which illustrates the movement of patients in our unit. The average age of these patients, 79, is clearly very high.

Table 11.1 Geriatric unit (1984 data)

No. patients admitted	695
Mean age	79.1 yr
Mean stay	16.5 days
Mortality	19.1%
Discharges with severe dependence	6%
Readmissions	21%

Table 11.2 shows the most common reasons for admission to the unit; although, logically, diseases such as heart failure or cerebral vascular accident hold first places, it can be seen that renal disease (renal failure and pre-renal failure) is in its own right the cause of a large number of admissions.

Table 11.2 Geriatric unit (1983–84), 1210 patients: reasons for admission

	No.	%
Heart failure	309	24.5
Cerebral vascular accident	257	19.6
Pneumonia	118	9.0
Chronic bronchopneumonopathy	106	8.1
Pre-renal and renal failure	100	7.6
Gastrointestinal haemorrhage	82	6.3
Deterioration of general condition	73	5.6
Programmed study	70	5.3
Diabetic decompensation	39	3.0
Pancreatitis	28	2.1
Jaundice	23	1.8
Other	105	8.0

Table 11.3 Geriatric unit (1983–84), 1310 patients: definitive diagnoses, by systems

	No.	%
Cardiovascular	608	51.0
Respiratory	488	37.3
Nephro-urologic	448	32.2
Nervous	393	30.0
Endocrine	388	29.6
Digestive	330	25.2
Locomotor	230	17.6
Blood	79	6.0
Other	198	15.0

Table 11.4 Geriatric unit (1983–84), 1310 patients: definitive diagnoses, by disease

	No.	%
Heart failure	390	29.8
Cerebral vascular disease	357	27.2
Chronic bronchopneumonopathy	281	21.5
Diabetes	235	17.9
Ischaemic heart disease	231	17.6
Renal insufficiency	201	15.3
Urinary infection	182	13.9
Pneumonia	164	12.5
Arterial hypertension	159	12.1
Arthrosis	144	11.1
Gallstones	102	7.8
Hiatal hernia	85	6.5
Neoplasias	80	6.1

Tables 11.3 and *11.4* give the final diagnoses of the patients admitted, classified by system and disease, respectively. Nephro-urologic disease shows as the third largest cause of disease in our patients. Upon considering specific diseases, renal failure (RF), with 201 patients, and urinary infections, with 182 patients, were clearly very common.

Renal pathology in a geriatric unit

Data are somewhat sparse in the literature on this particular aspect. Consequently, we will base our discussion mainly on our own case records. However, it is worth reviewing a few general studies.

Sourander *et al.* (1979), in his 5-year study of a Finnish community of 191 892 inhabitants of which 21 503 were over 65 (11 per cent), upon finding creatinine values over 2.6 mg/100 ml continued with a specialized study in which 70 per cent of the diagnoses were confirmed histologically. His conclusions are as follows: (a) uraemia was 10 times more common in the population aged over 65; (b) within this age group, the most usual aetiology was pyelonephritis in women (51 per cent) and post-renal obstruction in men (35 per cent); (c) no less than 30 per cent of the uraemias detected had a pre-renal origin; (d) interstitial nephritis was found in 15 per cent of the cases and glomerulonephritis in 3 per cent, with systemic diseases accounting for lower percentages; (e) mortality was over double the average in uraemic patients, with the exception of the over-80 age group, where it was identical.

Data can be collected from the findings of renal punctures/biopsies of elderly patients which cannot be extrapolated to the general population due to their being highly orientated towards the diagnosis of very specific pathologies. Moorthy and Zimmerman (1980), in a study of 115 biopsied patients aged over 60, found primary glomerular disease in 78 (65 per cent) (idiopathic glomerulonephritis in 19 cases, membranous glomerulonephritis in 15 cases, glomerulosclerosis in 16 cases) and systemic diseases with renal involvement in 27 (23 per cent) (the most prominent were vasculitis and amyloidosis). Out of 143 biopsies of patients over 60 years of age, Kingswood *et al.* (1984) found primary renal disease in 82 patients (57 per cent) (membranous glomerulonephritis in 24 cases, proliferative glomerulonephritis in 19 cases) and secondary renal diseases in 61 patients (43 per cent), amyloidosis and nephroangiosclerosis being the most frequent diagnoses in this group (see Chapters 15 and 21).

Turning to our own case records, we will briefly review renal disease from several viewpoints.

As cause of admission

It has already been noted in the general statistics that renal disease, essentially renal and/or pre-renal failure, was the cause of admission of 100 patients (7.6 per cent); if to this we were to add the cases where this failure was detected as a concomitant of other diseases, the figure increases to 262 patients (20 per cent). The main diseases are shown in order of frequency in *Table 11.5.*

Table 11.5 Patients with renal failure on admission: clinical pathology

1. Heart failure
2. Dehydration
3. Cerebral vascular accident
4. Metabolic decompensation
5. Haemorrhage
6. Sepsis
7. Pancreatitis

Dehydration and desalination is a common presentation in elderly patients (see Chapter 4); together with the causes that may occur at any age (e.g. vomiting, diarrhoea, treatments with laxatives or diuretics, fever, sweating), in geriatric patients, particular attention must also be paid to the mental (mainly senile dementia) and social conditions that may lead to any mundane illness developing into renal failure.

Other types of illness, genuine nephrological emergencies such as obstruction or septic shock, are referred to more specific departments (nephrology, intensive care) and therefore usually do not appear in our statistics.

As a finding during the aetiological study of the cause of admission

A previously undiscovered renal disease is often diagnosed during the examination of an eldery patient admitted to the GU. Sometimes, there exists a clear relationship with the cause of admission (e.g. the diagnosis of a hypernephroma in a patient with a sudden deterioration of his general condition or chronic renal failure in a patient with low haemoglobin counts); on other occasions, the relationship with the

Table 11.6 Geriatric unit (1983–84), 1310 patients: nephro-urologic disease in 448 patients

	No.	*%*	*Percentage of total admissions*
Renal failure	210	45	15.3
Urinary infection	182	40.6	13.8
Pre-renal failure	85	19	6.5
Adenoma of the prostate	70	15.6	5.3
Lithiasis	24	5.4	1.8
Renal cysts	20	5.4	1.5
Renal tumours	5	1.1	0.4
Other	22	4.6	1.6

symptoms is not so apparent. It was seen in *Table 11.3* that no fewer than 448 of the patients admitted to our unit were ill with diseases of the kidney and urinary tract. *Table 11.6* shows the main diseases found.

As a customary concomitant of diagnosed diseases

There is a whole series of diseases, which are very common in geriatric patients, that often affect the renal function. These are diabetes mellitus (18 per cent of our admissions), arterial hypertension (12 per cent), infections, uropathies, neoplasia and systemic diseases such as amyloidosis, lupus or myeloma.

Table 11.7 Geriatric unit (1983–84), 1310 patients: diabetes mellitus

No. patients	235 hospitalized elderly patients
Mean age	79 yr
Men	30%
Women	70%
Therapy:	
diet	40%
diet and OA*	37%
diet and insulin	23%
Disorder of renal function:	
moderate	30%
serious	10%

*OA, oral antidiabetic drugs

Table 11.7 details the data for diabetes mellitus, diagnosed in 235 of our patients. Obviously, in these patients, the diagnosis of impairment of the renal function was made exclusively on the basis of biochemical tests of blood and urine (see later). We will also briefly discuss in later sections some of the other diseases mentioned here.

As a complication during the patient's stay in hospital

More often than would be wished, patients without any previously discovered renal disease, even after routine analyses, develop renal failure during their stay in the hospital. Although there exists a large number of possible causes, we have listed below the most common in our experience with elderly patients:

(1) Septic clinical pictures presenting while in hospital presentation (e.g. pneumonias, pyelonephritis).

(2) Dehydration due to negative balances between supply and losses, especially in high risk patients (patients with cirrhosis or heart failure) treated with diuretics.
(3) States of hypotension of varying aetiology (e.g. myocardial infarction, pancreatitis, gastrointestinal haemorrhage).
(4) Use of nephrotoxic drugs, particularly aminoglycoside antibiotics.
(5) Heart failure, occasionally due to volume overload (transfusions, expanders, etc.).
(6) Contrast media.

In the survey carried out in Boston by Hou *et al.* (1983) on 2662 medical and surgical patients, 4.9 per cent developed some degree of renal failure during their stay in hospital. The main cause was the fall in renal perfusion (42 per cent) due to heart failure, shock, etc., followed by major surgery (18 per cent), contrast media (12 per cent) (Byrd and Sherman, 1979) and aminoglycosides (7 per cent). Overall mortality was 29 per cent and, in contrast with other studies (Kennedy *et al.*, 1973; Schrier, 1979), age had no significant effect on the evolution of the disease (see Chapter 20).

On the basis of a study of 143 patients in Sydney, who developed acute renal failure during their stay in hospital with aetiologies similar to those stated above and of whom 56 per cent were over 65, Rasmussen and Ibels (1982) also think that age is not a risk factor *per se,* while the existence of previous renal disease and arterial hypertension does constitute risk factors. Furthermore, there seems to be agreement on the importance of the conjunction of several associated risk factors in the same patient, such as dehydration and aminoglycoside therapy.

As a finding at autopsy

Some type of renal disease has been detected in 103 (79 per cent) of 130 autopsies performed on our patients in the past few years. Obviously, these autopsies were performed on patients with a wide variety of conditions, with special emphasis on

Table 11.8 Renal disease in 130 necropsies

	No.	*%*
Nephro-angiosclerosis	57	44
Chronic pyelonephritis	23	17
Renal cysts	18	14
Acute tubular necrosis	10	7.2
Renal infarct	10	7.2
Acute pyelonephritis	9	6.9
Hydronephrosis	9	6.9
Renal metastases	7	5.3
Lithiasis	6	4.6
Renal abscess	6	4.6
Renal carcinoma	3	2.3
Other	13	10

those cases of more complex diagnosis not necessarily related to renal disease. Hyaline arteriolar nephro-angiosclerosis was the most frequent diagnosis, followed by pyelonephritis and kidney cysts. The data from the autopsies are shown in *Table 11.8.*

Study method

As at any age, the study of a nephrological disease in an elderly patient must follow a series of steps (albeit perhaps slightly modified by the age parameter); these steps are described in the text below.

History and medical examination

These must be as detailed as possible, which is not always easy in elderly patients; often, the data will be obtained in later examinations and/or through relatives. The customary masked symptomatology of many diseases in geriatrics is well known. On the other hand, the existence of several diseases in the same patient may complicate the search for nephro-urological signs which are often specific, such as loss of appetite, asthenia and fever. Nevertheless, suggestive symptoms such as haematuria, frequency, dysuria and palpable masses such as adenoma of the prostate or nephromegaly are commonly detected in elderly patients (Rosen, 1976).

Laboratory tests

Urinalysis

We use the first urination of the morning, as this is more concentrated and has a more acid pH due to hypoventilation during sleep. When estimating the density–osmolarity, it should be borne in mind that the concentration capacity of elderly persons is lower, perhaps due to a higher water and solute load per nephron and also due to a reduction in interstitial and medullary osmolarity with a fall in the response to the antidiuretic hormone (Macias, 1983). A proteinuria over 150 mg in 24 h is abnormal and cannot be considered as a benign manifestation of the aging kidney. Should it persist after detection, a more complete study should be started on the patient (Hernando, 1980). Leucocyturia is found in up to 25 per cent of geriatric patients (Rosen, 1976) without it necessarily being accompanied by bacteriuria. The presence of haematuria and especially granular casts in the sediment is highly indicative of renal disease.

Glomerular filtration

It is generally accepted that the glomerular filtrate decreases with old age. The usual method of measurement is the 24 h creatinine clearance in the urine and up to 60 ml/min is considered as being a normal value. Due to the difficulties that geriatric patients often raise for the performance of this test, it can be replaced by the determination of creatinine in plasma which, with a few exceptions, is a valid parameter, especially for monitoring the evolution of the patient (Rowe *et al.*, 1976; Shock *et al.*, 1979).

Renal plasma flow

This can be determined by the para-aminohippurate (PAH) clearance, although these techniques are not usually used in geriatric patients.

Tubular function

Concentration and dilution tests are not always well tolerated by elderly patients, which consequently limits their use. However, urine electrolyte determination is routinely used, taking into account a number of physiological factors such as the presence of higher quantities of sodium (Epstein and Hollenberg, 1976) and the high nocturnal excretion of sodium and potassium by the elderly person (Berkland *et al.*, 1983). In fact, the determination of the fractional sodium excretion (see Chapters 4 and 20) is extremely useful for differentiating situations of pre-renal and renal failure (Espinel and Gregory, 1980).

Radiological studies

In addition to the abdominal X-ray which provides clear information on the size of the kidney and the presence of calcification and even masses, the following techniques are also available:

Intravenous urography

In principle, this should not be a routine test in elderly patients as it may induce acute renal failure. However, it provides excellent information and, on occasions, is absolutely indispensable.

Ultrasound scanning

Although not strictly a radiological test, it is very useful for evaluating the morphology of the kidney and neighbouring structures without having to use contrast material or ionizing radiation (Clayman *et al.*, 1984). As a non-invasive technique, its use is progressively increasing and it is widely indicated in geriatric patients.

Computed tomography

Normally used to obtain additional information after the ultrasound scan, it is a complex technique that gives highly specific images (Magilner and Ostrom, 1978) and is indispensable in any major hospital.

Renal arteriography

Logic indicates that this is not a technique for geriatric patients. With the approval of the consultant, however, it is indicated in cases of suspicion of stenosis of the renal arteries and in the diagnosis of masses which have not been sufficiently defined by the previous methods. The introduction of modern digital subtraction techniques has made its use more feasible in geriatric patients.

Table 11.9 Renal disease in 143 abnormal ultrasonic scans

	No.
Kidney stones	14
Renal cysts	14
Solid renal mass	4
Polycystic disease	2
Hydronephrosis	2
Renal atrophy	2
Renal abscess	2

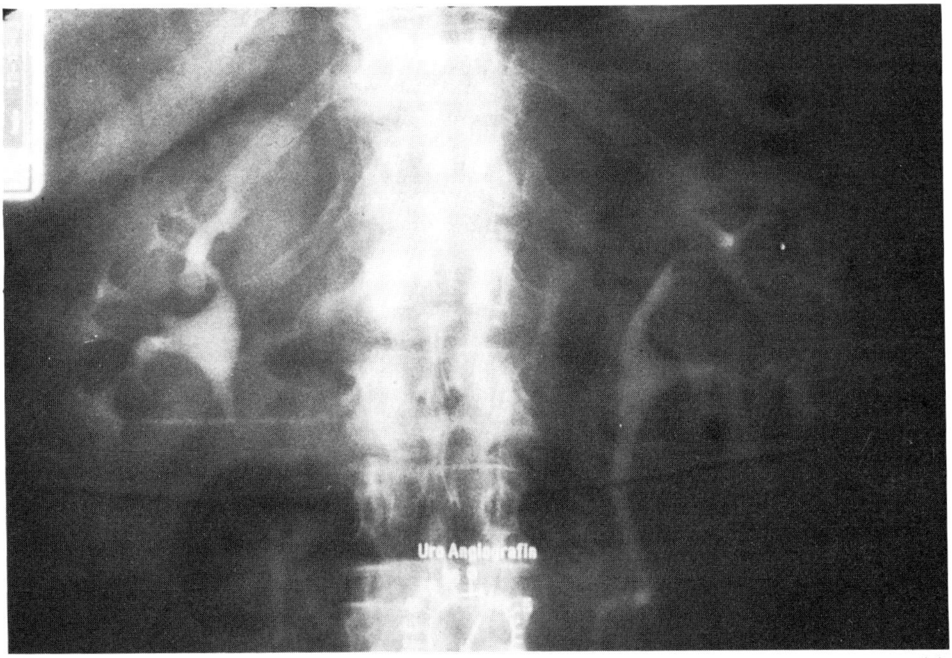

(a)

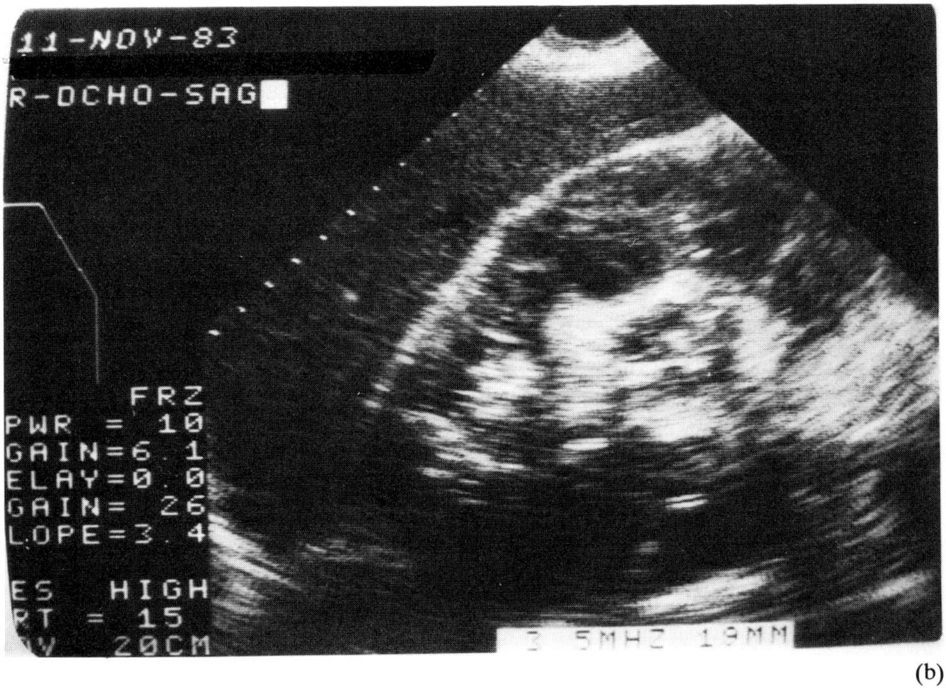

(b)

Figure 11.1 See caption opposite

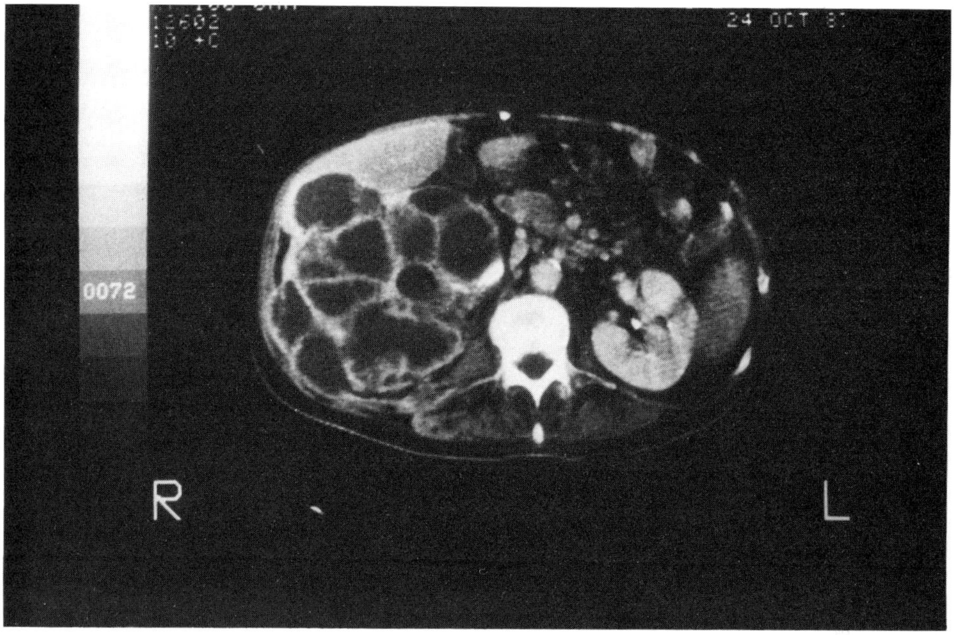

(c)

Figure 11.1 Comparison of three diagnostic imaging techniques in the same patient: (a) intravenous urography, which demonstrates cysts in the right kidney; (b) ultrasound scanning which shows that the cysts are not centrally echogenic; (c) computed axial tomography (CAT) which shows multiple, different-sized cysts in the right kidney

Of the 143 abdominal ultrasound scans performed in our department in the past year, renal disease was found in 42 cases, i.e. 30 per cent (*Table 11.9*); 42 urographies and 17 abdominal tomographies were also performed (*Figure 11.1*).

Renal biopsy

This too is not a customary technique in elderly patients. Its use is indicated whenever a justifiable cause of renal failure cannot be found, taking into account, of course, aspects such as life expectancy, prior condition of the patient and possibilities of an active treatment. It does not seem to be indicated in cases of acute renal failure, where the clinical diagnosis has a good chance of being correct and where, in any case, no changes are expected in the therapeutic approach (Mustonen *et al.*, 1984). We have already commented on the data from pathologic findings in renal biopsies of elderly patients (see Chapter 21).

Geriatric syndromes and renal disease

Dehydration and desalination (see also Chapters 4 and 20)

Volume depletion is by far the most common change in the fluid balance of elderly patients; generally, both water and electrolytes are lost. Many geriatric patients are admitted into hospital more because of this type of disorder than because of their main illness. There is considerable disagreement as to whether it is the disease, *per se*, which is associated with dehydration which constitutes a risk factor in the onset of acute renal failure (Rowe, Shock and de Fronzo, 1976; Rasmussen and Ibels, 1982), although the majority of medical opinion rejects this possibility. The main causes of dehydration in elderly patients are given in the following paragraphs.

Reduction of water intake

Together with disorders of the thirst mechanism, one must also consider mental, functional and social conditioning factors; sometimes, fear by the elderly patient's family of incontinence leads them to reduce the liquid intake (Brocklehurst, 1971). With regard to the hypodipsia mentioned above (Miller *et al.*, 1982), a number of hypotheses are put forward such as cortical dysfunction and disorders of the thyroid–pituitary axis (Robertson, Aynema and Zerbe, 1982); another mechanism would be the physiological reduction in the sensitivity to osmotic or volume stimuli, and it has been observed that the response of vasopressin to hypernatraemia is increased in the elderly (Phillips *et al.*, 1984). It is possible that the decrease of thirst, with the increase in vasopressin secretion, indicates a drop in osmoreceptor sensitivity. This sensitivity diminishes with age (Anderson, 1976) and there is also evidence of a decrease in osmoreceptor-mediated vasopressin release (Rowe *et al.*, 1982). In conclusion, the thirst mechanism is disturbed in the elderly person as is also the ability of his body to respond to the deprival of water.

Gastrointestinal losses

These are generally caused by vomiting, acute or chronic diarrhoea, fistulas, secreting adenomas and other diseases.

Cutaneomucosal losses

Large quantities of water may be lost during fever and sweating and also during intense dyspnoea.

Renal losses

This occurs during the diuretic phase of an acute tubular necrosis or during a post-obstructive nephropathy. Much more common as the cause of dehydration in the elderly person is the indiscriminate use of diuretics. However, most often, dehydration in elderly patients is the result of a conjunction of several of the above-mentioned causes.

Treatment of dehydration raises problems with respect to the rapidity of replacement. We replace 50 per cent of the deficit in the first few hours and the rest in the course of the following days in order to avoid problems in the brain area, as there exists the danger of oedema during correction (Feig and McCurdy, 1977) and also because of the risk of overload on the heart.

Infections (see Chapter 13)

Pyelonephritis is defined as any disorder which may occur as a result of the infection of the kidney (Kleeman, Hewitt and Gueze, 1960); some authors use the term to include non-infectious disease (see Chapters 13, 14 and 19). The importance of the problem of urinary infections in old people can be deduced from the following data: it affects 30 per cent of women and 7 per cent of men (Sourander, 1966); in autopsy studies, the incidence of chronic pyelonephritis can reach 20 per cent (Kimmelstiel *et al.*, 1961) and in our series it reached 17 per cent; infections of the middle tract associated with pyelonephritis account for 17 per cent (Gallagher, Montgomerie and North, 1965).

Obviously, the elderly person has specific risk factors that facilitate infection. Among them are: obstruction by stone or prostatic enlargement, neurological abnormalities of the bladder, diabetes and, especially, bladder catheters and their handling. The most common organism is *Escherichia coli,* although other Gram-negative bacteria are often found in hospitals. In the USA, out of 40 million hospitalized people, 1.5 per cent develop urinary infections (Center of Disease Control, 1982). Eighty per cent of these infections were attributed to the use of catheters (Turck and Stamm, 1981).

There are a number of different criteria for the diagnosis of urinary infection; it is not possible routinely to use the suprapubic approach to obtain urine samples (Turck and Stamm, 1981); our normal limit is the finding of 100 000 colonies/ml in the urine culture, while other authors prefer to use lower concentrations (Randall *et al.*, 1984). The normally masked nature of the symptoms, or modified by the low state of alertness of the patient, certainly does not make any easier the diagnosis of urinary infection, except in cases of contrasted sepsis (Stamm, Martin and Bennett, 1977).

It is thus clear that the placement of a catheter in an elderly patient is a risk factor and should be given careful thought. We are in favour of its use for short periods of time in acute clinical pictures which require close scrutiny of constants. Once the catheter is placed there is a 10:1 daily likelihood that the patient will develop *bacteriuria,* but only 2 per cent develop *symptomatic bacteraemia* (Warren, Platt and Thomas, 1978), usually by Gram-negative germs (Kreger *et al.*, 1980). The only justification for long-term placement is retention during the period that it is not possible to remove the obstacle surgically.

The major risk of urinary infection, and therefore of bladder catheterization, is septic shock, characterized by the existence of fever, disturbances of the state of mind and a decrease in arterial blood pressure. The shock is most often caused by *E. coli* or *Proteus mirabilis.*

The dilemma thus arises of whether or not to use antibiotics in catheterized patients (Warren *et al.*, 1982); we are against routine use, although it may be justified during changes of catheter and, of course, when signs of generalized infection appear (Norberg *et al.*, 1979).

Arterial hypertension (see also Chapters 5 and 12)

Arterial hypertension (AHT) is in fact a frequent phenomenon among the elderly population. According to our own case records (Guillén Llera and Martin Alvarez, 1976), for which a limit of 180/105 mmHg was established, 27 per cent of the study population over 65 years of age had AHT, although in two-thirds of the cases, only the systolic pressure was raised; 12.1 per cent of our hospitalized patients (see *Table 11.7*) were diagnosed with diastolic AHT. Although agreement on this matter is not universal (Babu *et al.*, 1977), it seems to be accepted that the limits for hypertension should be set at 160/95 mmHg, as in the adult. On the basis of this criterion, almost

40 per cent of the elderly population would be considered hypertensive (Kirkendall and Hammond, 1980).

It is generally admitted that the tolerance of AHT by the elderly person is good. The renal function is no exception to this rule and the effect of hypertension on it would be proportionately less in the elderly person than in the adult.

The incidence of secondary AHT in the elderly population is not clear. Although it is estimated at less than 5 per cent, some authors, such as Laugensen *et al.* (1983), claim that unilateral or bilateral renal disease may be the cause of up to 34 per cent of the cases of AHT in elderly patients.

The anatomical and functional changes that take place in the kidney during the aging process, such as the decrease in the plasma renin activity (Crane and Harris, 1976) are well known. According to Macias (1983), although these changes are similar to those found in the hypertensive adult, they should in no case be considered as a *cause* of AHT. Likewise, the fact that kidney damage is a frequent finding in elderly patients, as we saw in our data on necropsies, does not necessarily imply the presence of AHT, nor its direct relationship with AHT, should it exist.

Nevertheless, when faced with the sudden appearance of diastolic AHT in a previously normotensive elderly patient, the possibility of stenosis of the renal artery should be considered (Delin *et al.*, 1982). It should also be borne in mind that such common diseases of old age as pyelonephritis, obstructive uropathy and glomerulopathy may cause AHT in elderly people.

The treatment of arterial hypertension in old age, especially at ages over 70, is still a subject of debate (WHO, 1983). If treatment is given, the renal function must be monitored, as it may be affected by the antihypertensive treatment. Although we are convinced that AHT is also a major risk factor in geriatrics, we are not quite so sure of the beneficial effects of the treatment of it. The recent introduction of new antihypertensive drugs, such as the calcium antagonists (Guillén Llera, 1984), may enable us to hope that the scales that hold the balance between benefits and risks be finally tipped towards the former.

Diabetes mellitus (see also Chapters 15 and 21)

The incidence of diabetes is very high in the elderly population, reaching 30 per cent in the last decades of life (Williams, 1978). In our hospital the incidence was 17.9 per cent (see *Table 11.4*). Diabetic renal disease is a typical complication and is accepted as being related with the duration of the disease (over 20 years) and perhaps with the degree of insulin dependence and the quality of metabolic management of the disease (Camill, Etzwiller and Freinkel, 1976). The difference between 'old diabetes', which has been with the old person for very many years, and the more recent 'diabetes of od age' will be decisive in the generation of kidney disease.

For these reasons, many of our type II diabetic elderly patients do not have renal disease, as is seen in *Table 11.7*. Nevertheless, 40 per cent of our diabetic patients had renal disease, although it was classified as serious in only 10 per cent of the cases. Consequently, diabetic renal disease must be considered as a frequent aetiology of the advanced renal failures presented by the geriatric population. Although micro-angiopathy is the basic cause of the presence of renal failure in the elderly diabetic patient, one should not ignore other factors and, especially, the greater incidence of infection, particularly pyelonephritis. The sum of the effects of other associated diseases, such as AHT and arteriosclerosis, may lead the old person towards irreversible renal failure.

Systemic diseases (see also Chapters 15 and 21)

Apart from the diseases or syndromes mentioned so far, there is another group of diseases that normally affect the kidney. Omitting gout, whose relationship with renal disease is only too well known but poorly understood, we will briefly comment on some of these diseases.

Amyloidosis

Deposits of amyloid in various organs increase as the individual ages. In spite of this, it is a rare diagnosis, no doubt due to diagnostic difficulties in day-to-day clinical medicine, as it requires a histological study. The kidney may basically be affected by vascular and glomerular deposits (Hareda *et al.*, 1984); the tubule is generally respected. The clinical picture, which may begin with proteinuria and/or haematuria, usually develops towards a nephrotic syndrome and, in its advanced phase, towards renal failure.

Collagen diseases

Moorthy and Zimmerman (1980), in their series, found that 23 per cent of 115 renal biopsies showed systemic diseases. Of these, vasculitis, granulomatosis, lupus and scleroderma were the most common. Among the forms of vasculitis is included panarteritis which can maniffest as micro-infarcts, or chronic glomerulonephritis (see Chapter 16). Bolton and Couser (1979), apparently with good results, have used methyl prednisolone in the rapidly progressive forms of glomerulonephritis. They have also employed anticoagulants, platelet aggregability and inhibitors with acceptable results.

Multiple myeloma

The appearance of renal failure is attributed to the presence of Bence-Jones proteinuria associated with changes in urine pH and volume (de Fronzo *et al.*, 1978). Other factors are situations of hypercalcaemia, dehydration and infectious processes; its frequency in association with iodized contrast media does not seem to be as great as is stated in the literature (Cohen *et al.*, 1984). The clinical picture progresses towards renal failure and may require dialysis therapy. However, not all myelomas are accompanied by renal failure.

Liver diseases

Early and consistent disturbance of renal function is frequent during the course of chronic liver diseases. The renal disorders may follow an insidious course over a period of many years, passing through three clinical stages:

(1) The *subclinical* stage, where the surface blood perfusion decreases without the ischaemia affecting the overall blood flow or the glomerular filtration (Epstein, Schneider and Befeler, 1977).
(2) The *pre-uraemic* stage, where sodium and water retention may be detected in the tubules without affecting the serum levels of urea and creatinine.
(3) The *uraemic or renal dysfunction* stage; a large number of elderly cirrhotic patients, after a phase of functional disturbances, develop an established renal failure; 40–50 per cent of the cases show clear increases in creatinine and urea

levels in the last weeks of life (Reynolds, 1974); hyponatraemia, hypochloraemia and, above all, hyperkalaemia worsen the prognosis.

Upon observing a disturbance of the renal function in a cirrhotic patient, especially if he is elderly, it is vital to rule out reversible situations that can be given specific treatment such as haemorrhages, sepsis, spontaneous peritonitis and, of course, all types of dehydration.

Some specific renal disorders have been described as secondary to liver disease; among them are acute tubulo-interstitial nephropathy, suggesting a hyperbilirubinaemic aetiology, distal renal tubular acidosis (Golding, 1975) and mesangial or membranous glomerulopathies.

Acute renal failure (see also Chapter 20)

We have referred repeatedly to this disease throughout this chapter. We will now attempt to define some of the points most related the admission to a geriatric unit.

Pre-renal

This can occur in elderly patients with a previously intact renal function due to a low cardiac output or a sharp drop in plasma volume; the result is a reduction of the effective renal plasma flow. It is an extremely common situation in geriatric patients, and is best treated preventatively by a scrupulous monitoring of clinical data, especially the central venous pressure and urine volume. We have already commented that dehydration, heart failure and sepsis are its main causes in geriatrics (Kumar, Hill and McGeown, 1973).

Renal

Its aetiologies are innumerable and among them we will mention, in the old person, thrombosis of the renal artery or vein, glomerulonephritis, drug-induced interstitial nephritis (Richet and Mayaud, 1978) and hypercalcaemias in old people bedridden for long periods or with Paget's disease (Rosen, 1976). Of specific importance is the acute tubular necrosis caused by ischaemia or direct toxic effects.

Post-renal

As will be emphasized later, the main cause in the elderly person is the increased size of the prostate; there are other causes of retention, such as prolonged bedridden periods. Calculous lesions, neoplasia, especially of the bladder, and carcinomatosis must be considered as a frequent cause of this type of renal failure.

The prognosis of acute renal failure is very serious, attaining a mortality of 80 per cent (Cailer *et al.*, 1977) in the parenchymatous forms, generally due to septic complications, haemorrhages or heart failure. Of vital importance, therefore, is an early diagnosis through the medical history, the examination, the patient's evolution and the analyses of blood and urine (Espinel and Gregory, 1980). Therapy, directed to the primary disease if possible, can be taken as far as dialysis after consultation with the nephrology consultant.

Chronic renal failure (see also Chapters 21–23)

This is a common situation in geriatrics which can be defined as the persistent and progressive deterioration of glomerular and tubular functions, leading to an incapacity to maintain the balance of the internal milieu.

The priorities will be to recognize the primary renal disease, the degree of renal failure and the possibility of discovering exacerbating factors. These patients may also require strong support from the social and patient care services. We have thoroughly reviewed the diseases which may lead to chronic renal failure in the old. In addition to the symptomatic treatment, dilemmas may arise as to more direct therapies, such as dialysis and even renal transplant. Any such decision demands a complete knowledge of the aetiology and should be sufficiently reflected on and

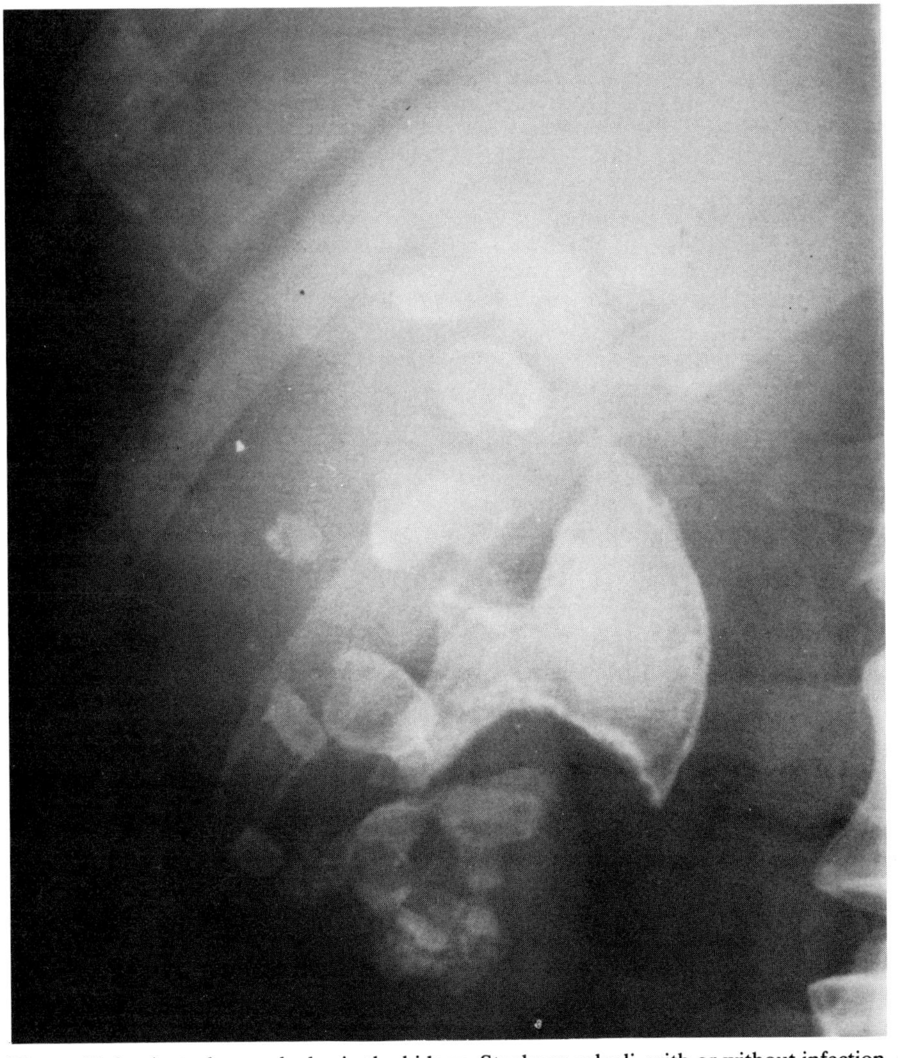

Figure 11.2 A staghorn calculus in the kidney. Staghorn calculi, with or without infection, are a common source of undiagnosed ill-health

discussed with the nephrologist. Obviously, the previous quality of life, life expectancy and the existence of concomitant illnesses may invalidate any theoretically correct line of action. On the other hand, neither heart failure nor arterial hypertension are contraindications. Cailer *et al.* (1977) propose therapy with dialysis, followed by transplantation (see Chapters 22 and 23).

Renal lithiasis

The formation of kidney and bladder stones increases with age and consequently they are common in the old (Blacklock, 1979). Thus, at 70 years of age, 14 per cent of men develop symptomatic calculi. In geriatric clinical medicine, it is not uncommon to find large asymptomatic staghorn calculi during a routine abdominal radiological examination (*Figure 11.2*) or to diagnose giant bladder lithiasis. Of all our inpatients, 1.8 per cent were diagnosed with lithiasis (see *Table 11.6*), while it was found in 4.6 per cent of the necropsies performed (see *Table 11.8*). The main complications of lithiasis are infection and obstruction of the urine flow, which are common diseases in geriatric clinical medicine.

Although the aetiopathogenic factors are extremely varied (environment, diet, geographical location, metabolism) (Castrillo, 1982), in geriatrics, perhaps special emphasis should be placed on four of them: hydronephrosis, the existence of renal cysts and, above all, urinary infection and immobilization, all of which are common events in elderly patients.

Consideration should also be given to primary or secondary hypercalciurias, hyperuricaemias and medicine intake, especially alkaline substances, vitamin D, uricosurics and ascorbic acid.

Clinically, the differences between adult and old person in the typical picture of pyelo-ureteral colic are not particularly marked, although in the latter, the pain may not be so spectacular and may be confused with vertebral algias. The existence of associated urinary infection may also modify the clinical manifestation.

The bilateral obstruction of urine flow, with the consequent anuria, is a common event among old patients. Although we have some experience of this condition (*Figure 11.3*), the patients are urgently referred to the urology department for appropriate specialized treatment.

Obstructive uropathy (see also Chapter 19)

Urinary obstruction means the blocking of urine flow by obstacles located between the renal calyces and the outside.

In geriatric clinical medicine, prostate disease is by far the main cause of 'low' obstructive uropathy in men. Other diseases which often cause it in elderly patients are lithiasis, bladder tumours, neurogenic bladder and abdominal and pelvic tumours.

We have already commented in the previous section on the acute picture of obstruction and anuria which require emergency treatment with external drainage (*Figure 11.4*). It should be stressed that the symptoms produced by vesicoprostatic obstructions are minimal, in spite of a clear dilatation of the urinary tract. When faced with any type of renal failure of unexplained origin in an old patient, the physician should consider the possibility of an obstructive uropathy, implementing the appropriate diagnostic techniques, among which the renal ultrasonic scan occupies a prominent place due to its safety, speed and efficiency. Obstructive

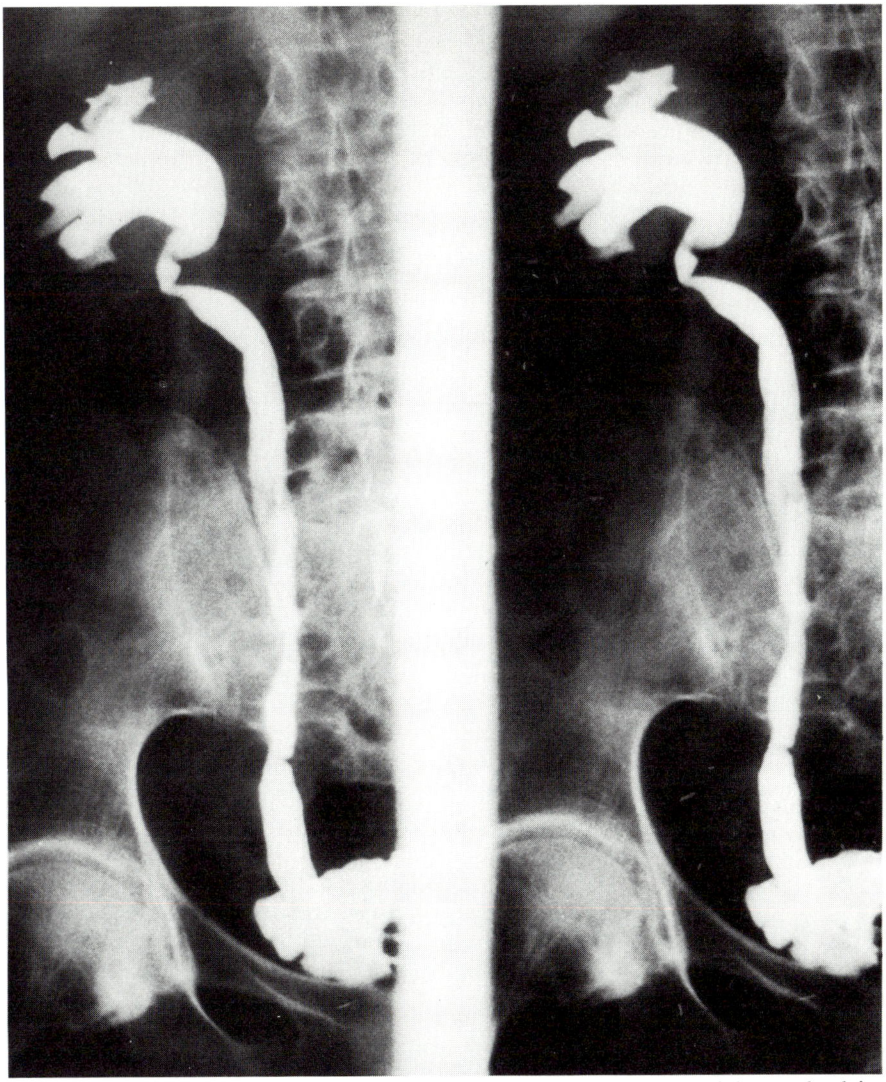

Figure 11.3 Intravenous urography. Ureteric dilatation and dilatation of the renal pelvis are seen, caused by an obstruction in the distal ureter

uropathy is a disease always to be kept in mind in geriatric clinical medicine, as it is initially reversible but can lead to irreversible renal failure.

Obviously, therapy will depend on aetiology. In elderly patients, a nephrostomy and/or the placement of a vesico-ureteral or suprapubic catheter may constitute an indispensable initial therapy, prior to a permanent solution, when possible.

Renal masses

These occupy a very interesting position within renal pathology in old age and require considered use of diagnostic techniques, which will be mainly based on radiology.

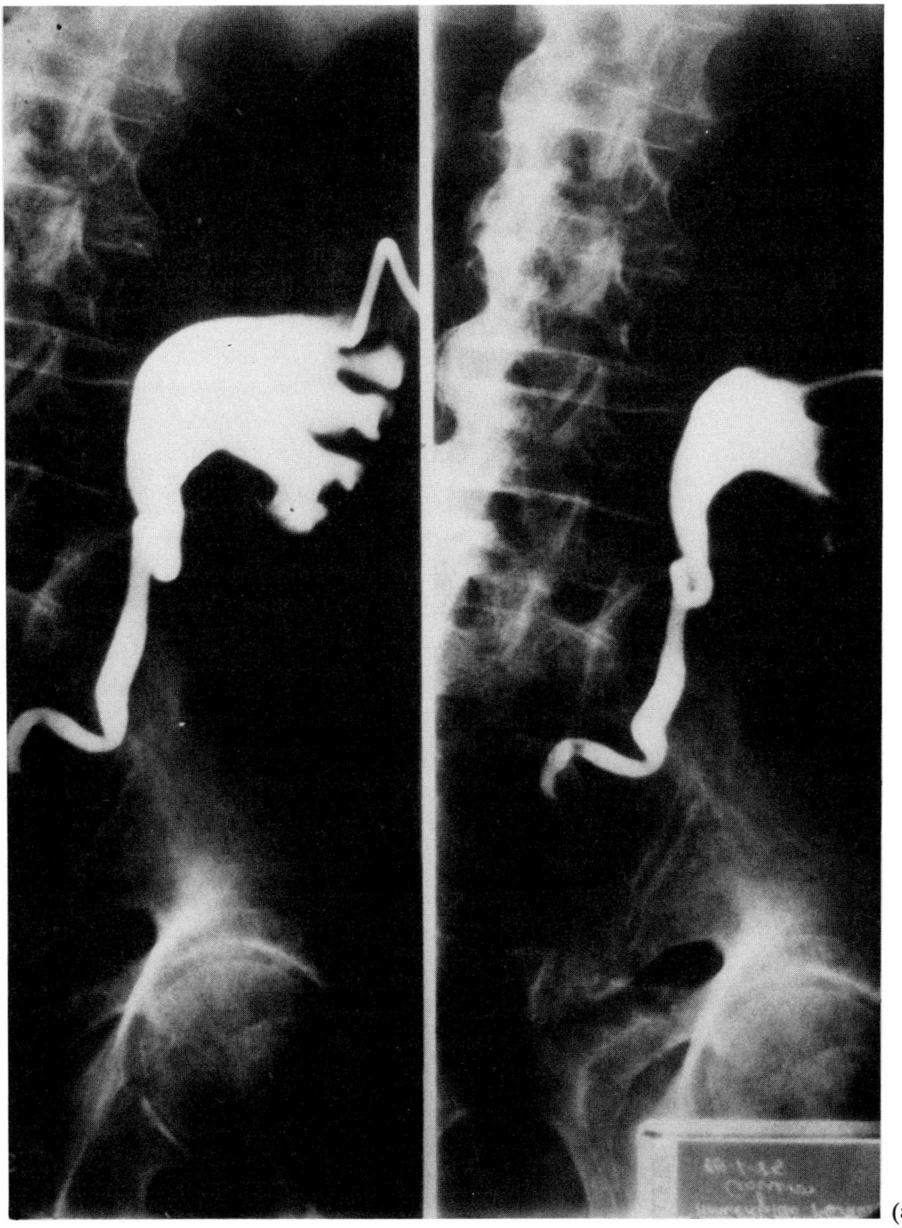

(a)

Figure 11.4 See caption opposite

The simple abdominal X-ray enables the detection of changes in the renal morphology, displacement of neighbouring organs and calcifications of difficult interpretation; these latter may be central, peripheral or mixed (Daniel *et al.*, 1972) and may correspond to simple blood cysts or calcified perinephritic abscesses (Holder and Bissada, 1977). Intravenous urography does not necessarily give definitive results; two-thirds of the renal adenocarcinomas diagnosed in the autpsy

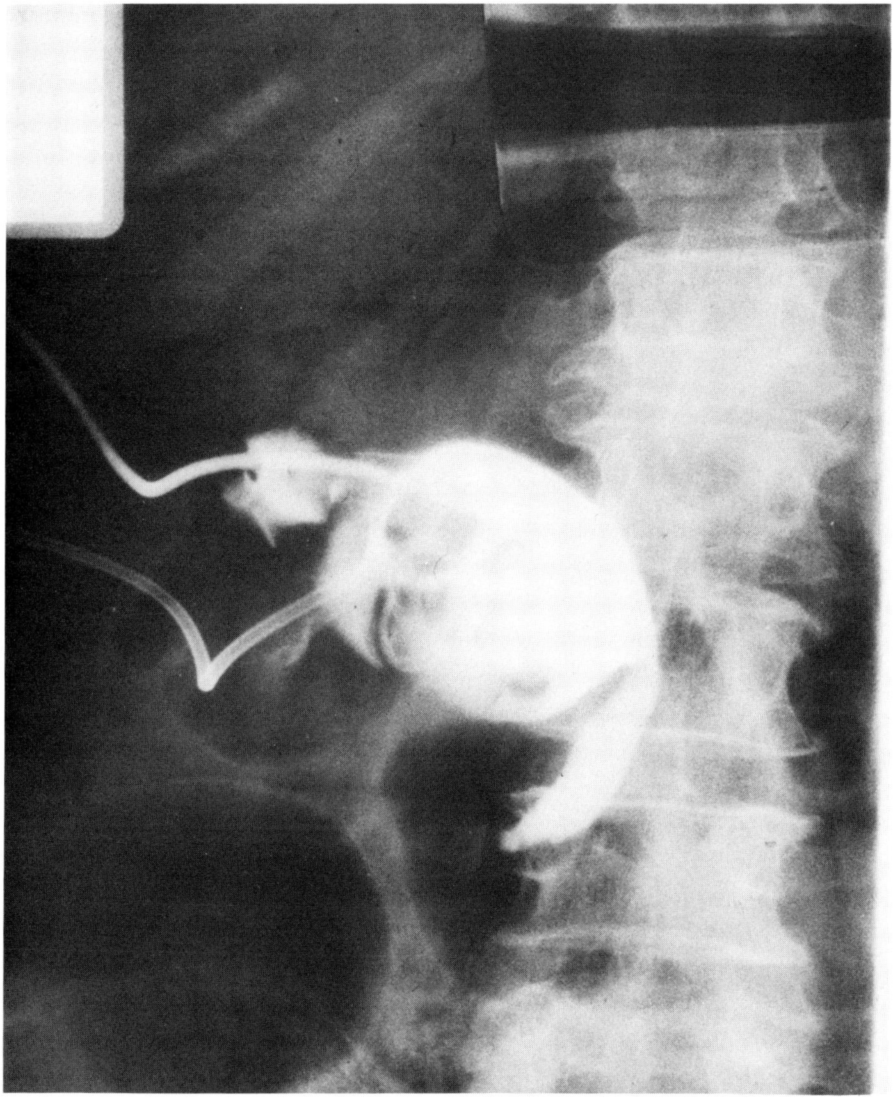

(b)

Figure 11.4 (a) A nephrostomy into an obstructed urinary tract, the obstruction being at upper mid-ureteric level; on the right the system has been drained. (b) A therapeutic nephrostomy drainage in a similar patient

had a normal urogram (Hadju and Thomas, 1967; Kass, Hricak and Davidson, 1983).

Tomography and, above all, ultrasonics may, when used jointly, obtain up to 98 per cent positive results (Goldberg and Pollack, 1971; Osteaux and Jeanmart, 1977; Mayayo *et al.*, 1978). We prefer to use computed tomography when the ultrasonic scan is not conclusive or when we require supplementary data.

A technique which, in specialized hands, is virtually risk free and yet may be conclusive is puncture aspiration under radiographic control, which enables the histological examination of the biopsied mass. Having diagnosed the existence of the mass, we use the technique almost routinely in the hospital when it presents diagnostic difficulties or when we need to define its histology.

The main renal masses seen in geriatrics are described in the following paragraphs.

Renal adenocarcinoma (Figure 11.5)

Only 10 per cent of the patients (Tueter, 1973) present with the classic triad of haematuria, pain and palpable mass, the metastases being very often the first clinical manifestation. The possibilities of therapy such as embolization, chemotherapy or surgery are remote in geriatrics, but even so they should be considered (see Chapter 18).

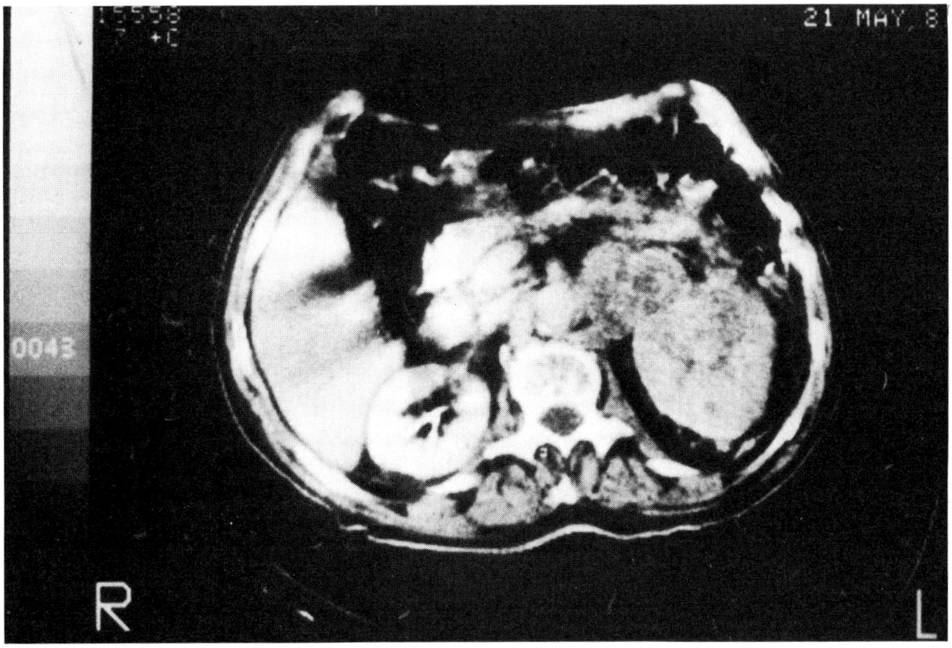

Figure 11.5 A cystic renal adenocarcinoma of the right kidney

Renal polycystic disease (Figure 11.6)

Some authors consider it to be a different phenomenon from the adult form. It is usually difficult to diagnose due to the lack of clear symptoms and the absence of biochemical changes. Not all cases show renal failure (Danovitch, 1976) and consequently it is often an autopsy finding. It may be associated with extrarenal cysts (mainly hepatic) and vascular abnormalities such as aneurysms in the circle of Willis, with an incidence between 4 and 16 per cent (see Chapter 17).

Solitary cyst

This manifests as a thin sac with squamous epithelium, mostly located in the lower renal pole. It is totally asymptomatic, being a radiologic or ultrasonographic finding, and is seen with considerable frequency in our patients (*Tables 11.6* and *11.8*).

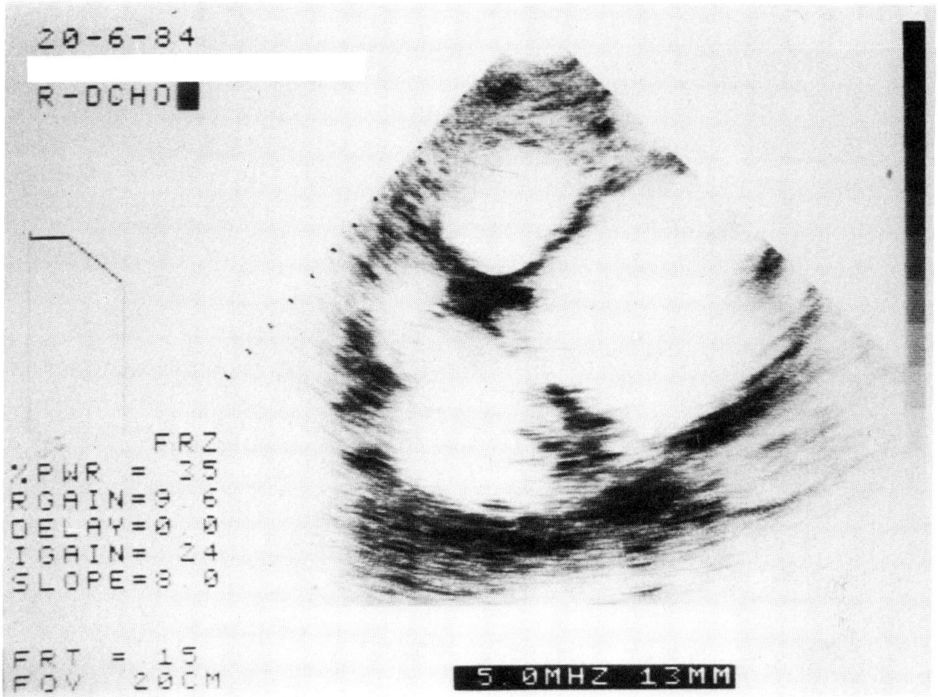

Figure 11.6 Echographic appearances of multiple cysts within the right kidney, also present in the liver (top)

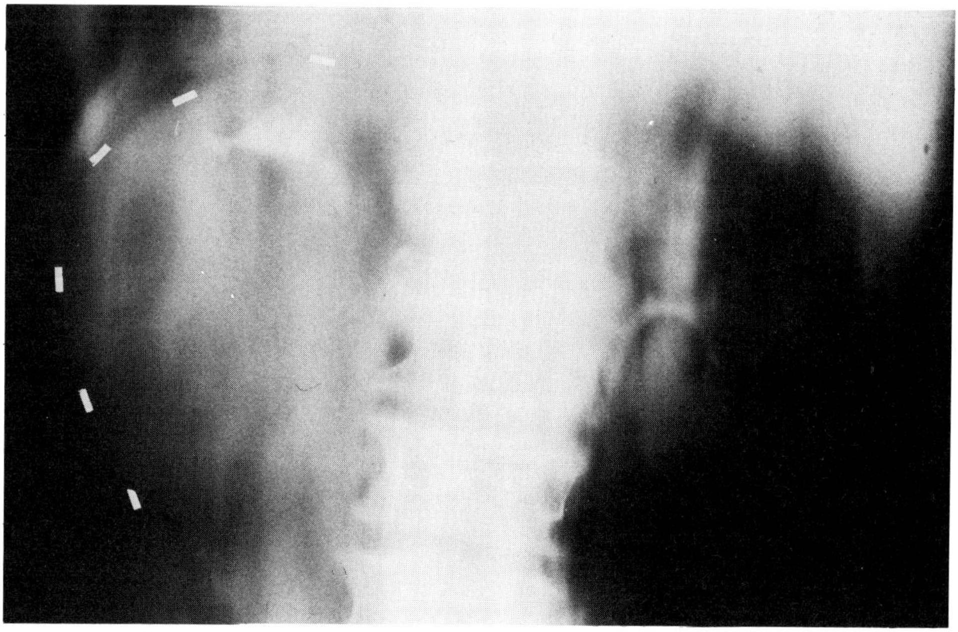

Figure 11.7 A perinephric abscess outlined on the right

Renal abscess

This is a collection of pus located in the renal parenchyma. The bacteria that mainly cause the infection are, at present, *Proteus* sp. and *Pseudomonas* sp. (Rives, Harty and Amin, 1980), displacing the traditionally accepted *Escherichia coli*. The process may become chronic, with perforation of the urinary tract or formation of a perinephric abscess (*Figure 11.7*) (Thorley, Jones and Sanford, 1974).

The clinical picture is that of a septic process on occasions indistinguishable from a pyelonephritis. In addition to the analytic data, the diagnosis is based on the ultrasound scan and computed tomography (Hoddick *et al.*, 1983) (*Figure 11.8*).

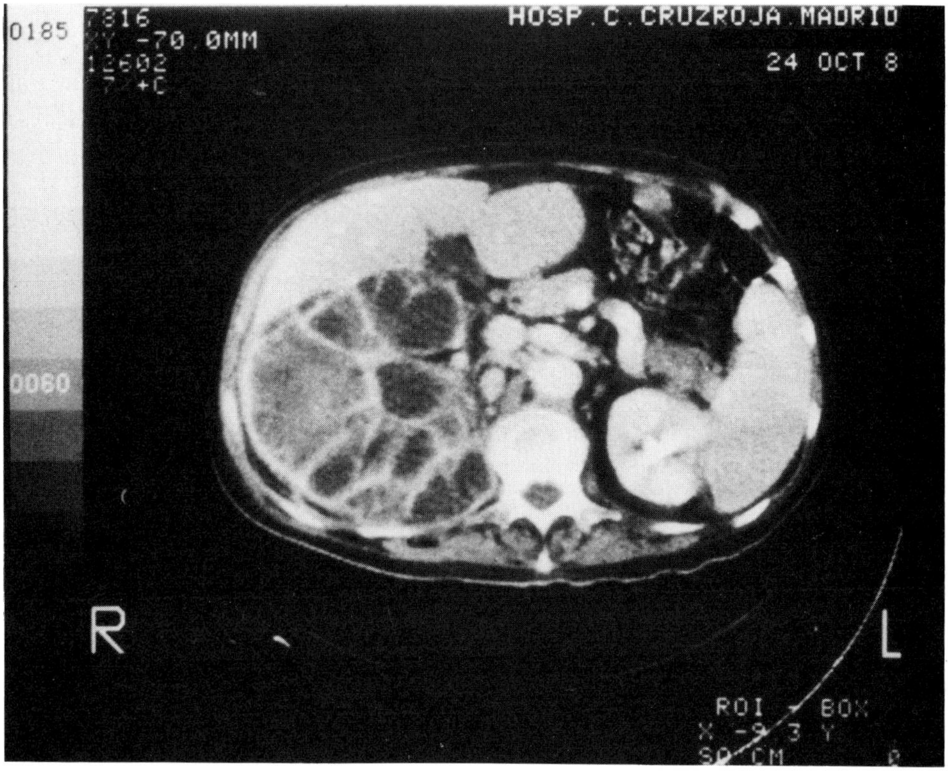

Figure 11.8 A CAT image of a pyonephrosis on the right, arising from obstruction; multiple dilated, pus-filled calyces can be seen

Although some authors such as Schiff *et al.* (1977) have obtained good results with antibiotics, current treatment consists of percutaneous drainage under radiological control (Cronan, Amis and Dorfman, 1984). This technique is perfectly usable in geriatric patients, even with serious impairment of the general condition.

Renal tuberculosis

Perhaps it is in the geriatric population that pulmonary and extrapulmonary tuberculous lesions (and specifically renal tuberculosis) may be most often found (*Figure 11.9*). Main clinical manifestations are dysuria and frequency and also

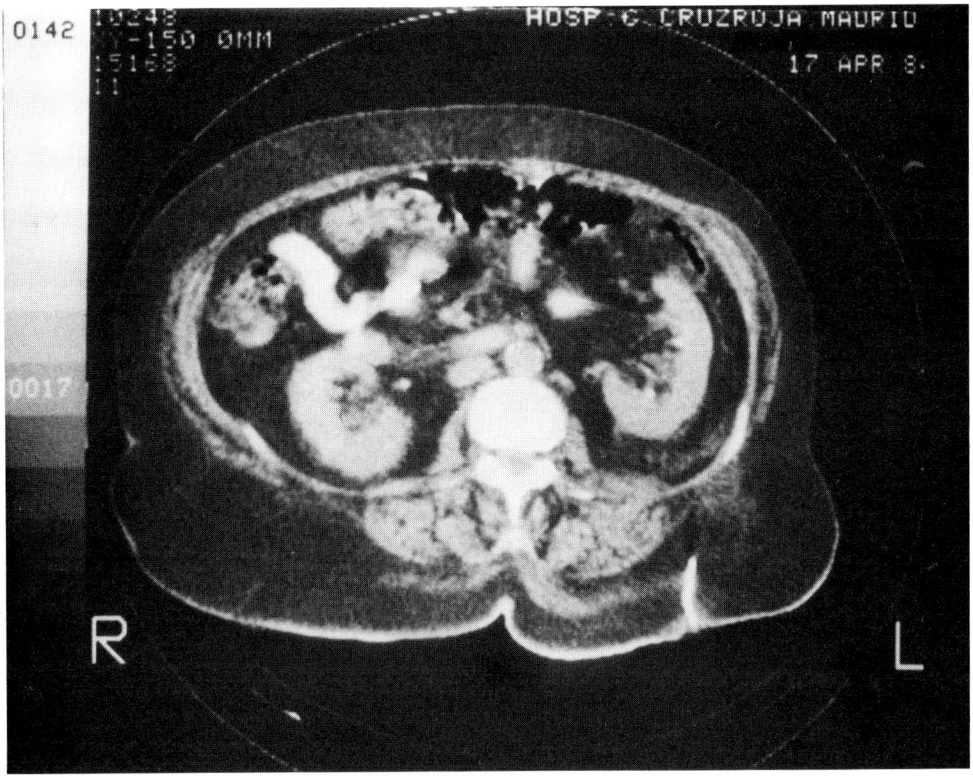

Figure 11.9 A tuberculous kidney on the left, demonstrated by CAT scanning. The irregular calyceal pattern can be seen, together with debris in the collecting system

fever, which may be the only manifestation. Sometimes, renal masses are involved in the diagnosis and it is not infrequent to find the production of papillary necrosis or associated cavitations (Simon *et al.,* 1977). The response to medical treatment is usually satisfactory although sometimes it may be necessary to resort to nephrectomy.

Iatrogenic renal disease

This is caused by a functional or structural impairment of the kidney due to a drug product. Very often, the lesion affects an already impaired kidney. Consequently, before beginning any treatment with a potentially nephrotoxic drug, it is absolutely vital that the prior state of the renal function be studied. If there coexist predisposing factors such as polypharmacy and disturbances of the fluid balance or renal flow, the chances of parenchymatous damage multiply.

The drugs that most often cause renal damage in geriatric clinical medicine are the *antibiotics.* They can cause several kinds of disorder such as acute tubular necrosis, interstitial nephritis, glomerulopathies caused by immune complexes and vasculitis (Appel and Neu, 1977). The nephrotoxicity of penicillins (Kovnato, Labovit and Levison, 1973; Colvin, Burton and Hyslop, 1974), aminoglycosides (Hewitt, 1973; Lisft, Patel and Moo, 1975), sulphonamides (Berglund, Killander and Pompeirs,

1975), polymyxin (Price and Graham, 1980) and amphotericin is well documented. However, there exists disagreement oncerning the nephrotoxicity of the cephalosporins (Hewitt, 1973). In any case, before using these antibiotics, the renal function should be studied and the dosage adjusted to its condition. There are many drugs used in geriatrics that may cause renal disease, including the anti-arrhythmic and psychotropic drugs.

Attention should be drawn to the use of analgesics, especially the non-steroid anti-inflammatory drugs, whose mechanism of action does not seem to be clear and which is assumed to be related with the synthesis of prostaglandins, without, however, this being able to account for the combination of disorders such as the nephrotic syndrome and interstitial nephritis (Brezin *et al.*, 1979; Abraham and Keane, 1984). There exists sufficient information on the nephrotoxicity of phenylbutazone (Greenstone, Hartley and Gabriel, 1981), fenoprofen (Finkelstein, Fraley and Stachura, 1982), indomethacin (Gary, Dodelson and Eisinger, 1980), and other drugs in this group. Also, the relationship between acetylsalicylic acid and necrotizing papillitis seems to be well established. Given the wide variety of drugs able to produce nephrotoxicity and the special vulnerability of elderly patients to this action, it is thus essential to study not only the toxic effects of the medication, but also the prior condition of the renal function and the various situations that predispose to this presentation. It should be remembered that the conjunction of several risk factors multiples the possibilities of toxic impairment of renal function.

Summary

Our short-stay geriatric unit admits elderly patients with a wide range of diseases. Our unit in the Central Red Cross Hospital in Madrid admits 695 patients per year, with a mean age of 79.1 years. The main causes of admission were heart failure and cerebral vascular accidents. Renal failures were the cause of admission in 7.6 per cent of the cases, either as sole disease or complicating primary diseases such as pneumonia or cerebral vascular accidents. Renal failure also accompanied mental impairments (mainly senile dementia) or unfavourable social situations.

In the final diagnosis, nephro-urological disease affects no less than 32.2 per cent of the patients, with renal failure and urinary infection holding first places. Equally definitive are the results of the autopsies performed by the department which reveal that no less than 79 per cent of patients have renal disease.

A geriatric unit is not a specialized nephrology department. Therefore, is often requires the assistance of this speciality. Nevertheless, there are a series of primary diseases common in geriatric clinical medicine that are accompanied by renal disease, such as diabetes, myeloma, etc. Of more importance are the clinical situations, such as heart failure, postoperative states and, above all, dehydration, which may develop acute renal failure or decompensate a previously existing dysfunction. Strict clinical vigilance is thus vital, with monitoring of the central venous pressure and diuresis during all critical moments of the evolution of the disease as, in the elderly person, any delay in the diagnosis of an incipient acute renal failure may make the process irreversible.

Chronic renal failure may be caused in many different ways, some of which have already been commented upon. We would particularly emphasize obstructive uropathy due to prostate disease, sometimes with very minor symptoms, which may lead to the situation of chronic renal failure.

Many other renal diseases are detected in a geriatric unit, such as tumours, abscesses, lithiasis, etc. With good back-up from the central diagnostic services, particularly radiology, and the co-operation of the urology and nephrology departments, it should be possible for the geriatric departments to obtain good management of renal disease in elderly patients.

References

ABRAHAM, P.A. and KEANE, W.F. (1984). Glomerular and interstitial disease induced by nonsteroidal antiinflammatory drugs. *American Journal of Nephrology,* **4,** 1–6

ANDERSON, W.F. (1976). *Practical Management of the Elderly.* Oxford, Blackwell

APPEL, G.B. and NEU, H.C. (1977). The nephrotoxicity of antimicrobial agents. *New England Journal of Medicine,* **296,** 663–670

BABU, T., NAZIR, F., RAO, D. and LOUISIADA, A. (1977). What is normal blood pressure in the aged? *Geriatrics,* **32**(1), 73–77

BERGLAND, K., KILLANDER, J. and POMPEIRS, R. (1975). The effect of trimethopim-sulfamethoxazole on the renal excretion of creatinine in man. *Journal D'Urologie,* **114,** 802–808

BERKLAND, C.M., LYE, M., LEVY, D.W. and BANERGEE, A.K. (1983). Patterns of urine flow and electrolyte excretion in healthy elderly people. *British Medical Journal,* **287,** 1665–1667

BLACKLOCK, N. (1979). Epidemiologics of renal lithiasis. In *Urinary Calculous Disease,* edited by S. Wickman, pp. 21–39. Edinburgh; Churchill Livingstone

BOLTON, W.K. and COUSER, W.G. (1979). Intravenous pulse methylprednisolone therapy of acute crescentic rapidly progressive glomerulonephritis. *American Journal of Medicine,* **66,** 495–502

BREZIN, J.H., KATZ, S.M., SCHWARTZ, A.B. and CHIMIZ, J.L. (1979). Reversible renal failure and nephrotic syndrome associated with nonsteroidal anti-inflammatory drug. *New England Journal of Medicine,* **301,** 1271–1273

BRITISH MEDICAL ASSOCIATION (1976). *Care of the Elderly.* London; BMA

BROCKLEHURST, J.C. (1971). The urinary tract. In *Clinical Geriatrics,* edited by Rossman, I., pp. 499–500. Philadelphia; Lippincott

BYRD, L. and SHERMAN, R.L. (1979). Radiocontrast-induced acute renal failure. A clinical review. *Medicine (Baltimore),* **58,** 270–279

CAILER, J., BECKER, H., KIENLEN, J. and BESSON, P. (1977). Bilan du traitment de 592 sujets de plus de 70 ans hospitalizés dans un service de réanimation. *Annales D'Anésthesiologie Française,* **18,** 486–491

CAMILL, G.F., ETZWILLER, D. and FREINKEL, V. (1976). Control and diabetes. *New England Journal of Medicine,* **294,** 1004–1005

CASTRILLO, J.M. (1982). Litiasis renal. *Medicine,* **36,** 2376–2386

CENTER OF DISEASES CONTROL (1982). National nosocomial infections study report. Annual Summary 1979. New York; CDC.

CLAYMAN, R.V., SURYA, V., MILLER, R.P., REINKE, D.B. and FRALEY, E.E. (1984). Pursuit of the renal mass: is ultrasound enough? *American Journal of Medicine,* **77,** 218–223

COHEN, D.J., SHERMANN, W.H., OSSERMAN, E.F. and APPEL, G.B. (1984). Acure renal failure in patients with multiple myeloma. *American Journal of Medicine,* **76,** 247–256

COLVIN, R.B., BURTON, J.R. and HYSLOP, N.T. (1974). Penicillin-associated interstitial nephritis. *Annals of Internal Medicine,* **81,** 404–405

CRANE, M.G. and HARRIS, J.J. (1976). Effects of aging on renin activity and aldosterone excretion. *Journal of Laboratory and Clinical Medicine,* **87,** 947–959

CRONAN, J.J., AMIS, E.S. and DORFMAN, G.S. (1984). Percutaneous drainage of renal abscess. *American Journal of Radiology,* **142,** 351–354

DANIEL, W.W., HARTMAN, G.W., WITTEN, D.M., FARROW, G.N. and KEALLIS, P.P. (1972). Calcified renal masses. A review of ten years' experience at the Mayo Clinic. *Radiology,* **103,** 503–508

DANOVITCH, G.A. (1976). Clinical features and pathophysiology of polycystic kidney diseases in man. In *Cystic Diseases of the Kidney,* pp. 125–135. New York; Wiley

DE FRONZO, R.A., COOKE, C.R., WRIGHT, J.R. and HUMPHREY, R.L. (1978). Renal function in patients with multiple myeloma. *Medicine (Baltimore),* **57,** 151–166

DELIN, K., AURELL, M., GRANERUS, B., HOLM, J. and SCHERSTEN, T. (1982). Surgical treatment of renovascular hypertension in the elderly patient. *Acta Medica Scandinavica,* **211,** 169–174

EPSTEIN, M. and HOLLENBERG, N.K. (1976). Age is a determinant of sodium conservation in man. *Journal of Laboratory and Clinical Medicine,* **89,** 411–417

EPSTEIN, M., SCHNEIDER, N. and BEFELER, B. (1977). Relationship of systemic and intrarenal hemodynamics in cirrhosis. *Journal of Laboratory and Clinical Medicine,* **89,** 1175–1187

ESPINEL, C.H. and GREGORY, A.W. (1980). Differential diagnosis of acute renal failure. *Clinical Nephrology,* **13,** 73–77

FEIG, F.U. and McCURDY, D.K. (1977). The hypertonic state. *New England Journal of Medicine,* **297,** 1444–1454

FINKELSTEIN, A., FRALEY, D.S. and STACHURA, I. (1982). Fenoprofen nephropathy: lipoid nephrosis and interstitial nephritis. *American Journal of Medicine,* **72,** 81–87

GALLAGHER, D.J.A., MONTGOMERIE, J.Z. and NORTH, J.D.K. (1965). Acute infection of the urinary tract and the urethral syndrome in general practice. *British Medical Journal,* **1,** 622–628

GARY, N.E., DODELSON, R. and EISINGER, R.P. (1980). Indomethacin-associated acute renal failure. *American Journal of Medicine,* **69,** 135–136

GOLDBERG, B. and POLLACK, H.H. (1971). Differentiation of renal masses using A-model ultrasound. *Journal of Urology,* **105,** 765–771

GOLDING, P.L. (1975). Renal tubular acidosis in chronic liver diseases. *Postgraduate Medical Journal,* **51,** 550–554

GREENSTONE, M., HARTLEY, B. and GABRIEL, R. (1981). Acute nephrotic syndrome with reversible renal failure after phenylbutazone. *British Medical Journal,* **282,** 950–951

GUILLEN LLERA, F. (1981). Unidad geriatrica. *JANO,* **465,** 90–94

GUILLEN LLERA, F. (1984). Efficacy and safety of nifedipine retard in elderly with mild arterial hypertension. Abstract. Mediterranean Symposium. Israel Heart Society. Jerusalem, October 1984

GUILLEN LLERA, F. and MARTIN ALVAREZ, M. (1976). Hipertensión arterial en Geriatría. Incidencia. Cifras limites. *Revista Española de Geriatria,* **11**(1), 5–20

HADJU, S.I. and THOMAS, A.G. (1967). Renal cell carcinoma at autopsy. *Journal of Urology,* **97,** 978–982

HAREDA, A., TONITA, Y., YAMAMOTO, H., ONOYAMA, K., OMEE, Y. and OH, Y. (1984). Renal amyloidosis associated with crescentic glomerulonephritis. *American Journal of Nephrology,* **4,** 52–55

HERNANDO, L. (1980). Sistemática del estudio analítico del enfermo renal. *Medicine (Edición española),* **45,** 15–22

HEWITT, W.L. (1973). The cephalosporines. *Journal of Infectious Diseases,* **128** (Suppl.), 312–319

HODDICK, W., JEFFREY, B.R., GOLDBERG, H.I., FEDERLE, M.P. and LAING, C.F. (1983). CT and sonography of severe renal and perirenal infections. *American Journal of Radiology,* **140,** 517–520

HOLDER, J.C. and BISSADA, N.K. (1977). Curvilinear calcification in renal cancers. Two etiologies. *Urology,* **9,** 701–704

HOU, S.H., BUSHINSKY, D.A, WISH, J.B., COHEN, J.T. and HARRINGTON, J.T. (1983). Hospital-acquired renal insufficiency; a prospective study. *American Journal of Medicine,* **74,** 243–248

KASS, A.D., HRICAK, H. and DAVIDSON, A.J. (1983). Renal malignancies with normal excretory urograms. *American Journal of Radiology,* **141,** 731–734

KENNEDY, A., BURTON, J., LUKE, R. *et al.* (1973). Factors affecting the prognosis in acute renal failure. *Quarterly Journal of Medicine,* **52,** 73–86

KLEEMAN, C.R., HEWITT, W.J. and GUEZE, L.B. (1960). Pyelonephritis. *Medicine (Baltimore),* **39,** 3–15

KIMMELSTIEL, P., KIM, O.J., BERES, J.A. and WEHMANNK, K. (1961). Chronic pyelonephritis. *American Journal of Medicine,* **30,** 589–597

KINGSWOOD, J.C., BANKS, R.A., TRIBE, C.R., OWEN-JONES, J. and MACKENZIE, J.C. (1984). Renal biopsy in the elderly: clinico-pathological correlations in 143 patients. *Clinical Nephrology,* **22,** 183–187

KIRKENDALL, W.H. and HAMMOND, J.J. (1980). Hypertension in the elderly. *Archives of Internal Medicine,* **140,** 1155–1161

KOVNATO, P., LABOVIT, E. and LEVISON, S. (1973). Antibiotics and the kidney. *Medical Clinics of North America,* **53,** 1045–1063

KREGER, B.E., CRAVEN, D.E., CARLING, P.C. and McCABE, W.R. (1980). Gram negative bacteremia. Reassessment of etiology, epidemiology and ecology in 612 patients. *American Journal of Medicine,* **68,** 332–343

KUMAR, R., HILL, C.M. and McGEOWN, M.G. (1973). Acute renal failure in the elderly. *Lancet,* **1,** 90–91

LAUGESEN, L.P., GADEGARD-HANSEN, A., JENSEN, H., PETERSEN, T. and TØNENSEN, K. (1983). The prevalence of secondary hypertension in elderly hypertensive patients. *Acta Medica Scandinavica,* **214** (Suppl.), 161–177

LISFT, F.C., PATEL, V. and MOO, N.Y. (1975). Experimental aminoglycoside nephrotoxicity. *Journal of Laboratory and Clinical Medicine,* **86,** 213–220

MACIAS NUÑEZ, J. (1983). Aspectos morfológicos, funcionales y patológicos del riñon del viejo. *Nefrología,* **3,** 1–7

MAGILNER, A.D. and OSTROM, B.J. (1978). Computed tomography in the diagnosis of renal masses. *Radiology,* **126,** 715–718

MAYAYO, T., MAGARTA, E., COVACO, F., MATEOS, J.A. and ESCUDERO, A. (1978). Nefrotomografía y ecografía en el estudio de masas renales. *Actas Urológicas Española,* **2,** 215–220

MILLER, P.D., KREBS, R.A., NEAL, B.J. and McINTYRE, D.O. (1982). Hypodipsia in geriatric patients. *American Journal of Medicine,* **73,** 354–356

MOORTHY, A.V. and ZIMMERMAN, S.W. (1980). Renal diseases in the elderly: clinicopathologic analysis of renal diseases in 115 elderly patients. *Clinical Nephrology,* **14,** 223–229

MUSTONEN, J., PASTERNACK, A., HELIN, H., PYSTYNEN, S. and TUOMINEN, T. (1984). Renal biopsy in acute renal failure. *American Journal of Nephrology,* **4,** 27–31

NORBERG, B., NORBERG, A., PARKETE, U., GIPPERT, H. and AKERMAN, H. (1979). The effect of short-term high-dose treatment with methenamine hippurate on urinary infection in geriatric patients with an indwelling catheter. *Uppsala Journal of Medical Sciences,* **84,** 67–74

OSTEAUX, M. and JEANMART, L. (1977). Nephrotomographie á haute dose et artériographies dans le diagnostic des tumeurs renales. *Journal de Radiologie d'Électrologie et de Médicine Nucléaire,* **58,** 279–286

PHILLIPS, M.B., PHILL, D., ROLLS, B.J., LEDINGHAM, J.G.G., FORSLING, M.L., MORTON, J.L., CROWE, M.J. and WOLLNER, L. (1984). Reduced thirst after water deprivation in healthy elderly men. *New England Journal of Medicine,* **311,** 753–759

PRICE, D.J.C. and GRAHAM, D.I. (1980). Effects of large doses of colistin sulphomethate sodium on renal function. *British Medical Journal,* **4,** 525–527

RANDALL, P., STARK, M.D., DENNIS, G. and MEKI, M.D. (1984). Bacteriuria in the catheterized patient. *New England Journal of Medicine,* **311,** 560–564

RASMUSSEN, H.H. and IBELS, L.S. (1982). Acute renal failure. *American Journal of Medicine,* **73,** 211–219

REYNOLDS, T.B. (1974). Hepatorenal syndrome. In *The Liver and Its Diseases,* edited by F. Schaffner, S. Sherlock and C.M. Leavy, pp. 307–319. New York; Intercontinental Medical Books

RICHET, G. and MAYAUD, C. (1978). The course of acute renal failure in pyelonephritis and other types of interstitial nephritis. *Nephron,* **22,** 124–127

RIVES, K.R., HARTY, I.J. and AMIN, M. (1980). Renal abscess: emerging concepts of diagnosis and treatment. *Journal of Urology,* **124,** 446–447

ROBERTSON, G.L., AYNEMA, D. and ZERBE, R.L. (1982). Neurogenic disorders of osmoregulation. *American Journal of Medicine,* **72,** 339–353

ROSEN, H. (1976). Renal diseases in the elderly. Symposium on geriatric medicine. *Medical Clinics of North America,* **60,** 1105–1119

ROWE, J.W., ANDRES, R., TOBIN, J.D., NORRIS, A.H. and SHOCK, N.W. (1976). The effect of age on creatinine clearance in man. A cross-sectional and longitudinal study. *Journal of Gerontology,* **31,** 155–163

ROWE, J.W., MINAKER, K.L., SPARROW, D. and ROBERTSON, G.L. (1982). Age-related failure of volume pressure-mediated vasopressin release. *Journal of Clinical Endocrinology and Metabolism,* **54,** 661–664

ROWE, R.J., SHOCK, N.W. and DE FRONZO, R.A. (1976). The influence of age in the renal response to water deprivation in man. *Nephron,* **17,** 270–278

SCHIFF, M., GLICKMAN, M., WEISS, R.M., AHERN, M.J., TOULOUKIAN, R.J., LITTON, B. and ANDREOLI, V.T. (1977). Antibiotic treatment of renal carbuncle. *Annals of Internal Medicine,* **87,** 305–308

SCHRIER, R.W. (1979). Acute renal failure. *Kidney International,* **15,** 205–216

SHOCK, N.W., ANDRES, R., HARRIS, A.H. and TOBIN, J.D. (1979). Patterns of longitudinal changes in renal function. In *Recent Advances in Gerontology,* edited by H. Orimo, K. Shimeda, M. Iriki and D. Maeda. International Congress Series 469, pp. 525–527. Amsterdam; Excerpta Medica

SIMON, H.B., WEINSTEIN, A.J., FASTERNAK, M.S., SWARTZ, M.N. and KUNZ, L.J. (1977). Genitourinary tuberculosis. *American Journal of Medicine,* **63,** 410–420

SOURANDER, L.B. (1966). Urinary tract infection in the aged. An epidemiological study. *Annales Medicinae Internae Fenniae,* **45**(Suppl.), 1–55

SOURANDER, L., KASANEN, A., PASTERNACK, A. and KMARSALO, E. (1979). Uremia in the aged in South Western Finland. A longitudinal study. In *Recent Advances in Gerontology,* edited by H. Orimo, K. Shimeda, M. Iriki and D. Maeda. International Congress Series 469, pp. 540–550, Amsterdam; Excerpta Medica

STAMM, W.E., MARTIN, S.M. and BENNETT, J.V. (1977). Epidemiology of nosocomial infections due to gram negative bacilli: aspects relevant to development and use of vaccines. *Journal of Infectious Diseases,* **128** (Suppl.), 136S–151S

THORLEY, J.D., JONES, S.R. and SANFORD, J.P. (1974). Perinephric abscess. *Medicine (Baltimore),* **53,** 441–445

TUETER, K.J. (1973). Unusual manifestations of renal carcinoma. A review of the literature. *Acta Chirurgica Scandinavica,* **139,** 401–408

TURCK, M. and STAMM, W. (1981). Nosocomial infection in the urinary tract. *American Journal of Medicine,* **70,** 651–656

UNITED NATIONS (1981). *Population Prospects in 1980.* Population Studies No. 78. New York; UN

UNITED NATIONS (1982). *Report of the World Assembly on Ageing.* UN Publication Sales No. E 82.1.16, pp. 61–66. New York; UN

WARREN, J.W., ANTHONY, W.C., HOOPAS, J.M. and MUNCIE, H.C. (1982). Cephalexin for susceptible bacteriuria in afebrile long-term catheterized patients. *Journal of the American Medical Association,* **248,** 454–458

WARREN, J.W., PLATT, R. and THOMAS, R.J. (1978). Antibiotic irrigation and catheter-associated urinary tract infections. *New England Journal of Medicine,* **299,** 570–573

WHO (1974). *Planning and Organization of Geriatric Services.* Technical Report Series, 548. Geneva; WHO

WHO (1983). *Treatment of mild hypertension.* Memorandum WHO–ISH, Bulletin 61, pp. 53–56. Geneva; WHO

WILLIAMS, T.F. (1978). Diabetes in the aged. In *Geriatric Endocrinology. Ageing,* edited by R.B. Greenblatt, pp. 103–133. New York; Raven Press

Chapter 12

Hypertension in the elderly: clinical aspects

José L. Rodicio, J.M. Alcazar and L.M. Ruilope

Introduction

This chapter complements and contrasts with Chapter 5, and should be read in conjunction with it.

In attempting to define the term 'arterial hypertension' in the elderly, one immediately encounters two difficult problems: first, to define what is 'elderly' and secondly, to settle the upper limit of normotension in this particular group of people. Most authors consider that 65 is the age above which a person can be considered as elderly, and for the purpose of this chapter we have followed this criterion. We are nevertheless aware that this age will change as a consequence of the augmented life expectancy in the general population (see the Preface). Blood pressure is a continuous variable, and so the level increases progressively with age. An extensive study by Master and Lasser (1961) revealed that after the age of 65, blood pressure does not exhibit a consistent rise, and they concluded that blood pressures higher than 160/100 mmHg should be considered as abnormal in elderly men, and levels in excess of 170/90 mmHg are abnormal in elderly women. The limit of 160/100 was later considered as adequate by other authors (Babu *et al.*, 1977) and will be employed in this chapter.

Hypertension in the elderly can be classified into two main groups: *isolated systolic hypertension,* defined by the finding of a systolic blood pressure higher than 160 mmHg, with a diastolic blood pressure of 95 mmHg or less, and both *systolic and diastolic hypertension.* This last group is frequently characterized by the coexistence of elevated diastolic blood pressure levels, and disproportionately augmented levels of systolic blood pressure.

Epidemiology and risk factors

In the USA, systolic blood pressure in women rises from a mean of 133 mmHg at age 50 to 165 mmHg at age 85, while in men the increase is from 128 mmHg to 154 mmHg during the same period (Gordon, 1964). Arterial hypertension affects 15–20 per cent of the general population, and its prevalence increases to 50 per cent in people older than 65 years (Östfeld, 1978). Isolated systolic hypertension occurs in about 5 per cent of the hypertensive population, and its prevalence is also higher in elderly people, affecting 15 per cent of the population between 65 and 74 years, and

27 per cent when the age is above 75 (National High Blood Pressure Education Program Coordinating Committee, 1980).

Of great theoretical and practical interest is the fact that in some primitive societies a rise in blood pressure with age does not occur (Page and Sidd, 1977). The initial observation was reported by Donnison (1929) who failed to find hypertensive patients among the native population of the Kavirondo district of Kenya. Furthermore, he could not show the rise in blood pressure with age observed among the European population. This finding was confirmed in some African populations, but not in others. Rural Zulus did not show an increase in their blood pressure with age, but individuals of the same population living in towns did present the usual European-type increase in blood pressure with age. The influences of the environment are far from clear, but dietetic habits and smoking may play a significant role in the development and complications of arterial hypertension (Editorial, 1980, 1981).

Sever *et al.* (1980), in a study carried out in Xhosa people of Southern Africa, were able to show that in the urban group, blood pressure significantly increased with age, but in the tribal group, blood pressure was lower and rose little with age. They found that indexes of obesity were greater and correlated well with blood pressure among the urban Xhosa. Also, dietary sodium and urine sodium:creatinine ratio were statistically higher in the urban group, although neither the dietary sodium nor the urine sodium:creatinine ratio correlated with blood pressure among Xhosa people living in towns.

Another important factor which increases the risk of cardiovascular events and strokes is smoking (MRC, 1985).

For many years it was thought that gradual elevation of blood pressure with age was 'necessary' to perfuse vital organs adequately. This concept was proved to be erroneous by the Framingham study (Kannel, 1974b; Kannel and Gordon, 1978; Kannel, Wolf and Dawber, 1978). This epidemiologic survey of 5209 men and women assessed a number of risk factors in the development of cardiovascular disease and showed that arterial hypertension constitutes the main risk for cardiovascular morbidity and mortality in elderly people. Increased systolic and/or diastolic hypertension were both associated with increased cardiovascular morbidity and mortality. The annual incidence of cardiovascular disease was 3–4 times greater in those patients between 65 and 74 years old who had blood pressure over 160/95 mmHg (Kannel, 1974a) (*Table 12.1*). The study revealed that compared with diastolic blood pressure, systolic pressure is the most potent contributor to cardiovascular complications (Rabkin, Mathewson and Tate, 1978). Other risk factors such as hypercholesterolaemia and smoking are less important in this age group.

Table 12.1 Risk of cardiovascular disease according to age in hypertension (After Kannel and Brand, 1985)

	Incidence per 1000		*Risk ratio**	
Age	*Men*	*Women*	*Men*	*Women*
45–54	23.6	9.7	2.7	3.6
55–64	43.9	23.7	2.8	3.9
65–74	51.0	35.6	3.0	4.1
All ages	35.7	20.6	2.8	3.5

*Risk ratio = $\frac{\text{Rate in hypertensives}}{\text{Rate in normotensives}}$

Among the cardiovascular complications, *stroke* is the major cause of mortality and a leading cause of disability in young as well as in elderly hypertensives. The Framingham study (Kannel *et al.*, 1976) reported an overall incidence of athero-embolic infarction 7 times greater in hypertensive individuals. The risk increased to 30 per cent for each 10 mmHg rise in blood pressure recorded in those persons over age 65. Likewise, the Hisayama study reported an increased incidence of stroke with age in 1621 individuals evaluated over a period of 13 years (Omae, Takeshita and Hirota, 1976). In addition, Ostfeld (1978) demonstrated an incidence rate for stroke twice as high in blacks as compared to whites. It seems clear that older, black, hypertensive individuals are more vulnerable to stroke and require particularly careful attention and appropriate treatment. These suggest that constitutional differences may account for the differences of the natural history of hypertension in blacks (Editorial, 1980).

Coronary events such as *angina pectoris, myocardial infarction* and *sudden death* are commonly observed in the hypertensive elderly patient. Men between the ages of 60 and 64 years, who have a diastolic blood pressure of 95 mmHg or above, have an annual risk of a major coronary event that is 3.7 times greater than those age-matched individuals with a pressure less than 80 mmHg (Pooling Project Research Group, 1978). Similarly, in men and women between 65 and 74 years of age, the presence of left ventricular hypertrophy predicted a 10-fold increase in the risk of congestive cardiac failure as compared with subjects without evidence of left ventricular hypertrophy (Kannel *et al.*, 1972). The level of systolic pressure correlated best with the development of ventricular hypertrophy. Indeed, isolated systolic hypertension has been associated with an increased incidence of myocardial infarction or ischaemia (Gubner, 1962; Sellers, 1966; Tarazi, 1978).

A systolic blood pressure greater than 180 mmHg predicted an increased risk with electrocardiographic signs of myocardial infarction or ischaemia (Shekelle, Ostfeld and Dawans, 1985). It remains to be demonstrated, however, that these relationships are cause and effect (Gifford, 1982). Isolated systolic pressure and systolic–diastolic hypertension are detrimental to the cardiovascular system; it is important to show that treatment will decrease the risk associated with hypertension. Several long-term therapeutic studies that have included elderly patients have looked into this question.

Pathophysiology of arterial hypertension in the elderly (see also Chapter 5)

The aging process is characterized by the progressive establishment of a series of changes influencing most of the systems that maintain normal cardiovascular homeostasis. Aging is associated with a progressive increase in the rigidity of the aorta and peripheral arteries due to loss of elastic fibres in the media, and to the increase of calcium and collagen content of the arterial wall (Hass, 1943). These changes have the functional consequence that the vessels behave like rigid tubes. The systolic pressure generated in the left ventricle is then transmitted with very little buffering to the arterial tree, causing an increase in the systolic blood pressure (O'Malley and O'Callaghan, 1982). The increase of systolic blood pressure takes place in the face of a diminished cardiac output, due in turn to the diminution of both myocardial contractility and blood volume (Lakatta, 1973). Meanwhile, and through mechanisms not completely understood, aging is accompanied by an elevation of the peripheral resistance (Amery *et al.*, 1978).

The aging process is also characterized by a diminution of the functional renal tissue and of renal vasculature (Hollenberg *et al.*, 1974; Macias Nuñez, 1983). These changes induce a progressive diminution of both renal plasma flow and glomerular filtration rate (Watkin and Shock, 1955; Darmady *et al.*, 1973). An incapacity of the aging kidney to retain sodium has also been described (Macias Nuñez *et al.*, 1983), together with a diminished activity of the renin–angiotensin–aldosterone system (Weidmann *et al.*, 1975).

Plasma norephinephrine levels have been shown to be increased in elderly people (Lake *et al.*, 1977; Sever *et al.*, 1977). This fact is accompanied by a reduced sensitivity of the baroreceptor area (Gribbin *et al.*, 1971) and by a diminution of the vascular sensitivity to catecholamines (Vestal *et al.*, 1979).

All these characteristics of elderly people induce derangements of the cardiovascular mechanisms of adaptation to low or high blood pressure levels. In fact, the tachycardia and vasoconstriction that usually accompany a decrease of blood pressure are impaired. The opposite, i.e. blood pressure elevation, is not associated with bradycardia and vasodilatation.

Pathophysiology of systolic and diastolic blood pressure in the elderly (see also Chapter 5)

It has been suggested that this type of hypertension has distinctive characteristics in the elderly that differentiate it from that in younger people (Swales, 1979; O'Malley and O'Brien, 1980; Niarchos and Laragh, 1984). A recent study by Messerli (1983) has confirmed this statement. These authors have shown that, when compared with that of younger patients, arterial hypertension in the elderly can be characterized by lower values of cardiac output, heart rate, ejection fraction and intravascular volume, renal blood flow and plasma renin activity. Together with this, elevated levels of peripheral and renal resistance have been found. The appearance of both systolic and diastolic hypertension in elderly people is accompanied by an exaltation of the haemodynamic changes that normally take place during the aging process. Although the levels of renin are usually lower than in younger hypertensives, a dependency of the systolic blood pressure on the levels of renin has recently been described in some of these patients (Niarchos and Laragh, 1984).

It has been suggested that salt intake can contribute to the development of arterial hypertension in younger people. An elevated salt ingestion would favour the elevation of blood pressure levels through a defect in the renal sodium handling causing salt retention. The renal inability of elderly people to retain sodium contradicts this possibility (Macias Nuñez, 1983). Nevertheless, we and others (Niarchos *et al.*, 1984) have observed that a restriction of sodium intake is enough to attain an adequate control of blood pressure in a large proportion of elderly people. This last observation indicates a definite role of sodium, at least, in the maintenance of the elevated blood pressure levels.

The possible participation of the autonomic nervous system remains incompletely studied. Nevertheless, the attenuated cardiovascular response to stress (O'Malley and O'Brien, 1980) and to catecholamines (Vestal *et al.*, 1979) in aged patients makes this possibility unlikely. On the other hand, a diminution of baroreflex function in response to the increased levels of norepinephrine has been attributed to a decreased number of beta-adrenoceptors (Bristow *et al.*, 1969; Vestal *et al.*, 1979).

Pathophysiology of isolated systolic hypertension in the elderly

As previously mentioned, aging is usually accompanied by a loss of elasticity of the aorta and peripheral arteries (Hass, 1943; Hollander, 1976). The reason for elevation of systolic blood pressure in the elderly lies in the loss of distensibility of the aorta and large arteries. As the aortic wall becomes rigid, the pulse generated during left ventricular contraction is transmitted to the aorta relatively unchanged. Pulse pressure then widens mainly as a consequence of the augmentation of systolic blood pressure, with little or no variations of diastolic blood pressure. The study of Colandrea *et al.* (1970) illustrates the pathophysiology of this process, showing that 44 per cent of the patients having isolated systolic hypertension had aortic calcifications at the beginning of the study.

Haemodynamic studies of isolated systolic hypertension in the elderly have shown, in opposition to data from younger hypertensives, that heart rate and cardiac output are not increased (Adampoulos *et al.*, 1975). At the same time, peripheral resistances are increased and plasma volume tends to be low. As cardiac work is related to systolic blood pressure, any increase in this parameter will induce parallel changes in left ventricular work load. This fact, together with the usual diminution of oxygen blood supply through the coronary arteries in elderly people, makes the appearance of the left ventricular failure common in these patients.

The debate about isolated systolic hypertension lies in whether it constitutes *per se* a risk factor promoting vascular disease, as opposed to the alternative hypothesis, that systolic hypertension is only a secondary manifestation of an already established vascular disease (Swales, 1979; Brest and Majdan, 1981; Gifford, 1982). As already mentioned, the elevation of systolic blood pressure is associated with increased morbidity and mortality (Gubner, 1962; Sellers, 1966; Tarazi, 1978). The fact that this statement is also true for younger hypertensives, points to a definite role of isolated systolic hypertension in the induction of cardiovascular damage.

Clinical aspects of arterial hypertension in the elderly

Measurement of blood pressure

In patients over 60 years of age, a difference between the blood pressure measured by intra-arterial and conventional indirect methods can be observed (Spence *et al.*, 1978). The so-called 'pseudohypertension' in the elderly is a consequence of the rigid vessels which cannot be adequately occluded when the sphygmomanometer cuff is inflated. This gives rise to the appearance of falsely elevated pressure levels.

Although small, differences can appear in as much as 80 per cent of patients for systolic and 50 per cent for diastolic blood pressure (Rosenfeld, 1983) with the conventional method of measurement. Few cases of real pseudohypertension are described in the literature (Nielsen, 1982), but the importance of this finding lies in the deleterious consequences that hypotensive drugs, when inappropriately employed, can induce in elderly people. To avoid this problem we recommend the palpation of the pulseless brachial artery, distal to the cuff, in order to demonstrate calcified arteries. The blood pressure should also be taken in both arms (Messerli, Ventura and Anrodeo, 1985).

Another problem to bear in mind when measuring blood pressure in elderly people is the fairly common underestimation of systolic blood pressure, due to an auscultatory gap. This problem is avoided if the cuff is inflated to higher than 250 mmHg, and then deflated slowly.

Finally, greater variability in resting blood pressure in the elderly has been reported (Rowlands, Stolland and Litter, 1984), so that blood pressure should be evaluated over a period of weeks or perhaps monthly before instituting treatment.

Evaluation of the hypertensive patient

Once the diagnosis has been confirmed through at least three separate blood pressure readings, a thorough investigation of clinical history directed at detecting evidence of possible *target organ damage* should be obtained. *Table 12.2* contains our experience of the symptomatology at the beginning of the study in a group of 125 elderly hypertensive patients. The patients were divided into those having isolated

Table 12.2 Symptomatology at the beginning of a study in a group of 125 elderly hypertensive patients and 400 essential hypertensive patients younger than 60 years

	n	*None* (%)	*Cardiac* (%)	*Neurological* (%)	*Peripheral artery disease* (%)
1. Systolic and diastolic hypertension	75	13	44	38	5
2. Isolated systolic hypertensives	50	0	37	24	39*‡
3. Essential hypertension (age <60 yr)	400	49†	33	15	3

Statistical analysis performed by means of the chi-square test.
* $P<0.01$ vs. 3.
† $P<0.01$ vs. 1 and 2.
‡ $P<0.01$ vs. 1 and 3.

systolic hypertension or those with both systolic and diastolic hypertension. The results were compared with similar tests in younger hypertensive people. The percentage of asymptomatic patients was very low in elderly people, with more frequent symptoms of neurological or peripheral artery disease.

Physical examination also is directed towards assessing both the severity of the hypertension and target organ damage. Fundoscopy, vascular palpation, vascular bruits, cardiac enlargement, signs of congestive cardiac failure, arrhythmias or thyroid disease are important, and neurological examination may reveal deficits secondary to the vascular problem, e.g. signs of former cerebrovascular accidents.

The initial *laboratory investigation* should comprise a full blood count, urinalysis with microscopic examination, and the determination of the serum levels of creatinine, glucose, uric acid, cholesterol, triglycerides and potassium. An electrocardiogram and chest roentgenogram should also be performed. Echocardiography is cheap, non-invasive and informative. As can be seen in *Table 12.3*, the biochemical aspects in the initial study of our group of elderly hypertensives showed significantly higher values of creatinine and glucose and lower uric acids in elderly patients with isolated systolic hypertension, than in those with both systolic and diastolic hypertension. When compared with younger essential hypertensive patients, isolated systolic hypertension again showed higher values of creatinine and glucose ($P<0.05$). The values of creatinine were also higher in elderly patients with both systolic and diastolic hypertension than in younger patients ($P<0.05$).

Table 12.3 Biochemical aspects in arterial hypertension of the elderly compared with a group of 400 younger essential hypertensives

	Aged patients				*Young*
	Systolic and diastolic hypertension ($n = 75$)		*Isolated systolic hypertension* ($n = 50$)		*essential hypertension* ($n = 400$)
Serum creatinine (mmol/l)	101.6 ± 35.3	$P<0.05$	114.9 ± 61.8	$P<0.05$	96 ± 38*
Serum sodium (mmol/l)	138 ± 4		139 ± 3		141 ± 3.8
Serum potassium (mmol/l)	4.0 ± 0.5		4.2 ± 0.7		4.1 ± 1.1
Serum chloride (mmol/l)	101 ± 9		105 ± 7		100 ± 8.8
Serum glucose (mmol/l)	5.55 ± 1.27	$P<0.001$	8.65 ± 5.5	$P<0.001$	5.38 ± 1.1
Serum cholesterol (mmol/l)	5.24 ± 1.11		5.68 ± 1.24		5.37 ± 1.2
Serum triglycerides (g/l)	1.56 ± 1.26		1.47 ± 0.90		1.53 ± 0.67
Serum uric acid (mmol/l)	0.42 ± 0.11	$P<0.05$	0.35 ± 0.12		0.39 ± 0.1

Values expressed as $\bar{X}$ ± S.D.
Statistical analysis performed by means of Student's *t* test for impaired data.
* $P<0.05$ vs. systolic and diastolic.

Among the secondary origins of arterial hypertension, *renovascular* and *renal parenchymatous disease* (both unilateral and bilateral) have been described as fairly common in the elderly hypertensives. Laugesen *et al.* (1982) described a frequency of 6 per cent of renin-dependent hypertension (unilateral renal artery stenosis with elevated peripheral plasma renin activity and a positive ratio of plasma renin concentration from the renal veins), the frequency being 13 per cent for unilateral kidney disease and 21 per cent for bilateral chronic nephropathy, respectively. In our experience, renovascular hypertension in elderly people represents one-third of all our series of cases with an atherosclerotic origin (15 out of 45 patients). These patients had some distinctive features, as can be seen in *Table 12.4* (see also Chapter 5). They had a higher degree of renal failure, with similar levels of visceral damage in the heart and retina.

The presence of a grade 3–4 retinopathy, of vascular murmurs over the abdomen and the findings of abnormalities will force the performance of further studies in these patients. A plain abdominal film may show a marked difference of kidney size, and the performance of an isotope renogram could confirm the suspicion of

Table 12.4 Clinical and biochemical characteristics of renovascular hypertension in elderly people; the aetiology of all cases was atherosclerosis

	Age below 65	*Age above 65*	*P*
n	30	15	—
Retinopathy grade 3–4	40%	46%	NS
Male/female	28/2	14/1	NS
Systolic blood pressure (mmHg)	218 ± 16	221 ± 14	NS
Diastolic blood pressure (mmHg)	116 ± 8	119 ± 10	NS
Serum creatinine (μmol/l)	216.4 ± 79.5	335.9 ± 97.2	<0.01
Creatinine clearance (ml/min)	65 ± 20	38 ± 29	<0.02
Left ventricular enlargement on ECG	20 (66%)	12 (80%)	NS
Previous episode(s) of:			
stroke	8 (26%)	7 (46%)	NS
angina	16 (53%)	4 (26%)	NS
intermittent claudication	13 (43%)	9 (60%)	NS

Values expressed as X ± S.D.
Statistical studies performed by Student's *t* test for impaired data and chi-squared test.

abnormalities in the renal arteries. Further studies using radiocontrast media, such as an intravenous pyelogram or a renal arteriogram, should be performed cautiously due to the elevated risk of renal damage in these particular patients (Byrd and Sherman, 1979). Their performance is indicated when the condition of the patient permits consideration of later surgical treatment or percutaneous transluminal angioplasty. In our opinion, further investigations are necessary when grade 3–4 retinopathy is present, when rapidly developing renal failure appears, and in patients with a poor response to medical treatment even in the absence of these clinical characteristics. Following these criteria, the prevalence of the arterial hypertension of secondary origin in elderly people is in our experience 32 per cent (58 out of 183), in accordance with previous reports. Renovascular hypertension represents 8.2 per cent of the total, and arterial hypertension accompanying chronic renal parenchymatous diseases represents 26.7 per cent.

Prognosis and hypertension

The prognosis of those aged 65–74 is discussed in relation to treatment in the section on trials below. The prognosis of those *patients above 75 years* is not as clear. Rajala *et al.* (1983) studied a group of 559 persons (83 per cent above 85 years) over a period of 11 years. These authors showed an *inverse* correlation between the levels of systolic and diastolic blood pressure and mortality, suggesting that in the very old, mortality *decreases* in parallel with the increase of blood pressure. Sprackling *et al.* (1981), studying patients between 75 and 94 years, also observed that the *higher* the blood pressure, the *lower* the mortality (Sprackling *et al.*, 1981; Mitchell, 1983). Further studies are needed in order to know whether or not in very old patients blood pressure loses its predictive values for morbidity and mortality.

The influence of treatment on the prognosis of *isolated systolic hypertension* is less clear also, because of the lack of prospective therapeutic trials, or because therapy was associated with severe side effects when attempted (Traub *et al.*, 1974).

Treatment

Non-pharmacological treatment of hypertension in the elderly

Any approach to the management of hypertension in the elderly must begin with simple, non-pharmacological measures, such as correction of obesity if present, avoiding smoking if possible, adjustment of dietary sodium and potassium intake, reducing alcohol consumption and the institution of regular exercise. However, salt restriction must be carefully watched because of the impairment of the aging kidney in retaining sodium (see Chapter 4). Reduction of sodium intake must be in the range of 30–80 mmol/day (approximately 3–5g of salt) (MacGregor, 1983). Greater reductions are followed only by a few patients in practice, and may be dangerous if any intercurrent illness causing loss of appetite or water and/or electrolyte losses appears in the course of the treatment of hypertension with drastic reduction of salt intake in an old person.

Potassium has been a matter of controversy, as to whether to include it in the treatment of hypertension either alone, or in order to prevent the undesirable effects of diuretic-induced hypokalaemia (MacGregor, 1983; Editorial, 1985a; Kaplan *et al.*, 1985). It is believed that moderate salt restriction and potassium supplementation produces a small but significant fall in blood pressure (MacGregor, 1983). Behaviour modification, informal or formal, can also be useful (see also Chapter 5).

Pharmacological treatment of hypertension in the elderly

Advanced age is usually accompanied by changes in drug kinetics and metabolism (Vestal, 1978; O'Malley *et al.*, 1980) (see Chapter 9) that favour an elevated incidence of side effects in aged patients (Hurwitz, 1969). Thus, in any treatment regimen it is necessary to use low initial doses, and increase them very gradually.

Trials of treatment in hypertension of the elderly

The first controlled trial to examine the effects of therapy on cardiovascular morbidity and mortality was the Chelmsford study reported by Hamilton, Thompson and Wisniewski (1964). Sixty-one patients with moderate to severe hypertension (diastolic blood pressure over 110 mmHg) clearly demonstrated a distinct benefit from therapy. Similar results were obtained in 143 male veterans by the first Veterans Administration Cooperative Study published in 1967. A more detailed study of 380 patients, 81 of them over the age of 60, with diastolic pressure between 90 and 114 mmHg was published in 1970 by the Veterans Administration (Veterans Administration, 1970, 1972). This study showed an unquestionable decrease in the incidence of morbid cardiovascular events in patients with diastolic pressures ranging from 105 to 114 mmHg who were successfully treated. In those with a diastolic pressure in the 90–104 mmHg range there was a protective trend, but this was not statistically significant. In particular, no benefits from coronary events were noted in the group with mild hypertension. These results created much speculation as to whether mild hypertension should be treated or not. In view of this, several studies in patients with mild hypertension were initiated.

Table 12.5 Treatment outcome in patients with diastolic hypertension after age 60

Study	*Year*	*Diastolic blood pressure*	*No. patients over 60 yrs*	*Design control-active*	*Outcome per 1000 patient years*	
					Mortality active: SC	*Mortality placebo: RC*
HDFP	1979	≧90	2376	RC–SC	25	30
ANS	1980	95–109	582	Placebo–SC	6	8

ANS, Australian National Study; HDFP, Hypertension Detection and Follow-up Program; RC, referred care; SC, stepped care.

The studies on mild hypertension were conducted by Public Health Services in the United States, in 1972, and one performed in Chelmsford, England (Johnson, Pearce and Hamilton, 1978). They included a small number of patients, which made analysis of data less reliable. Recently, two large-scale trials have been published in Australia and the USA (*Table 12.5*). The Australian trial (Australian National Blood Pressure Study Management Committee, 1979) examined 3427 patients aged 30–69 years for an average study duration of 4 years. All cases had diastolic blood pressures between 95 and 109 mmHg and were treated with placebo or diuretics followed by beta-blockers. There was a significant reduction of stroke and deaths from all causes; there was also a reduction in fatal ischaemic significance which did not attain statistical significance. This study demonstrated that therapeutic blood pressure reduction was much more important in preventing complications than the initial value of blood pressure. Also, a 39 per cent reduction in complications was observed in those patients over 60 years of age at entry.

The Hypertension Detection and Follow-up Program Cooperative Group (1979a, 1979b) included 11 000 hypertensive patients in 14 centres followed for 5 years. Patients were randomized to either stepped care (SC) or referred care (RC) groups. The SC patients attended special clinics where they received special therapeutic intervention and counselling; the RC patients were referred to their private physician for usual care. The findings indicated that the 5-year mortality rates from all cardiovascular causes were significantly lower in the SC group, and this was largely due to reduction in stroke and non-cardiovascular deaths.

The incidence of myocardial infarction was less in patients with mild hypertension than in those with higher levels of blood pressure. A subgroup of 2376 patients aged 60–69 also benefited greatly from therapy. The overall mortality in the elderly SC group was 16.4 lower than the RC group, with marked reduction in both fatal and non-fatal stroke. A recent report of this programme shows that left ventricular hypertrophy, a predictor of poor prognosis, can be prevented and reversed by systemic antihypertensive treatment (Hypertension Detection and Follow-up Program Cooperative Group, 1985). *Table 12.5* shows two important studies carried out in elderly patients with mild hypertension. These studies invariably demonstrated that elderly patients with mild or severe hypertension must be treated to avoid catastrophic cardiovascular events.

Whereas no doubts may exist as to the treatment of diastolic hypertension, serious questions have been raised about the benefit of the treatment of *isolated systolic hypertension* in the elderly. As mentioned earlier, systolic hypertension correlates best with increased cardiovascular morbidity and mortality. Data from several epidemiological surveys are consistent with this observation (Gubner, 1962; Sellers, 1966; Colandrea *et al.*, 1970; Shekelle, Ostfeld and Dawans, 1985; Tarazi, 1978). In addition, a recent Framingham report of 1254 untreated persons surviving after age 65 supports the univariate relationship of several measures of systolic blood pressure over time with increased risk of cardiovascular disease (Harris *et al.*, 1985).

On the other hand, if systolic hypertension indicates rigidity of large arteries, reduction of systolic blood pressure may not decrease the risk of cardiovascular events since therapy could lead to an unacceptable decrease in diastolic blood pressure and the side effects of treatment would mitigate against the use of antihypertensive agents. Nevertheless, it it generally believed that systolic hypertension exceeding 180 mmHg should be treated (Priddle *et al.*, 1968).

In an attempt to answer these questions better, the European Working Party on High Blood Pressure in the Elderly (EWPHBPE) has established a double blind, multicentre trial in patients over the age of 60 years (Amery *et al.*, 1978). Patients were receiving hydrochlorothiazide together with triamterene or placebo. If blood pressure remained above the pre-established limit, methyldopa was added to the active therapy and placebo in the placebo group.

Final results of this study show that the total mortality rate was not influenced by active drug treatment. Cardiovascular mortality was reduced in the treated group, due to a reduction in cardiac deaths, but cerebrovascular terminating complications were not affected by treatment. Non-terminating cerebrovascular events were lower in the active treated group, although non-terminating cardiac events were not. The terminating events were: death, non-fatal or subarachnoid haemorrhage, development of hypertensive retinopathy grade III or IV, dissecting aneurysm, congestive heart failure not controllable without diuretics or antihypertensive drugs, hypertensive encephalopathy, severe increase in left ventricular hypertrophy and a rise of blood pressure exceeding the defined limits. The treatment produced a decrease in glucose tolerance and an increase in uric acid and creatinine in patients on diuretics (Amery *et al.*, 1985). These ancillary effects of treatment were also present in our own series.

The MRC trial of treatment in mild hypertension is an impressive large-scale study composed of 17 354 hypertensive patients. It was designed to determine if drug treatment of mild hypertension (diastolic hypertension 90–109 mmHg) reduced the rates of strokes and coronary events in men and women aged 35–64 years. The drugs used were diuretics (bendrofluazide) in a dose of 10 mg and beta-blockers (propranolol to a maximum of 240 mg/day) or matched placebo.

The main conclusions are that the rate of mortality from all causes was equal in the drug-treated and placebo groups, although a sex difference was obtained. The death rate decreased in men but increased in women, owing to non-cardiovascular deaths, principally malignancies. The stroke rate was reduced in the treated group. The overall rates of coronary events were similar in both groups. Nevertheless, the non-smoker mild hypertensive men on propranolol had an extremely low incidence in coronary events. The smoker hypertensives did not show this 'protective' effect of propranolol on cardiac complications. Propranolol was more effective in lowering blood pressure in the young than in the older population. Bendrofluazide reduced the rate of strokes in smokers and non-smokers, but propranolol in the non-smokers only (MRC trial, 1985).

The International Prospective Primary Prevention Study in Hypertension, in a randomized study of 6537 patients treated with beta-blockers (oxprenolol) and regimens which did not include beta-blockers, concluded that the two groups exhibited a similar prevalence of sudden deaths, cerebrovascular accidents and myocardial infarction (IPPPSH Collaborative Group, 1985).

Treatment of hypertension in the elderly in practice

Thus, results of the MRC trial, the IPPPSH trial, and particularly the EWPHBPE, show that pharmacological treatment does *not* influence the *survival* of the mild hypertensive aged over 60, although the prevalence of strokes is diminished by antihypertensive drugs. So far, it is not at all clear if mild hypertension should be pharmacologically treated in the elderly, without a non-pharmacological approach to the problem first (Breckenridge, 1985; Editorial, 1977; Editorial, 1985b, 1985c). Questions that doctors involved in the treatment of mild hypertension in the elderly should always keep in mind before starting any pharmacological antihypertensive therapy in the elderly are: is the risk associated with mild hypertension in the elderly reversible with therapy; how justified is it to treat symptomless mild hypertension in the elderly?

When hypertension is severe and/or target organs are damaged (heart, kidney and brain), patients will almost certainly obtain benefit from active treatment. The use of drugs in the therapy of elevated blood pressure in the aged patient has limitations, due to the previously described characteristics of this clinical group. Drugs acting as peripheral and central adrenergic inhibitors should not be used, because of the high risk of central nervous system side effects, and because of the susceptibility of elderly people to hypotension (Rosenfeld, 1983; O'Malley and O'Brien, 1980). Nevertheless, some studies have shown a good tolerance of methyldopa (Amery *et al.*, 1978; Sprackling *et al.*, 1981).

The most widely used drugs in general for the treatment of arterial hypertension in the elderly have been the diuretics and the beta-adrenoceptor blocking agents. The *thiazide diuretics* are effective in most of the patients in the absence of major clinical or biochemical disturbances (Priddle *et al.*, 1968; Amery *et al.*, 1978). Postural hypotension occurred with diuretics in only 4.6 per cent, compared with 3.4 per cent in non-treated men of similar age in the series of Myers *et al.* (1978). One of the principal problems in using thiazide diuretics is the appearance of hypokalaemia (Kassirer and Harrington, 1977). Low plasma potassiums are frequently found in elderly people in the absence of any treatment (Macias Nuñez, 1983). The combination of thiazides or amiloride is effective in avoiding this complication.

Table 12.6 Five-year evolution of blood pressure and some serum biochemical parameters in a group of 75 elderly patients with both systolic and diastolic hypertension*

	Group 1 (n=20)		*Group 2 (n=25)*		*Group 3 (n=15)*		*Group 4 (n=15)*	
	Initial	*60 mths*	*Initial*	*60 mths*	*Initial*	*60 mths*	*Initial*	*60 mths*
Potassium (mmol/l)	4.3±0.3	4.3±0.4	4.2±0.6	4.0±0.3	3.9±0.5	3.8±0.5	4.0±0.4	4.2±0.3
Creatinine (µmol/l)	88±39	88±33	97±30	99±35	91±17	121±17†	97±28	101±26
Glucose (mmol/l)	5.3±0.8	5.6±0.9	5.7±0.6	6.1±1.1‡	5.7±1.3	6.9±1.6‡	6.1±2.0	6.6±0.9
Cholesterol (mmol/l)	5.4±0.9	5.4±0.3	4.7±1.0	5.7±1.1†	5.0±1.2	5.8±0.7‡	5.4±0.9	5.6±0.5
Triglycerides (g/l)	1.3±0.5	1.2±0.3	1.4±0.4	1.3±0.4	1.7±1.1	1.4±0.5	1.7±0.7	1.3±0.6‡
SBP (mmHg)	170±20	149±16†	183±29	151±25†	205±39	151±25†	185±26	151±11†
DPB (mmHg)	102±8	88±8†	113±16	92±12†	122±23	92±12†	111±14	89±12†

Values expressed as $\overline{X}$ ±S.D.
SBP, systolic blood pressure.
DBP, diastolic blood pressure.
Statistical analysis performed by means of Student's *t* test for paired data.
*Patients are classified by the treatment maintained during the follow-up period in four groups: (a) low salt diet alone (group 1); (b) diuretic (hydrochlorothiazide + amiloride (group 2); (c) same as group 2 + propranolol (group 3); (d) propranolol alone (group 4)
†$P<0.01$ vs. initial values.
‡$P<0.05$ vs. initial values.

The appearance of significant glucose intolerance has also become evident with the use of diuretics in elderly people (Amery *et al.*, 1978). *Table 12.6* contains our experience with a group of 75 elderly hypertensive patients followed for 5 years and treated with a low salt diet, with a diuretic or a beta-blocker or with a combination of both drugs. A derangement of renal function was observed in the group treated with the association of a diuretic and a beta-blocker. An increase of the plasma levels of glucose and cholesterol was also seen whenever the diuretic alone or in combination was used. These results are again in accordance with those of Amery *et al.* (1978).

Beta-adrenoceptor blocking agents have been used in the treatment of hypertension in the elderly (Rosenfeld, 1983; Miranda *et al.*, 1984). Nevertheless, many aspects of the pharmacology of these drugs are different in the aged. Plasma levels of propranolol are higher in the elderly (Castleden and George, 1979) and the incidence of side effects due to its use is higher (Greenblatt and Koch-Weser, 1973). Furthermore, a decrease in the response of the sympathetic nervous system to beta-blockers in aged people has been shown (Vestal, 1978; Dillon *et al.*, 1980).

The 'stepped-care' drug regimen, using a diuretic or beta-blocker as the first drug and adding the other if necessary in a second step, can be equally effective in older as in younger hypertensives (National High Blood Pressure Education Program Coordinating Committee, 1980). Vasodilators such as hydralazine can be used as a third-step drug when needed. Such a regimen has been found in our experience to be adequate for the control of blood pressure in elderly people.

The therapeutic approach to *isolated systolic hypertension* has used the stepped-care regimen (Chobanian, 1981), based on the haemodynamic characteristics of the disease (Adamapoulos *et al.*, 1975; Simon *et al.*, 1979). Recent reports have shown that salt restriction and/or a thiazide diuretic are effective antihypertensive means in most patients with isolated systolic hypertension (Miranda *et al.*, 1984; Niarchos *et al.*, 1984).

The new hypotensive drugs such as *converting-enzyme inhibitors* and *calcium channel blockers* look promising (Bellani *et al.*, 1983; Storstein *et al.*, 1984; Ferroni and Pacianori, 1984). Captopril is generally well tolerated, if initial treatment is started with low doses. The antihypertensive effect is maintained over the long term (Groel *et al.*, 1983). Although its use has been largely limited because of safety considerations, the recent reports using lower doses suggest that antihypertensive efficacy is maintained in the absence of side effects (Frolich *et al.*, 1984; Veterans Administration Cooperative Study Group on Antihypertensive Agents, 1984). The efficacy of captopril in the treatment of congestive heart failure (Chatterjee *et al.*, 1981) favours its use in the elderly hypertensive patients presenting with symptoms of heart failure.

Calcium channel blockers have also been used successfully in the treatment of essential hypertension. These drugs are usually well tolerated and the appearance of important side effects during their use is rare (Spivack *et al.*, 1983; Lewis, 1983). The simultaneous role of these drugs in the prevention of myocardial ischaemia makes them a theoretically valuable tool for the treatment of hypertension in elderly people. Calcium channel blockers have recently been recommended for the treatment of hypertension in elderly people (Müller *et al.*, 1984). These authors found a positive response in 80 per cent of hypertensive patients above 60 years. This figure compared with only 25 per cent controlled with beta-blockers.

The treatment of *renovascular hypertension* has some distinct characteristics in the elderly. The medical treatment is similar to that of younger people. Converting-enzyme inhibitors may be the elective drug in unilateral renal artery stenosis (Frolich *et al.*, 1984). Surgical revascularization is necessary when the atheromatous lesion involves only the renal artery, and also in those cases with systemic atherosclerosis in which progressive renal failure takes place (Libertino *et al.*, 1980; Alcazar and Ruilope, 1983).

Percutaneous transluminal angioplasty of the renal artery constitutes an alternative method of treatment for renovascular hypertension. This technique has the advantage of safety and simplicity. Nevertheless, when atherosclerosis is the cause of the renal vascular damage, it has the disadvantage of frequent relapse of the stenoses (Alcazar and Ruilope, 1983; Martin and Cassarella, 1984), which limits the effectiveness of this method in elderly renovascular hypertension. The prognosis of renal function when medical treatment is used in patients with progressive shrinkage of the renal size (Dean *et al.*, 1981) can enhance the performance of more aggressive therapies. Renal angioplasty will probably show better results if the inclusion criteria are carefully worked out and adhered to (Martin and Cassarella, 1984), and surgical revascularization should be employed when renal angioplasty is not technically performable, or when this technique fails.

Whenever *renal insufficiency* is present, the medical treatment of elderly hypertensives is also similar to that in younger patients. Frusemide is usually employed if renal function falls below 50 per cent of normal, especially if arterial hypertension is accompanied by oedema or cardiac failure. Potassium-sparing agents should be avoided in this particular situation. When needed, a second drug should be added to the diuretic. Commonly, beta-blockers are used in the second step, but again calcium antagonists or converting-enzyme inhibitors are increasingly being used.

References

ADAMOPOULOS, P.N., CHRYSANTHAKOPOULIS, S.G. and FROLICH, E.D. (1975). Systolic hypertension: nonhomogeneous diseases. *American Journal of Cardiology,* **36,** 697–701

ALCAZAR, J.M. and RUILOPE, L.M. (1983). Tratamiento de la hipertension vasculorrenal. *Nefrologia,* **3,** 149–152

AMERY, J.M., BERTHAUX, P., BULPITT, C., DERNYTTERE, M., DE SCHAEPDRYVER, A., DOLLERY, C. *et al.* (1978). Glucose intolerance during diuretic therapy: results of trial by the European Working Party on high blood pressure (EWPHE). *Lancet,* **1,** 681–683

AMERY, A., BRIXKO, P., CLEMENT, D., DE SCHAEPDRYVER, A., FAGARD, R., FORTE, J. *et al.* (1985). Mortality and morbidity results from the European working party of high blood pressure in the elderly trial. *Lancet,* **1,** 1349–1354

AMERY, A., WASIR, H., BULPITT, C., CONWAY, J., FAGARD, R., LIJEN, P. *et al.* (1978). Ageing and the cardiovascular system. *Acta Cardiologica,* **33,** 443–467

AUSTRALIAN NATIONAL BLOOD PRESSURE STUDY MANAGEMENT COMMITTEE (1979). Initial results of the Australian Therapeutic Trial in mild hypertension. *Clinical Science,* **57,** 449s–454s

BABU, T.N., NAZIR, F., RAO, D. and LUISADA, A.A. (1977). What is normal blood pressure in the aged? *Geriatrics,* **32,** 73–76

BELLANI, M., MEREGALLI, M., GUFFANI, E., BARTUCCI, F., FIORELLA, G., CHIERICHETTI, S.M. *et al.* (1983). Treatment of hypertension in the elderly: a controlled clinical trial of dihydroergotoxine mesilate in comparison with nifedipine. *Current Therapeutic Research,* **34,** 1014–1022

BRECKENRIDGE, A. (1985). Treating mild hypertension. *British Medical Journal,* **291,** 89–90

BREST, A.N. and MAJDAN, J. (1981). Hypertension in the elderly. In *Geriatric Cardiology,* edited by A.N. Brest, R.J. Woble and D.A. Rothbaum, pp. 161–167. Philadelphia; Davis

BRISTOW, J.D., HONOUR, A.K., PICKERING, G.W., SLEIGHT, P. and SMITH, H. (1969). Diminished baroreceptor sensitivity in high blood pressure. *Circulation,* **39,** 48–54

BYRD, L. and SHERMAN, R.L. (1979). Radiocontrast-induced acute renal failure. A clinical review. *Medicine (Baltimore),* **58,** 270–279

CASTLEDEN, C.M. and GEORGE, C. (1979). The effects of ageing on hepatic clearance of propranolol. *British Journal of Clinical Pharmacology,* **7,** 49–54

CHATTERJEE, K., ADER, R. and PARMELEY, W.W. (1981). Angiotensin converting enzyme inhibitors in congestive heart failure. In *Angiotensin Converting Enzyme Inhibitors. Mechanisms of Action and Clinical Implications,* edited by Z.P. Horovitz, pp. 285–300. Baltimore; Urban and Schwarzenberg

COLANDREA, M.A., FRIEDMAN, G.D., NICHAMAN, M.Z. and LYND, C. (1970). Systolic hypertension in the elderly: an epidemiological assessment. *Circulation,* **41,** 239–245

CHOBANIAN, A.V. (1981). Therapeutic decision-making in systolic hypertension. *Geriatrics,* **36,** 36–43

DARMADY, A.M., OFFER, J. and WOODHOUSE, M.A. (1973). The parameters of the aging kidney. *Journal of Pathology,* **109,** 182–195

DEAN, R.H., KIEFFER, R.W. and SMITH, B.M. (1981). Natural history of renovascular hypertension: changes in renal function during medical therapy. Abstract Program of the International Cardiovascular Society, 29th Scientific Meeting, the Hyatt Regency. Dallas, Texas, 11–13 June

DILLON, N., CHUNG, S., KELLY, J. and O'MALLEY, K. (1980). Age and beta-adrenoceptor function. *Clinical Pharmacology and Therapeutics,* **27,** 769–772

DONNISON, C.P. (1929). Blood pressure in the African native: its bearing upon aetiology of hyperplasia and arteriosclerosis. *Lancet,* **1,** 6–7

EDITORIAL (1977). Hypertension in the elderly. *Lancet,* **1,** 684–685

EDITORIAL (1980). Hypertension in Blacks and Whites. *Lancet,* **1,** 73–74

EDITORIAL (1981). Why does blood-pressure rise with age? *Lancet,* **1,** 289–290

EDITORIAL (1985a). Dietary potassium and hypertension. *Lancet,* **1,** 1308–1309

EDITORIAL (1985b). Treatment of hypertension in the over-60s. *Lancet,* **1,** 1369–1370

EDITORIAL (1985c). Treatment of hypertension: the 1985 results. *Lancet,* **2,** 645–647

FERRONI, C. and PICCARONI, E. (1984). L'Ace-inhibitore captopril nel tratamento della ipertensione arteriosa dell'anziano (Abstract). Le Basi Razionale della Terapia, **14,** 387

FROLICH, E.D., COOPER, R.A. and LEWIS, E.J. (1984). Review of the overall experience of captopril in hypertension. *Archives of Internal Medicine,* **144,** 1441–1444

GIFFORD, R.W. (1982). Isolated systolic hypertension in the elderly. Some controversial issues. *Journal of the American Medical Association,* **247,** 781–785

GORDON, T. (1964). Blood pressure of adults by age and sex, United States 1960–62. *National Center for Health Statistics PHS Publ. 1000,* ser. 11, no. 4

GREENBLATT, D.J. and KOCH WESER, J. (1973). Adverse reactions to propranolol in hospitalized medical patients: a report from the Boston Collaborative Drug Surveillance Program. *American Heart Journal,* **86,** 478–484

GRIBBIN, B., PICKERING, T.G., SLEIGHT, P. and PETO, R. (1971). Effect of age and high blood pressure on baroreflex sensitivity in man. *Circulation Research,* **29,** 424–431

GROEL, J.T., TADROS, S.S., DRELINSKI, G.R. and JENKINS, A.C. (1983). Long-term antihypertensive therapy with captopril. *Hypertension,* **5,** Suppl. III, 145–151

GUBNER, R. (1962). Systolic hypertension: pathogenic entity. Significance and therapeutic considerations. *American Journal of Cardiology,* **9,** 773–777

HAMILTON, M., THOMPSON, E. and WISNIEWSKI, T.K.M. (1964). The role of blood pressure control in preventing complications of hypertension. *Lancet,* **1,** 235–238

HARRIS, T., FRANCIS COOK, E., KANNEL, W., SCHATZKIN, A. and GOLDMAN, L. (1985). Blood pressure experience and risk of cardiovascular disease in the elderly. *Hypertension,* **7,** 118–124

HASS, G.E. (1943). Elastic tissue. III. Relationship between structure of the ageing aorta and the properties of the isolated aortic elastic tissue. *Archives of Pathology,* **35,** 29–45

HOLLANDER, W. (1976). Role of hypertension in atherosclerosis and cardiovascular disease. *American Journal of Cardiology,* **38,** 786–800

HOLLENBERG, N.K., ADAMS, D.F., SOLOMON, M.H., RASHIO, A., ABRAMS, M.I. and MERRILL, J.P. (1974). Senescence and the renal varsculature in normal man. *Circulation Research,* **34,** 309–316

HURWITZ, N. (1969). Predisposing factors in adverse reaction to drugs. *British Medical Journal,* **i,** 535–539

HYPERTENSION DETECTION AND FOLLOW-UP PROGRAM COOPERATIVE GROUP (1979a). Five years finding of the hypertension detection and follow-up program. I. *Journal of the American Medical Association,* **242,** 2562–2571

HYPERTENSION DETECTION AND FOLLOW-UP PROGRAM COOPERATIVE GROUP (1979b). Five years finding of the hypertension detection and follow-up program. II. Mortality by race, sex and age. *Journal of the American Medical Association,* **242,** 2572–2577

HYPERTENSION DETECTION AND FOLLOW-UP PROGRAM COOPERATION GROUP (1985). Five years finding of the hypertension detection and follow-up program. Prevention and reversal of left ventricular hypertrophy with antihypertensive drug therapy. *Hypertension,* **7,** 105–112

HYPERTENSION-STROKE COOPERATIVE GROUP (1974). Effect of antihypertensive treatment on stroke recurrence. *Journal of the American Medical Association,* **229,** 409–418

IPPSH COLLABORATIVE GROUP (1985). Cardiovascular risk and risks factors in a randomized trial of treatment based on the beta-blocker oxprenolol. The International Prospective Primary Prevention Study in Hypertension (IPPPSH). *Journal of Hypertension,* **3,** 379–392

JOHNSON, H.B., PEARCE, V.R. and HAMILTON, M. (1978). Treatment of mild hypertension. An attempted controlled therapeutic trial. *Journal of Chronic Diseases,* **31,** 513–519

KANNEL, W.B. (1974a). Role of blood pressure in cardiovascular morbidity and mortality. *Progress in Cardiovascular Disease,* **17,** 5–24

KANNEL, W.B. (1974b). Some lessons in cardiovascular epidemiology from Framingham. *American Journal of Cardiology,* **37,** 269–282

KANNEL, W.B. and BRAND, F.N. (1985). In *Principles of Geriatric Medicine,* edited by R. Andres, E. Bierman and W.R. Hazzard. New York; McGraw-Hill

KANNEL, W.B., CASTELLI, W.P., NAMARA, P., McKEE, P.A. and FEINLEIB, M. (1972). Role of blood pressure in the development of congestive heart failure. The Framingham Study. *New England Journal of Medicine,* **287,** 781–787

KANNEL, W.B. and GORDON, T. (1978). Evaluation of cardiovascular risk in the elderly. The Framingham Study. *Bulletin of the New York Academy of Medicine,* **54,** 573–591

KANNEL, W.B., WOLF, P. and DAWBER, T.R. (1978). Hypertension and cardiac impairments increase stroke risk. *Geriatrics,* **33,** 71–83

KAPLAN, N.M., CARNEGIE, A., RASKIN, P., HELLER, J.A. and SIMMONS, M. (1985). Potassium supplementation in hypertensive patients with diuretic-induced hypokalaemia. *The New England Journal of Medicine*, **312**, 746–749

KASSIRER, J.P. and HARRINGTON, J.T. (1977). Diuretics and potassium metabolism: a reassessment of the need, effectiveness and safety of potassium therapy. *Kidney International*, **11**, 505–515

KASSIRER, J.P. and HARRINGTON, J.T. (1985). Fending off the potassium pushers. *The New England Journal of Medicine*, **312**, 785–787

LAKATTA, E. (1973). Alterations in the cardiovascular system that occur in advanced age. *Federation Proceedings*, **38**, 163–167

LAKE, C.R., ZIEGLER, M., COLEMAN, M.G. and KOPIN, I.J. (1977). Age adjusted plasma norepinephrine levels are similar in normotensives and hypertensive subjects. *New England Journal of Medicine*, **296**, 208–209

LAUGESEN, L.P., GADEGÅRD-HANSEN, A., JENSEN, H., PETERSEN, T. and TØNENSEN, K.H. (1982). The prevalence of secondary hypertension in elderly hypertensive patients. *Acta Medica Scandinavica*, Suppl. 676, 161-177

LEWIS, J.G. (1983). Adverse reactions to calcium antagonists. *Drugs*, **25**, 196–222

LIBERTINO, J.A., ZINMAN, L., BRESLIN, D.J., SWINTON, N.W. and LEGG, M.A. (1980). Renal artery revascularization restoration or renal function. *Journal of the American Medical Association*, **244**, 1340–1342

MacGREGOR, G.A. (1983). Dietary sodium and potassium intake and blood pressure. *Lancet*, **2**, 750–753

MACIAS NUÑEZ, J.F. (1983). Aspectos morfologicos, funcionales y pastologicos del riñon del viejo. *Nefrologia*, **3**, 1–4

MARTIN, E.C. and CASARELLA, W.J. (1984). Percutaneous tranluminal angioplasty in renovascular hypertension. In *Renovascular Hypertension*, edited by J.C. Stanley, C.B. Ernst and W.J. Fry, pp. 254–274. Philadelphia; Saunders

MASTER, A.M. and LASSER, R.P. (1961). Blood pressure elevation in the elderly patients. In *Hypertension: Recent Advances*, edited by A.N. Brest and J.H. Moyer, pp. 24–38. Philadelphia; Lea and Febiger

MESSERLI, F.H., SUNDGAARD-RIISE, K., VENTURA, P.O., DUNN, F.G., GLADE, L.B. and FROLICH, E.D. (1983). Essential hypertension in the elderly: hemodynamics, intravascular volume, plasma renin activity and circulating catecholamine levels. *Lancet*, **2**, 983–985

MESSERLI, F.H., VENTURA, H.D. and ANDRODEO, C. (1985). Osler's maneuver and pseudohypertension. *New England Journal of Medicine*, **312**, 1548–1550

MIRANDA, B., ALCAZAR, J.M., RUILOPE, L.M., NIETO, J., DIAZ ROLON, J.A. *et al.* (1984). Diferentes tipos de hipertension arterial en la tercera edad (Abstract). *Nefrologia*, Suppl. I, **22**

MITCHELL, J.R.A. (1983). Blood pressure and mortality in the very old (Letter). *Lancet*, **2**, 1248

MORGAN, T., ADAM, W., CARNEY, S., GIBBARD, R., BROWN, S. and WHEELER, D. (1979). Treatment of mild hypertension in elderly males. *Clinical Science*, **27**, 355s–357s

MRC (1985). Trial of treatment of mild hypertension: principal results. *British Medical Journal*, **291**, 97-104

MÜLLER, F.B., BOLLI, P., ERNE, P., KIOWSKI, W. and BUHLER, F.R. (1984). Use of calcium antagonists as monotherapy in the management of hypertension. *American Journal of Medicine*, **77**(2B), 11–15

MYERS, M.G., KEARNS, P.M., KENNEDY, D.S. and FISHER, R.H. (1978). Postural hypotension and diuretic therapy in the elderly. *Canadian Medical Association Journal*, **119**, 581–584

NATIONAL HIGH BLOOD PRESSURE EDUCATION PROGRAM COORDINATING COMMITTEE (1980). *Statement on Hypertension in the Elderly*. Bethesda, Md.; High Blood Pressure Information Center, National Institutes of Health

NIARCHOS, A.P. and LARAGH, J.H. (1984). Renin dependency of blood pressure in isolated systolic hypertension. *American Journal of Medicine*, **77**, 407-414

NIARCHOS, A.P., WEINSTEIN, D.L. and LARAGH, J.H. (1984). Comparison of the effects of diuretic therapy and low sodium intake in isolated systolic hypertension. *American Journal of Medicine*, **77**, 1061–1068

NIELSEN, P.E. (1982). The accuracy of auscultatory blood pressure measurement in the elderly. *Acta Medica Scandinavica*, Suppl. 676, 39–44

OMAE, T., TAKESHITA, M. and HIROTA, Y. (1976). The Hiriyama study and joint study on cerebrovascular diseases in Japan. In *Cerebrovascular Diseases* (16th Princeton Conference), edited by P. Scheinberg, pp. 255–265. New York; Raven Press

O'MALLEY, K., JUDGE, T. and CROOKS, J. (1980). Geriatric clinical pharmacology and therapeutics. In *Drug Treatment: Principles and Practice of Clinical Pharmacology and Therapeutics*, edited by G. Avery, pp. 158–181. Sydney; ADIS Press

O'MALLEY, K. and O'BRIEN, E. (1980). Management of hypertension in the elderly. *New England Journal of Medicine*, **302**, 1397–1401

O'MALLEY, K. and O'CALLAGHAN, W. (1982). Hypertension in the elderly: an overview. *Current Medical Research and Opinion*, **7**, Suppl. I, 53–62

OSTFELD, A.M. (1978). Elderly hypertensive patients. Epidemiologic review. *New York State Journal of Medicine*, **78**, 1125–1129

PAGE, L.B. and SIDD, J.J. (1977). Medical management of arterial hypertension. *New England Journal of Medicine,* **287,** 960–963

POOLING PROJECT RESEARCH GROUP (1978). Relationship of blood pressure, serum cholesterol, smoking habit, relative weight and ECG abnormalities to the incidence of major coronary events. Final report of the pooling project. *Journal of Chronic Diseases,* **31,** 201–306

PRIDDLE, W.W., LIN, S.F., BREITHAUPT, D.J. and GRANT, P.G. (1968). Amelioration of high blood pressure in the elderly. *Journal of the American Geriatric Society,* **16,** 887–892

RABKIN, S.W., MATHEWSON, F.A.L. and TATE, R.B. (1978). Predicting risk of ischemic heart disease and cerebrovascular disease from systolic and diastolic blood pressure. *Annals of Internal Medicine,* **88,** 342–345

RAJALA, S., HAAVISTO, M., HEIKINHEIMO, R. and MATTILA, K. (1983). Blood pressure and mortality in the very old. *Lancet,* **2,** 520–521

ROSENFELD, J. (1983). Hypertension in the elderly. *Kidney International,* **23,** 540–547

ROWLANDS, B.D., STOLLARD, T.J. and LITTLE, W.A. (1984). Continuous ambulatory monitoring of blood pressure and assessment of cardiovascular refluxes in the elderly hypertensive. *Journal of Hypertension,* **2,** 615–622

SELIGMANN, A.W., ALDERMAN, M.H. and DAVIS, T.K. (1979). Systolic hypertension: occurrence and treatment in a defined community. *Journal of the American Geriatric Society,* **97,** 135–138

SELLERS, A.M. (1966). Significance and management of systolic hypertension. *American Journal of Cardiology,* **17,** 648–652

SEVER, P.S., OSIKAWA, B., BIRCH, M. and TURNBRIDGE, R.B.C. (1977). Plasma noradrenaline in essential hypertension. *Lancet,* **1,** 1078–1081

SEVER, P.S., PEART, W.S., GORDON, D. and BEIGHTON, P. (1980). Blood-pressure in urban and tribal Africa. *Lancet,* **2,** 58–64

SHEKELLE, R.B., OSTFELD, A.M. and DAWANS, H.L. Jr. (1985). Hypertension and risk of stroke in an elderly population. *Stroke,* **5,** 71–75

SIMON, A.C., SAFAR, M.A., LEVENSON, J.A., KHEDER, A.M. and LEVY, B.I. (1979). Systolic hypertension. Hemodynamic mechanism and choice of antihypertensive treatment. *American Journal of Cardiology,* **44,** 505–511

SPENCE, J.D., SIBBALD, W.J. and CAPE, R.D. (1978). Pseudohypertension in the elderly. *Clinical Science and Molecular Medicine,* **55,** 399–402

SPIVACK, C., OCKEN, S. and FRISHMAN, W.H. (1983). Calcium antagonists. Clinical use in the treatment of systemic hypertension. *Drugs,* **25,** 154–177

SPRACKLING, M.E., MITCHELL, J.R.A., SHORT, A.H. and WATT, G. (1981). Blood pressure reduction in the elderly: a randomised controlled trial of methyldopa. *British Medical Journal,* **283,** 1151–1153

STORSTEIN, L., LASRSEN, A., MIDTBO, K. and VAREID, L. (1984). Pharmakokinetics of calcium channel blockers in patients with renal insufficiency and geriatric patients. *Acta Medica Scandinavica,* Suppl. 681, 25–30

SWALES, J.D. (1979). Pathophysiology of blood pressure in the elderly. *Age and Ageing,* **8,** 104–109

TARAZI, R.C. (1978). Clinical importance of systolic hypertension (Editorial note). *Annals of Internal Medicine,* **88,** 426–427

TRAUB, Y.M., AYGEN, M.M. and ROSENFELD, J.G. (1979). Hazards of the treatment of systolic hypertension. *American Heart Journal,* **97,** 174–177

VESTAL, R.E. (1978). Drug use in the elderly: a review of problems and special considerations. *Drugs,* **16,** 358–382

VESTAL, R.E., WOOD, A.J.J. and SHAND, D.G. (1979). Reduced beta-adrenoceptor sensitivity in the elderly. *Clinical Pharmacology and Therapeutics,* **26,** 181–186

VETERANS ADMINISTRATION COOPERATIVE GROUP ON HYPERTENSIVE AGENTS (1970). Effects of treatment on morbidity in hypertension. II. *Journal of the American Medical Association,* **213,** 1143–1152

VETERANS ADMINISTRATION COOPERATIVE STUDY ON ANTIHYPERTENSIVE AGENTS (1972). Effects of treatment on morbidity in hypertension. III. *Circulation,* **45,** 991–1004

VETERANS ADMINISTRATION COOPERATIVE STUDY GROUP ON ANTIHYPERTENSIVE AGENTS (1984). Low dose captopril for the treatment of mild to moderate hypertension. I. Results of a 14 week trial. *Archives of Internal Medicine,* **144,** 1947–1953

WATKIN, D.M. and SHOCK, N.W. (1955). Age wise standard values for Cin, CPAH and TmPAH in adult males. *Journal of Clinical Investigation,* **34,** 969

WEIDMANN, P., DEMYTTENAERE-BURSZTEIN, S., MAXWELL, M.H. and DE LIMA, J. (1975). Effect of ageing on plasma renin and aldosterone in normal male. *Kidney International,* **8,** 325–333

Chapter 13

Urinary tract infection in old age

S.L. Choudhury and J.C. Brocklehurst

Introduction

Urinary tract infection (UTI) is common at all ages, but its prevalence increases with advancing age, with institutionalization and with the female sex (Sourander, 1966; Brocklehurst *et al.*, 1968a; Akhtar *et al.*, 1972; Sourander and Kasanen, 1972; Brocklehurst *et al.*, 1977; Kass *et al.*, 1978; Asscher, 1980a; Kasviki-Charvati *et al.*, 1982; Heinamaki *et al.*, 1984). In the elderly, clinical presentation is often unusual — for instance, with the symptoms of mental confusion or incontinence. Also, much infection is asymptomatic and when discovered its management poses problems.

Terminology and classification

Significant bacteriuria refers to the quantitative estimation of bacteria by the method of Kass (1955, 1956, 1957) when more than 100 000 organisms per ml of urine are present. Lower numbers are regarded as contaminants, although counts between 10^3/ml and 10^5/ml are usually regarded as of uncertain significance and require repeating. It must be emphasized, however, that no absolute count precisely identifies or excludes the diagnoses of a UTI. Quantitation of urine depends on a number of factors, including the method of collection and processing of the sample, state of hydration and frequency of urination, the presence of obstruction and the administration of antimicrobial agents (Roberts, Robinson and Beard, 1967).

A clinical classification involving four categories was proposed by Kaye (1972) as follows: symptomatic infection; asymptomatic (covert) bacteriuria; relapse (or bacterial persistence); reinfection. Symptomatic infection indicates a new infection or one in which there is insufficient information to determine whether it may be a relapse or reinfection. Similar qualifications apply to asymptomatic bacteriuria. In relapse, the pretreatment pathogens are temporarily eliminated from the urine following chemotherapy, but survive within the urinary tract and subsequently initiate a recurrent infection. Reinfection, again developing after chemotherapy, represents a recurrent bacterial infection caused by an organism different from that initiating the original infection.

Prevalence

The prevalence of UTI in non-institutionalized old people is illustrated in *Figure 13.1,* where it is compared with prevalence in younger age groups. Overall the

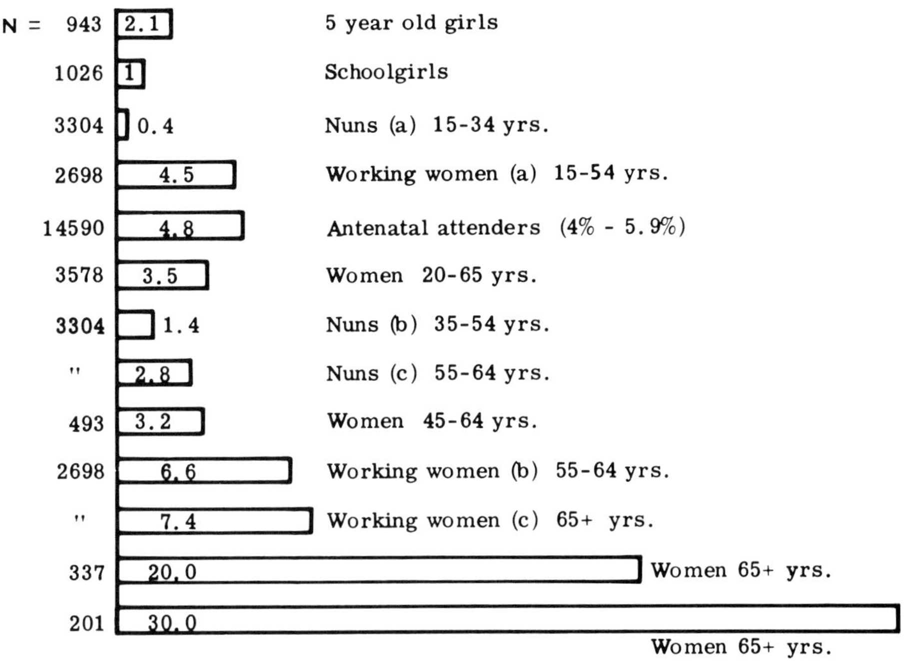

Figure 13.1 Prevalence of urinary infection in females

prevalence in old people living in the community is between 15 per cent and 20 per cent. This figure increases among the institutionalized and especially the group of old people living in long-stay hospital wards (who are likely to be among the most physically and mentally disabled in our society). Here, it may be over 30 per cent (Gibson and Pritchard, 1965; Sourander, Ruikka and Gronroos, 1965; Sourander, 1966; Walkey *et al.*, 1967; Brocklehurst *et al.*, 1968a, 1968b; Moore-Smith, 1971; Akhtar *et al.*, 1972; Brocklehurst *et al.*, 1977). The hospital environment is an important determinant of the nature of the bacterial flora in hospitalized patients which will probably differ from that in community patients (Kaitz and Williams, 1960; Kass, 1960; Rocha, 1972; McMillan, 1972; Asscher, 1980f).

Shortness of the female urethra and lack of prostatic secretion and prolapse of the uterus and vagina are all factors which have been implicated in accounting for the higher prevalence of UTI in females (Sourander *et al.*, 1965) and so has faecal incontinence (Brocklehurst *et al.*, 1977).

Localization of infection

Techniques to localize the site of UTI may be direct (or invasive) or indirect (and non-invasive) (Gleckman, 1982). The former includes renal biopsy, ureteric catheterization, bladder washout techniques and differential culture of prostatic secretions. Indirect methods include the clinical examination, microscopic examination of urine, maximum urine osmolality, water loading test, measurement of urinary β_2 microglobulin and muramidase, measurement of urinary enzymes, serum antibody determination, pattern of response to therapy, radiographic techniques and antibody-coated bacteria (ACB) immunofluorescence. Excellent reviews of the available tests to identify the site of the UTI are those of Kunin (1979a) and (Gleckman (1982).

Infection may develop at any point between the para-urethral glands and the kidneys, and indeed may be localized at more than one site. Because of differences in management, an attempt at localization should be made in every case. Most methods of localization depend on sampling urine at multiple sites in order to establish its level.

Direct techniques

While culture of renal biopsy specimens would be the most direct way of establishing a diagnosis of pyelonephritis, it is too dangerous to be used for this purpose. Bilateral ureteric catheterization following bladder washouts to sterilize the bladder urine can localize renal infection with relative safety (Stamey, Govan and Palmer, 1965). There is, however, a risk of bacteraemia, the method is lengthy, uncomfortable and expensive, and a false positive bladder reading may be obtained if the infection is bilateral. Isolation of organisms from the ureter implies bacterial pyelonephritis, not simply pyelitis (Whitworth *et al.*, 1974).

A method not requiring ureteric catheterization (Fairley *et al.*, 1967) involves collecting an initial bladder specimen of urine, washing out the bladder with neomycin and a fibrinolytic enzyme (Elase), then taking three consecutive 10-min samples. If one or more of these shows infection the assumption is that this has come from one or other kidney. It may, however, provide false negative results if the discharge of infected urine from the renal parenchyma is intermittent (Fairley and Butler, 1970). A later modification, substituting 0.5 per cent gentamicin sulphate, has been useful in the evaluation of women with recurrent UTIs (Ronald, Boutros and Mourtada, 1976) and indeed the method is occasionally therapeutically successful.

If urethral or prostatic infection is suspected in males, the following technique may be employed. The urine is collected in two containers during micturition (the first 5–10 ml representing the urethral sample and the second a mid-stream portion representing the bladder urine). Micturition is stopped just before it is complete, the prostate massaged and the prostatic expressate (a few drops) collected. If no prostatic specimen results, the final residue of voided urine is collected (the post-prostatic specimen). Infection in the urethral but not bladder urine indicates urethritis. If the bacterial count in the expressed prostatic fluid or post-prostatic specimen is two or more times higher than that of the urethra or bladder urine, a diagnosis of bacterial prostatitis is made (Drach, 1975). These methods are time consuming and require patience and co-operation on the part of the patient.

Indirect techniques

Clinically it may be difficult to localize UTI, although loin pain and fever suggest renal involvement. Attempts to measure excretion rates, staining properties, cast formation and response of urinary white cells to provocative stimuli have largely been abandoned having proved ineffective (Gleckman, 1982). Bacterial pyelonephritis but not lower UTI is associated with decreased urine concentrating ability which is reversible with effective antimicrobial therapy (Turck, 1975).

Measurement of maximum urinary osmolality has not proved to be a sensitive method of localizing the site of infection (Ronald, Cutler and Turck, 1969).

Attempts to provide a natural (endogenous) washout method which is non-invasive have involved attempts to increase the rate of urine flow rapidly (Cattell *et al.*, 1972), in some cases by using a 'water loading test' (Papanayiotou and Dontas, 1972) or frusemide (Dontas *et al.*, 1974). During a diuresis the bacterial excretion rate may diminish markedly, may increase or may retain a steady state. In the latter two cases, a renal infection may be suspected. Indeed, a proportion of subjects with negative initial urine cultures respond to diuresis with a transient bacteriuria and would otherwise comprise false negative results. Dontas and Kasviki-Charvati (1976) suggest this may occur in one-fifth of non-bacteriuric elderly subjects.

Attempts to correlate the site of infection in these direct and indirect methods have not been very successful (Prát *et al.*, 1977) and thus question the value of the water loading test.

Increased concentration of urinary fibrin degradation products (FDP) have been detected in numbers of renal diseases, including bacterial pyelonephritis (Whitworth *et al.*, 1973). This may be a useful test to exclude bacterial cystitis as the site of UTI, although a negative test does not exclude a renal source of infection.

Measurement of urinary concentration of two low molecular weight proteins — β_2-microglobulin and lysozyme (Bonadio, Donadio and Catania, 1979; Schardijn *et al.*, 1979) — may distinguish bacterial cystitis from pyelonephritis. An increased excretion of these substances has been reported in association with numerous renal diseases characterized by tubular injury as well as in shock, fever and the administration of nephrotoxic agents such as gentamicin.

Determination of various urinary enzymes in the hope that an abnormally high density or quantity excreted per day might indicate a renal source of UTI have been disappointing because of the large spread of values even in normal subjects. These included lactic dehydrogenase (Rosalki and Wilkinson, 1959; Wacker and Dorfman, 1962), alanine aminopeptidase, betaglucuronidase (Bank and Bailine, 1965; Ronald *et al.*, 1971; Turck, 1975) and LDH isoenzymes (Carvajal *et al.*, 1975). Elevated concentrations of LDH isoenzymes have been described as originating from renal cortical tissue damaged by pyelonephritis or acute tubular necrosis and forming a highly sensitive test identifying upper UTI (Fries *et al.*, 1977; Devaskar and Montgomery, 1978; Lorentz and Resnick, 1979; Brouhard and Cunningham, 1981). The specificity of this test may be impaired by a number of factors including the use of nitrofurantoin, slow freezing and thawing of the urine repeatedly, and exposure of the urine to room temperature for a number of hours.

Immunological techniques have been used in an attempt to identify patients with bacterial pyelonephritis (Brumfitt and Percival, 1965; Brenner, Fairley and Kincaid-Smith, 1969; Scarpelli, Lamanna and Bigioli, 1979) and tests such as immunofluorescence and solid phase radioimmunoassay are currently being assessed (Sanford, Thomas and Forland, 1978).

A renal glycoprotein (Tamm–Horsfall protein) is a primary constituent of urinary casts, and elevated serum IgG antibodies to this protein have recently been identified in girls with acute pyelonephritis. It is suggested that elevated serum levels of this protein should raise suspicion of infection superimposed on obstruction (Marier *et al.*, 1978).

If relapse occurs, the rate at which this happens has been compared with direct techniques to establish the tissue source of infection and showed that the pattern of recurrence may identify the site of infection in approximately 80 per cent of cases

(Turck, Ronald and Petersdorf, 1968; Ronald, Boutros and Mourtada, 1976). Relapse occurring within 2 weeks of the cessation of drug treatment usually signifies bacterial pyelonephritis, whereas reinfection usually indicates bacterial cystitis.

Imaging techniques (including excretory urography and gallium citrate scanning) often fail to identify accurately the site of infection in patients experiencing recurrent disease (Fries *et al.*, 1977).

The preferred method of determining the tissue source of a urinary tract infection at the present time is the antibody-coated bacterial immunofluorescence test (ACB) (Jones, Smith and Sanford, 1974; Thomas, Shelokov and Forland, 1974). This depends on the renal or prostatic tissue producing antibody directed against the bacterial surface antigen (Smith, Jones and Kaijser, 1977). Direct immunofluorescence is used for visualizing antibody which is complexed with bacteria in the patient's urine sediment. With tissue invasion (as in bacterial pyelonephritis or prostatitis), antibody is synthesized and a positive antibody-coated bacterial test results. In most cases of cystitis the infection appears limited to the mucosa and tunica propria and a negative ACB results (Jones, Smith and Sanford, 1974; Thomas, Shelokov and Forland, 1974). This technique is one of the methods of choice among indirect methods of localizing UTI (Jones, 1979). It is non-invasive, inexpensive and reproducible, and results can be available within hours (Rubin *et al.*, 1980). The ACB test appears more sensitive than serum antibody titration in distinguishing pyelonephritis from cystitis (Jones, Smith and Sanford, 1974; Thomas, Shelokov and Forland, 1974). Animal experiments have shown 10–16 days to elapse before a positive ACB result occurs following an initial infection (Smith, Jones and Kaijser, 1977; Rubin *et al.*, 1980). Reinfection, however, will result in a positive ACB assay within 2–5 days.

Despite initial enthusiasm for the ACB test, there is still no real agreement about what constitutes a positive result and the accuracy of the test. Thomas, Shelokov and Forland (1974) considered the test positive when more than 25 per cent of the bacteria in the urinary sediment fluoresced. However, a number of false negative results have been reported among patients with acute bacterial pyelonephritis (Jones, 1976; Rumans and Vosti, 1978) and caution is also required in subjects over 75 following antibiotic therapy or if the bacterial count is less than 10^5 per ml (Giamarellou *et al.*, 1983). The accuracy has also been questioned in women with recurrent UTI (Prát, Bohuslav and Hatala, 1977). Opposing views on the status of this test continues to be held (e.g. Jones, 1979; Mundt and Polk, 1979).

Recurrent UTI

Males

In men, recurrent UTI is almost exclusively a problem of the over 50s and is found particularly with coexisting medical disease including diabetes mellitus and essential hypertension. Radiographic studies identify structural abnormalities in the kidneys in approximately half of these patients, including pyelonephritic scarring and renal calculi. *Escherichia coli* causes the great majority of recurrent urinary tract infections which develop in men in the absence of urethral catheters or ileal loop bladders (Gleckman, 1982).

Patients with recurrent infection invariably demonstrate a bacteriological response to drug treatment prescribed in accordance with the *in vitro* sensitivity of the pretreatment organisms and superinfection appears to be an infrequent occurrence (Gleckman, 1982). Structural abnormality in the kidney or prostate contributes to the inability of drugs to eradicate infections and poorly defined host factors undoubtedly also explain some therapeutic failure (Stamey and Pfau, 1963). Relapse rather than reinfection is the more prevalent pattern of recurring infection experienced by men (Gleckman, Crowley and Natsios, 1979, 1980b). The organisms remain susceptible to the antimicrobial agent exhibited, thus excluding the development of drug resistance as the cause of the therapeutic failure (Gleckman, 1982).

Infection stones (triple phosphate or struvite stones) may occur in association with infections, principally with *Proteus mirabilis* (Griffith, 1978). They form as a consequence of urease-induced hydrolysis of urea and are a mixture of struvite (magnesium ammonium phosphate) and carbonate apatite. They contain bacteria incorporated within the stone substance and therefore antibiotics are unable to sterilize the urine in their presence. They may be responsible for a high relapse rate. They must be removed or dissolved and at the same time therapy be directed towards urease-producing bacteria, either by antibiotics or by a urease inhibitor such as acetohydroxamic acid (Griffith, Moskowitz and Carlton, 1978).

An association has also been noted between bacterial relapse and the presence of prostatic calculus (Freeman *et al.*, 1975; Gleckman, Crowley and Natsios, 1980b). In fact, on rare occasions bacteria embedded in the substance of a prostatic calculus produced a situation similar to that described above (Eykyn *et al.*, 1974; Meares, 1974). Infected prostatic calculi, however, are usually caused by *E. coli* rather than *P. mirabilis.* Antibiotics fail to produce a permanent cure and total prostatectomy offers the best likelihood of eradicating the recurrent UTI (Gleckman, 1982).

Meares and Stamey (1968) claim that chronic bacterial prostatitis explains most bacterial relapses in males, possibly because of inadequate antibiotic penetration within the infected prostate (Gleckman, 1982). Recurrent UTI secondary to chronic bacterial prostatitis should be treated with an extended course of antibiotic (Meares, 1975).

The optimum duration of therapy for patients with recurrent UTI remains controversial. A 10–14-day course of trimethoprim sulphamethoxazole is often unsuccessful in sterilizing the urinary tract in men with recurrent invasive UTI (Gleckman, Crowley and Natsios, 1979). Analogy between this condition and subacute bacterial endocarditis has been suggested (Turck, 1972) and a prolonged course of therapy proposed. It may be that this is often effective because it is in fact treating chronic bacterial prostatitis (Meares, 1975).

It has been postulated that bacterial relapse results from the ability of microbial variants, known as cell-wall defective bacteria, to remain in the kidney during chemotherapy and then revert to the parent bacteria when therapy is discontinued. However, this theory is still unproven (Watanakunakorn, 1979; Gleckman *et al.*, 1980a).

The possibility of long-term therapy preventing recurrent urinary tract infection in men was investigated in a trial in which antibiotic therapy was followed by sulphamethiazole, nitrofurantoin or methenamine mandelate (Freeman, Smith and Richardson, 1975). Continued therapy did result in significantly fewer bacterial recurrences, but was ineffective in the presence of renal or prostatic calculi or radiographic abnormalities consistent with pyelonephritis. Recurrences tend to re-emerge after 2 years of such prophylaxis or sooner if it is discontinued. It was suggested that persistent bacteriuria unaccompanied by obstructive uropathy did not lead to deterioration of renal function and also that there was an increased mortality rate in those patients receiving sulphamethiazole; the use of sulphonamides for prolonged therapy was advised against. However, the design of this study is open to criticism on a number of grounds (arbitrary therapeutic criteria, no account of compliance, relapse not distinguished from reinfection, no tests to define tissue source of the infection and symptomatic exacerbations were treated with antibiotics without being microbiologically confirmed).

Most men who experience recurrent UTI should not be considered for prolonged continuous prophylactic medication. This may, however, be appropriate for those men with multiple recurrent symptomatic UTI in the absence of surgically remediable lesions such as infection stones. Methianine or trimethoprim may be the preferred drugs (Kass, 1979; Kunin, Craig and Uehling, 1978), the latter particularly if there is evidence of renal insufficiency.

Females

In women, most recurrence is caused by *E. coli* and appears to be reinfection rather than relapse (Harrison *et al.*, 1974) and the bladder is the usual site of infection (Turck, Ronald and Petersdorf, 1968). Recurrence usually occurs within 6 months of the previous infection and is invariably symptomatic (McGeachie, 1966; Kraft and Stamey, 1977; Stamm *et al.*, 1980). Factors associated with recurrent UTI include infrequent voiding, uninhibited neurogenic bladder, persistent colonization of the introitus and vaginal vestibule with enterobacteria possibly in association with thinning and atrophic changes of the vaginal–periurethral epithelia, a relatively high pH of vaginal secretion in post-menopausal women, enhanced adherence of the organisms to the mucosal cells of the introitus and the absence of cervicovaginal antibody (Lapides, Costello and Zierdt, 1968; Stamey *et al.*, 1978; Addato *et al.*, 1979; Kunin, 1982). It seems that recurrent UTI tends to occur in clusters and the longer the interval between infections the less likely that recurrence will develop (Kraft and Stamey, 1977).

There is no convincing evidence that extending the duration of therapy or increasing the intensity of drug treatment will reduce the incidence of reinfection in women, particularly when the infection is confined to the bladder (Fair *et al.*, 1980). There is, however, some evidence that prophylactic low dose antimicrobial therapy can reduce the incidence of recurrent UTI in susceptible women (Gleckman, 1982). Agents that may be used include nitrofurantoin, methenamine mandalate, trimethoprim and cotrimoxazole (Stamm, Wagner and Amsel, 1980). However, these will not eradicate the biological defects which predispose to recurrent infection and, in view of the cost and potential risk of adverse side effects, should only be used in women who experience multiple disabling symptomatic flare-ups.

It is generally agreed that the preventative effect of drug treatment disappears within a month of discontinuation. This is particularly likely in women who have a previous history of multiple infections (Stamm, Wagner and Amsel, 1980). This includes 4 or more infections during the year prior to treatment. However, prolonged administration of nitrofurantoin and sulphonamides have been incriminated in serious side effects such as peripheral neuropathy, interstitial pneumonitis and irreversible liver damage, and coronary artery disease (Freeman, Smith and Richardson, 1975; Gleckman *et al.*, 1979; Sharp, Ishak and Zimmerman, 1980; Holmberg *et al.*, 1980).

Local antimicrobial treatment has been prescribed in this condition (Motzkin, 1972), but the value of this treatment is still uncertain. Intravaginal oestrogens have been used successfully in the treatment of recurrent UTI in post-menopausal females (Parsons and Schmidt, 1982). Cystitis (if present) is first treated and the patient put on suppressive therapy appropriate to the organism colonizing the vagina. This treatment is continued while oestrogens are given in a unit dose delivering 0.3 mg oestroen per gram. This is given daily for 7 days (intravaginally) then every second day for 7 days, then every third day until vaginal culture reverts to the normal flora seen in pre-menopausal women. The dose is then titred to the lowest necessary to maintain a vaginal pH of 4–4.6 (usually 1 dose every 4–7 days).

The point of this treatment is that *E. coli* in the vaginal introitus rarely occurs at pHs of less than 4.5 (the normal vaginal pH in pre-menopausal women is about 4.0). The source of recurent UTI is colonization from the rectum, the whole vagina and urethral area being infected as a unit.

Although surgical procedures such as urethral dilatation and internal urethrotomy have been claimed to be successful, there is as yet no clear evidence for these (Kraft and Stamey, 1977).

Relapsing infection is reported in women with pyelonephritis following discontinuation of drug therapy (Gutman *et al.*, 1978). It is not clear whether this is due to bacterial persistence in the kidney or the emergence of a new infection by the same organism residing in the urethra or vaginal introitus. Those developing within 2 weeks of discontinuing treatment have been considered as persistent renal parenchymal infection, whereas those developing more than a month later probably indicate reinfection from entobacteria in the urethra and vaginal introitus (Levinsen and Kaye, 1972). Renal calculi, renal scarring and papillary necrosis may account for some persistent bacterial pyelonephritis (Nanra *et al.*, 1970; Cattell *et al.*, 1973; Gutman *et al.*, 1978).

The conventional two-week course of chemotherapy for women with bacterial pyelonephritis is often unsuccessful and relapse occurs (Nanra *et al.*, 1970; Gutman *et al.*, 1978). However, an extended course of treatment may be successful (Motzkin, 1972).

Relapse following treatment of bacterial cystitis (Cattell *et al.*, 1973; Gutman *et al.*, 1978) may reduce the value of this therapeutic response as a means of localizing the site of UTI. No evidence has been established on the role of cell-wall defective bacteria in females (Gutman *et al.*, 1978).

Diagnosis of UTI

Bacteriuria is often asymptomatic and its importance then requires careful consideration. Cystitis in the elderly may present with the classical symptoms of pain and burning on micturition, urgency, frequency and possibly incontinence. Pyelonephritis may present with fever, rigors, loin pain and dysuria or haematuria. However, both upper and lower urinary tract infection in old people often presents in quite a non-specific way with mental confusion, fatigue, dizziness or simply increasing immobility.

Some population studies among the elderly have shown that a number of the dysuric symptoms do not have a statistically significant correlation with bacteriuria. In women, these include incontinence, stress incontinence and nocturnal frequency and, in males, precipitancy, nocturnal frequency, incontinence, difficulty in passing urine (Brocklehurst, 1978). In women, a statistical correlation has been shown between bacteriuria and precipitancy, and bacteriuria and difficulty in passing urine (Brocklehurst, 1978). Of course, individual patients may manifest the infection with any of these symptoms. In these correlations account has to be taken of both the large number of causes other than infection and also of the differences between old people in different locations. For instance, in long-stay geriatric wards there is a close correlation between incontinence and urinary tract infection (Brocklehurst *et al.*, 1977).

Incontinence (urinary and faecal) is closely associated with mental impairment. Increasing degrees of incontinence and mental impairment go hand in hand (Isaacs and Walkey, 1964; Brocklehurst *et al.*, 1977; James, 1979). A common factor linking these three may be faecal soiling of the perineum and another common factor is the presence of an uninhibited neurogenic bladder in patients with chronic brain failure which in turn is associated with a degree of residual urine forming a reservoir for organisms.

Very occasionally the first evidence of an asymptomatic bacteriuria may be spontaneous haematogenous dissemination (Gleckman, 1982). Such a dissemination may cause vertebral osteomyelitis, septic arthritis, endocarditis, septic pulmonary embolus, subdural empyema and endophthalmitis. However, these events have invariably followed in the wake of urological procedures performed in the bladder, prostate or urethra (Siroky *et al.*, 1976).

Other factors in the history

There is evidence of a good correlation between a past history of UTI and the presence of significant bacteriuria (Hagenfeldt *et al.*, 1962; Sourander, 1966; Sussman *et al.*, 1969). In long-stay geriatric patients, bacteriuria correlated with mobility rather than immobility (perhaps because the more mobile represented those suffering from dementia who may also have impaired perineal hygiene associated with faecal incontinence). In this same study, the bacteriuria was associated with the presence of faecal incontinence (Brocklehurst *et al.*, 1977). No correlation between bacteriuria and socioeconomic factors in the elderly have been demonstrated (Sourander, 1966).

Proteinuria and haematuria

The absence of proteinuria does not rule out UTI. However, most patients with UTI excrete an amount of protein which varies between the upper limit of normal (100 mg/day) and 1–2 g/day (Cobbs, 1972). Microscopic haematuria is not a useful indicator of bacterial infection.

Casts

The finding of 'white cell casts' (i.e. casts which include polymorphonuclear leucocytes) is fairly good evidence of inflammatory disease in the upper urinary tract, but neither these nor granular casts are in any way specific for infection. Such casts are often absent in the presence of active pyelonephritis. In enumerating casts it is essential to examine a freshly voided specimen of urine (Cobbs, 1972).

Haematology

Mean haemaglobin is not usually affected by UTI. An elevated ESR is also uncertain evidence of UTI (Sourander, 1966; Sussman *et al.*, 1969).

Urine samples — collection and culture

The urine specimen most commonly examined is the mid-stream specimen preceded by external washing with soap and water or sterile water. In elderly females, it is not unreasonable to insert a catheter with full sterile precautions if it is difficult to obtain a satisfactory specimen otherwise. An Alexa bag may also be used. Suprapubic bladder aspiration is a difficult procedure in elderly patients and has not proved generally practicable.

Unless the urine can be cultured immediately after it is passed, it must be stored in a refrigerator. If it stands at room temperature for a period exceeding 2 h, more than one organism is often grown. If it is not practicable to deliver the specimen within this time, alternative procedures include the use of a maintenance preservative, boric acid (Porter and Brodie, 1969) being the only serious contender in this class, or of dip-inoculation cultures (dip-inoculum transport medium outfit of Mackey and Sandy, 1965; dip slide technique of Guttman and Naylor, 1967).

There are several different culture methods allowing the enumeration of bacteria (Bradley and Little, 1963). The poured plate method consists of adding 0.1 ml of well-mixed urine to 9.9 ml sterile water and discharging 0.1 ml of the diluted urine onto a sterile Petri dish, mixing with 10–20 ml nutrient agar. Each colony identified represents 1000 viable organisms in the original sample. The streak plate method uses 0.001 ml on a calibrated loop and each colony identified represents 1000 organisms per ml^{-1} in the original specimen. Dip-inoculation tests appear to provide reliable information and are technically less demanding (Mann and Sandys, 1978).

Automated screening procedures are available (Isenberg *et al.*, 1979; Nicholson and Koepke, 1979; Jenkins, Hale and Matsen, 1980) but are not entirely reliable, and conventional urine processing remains essential when patients are receiving antibiotics, harbour polymicrobic bacteria, are subject to suprapubic bladder aspiration or diagnostic catheterization, or are being assessed for evidence of chronic prostatitis.

Specimens should be cultured on a medium which reliably grows all the known urinary pathogens as well as commensals which if present in a mixed culture indicate contamination. It should identify lactose fermentation by a colour change and inhibit the swarming of *Proteus* species. The medium currently available which best fulfils these requirements is cystine–lactose–electrolyte deficient (CLED) agar.

Further developments in laboratory technique include testing for the presence of slow-growing CO_2-dependent organisms (Maskell, 1980) and of obligatory anaerobes (Gargan, Brumfitt and Hamilton-Miller, 1978; Meijer-Severs *et al.*, 1979), although there is little evidence that the latter have a pathogenic role. The pad culture method (Microstix, Ames) combines bacteriological and chemical methods. The strip contains two areas with dehydrated culture media, one for total bacteria and one for Gram-negative bacteria, as well as a nitrite–nitrate pad for quick appraisal (Griess chemical screening technique to identify significant bacteriuria).

Other chemical methods to detect bacterial metabolizing activity and significant bacteriuria include gas–liquid chromatography to detect microbial metabolites and quantify bacteria (Barrett, Lynam and Trustey, 1978; Coloe, 1978) and measurement in urinary impedance (Throm *et al.*, 1977; Cady *et al.*, 1978). These are for the future.

Significant bacteriuria

The predictive value of a significant bacteriuria in one, two or three consecutive specimens has been reported by numbers of workers with close agreement. On a single MSU it is approximately 80 per cent; this was increased to 90–96 per cent when the same results were obtained in a second specimen and between 95 and 100 per cent when three consecutive specimens were positive with the same organisms (Kass, 1962; Andriole, 1972; Association of Clinical Pathologists, 1973; Kunin, 1979a; Asscher, 1980d). However, single clean-void urine culture can be diagnostic in man (Craig, 1977; Kunin, 1979a; Gleckman *et al.*, 1979).

White blood cells in urine

Although urinary infection is defined by bacterial counting, the detection of increased white cell excretion indicating inflammation within the urinary tract is also important, and an association between leucocyturia and urinary infection has long been recognized. A white cell excretion of more than 10 per cubic millimetre is considered abnormal (Little, 1964; Brumfitt, 1965; Association of Clinical Pathologists, 1973; Musher, Thorsteinsson and Airola, 1976), and the close correlation between white cell count and bacterial count has been reported by many workers (McGeachie and Kennedy, 1963; Brocklehurst *et al.*, 1968a; Musher, Thorsteinsson and Airola, 1976). Renal and bladder epithelial cells, however, may be confused with polymorphonuclear leucocytes and their positive identification may be facilitated by appropriate staining.

A sterile pyuria, of course, may be present shortly after treatment with antibiotics or chemotherapeutic agents. It must also alert to the possibility of renal tuberculosis, calculi, analgesic abuse, infection with micro-aerophilic and anaerobic bacteria and almost any injury to the urinary tract from chlamydial urethritis to glomerulonephritis and nephrosis.

Urinary tract infection without pyuria may occur in leucopenia resulting from drugs, aplastic anaemia, etc., and in patients with infectious processes remote from the kidney's collecting system (e.g. renal cortical abscess) or occasionally in obstructive uropathy.

Leucocyturia is not a constant feature and cell counts are known to vary in successive specimens (Stansfield and Webb, 1953). Its absence from any single specimen therefore cannot be taken as evidence of the absence of bacteriuria. Pyuria is dependent on urine flow and pH of the urine (Kunin, 1979b). Bacterial counts also may vary at different time of the day and generally speaking the early morning specimen of urine is the preferred specimen for examination (Roberts, Robinson and Beard, 1967; Kunin, 1979a; Asscher, 1980d).

Organisms

Undoubtedly the commonest infecting organisms both in hospital and in the community are the Gram-negative bacilli. *Escherichia coli* tops the list, closely followed by *Klebsiella pneumoniae* and *Proteus mirabilis,* although there are differences of balance between community and hospitalized patients (*Table 13.1*). In general, these are aerobic bacteria from the bowel which may be pathogenic when they are introduced into the urinary tract. *Proteus* spp. is a common organism in aged males and it is interesting that it is also frequently found in UTI in boys but is rare during adulthood (Maskell, Pead and Hallett, 1975). It is suggested that the prostatic secretion may play a part in diminishing the survival of this particular organism and this may explain the significant correlation between old men with

Table 13.1 Organisms commonly causing UTI in the elderly

General practice
90% *E. coli*
Hospital (hospital-acquired infections tend to be due to drug-resistant bacteria)
47% *E. coli*
In addition to *E. coli,* nosocomial infections are caused by a wide variety of less frequently occurring organisms than those which occur commonly in the community, such as:
Klebsiella
Proteus spp.
Pseudomonas
Strep. faecalis
Staph. aureus
Staph. albus
Acinetobacter
Alcaligenes
Providencia
Mixed organisms

(Data from Montgomerie *et al.*, 1970; McAllister *et al.*, 1971; McMillan, 1972; Asscher, 1980f).

prostatectomies and others — the former having a higher prevalence of UTI (Brocklehurst *et al.*, 1968a).

Numbers of coagulase-negative staphylococci may colonize the bladder, usually in elderly patients who are catheterized. They form part of the commensal flora of the distal urethra and gain access to the bladder via the moist surface of the indwelling catheter. Under normal conditions they are non-pathogenic (Maskell, 1980). Another organism with circumscribed age and sex incidence is *Staphylococcus saprophyticus* (formerly known as *Micrococcus*). It is now recognized as the second commonest urinary pathogen after *E. coli* in young women, but it is rarely isolated from elderly individuals of either sex (Sellin *et al.*, 1975; Pead, Crump and Maskell, 1977; Wallmark, Arremark and Telander, 1978; Lewis *et al.*, 1982; Marrie *et al.*, 1982).

It is now becoming apparent that anaerobic bacteria which are a commensal of the normal vaginal flora may occasionally cause UTI, particularly in the setting of structural abnormalities. Additionally, fastidious organisms which do not grow after overnight culture in air may cause some urinary symptoms and pyuria. Incubation for 48–72 h in 7 per cent CO_2 may yield pure growths of micro-aerophilic or CO_2-requiring organisms such as Lactobacilli, *Streptococcus milleri* or *Corynebacterium* spp. (Maskell, Pead and Allen, 1979).

The place of the L-form of bacteria in chronic urinary tract infection, particularly in recurrent pyelonephritis, requires consideration. The L-forms are bacterial cells without solid wall structure. Bacteria can change into L-forms after being exposed to agents which damage the surface (e.g. antibiotics or natural defensive mechanism acting through antibody–complement–lysozyme enzymes). L-forms do not grow in common broth and need their own cultivation techniques. Hypertonic conditions in the renal medulla favour their survival. During cultivation they return to their normal forms. Virulence of the L-forms is low, but after returning to the normal bacterial form virulence is restored. L-forms may survive in tissue for long periods and have been isolated in many cases in old people with chronic urinary infections, often with severe underlying disease (Gutman *et al.*, 1965; Conner *et al.*, 1968).

Candida organisms are occasionally isolated from specimens of clean-voided urine — often in pure culture — and their presence rarely gives rise to concern (Haley, 1965), although their clinical significance is uncertain.

Candida albicans is a yeast-like fungus, usually of low pathogenicity, most commonly carried as a symptomless commensal on the skin and various mucous membranes. It may act as an opportunistic pathogen in various conditions which reduce host resistance. Blood-borne *Candida* may localize in the kidneys. Bulky mycelia may produce vascular obstruction so that the condition may present with haematuria, loin pain and tenderness due to renal infarcts. Systemic infection may also produce a mycetoma or perinephric abscess and mycelia may lead to obstructive uropathy. *Candida* infection may also reach the urinary tract by ascent in the presence of indwelling catheters and in this case the presence of *Candida* in large numbers is not usually associated with tissue invasion (Thornton, Lytton and Andriole, 1966). Nevertheless, repeated isolation of pure cultures of yeast from the urine of symptomatic patients or those with primary debilitating diseases may reflect invasion of the urinary tract by these organisms (Louria and Finkel, 1965). The problem is compounded because there are as yet no criteria to establish the diagnosis of renal candidiasis by quantitation of mid-stream clean-void urine. It has been suggested that more than 10 000 *Candida* per ml^{-1} from a catheterized specimen provides a useful criterion distinguishing colonization from infection (Kozinn *et al.*, 1978).

In all cases of *Candida* infection of the urinary tract, fungal threads are found in the urine and in the absence of a local source (e.g. vaginal thrush) the organism should be looked for in the blood stream and an excretion urogram performed.

In contrast, the isolation of *Histoplasma capsulatum, Coccidioides immites, Blastomyces dermatitidis* and other primary pathogenic fungi, regardless of the colony count, would suggest true infection (Andriole, 1972).

When urinary tract tuberculosis is suspected, direct examination of the urine for acid-fast bacilli has little value and culture on appropriate media is required. Other acid-fast bacilli (e.g. *Mycobacterium hominis*) may be found in the urine of healthy adults. The disease often presents with frequency of micturition and nocturia.

Viruses have very rarely been implicated as causing urinary lesions (Jenson, 1967; Minkowitz *et al.*, 1968; Editorial, 1968). The lining of the urinary tract, unlike that of the respiratory tract, is very resistant to viral invasion. Exceptions include smallpox, haemorrhagic fever, herpes zoster (Gibbon, 1956); chickenpox (Amar, 1966), etc.

Ureaplasma and *Chlamydia* sp. are known to be involved in urethritis in males and possibly also in females, but facilities for their isolation are in general only available to venereologists at the present time and are not routinely available (Maskell, 1980). Renal lesions due to *Schistosoma* and other parasites must be kept in mind.

Mixed infections

Infection due to more than one organism nearly always occurs in the presence of underlying structural abnormality or with indwelling Foley or suprapubic catheters. It is often dismissed as an indication that the urine has been contaminated, but if consistently confirmed would suggest the possibility of structural abnormality, bladder calculus, diverticulum or the uninhibited neurogenic bladder. Such a mixed culture may lead to Gram-negative bacteraemia (Gross, Flower and Barden, 1976).

Management of UTI

As with many conditions in old age the symptoms of UTI are often atypical and may not be taken as a reliable indicator of infection. They frequently do not relate to the urinary tract (Esposito *et al.*, 1980) and bacteriuria constitutes the only accurate indicator of bacterial UTI. The high prevalence of significant bacteruria in elderly people both in the community and in institutions suggests that it is impracticable to treat and continue treating all such patients. In particular, there is a strong body of opinion that asymptomatic bacteriuria in old people should not be treated, that it is a relatively benign condition not affecting renal function nor diminishing life expectancy (Petersdorf, 1966; Sourander, 1966; Akhtar *et al.*, 1972; Gleckman, 1976; Brocklehurst *et al.*, 1977; Brocklehurst, 1978; Carty, Brocklehurst and Carty, 1981). The toxic side effects of drugs, the risk of superinfection, the cost and the high failure rate of therapy all argue against treatment of asymptomatic urinary infection in this group (Levison and Kaye, 1972). Among disabled long-term care patients in institutions in particular, there is a 50 per cent chance of developing bacteriuria at some time within 1 year and of relapse or reinfection following treatment (Brocklehurst *et al.*, 1968b; Levison and Kaye, 1972).

The symptom of incontinence in particular poses problems. Acute cystitis may present with incontinence and treatment cure the symptom. At the same time, bacteriuria may be a secondary phenomenon in other conditions which are the primary cause of incontinence (e.g. uninhibited neurogenic bladder particularly if associated with faecal soiling or any condition associated with a degree of residual urine).

Having all these problems in mind, it is suggested (Brocklehurst, 1978) that a single-term course of therapy should be given in all patients in whom bacteriuria is encountered fo the first time whether they are symptomatic or otherwise. If symptoms are relieved by therapy, then further treatment may be vindicated should reinfection or relapse occur. If therapy produced no effect on symptoms or if the patient is asymptomatic, no further courses of treatment should be given even in the presence of reinfection or relapse. This principle, of course, is a generalization and should there be other indications for repeated or continued therapy (e.g. progressive impairment of renal function), then such cases must be regarded individually. In particular, patients with indwelling catheters on a long-term basis will inevitably show infection and possibly mixed infection and it is likely that this will involve the kidney in due course of time (Carty, Brocklehurst and Carty, 1981). However, short courses of antimicrobial therapy or long courses of urinary antiseptics do not prevent reinfection or relapse and should not be used in asymptomatic patients.

Dontas (1984) has proposed three conditions where UTI in the elderly should be aggressively treated, as follows:

(1) Patients with a proved bladder infection if it is the initial episode.
(2) Patients with advanced renal involvement (creatinine clearance less than 40 ml/min or active glomerular damage (proteinuria).
(3) Febrile patients with symptoms of upper UTI, particularly if lithiasis is present.

In addition to specific antimicrobial therapy, a very high fluid intake should be aimed at with frequent voiding. These will contribute to dilution of the bacteriuria and ‘washout’ of the organisms. Water diuresis diminishes medullary hypertonicity and so increases leucocyte migration activity in the medulla as well as inhibiting the formation of cell-wall-defective bacteria. On the other hand, the larger urinary flow will dilute urinary antibacterial substances such as urea and reduce medullary concentration of antimicrobial agents.

Numbers of drugs are enhanced in an alkaline urine (aminoglycosides and erythromycin). On the other hand, urinary antiseptics like methenamine are effective in an acid urine.

Obstruction to urinary flow from whatever cause impedes successful eradication of a bacterial UTI and obstructions must be removed before successful treatment can be accomplished (Gleckman, 1982).

Duration of therapy

Optimum length of antimicrobial therapy depends on the nature of the infection. One-day therapy is adequate for women with acute symptomatic community acquired bacterial cystitis (Fang, Tolkoff-Rubin and Rubin, 1978), although three-day therapy has been suggested as superior to one-day treatment and also no better than 10-day treatment in women of this type (Charlton, 1980). An extended course of therapy of at least 6 weeks achieves a higher cure rate in elderly men with recurrent invasive UTI (Gleckman, Crowley and Natsios, 1979) and some patients who experience bacterial relapse appear to benefit from an extended course of therapy (Turck, Ronald and Petersdorf, 1968; Stamey, 1980, in 'Discussion' on paper of Grüneberg, 1980).

Patients experiencing acute symptomatic community acquired bacterial pyelonephritis should be treated for 10–14 days, although the length of treatment for this condition has not yet been evaluated from prospective control studies.

Specific principles of drug therapy

(1) A strong correlation exists between the immediate eradication of bacteriuria and *in vitro* antibiotic susceptibility. Without initial sterilization of the urine, successful therapy rarely follows (Gleckman, 1982), and urine which is not sterile within 2 days of treatment indicates incorrect therapy (Stamey, 1967).

(2) The therapeutic goal has been achieved when symptoms resolve, the organisms have been eradicated and the urine remains sterile for a minimum of 6 weeks after the cessation of drug therapy. Symptomatology, if used exclusively, constitutes an inadequate indicator of therapeutic cure (Gleckman, 1982).

(3) No evidence exists that bactericidal compounds produce more effective cure than bacteriostatic agents in patients with UTI (Gleckman, 1982). In fact trimethoprim, a bacteriostatic compound, compares favourably with bactericidal antibiotics such as ampicillin and cephalexin in women with acute symptomatic and recurrent UTI caused by *E. coli* (Brumfitt and Pursell, 1972).

(4) There is no evidence to support the prescription of multiple antibicrobials simultaneously as a method of producing a higher cure rate (McCabe and Jackson, 1960; Acar and Brisset, 1975). No study has so far demonstrated conclusively that trimethoprim/sulphamethoxazole is a more effective chemotherapeutic agent than trimethoprim in the treatment of females with acute symptomatic or recurrent UTI.

(5) The choice of drug and duration of therapy depends on the tissue source of infection and the nature of complications (Naumann, 1978). Patients with acute uncomplicated bacterial cystitis should be treated with a drug that achieves therapeutic concentration in the urine. Those with acute symptomatic and recurrent

pyelonephritis and those experiencing bacteraemia should be treated with medications resulting in therapeutic concentrations in the urine and the serum. Patients with recurrent pyelonephritis associated with structural abnormalities or renal insufficiency should be treated with an agent that achieves effective serum and tissue concentrations (Naumann, 1978).

Parenteral antibiotics are required for patients with suspected bacteraemia and for those with pyelonephritis associated with shaking chills, sweats, fever and tachypnoea. The antibiotic to be used will depend upon the organism, any history of drug allergies and the nature of concomitant diseases. Community acquired Gram-negative aerobic bacilli indicate a cephalosporin (effective against *E. coli, Proteus mirabilis* and *Klebsiella* spp.). If the infection develops in a recently catheterized subject or one who has had a urological procedure or recurrent UTIs, aminoglycocides are indicated (e.g. gentamicin, tobramycin, amikacin). Once the infecting organism and its susceptibility have been established, a potentially less toxic drug should be substituted if possible.

Those patients with acute pyelonephritis who experience bacteraemia or remain febrile more than 96 h after the onset of antibiotic treatment should be suspected of obstructive uropathy or perinephric abscess and require urological and radiological evaluation (Thorley, Jones and Sanford, 1974) (see Chapters 11 and 19).

Management of reinfection

Since the intervals between successive attacks of symptomatic reinfection are longer than those between symptomatic relapses, it is seldom justified to institute long-term suppressive treatment and the following procedure is recommended. The patient should be supplied with an antibacterial agent to which the original infecting organism is sensitive and with a dip-inoculum transport medium apparatus. At the very first evidence of recurrence he should send the dip-inoculated transport media immediately to the laboratory and start on the treatment with which he has been supplied. Symptoms may thus be minimized while bacteriological supervision is maintained. A high fluid intake and complete bladder emptying are also important (Asscher, 1980e).

Management of infection associated with urethral manipulation

Bacteraemia immediately following genito-urinary tract manipulation is the most common definable cause of Gram-negative sepsis and endotoxic shock in hospital. However, the question of prophylactic antimicrobial therapy or bladder irrigation remains controversial.

Kunin (1979c) suggests the following routine. All patients about to undergo urological studies or procedures should have a urine culture carried out and those with infection treated with a specific antimicrobial, deferring instrumentation if necessary until the urine is sterile. Bacteraemia following instrumentation in non-infected patients is usually transient and without sequelae. In this non-infected group, therefore, only higher risk patients require prophylactic treatment for 2–3 days before the procedure (ampicillin, sulphonamide, tetracyclin, nitrofurantoin or co-trimoxazole may all be appropriate). If the elderly patient has a heart murmur he should be started on a combination of penicillin G or ampicillin together with an aminoglycoside. No good procedure is available for patients allergic to penicillin, since the cephalosporins are not effective against Enterococci and vancomycin is probably too toxic for routine use. The value of erythromycin is not established in this situation.

Management of indwelling catheters

Indwelling urinary catheters are used as an acceptable method of controlling urinary incontinence in the small group of patients with a disorder of the central nervous system thoroughly investigated, in whom other treatment has failed and life expectancy is limited to 2 or 3 years; or men with prostatic obstruction in whom surgery is contraindicated. In the former group, intermittent self-catheterization is much to be preferred if it is possible.

However, many patients on prolonged catheter drainage have evidence of upper urinary tract infection by antibody-coated bacterial test (Gonik *et al.*, 1975) and the *Limulus test* for circulating endotoxin is often positive as well (Garibaldi *et al.*, 1973). Renal infection is also more frequent in catheterized patients than in other infected patients or non-infected patients (Carty, Brocklehurst and Carty, 1981).

A closed sterile system may generally be maintained for up to a week, but it is virtually impossible to maintain sterility in indwelling catheters thereafter. Under optimal care the risk of bacteriuria has been described as increasing by 5 per cent daily (Kass, 1983). Nevertheless, the breaks in continuity between the drainage tube and the collecting bag should be reduced to a minimum. The collecting bag should be protected from outside contamination and must itself be regarded as a source of infection and handled by staff with appropriate preventative techniques. Approximately half a million catheter-associated nosocomial urinary tract infections per year have been described in the USA (quoted from Platt *et al.*, 1983).

A good renal flow is desirable and while bladder washout systems will not diminish the presence of infection they will diminish debris formation and catheter blockage (Brocklehurst and Brocklehurst, 1978). In women with catheters, organisms may be introduced from the introitus into the bladder as a result of catheter movement through the lumen of catheter, along with air bubbles (Gillespie *et al.*, 1960, 1967), or in the film of fluid which forms between the outside of the catheter and the urethral mucosa (Kass and Schneiderman, 1957), and urethral trauma may allow tissue penetration and bacteraemia.

Management of complicated infection

The medical treatment of patients with complicated infection (obstruction, stones, catheters, structural or neurological abnormalities of the urinary tract, etc.) should only be on a short-term basis for acute episodes which may arise. The surgical relief of obstructive lesions, removal of stones and removal of infected non-functioning kidney is indicated wherever these are present.

There is no place for prophylactic antimicrobial therapy (nor continuous urinary antiseptic therapy) in the prevention of UTI in patients on long-term indwelling catheters (Brocklehurst and Brocklehurst, 1978). Symptomatic infections, of course, must be treated. There is no justification for regular laboratory testing of urine for UTI in old people with indwelling catheters who are asymptomatic.

Drugs for long-term prophylaxis

There are few situations in which long-term prophylaxis against UTI has been shown to be indicated in old people. The exception would be multiple, disabling symptomatic flare-ups and in relation to indwelling catheters, but no successful method of prophylaxis has so far emerged. Drugs that might be considered are nitrofurantoin, which does not alter rectal carriage of *E. coli* and produces only modest reduction in vaginal and peri-urethral cultures, but trimethoprim or trimethoprim–sulphamethoxazole, which eliminate *E. coli* from the rectum, urethra and vagina, have been shown to be effective in this regard (Stamm *et al.*, 1980). Co-trimoxazole treatment has shown a marked reduction in the number of aerobic bowel flora (Gruneberg *et al.*, 1975) and very little generation of resistance to sulphonamides or trimethoprim among surviving bacteria (Gruneberg *et al.*, 1975, 1979). However, the use of co-trimoxazole in this way should be reserved for high risk patients (Stamey, Condy and Mihara, 1977).

Treatment of prostatic infection

Chronic bacterial prostatitis is a common source of UTI in males and is difficult to eradicate since many of the commonly used antibacterial agents fail to penetrate prostatic fluid and if they do it may not be effective there because of its high acidity. Erythromycin, oleandomycin, co-trimoxazole, tetracycline and clindamycin are the main antibiotics which reach high enough concentrations in prostatic fluid to suggest any therapeutic potential (Winningham, Nemoy and Stamey, 1968; Winningham and Stamey, 1970; Reeves *et al.*, 1973).

Treatment of UTI in kidney failure

The problems that arise in attempting to treat UTI in the presence of renal failure have been well summarized by Asscher (1980e). The infection is usually hospital acquired and thus more likely to be due to resistant organisms; therapeutic urinary concentrations of antibacterial agents may be difficult to attain without systemic toxicity; the therapeutic urinary concentration of antibacterial agents is more slowly established and drug resistance may therefore develop more readily during treatment; urinary acidification is difficult to achieve and disparity of functional impairment between the two kidneys may lead to unequal excretion of antibacterial agents and persistence of infection in the kidney with diminished function. The adjustment of dose to avoid accumulation of drug in renal failure will also result in reduced concentration in the urine, and so the need to restrict doses of potentially toxic agents also restricts their therapeutic effectiveness.

Ampicillin, cephalosporins, nalidixic acid, co-trimoxazole and gentamicin are excreted in uraemic patients in adequate urinary concentration without systemic toxicity. Most other penicillin and cephalosporin derivatives may also achieve adequate urinary concentration if doses are not reduced. Cephaloridine, however, is contraindicated in uraemic patients because of its nephrotoxic potential. Co-trimoxazole may produce therapeutically adequate concentration. The sulphonamide moiety of co-trimoxazole is well excreted despite the presence of advanced renal failure (Sharpstone, 1969). In general, tetracyclines (with the exception of doxycycline), sulphonamides, nitrofurantoins and chloramphenicol should be avoided in patients with renal failure. In patients on dialysis, the drug half-life should be determined in the same patient during and between haemodialysis or peritoneal dialysis.

In aged patients with impaired renal function, the duration of treatment should be for not less than 3 weeks (Dontas, 1984).

Treatment of tuberculosis of the kidney and urinary tract

Accurate initial assessment of the extent of the disease, the presence of obstructive uropathy and the state of renal function is essential. Multiple drug therapy is used to delay emergence of strains of organism resistant to drugs and to achieve a synergistic therapeutic effect. Until the sensitivity of the tubercle bacilli is known, chemotherapy should be started with a triple-drug regimen from the following drugs — isoniazid (INH), ethambutol or sodium aminosalicylate (PAS), streptomycin or rifampicin. In the elderly, in the presence of impaired renal function extreme care must be taken over the use of streptomycin and ethambutol. Treatment generally requires to be continued for at least 1–2 years. Surgery may be necessary to relieve obstruction. Nephrectomy is rarely necessary.

Treatment of candidiasis

The treatment of urinary candidiasis is that of the underlying predisposing disease. At the same time, fluorocytosine and/or amphotericin B should be started (although this latter must be avoided in the presence of renal functional impairment). If the disease is confined to the bladder, irrigation with nystatin solution or amphotericin B may be sufficient.

Effects of UTI

While there is no doubt that infection associated with pyelonephritis will impair renal function in old as in young people, there is a controversy as to the effect of asymptomatic bacteriuria on renal function. A number of papers have described no change (Freedman and Andriole, 1969; Asscher *et al.*, 1973; Freeman *et al.*, 1975; Kunin, 1975; Gower, 1976; Carty, Brocklehurst and Carty, 1981) and others have reported a deterioration (Dontas *et al.*, 1966, 1968; Dontas, Marketos and Papanayiotou, 1972). An increase in mortality among elderly persons with UTI has been described (Sourander and Kasanen, 1972; Dontas *et al.*, 1981). There is also controversy as to a relationship between raised blood pressure and UTI in the elderly. Marketos and colleagues (Marketos *et al.*, 1970) described a positive relationship in hospitalized patients, but not in old people at home.

It must be remembered that analgesic nephropathy may be a more common cause of progressive renal damage in elderly people without obstructive nephropathy than is generally realized (Gower, 1976).

In old age, bacteriuria is associated with significant deficit of tubular and renovascular functions. The disturbed medullary integrity and the specific epithelial impairment of the distal collecting tubule are evident from the elderly bacteriuric's inability to concentrate or dilute urine during periods of hydropenia or water-loading, respectively (Turck, 1975). A sex difference between impairment of glomerular filtration rate (GFR) and renal plasma flow (RPF) in the presence of bacteriuria has been described (Dontas, 1984) and this may represent an aggravation by the infection of the effects of mechanical and hormonal factors on certain renal function in the aged male.

Longitudinal studies have shown a more rapid decline in renovascular function (GFR and RPF) in bacteriuric subjects than in non-infected controls of the same age (Marketos, Papanayiotou and Dontas, 1969). It is not necessarily certain that these changes in function in association with infection are a direct effect of the infection or whether they provide a favourable background for the development of infection. It would appear nevertheless that the nephrosclerotic changes of old age are markedly accelerated by long-standing asymptomtic UTI (Weiss and Parker, 1939).

The relationship between bacteriuria and hypertension is also uncertain. For instance, in hospitalized patients both conditions are very common and it is hard to decide whether or not there is a causal relationship. In ambulant clinically healthy subjects in a study by Marketos *et al.* (1970), bacteriuria did not appear to be a causative factor in the emergence of hypertension in the elderly. There may, of course, be a selective screening out by death or hospitalization of elderly hypertensive pyelonephritic patients.

Mortality and UTI

From a 10-year follow-up of 342 ambulant residents of a residential home for the elderly, it was shown that median survival for the 76 who were bacteriuric at entry was significantly less than for the non-infected (Dontas *et al.*, 1981). There were no differences at entry between the two groups in several risk factors including blood pressure, serum cholesterol and smoking habits and the differences have been attributed to the presence of bacteriuria. Uraemia, however, did not contribute substantially to the increased mortality of the bacteriuric group, nor did Gram-negative septicaemia (Dontas, 1984). It is not certain whether this relationship is causal, since a major factor in population studies of this type in a condition which may be intermittent, is the possibility that the presenting characteristic may be transient. Thus, a significant number of subjects non-bacteriuric at entry may have later become infected and a study of the persistence of bacteriuria rather than its spot prevalence should be more sensitive in detecting possible effects on survival. Surveys carried out in Jamaica and Wales on women aged 15–84 years (Evans *et al.*, 1982) showed that the duration of exposure to bacteriuria had a bearing on its ultimate effect on mortality.

These two long-term studies do complement each other but do not clarify the mode by which asymptomatic UTI increases the risk of death. A causal relationship could be supported if bacteriuria could be shown to induce bacteraemia, accelerated development of renal failure or elevation of blood pressure in these patients. Of these possibilities, disseminated infection from Gram-negative rods is not often recognized in the community and most such recorded deaths occur in hospitals. As regards hypertension, when the Jamaican/Welsh data were analysed with blood pressure as an additional variable, bacteriuria still remained significantly associated with increased mortality, but less strongly so than when it was the only variable. Finally, although GFR declines faster in infected subjects, frank uraemia has been only rarely identified as a chief cause of death in either of the above studies (Dontas, 1984).

It is possible that other factors such as diseases of the central nervous system, brain failure or any debilitating illness could account for both the reduced life expectancy and the bacteriuria. For instance, patients with dementia usually have a lower level of personal hygiene so that mental impairment, incontinence of faeces and bacteriuria may be correlated (Brocklehurst *et al.*, 1977; James, 1979).

What is it about moderate and covert renal infection in old age which may hasten death? Frank renal insufficiency is certainly not the chief cause of death, as it would be recognized and recorded. It may represent, however, a significant contributory factor during respiratory infections or complications of diabetes by impeding the capacity of the kidney to retain plasma tonicity or correct sudden disturbances of homeostasis. Thus the immediate cause of death may be classified as non-renal, but the decisive factor in the non-recovery of the patient will have been the kidney's incapacity to maintain a stable environment (Dontas, 1984). While in a generally younger population a potentially lethal but infrequent characteristic may not influence the rate of mortality to a decisive extent, if the same characteristic were present at an age when the forces of death are much stronger, its effect might become apparent. It is also probable that the duration of exposure to bacteriuria is longer in old age, so that cumulative exposure of the individual to it might be an important discriminating factor (Dontas, 1984).

References

ACAR, J.F. and BRISSET, J.M. (1975). Combinations of antibiotics in urinary tract infections. In *Clinical Use of Combinations of Antibiotics,* edited by J. Klastersky, pp. 126–134. New York; Wiley

ADDATO, K., DOEBELE, K.G., GALLAND, L. *et al.* (1979). Behavioural factors and urinary tract infection. *Journal of the American Medical Association,* **241,** 2525–2526

AKHTAR, A.J., ANDREWS, G.R., CAIRD, F.I. and FALLON R.J. (1972). Urinary tract infection in the elderly: a population study. *Age and Ageing,* **1,** 48–54

AMAR, A.D. (1966). Haematuria caused by varicella lesions in the bladder. *Journal of the American Medical Association,* **196,** 450

ANDRIOLE, V.T. (1972). Diagnosis of urinary tract infection by urine culture. In *Urinary Tract Infection and Its Management,* edited by D. Kaye, pp. 28–42. St. Louis; Mosby

ASSCHER, A.W. (1980a). The problems. In *The Challenge of Urinary Tract Infection,* pp. 13–21. London; Academic Press

ASSCHER, A.W. (1980b). Pathogens of ascending infection. In *The Challenge of Urinary Tract Infection,* pp. 41–51. London; Academic Press

ASSCHER, A.W. (1980c). Covert infections. In *The Challenge of Urinary Tract Infection,* pp. 52–73. London; Academic Press

ASSCHER, A.W. (1980d). Terminology. In *The Challenge of Urinary Tract Infection,* pp. 7–12. London; Academic Press

ASSCHER, A.W. (1980e). Treatment. In *The Challenge of Urinary Tract Infection,* pp. 129–145. London; Academic Press

ASSCHER, A.W. (1980f). NosoLIASH, H. (1962). The incidence of urinary tract infection in hospitalized patients. *Scandinavian Journal of Clinical & Laboratory Investigation,* Suppl. 64, 77–83

ASSCHER, A.W., CHICK, S., RADFORD, N., WATERS, W.E., SUSSMAN, M., EVANS, J.S., McLACHLAN, M.S.F. and WILLIAMS J.E. (1973). Natural history of asymptomatic bacteriuria (ASB) in non pregnant women. In *Urinary Tract Infection,* edited by W. Brumfitt and A.W. Asscher, pp. 51–60.London; Oxford University Press

ASSOCIATION OF CLINICAL PATHOLOGISTS (1973). Estimation of bacteria and white cells in the urine. Broadsheet 80. London; ACP.

BANK, N. and BAILINE, S.H. (1965). Urinary betaglucuronidase activity in patients with urinary tract infection. *New England Journal of Medicine,* **272,** 70–75

BARRETT, E., LYNAM, G. and TRUSTEY, S. (1978). Gas liquid chromatography for detection of bacteriuria: examination for volatile acidic and neutral compounds. *Journal of Clinical Pathology,* **31,** 859–865

BONADIO, M., DONADIO, C., CATANIA, B. *et al.* (1979). Lysozymuria and upper-urinary tract infection. *New England Journal of Medicine,* **301,** 1065–1066

BRADLEY, J.M. and LITTLE, P.J. (1963). Quantitative urine culture. *British Medical Journal,* **ii,** 361–363

BRENNER, D.A., FAIRLEY, K.F. and KINCAID-SMITH, P. (1969). The serum antibody response in renal and bladder infections. *Medical Journal of Australia,* **1,** 1069–1071

BROCKLEHURST, J.C. (1978). A geriatrician's view of the laboratory examination of urine. In *The Bacteriological Examination of Urine: Report of a Workshop on Needs and Methods,* edited by P.D. Meers, Public Health Service Monograph, Series 10, pp. 65–69. London; HMSO

BROCKLEHURST, J.C. and BROCKLEHURST, S. (1978). Management of indwelling catheters. *British Journal of Urology,* **50,** 102–105

BROCKLEHURST, J.C., BEE, P., JONES, D. and PALMER, M. (1977). Bacteriuria in geriatric hospital patients: its correlates and management. *Age and Ageing*, **6**, 240–245

BROCKLEHURST, J.C., DILLANE, J.B., GRIFFITHS, L. and FRY, J. (1968a). The prevalence of symptomatology of urinary infection in an aged population. *Gerontologia Clinica*, **10**, 242–253

BROCKLEHURST, J.C., DILLANE, J.B., GRIFFITHS, L. and FRY, J. (1968b). A therapeutic trial in urinary infection of old age. *Gerontologia Clinica*, **10**, 345–347

BROUHARD, B.H. and CUNNINGHAM, R.J. (1981). Single-dose antibiotics for urinary infections. *The Lancet*, **i**, 331

BRUMFITT, W. (1965). Urinary cell counts and their value. *Journal of Clinical Pathology*, **18**, 550–555

BRUMFITT, W. and PERCIVAL, A. (1965). Serum antibody response as an indication of renal involvement in patients with significant bacteriuria. In *Progress in Pyelonephritis*, edited by E.H. Kass, pp. 118–128. Philadelphia; Davis

BRUMFITT, W. and PURSELL, R. (1972). Double blind trial to compare ampicillin, cephalexin, co-trimoxazole and trimethoprim in treatment of urinary infection. *British Medical Journal*, **2**, 673–676

CADY, P., DUFOUR, S.W., LAWLESS, P. *et al.* (1978). Impedimetric screening for bacteriuria. *Journal of Clinical Microbiology*, **7**, 273–278

CARTY, M., BROCKLEHURST, J.C. and CARTY, J. (1981). Bacteriuria and its correlates in old age. *Gerontology*, **27**, 72–75

CARVAJAL, H.F., PASSEY, R.B., BERGER, M. *et al.* (1975). Urinary lactic dehydrogenase isoenzyme 5 in the differential diagnosis of kidney and bladder infections. *Kidney International*, **8**, 176–184

CATTELL, W.R., CHARLTON, C.A., FRY, I.K., McSHERRY, A. and O'GRADY, F. (1972). Predictive value of endogenous wash-out test and uroradiology in assessing likely response of urinary tract infection to treatment. *The Lancet*, **ii**, 199–201

CATTELL, W.R., CHARLTON, C.A.C., McSHERRY, A. *et al.* (1973). The localization of urinary tract infection and its relationship to relapse, reinfection and treatment. In *Urinary Tract Infection*, edited by W. Brumfitt and A.W. Asscher, pp. 206–214. London; Oxford University Press

CHARLTON, C.A.C. (1980). Ultra short treatment of urinary tract infection. In *The Management of Urinary Tract Infection. An International Symposium*, edited by A.W. Asscher, pp. 81–84. Oxford; The Medicine Publishing Foundation

COBBS, C.G. (1972). Presumptive test for urinary tract infection. In *Urinary Tract Infection and its Management*, edited by D. Kaye, pp. 43–51. St. Louis; Mosby

COLOE, P.J. (1978). Headspace gas liquid chromatography for rapid detection of *Escherichia coli* and *Proteus mirabilis* in urine. *Journal of Clinical Pathology*, **31**, 365–369

CONNER, J.F., COLEMAN, S.E., DAVIS, J.L. and McGAUGHEY, F.S. (1968). Bacterial L-forms from urinary tract infections in a veterans' hospital population. *Journal of the American Geriatrics Society*, **16**, 893–900

CRAIG, W.A. (1977). Urinary tract infections: regimens to avoid recurrence. *Medical Times*, **105**, 49–61

DEVASKAR, U. and MONTGOMERY, W. (1978). Urinary lactic dehydrogenase isoenzyme IV and V in the differential diagnosis of cystitis and pyelonephritis. *Journal of Paediatrics*, **93**, 789–791

DONTAS, A.S. (1984). Urinary tract infection and their implications. In *Urology in the Elderly*, edited by J.C. Brocklehurst, pp. 162–192. Edinburgh; Churchill Livingstone

DONTAS, A.S. and KASVIKI-CHARVATI, P. (1976). Significance of diuresis-provoked bacteriuria. *Journal of Infectious Diseases*, **134**, 174–180

DONTAS, A.S., KASVIKI-CHARVATI, P., PAPANAYIOTOU, P.C. and MARKETOS, S.G. (1981). Bacteriuria and survival in old age. *New England Journal of Medicine*, **304**, 939–943

DONTAS, A.S., MARKETOS, S.G. and PAPANAYIOTOU, P. (1972). Mechanisms of renal tubular defects in old age. *Postgraduate Medical Journal*, **48**, 295–303

DONTAS, A.S., MARKETOS, S.G., PAPANAYIOTOU, P.C., TSEKOS, G.N. and MALAMOS, B.K. (1974). Simplified water-loading test in bacteriuria. *Nephron*, **12**, 121–128

DONTAS, A.S., PAPANAYIOTOU, P., MARKETOS, S. and PAPANICOLAOU, N. (1968). The effect of bacteriuria on renal function patterns in old age. *Clinical Science*, **34**, 73–81

DONTAS, A.S., PAPANAYIOTOU, P.C., MARKETOS, S., PAPANICOLAOU, N. and ECONOMOU, P. (1966). Bacteriuria in old age. *The Lancet*, **2**, 305–306

DRACH, G.W. (1975). Prostatitis: man's hidden infection. *Urologic Clinics of North America*, **2**, 499–520

EDITORIAL (1968). Viruses and renal disease. *Journal of the American Medical Association*, **204**, 219

ESPOSITO, A.L., GLECKMAN, R.A., CRAM, S. *et al.* (1980). Community-acquired bacteriuria in the elderly: analysis of one hundred consecutive episodes. *Journal of the American Geriatrics Society*, **28**, 315–319

EVANS, D.A., HENNEKENS, C.H., MIAO, L., MIALL, W.E. *et al.* (1982). Bacteriuria and subsequent mortality in women. *The Lancet*, **i**, 156–158

ELKYN, S., BULTITUDE, M.I., MAYO, M.E. *et al.* (1974). Prostatic calculi as a source of recurrent bacteriuria in males. *British Journal of Urology,* **46,** 527–532

FAIR, W.R., CRANE, D.B., PETERSON, L.J. *et al.* (1980). Three-day treatment of urinary tract infections. *Journal of Urology,* **123,** 717–721

FAIRLEY, K.F., BOND, A.G., BROWN, R.B. and HABERSBERGER, P. (1967). Simple test to determine the site of a urinary tract infection. *The Lancet,* **ii,** 427–428

FAIRLEY, K.F. and BUTLER, H. (1970). Sterile pyuria as a manifestation of occult bacterial pyelonephritis with special reference to intermittent bacteriuria. In *Renal Infection and Renal Scarring,* Proceedings of an International Symposium on pyelonephritis vesico-ureteric reflux and renal papillary necrosis held at Royal Melbourne Hospital, 1970, edited by P. Kincaid-Smith and K.F. Fairley, 2nd edn, pp. 51–67. Melbourne; Mercedes Publishing Services

FANG, L.S.T., TOLKOFF-RUBIN, N.E. and RUBIN, R.H. (1978). Efficacy of a single dose and conventional amoxycillin therapy in urinary tract infection localised by the antibody-coated bacteria technique. *New England Journal of Medicine,* **298,** 413–416

FREEDMAN, L.R. and ANDRIOLE, V.T. (1969). A long-term study of women with urinary tract infections. In *Abstracts IVth International Congress on Nephrology,* Vol. I, p. 386, Stockholm

FREEMAN, R.B., SMITH, M.W., RICHARDSON, J.A., THURM, R.H. *et al.* (1975). Long-term therapy for chronic bacteriuria in men (U.S. Public Health Service co-operative study). *Annals of Internal Medicine,* **83,** 133–147

FRIES, D., DELAVELLE, F., SIMONET, M. *et al.* (1977). Diagnostic topographique de l'infection urinaire par dosage de la fraction 5 de la lacticodeshydrogenase. *Nouvelle Press Medicale,* **6,** 3815–3818

GARGAN, R.A., BRUMFITT, W. and HAMILTON-MILLER, J.N.T. (1978). Do anerobes cause urinary infection? (letter). *The Lancet,* **i,** 37

GARIBALDI, R.A., ALLMAN, G.W., LARSEN, D.H. *et al.* (1973). Detection of endotoxemia by the limulus test in patients with indwelling urinary catheters. *Journal of Infectious Disease,* **128,** 551–554

GIAMARELLOU, H., PAPAPETROPOULOU, M., DONTAS, A.S. and DAIKOS, K. (1983). Antibody-coated bacteria in urine: long follow-up and the effect of antibiotics. *Chemiotarapia,* **2,** 131–136

GIBBON, N. (1956). A case of herpes zoster with involvement of the urinary bladder. *British Journal of Urology,* **28,** 417–421

GIBSON, I.I.J.M. and PRITCHARD, J.G. (1965). Screen investigation in the elderly. *Gerontologia Clinica,* **7,** 330–342

GILLESPIE, W.A., LENNON, G.G., LINTON, K.B. and PHIPPEN, G.A. (1967). Prevention of urinary infection by means of closed drainage into a sterile plastic bag. *British Medical Journal,* **3,** 90–92

GILLESPIE, W.A., LINTON, K.B., MILLER, A. and SLADE, N. (1960). The diagnosis, epidemiology and control of urinary infection in urology and gynaecology. *Journal of Clinical Pathology,* **13,** 187–194

GLECKMAN, R. (1976). A controversy of treatment of asymptomatic bacteriuria in non-pregnant women — resolved. *Journal of Urology,* **116,** 776–777

GLECKMAN, R.A. (1982). Urinary tract infection in adults: selective clinical, microbiological and therapeutic considerations. In *Medical Microbiology,* Vol. I, edited by C.S.F. Easmon and J. Jeljaszewicz, pp. 267–326. London; Academic Press

GLECKMAN, R., CROWLEY, M. and NATSIOS, G.A. (1979). Therapy of recurrent invasive urinary tract infections of men. *New England Journal of Medicine,* **301,** 878–880

GLECKMAN, R.A., CROWLEY, M.M. and NATSIOS, G.A. (1980a). Recurrent urinary tract infections in men: a role for aberrant bacterial forms? *Journal of Clinical Microbiology,* **II,** 650–653

GLECKMAN, R., CROWLEY, M. and NATSIOS, G.A. (1980b). Recurrent urinary tract infections in men: an assessment of contemporary treatment. *American Journal of Medical Science,* **279,** 31–36

GLECKMAN, R., ESPOSITO, A., CROWLEY, M. and NATSIOS, G.A. (1979). Reliability of a single urine culture in establishing diagnosis of asymptomatic bacteriuria in adult males. *Journal of Clinical Microbiology,* **9,** 596–597

GONIK, P., FALKNER, B., SCHWARTZ, A. *et al.* (1975). Bacteriuria in catheterized patients. *Journal of the American Medical Association,* **233,** 253–255

GOWER, P.E. (1976). A prospective study of patients with radiological pyelonephritis, papillary necrosis and obstructive atrophy. *Quarterly Journal of Medicine,* **178,** 315–349

GRIFFITH, D.P. (1978). Struvite stones. *Kidney International,* **13,** 372–382

GRIFFITH, D.P., MOSKOWITZ, P.A. and CARLTON, C.E. Jr. (1978). Adjunctive chemotherapy of infection-induced staghorn calculi. *Transactions of the American Association of Genito-Urinary Surgeons,* **70,** 25–29

GROSS, P.A., FLOWER, M. and BARDEN, G. (1976). Polymicrobic bacteriuria: significant association with bacteremia. *Journal of Clinical Microbiology,* **3,** 246–250

GRÜNEBERG, R.N. (1980). Extended treatment of urinary tract infection. In *The Management of Urinary Tract Infection: An International Symposium,* edited by A.W. Asscher, pp. 73–80. Oxford; The Medicine Publishing Foundation

GRÜNEBERG, R.N., LEAKEY, A., BENDALL, M.J. and SMELLIE, J.M. (1975). Bowel flora in urinary tract infection: effects of chemotherapy with special reference to co-trimoxazole. *Kidney International,* Suppl. 4, S122–129

GRÜNEBERG, R.N., SMELLIE, J.M., LEAKEY, A. and ATKIN, W.S. (1979). Trimethoprim-sulphamethoxazole for treatment of urinary tract infections: some bacteriological considerations. In *Infections of the Urinary Tract,* edited by E.H. Kass and W. Brumfitt, pp. 74–77. Chicago; University of Chicago Press

GUTMAN, L.T., HOLMES, K.K., WIESNER, P.J. *et al.* (1978). Recurrent bacteriuria in women: urologic abnormalities, perineal flora and bacterial variants in relation to site of infection and outcome of treatment. In *Infections of the Urinary Tract,* edited by E.H. Kass and W. Brumfitt, pp. 171–176. Chicago; University of Chicago Press

GUTMAN, L.T., TURCK, M., PETERSDORF, R.G. and WEDGEWOOD, R.J. (1965). Significance of bacterial variants in urine of patients with chronic bacteriuria. *Journal of Clinical Investigation,* **44,** 1945–1952

GUTTMAN, D. and NAYLOR, G.R.E. (1967). Dip slide: an aid to quantitative urine culture in general practice. *British Medical Journal,* **3,** 343–345

HAGENFELDT, L., WESTER, P.O., LITHANDER, A. and ELIASH, H. (1962). The incidence of urinary tract infection in hospitalized patients. *Scandinavian Journal of Clinical and Laboratory Investigation,* Suppl. 64, 77–83

HALEY, L.D. (1965). Yeast infections of the lower urinary tract. 1 — *In vitro* studies of the tissue phase of *Candida albicans. Sabouraudia,* **4,** 98–105

HARRISON, W.O., HOLMES, K.K., BELDING, M.E. *et al.* (1974). A prospective evaluation of recurrent urinary tract infection in women. *Clinical Research,* **22,** 125A

HEINAMAKI, P., HAVISTO, M., MATTILA, K. and RAJALA, S. (1984). Urinary characteristics and infections in the very aged. *Gerontologia Clinica,* **30,** 403–407

HOLMBERG, L., BOMAN, G., BOTTIGER, L.E. *et al.* (1980). Adverse reactions to nitrofurantoin. Analysis of 921 reports. *American Journal of Medicine,* **69,** 733–738

ISAACS, B. and WALKEY, F.A. (1964). A survey of incontinence in the elderly. *Gerontologia Clinica,* **6,** 367–376

ISENBERG, H.D., GAVAN, T.L., SONNENWIRTH, A. *et al.* (1979). Clinical laboratory evaluation of automated microbial detection/identification system in analysis of clinical urine specimens. *Journal of Clinical Microbiology,* **10,** 226–230

JAMES, M.H. (1979). Disorders of micturition in the elderly. *Age and Ageing,* **8,** 285–288

JENKINS, R.D., HALE, D.C. and MATSEN, J.M. (1980). Rapid semiautomated screening and processing of urine specimens. *Journal of Clinical Microbiology,* **11,** 220–225

JENSEN, M.M. (1967). Viruses and kidney disease. *American Journal of Medicine,* **43,** 897–911

JONES, S.R. (1976). Antibody-coated bacteria in urine (letter). *New England Journal of Medicine,* **295,** 1380

JONES, S.R. (1979). The current status of urinary tract infection localization by the detection of antibody-coated bacteria in urine sediment. In *Infectious Diseases: Current Topics,* edited by D.N. Gilbert and J.P. Sanford, pp. 97–106. New York; Grune and Stratton

JONES, S.R., SMITH, J.W. and SANFORD, J.P. (1974). Localization of urinary tract infections by detection of antibody-coated bacteria in urine sediment. *New England Journal of Medicine,* **290,** 591–593

KAITZ, A.L. and WILLIAMS, E.J. (1960). Bacteriuria and urinary tract infection in hospitalized patients. *New England Journal of Medicine,* **262,** 425–430

KASS, E.H. (1955). Chemotherapeutic and antibiotic drugs in the management of infections of the urinary tract. *American Journal of Medicine,* **18,** 764–781

KASS, E.H. (1956). Asymptomatic infections of the urinary tract. *Transaction of the Association of American Physicians,* **69,** 56–64

KASS, E.H. (1957). Bacteriuria and the diagnosis of infections of the urinary tract. *Archives of Internal Medicine,* **100,** 709–714

KASS, E.H. (1960). The role of asymptomatic bacteriuria in the pathogenesis of pyelonephritis. In *Biology of Pyelonephritis,* edited by E.L. Quinn and E.H. Kass, pp. 399–412. Boston; Little, Brown

KASS, E.H. (1962). Bacilluria in pregnancy (letter). *The Lancet,* **i,** 46

KASS, E.H. (1979). An approach to the management of resistant urinary infections (Clinical Conference). *Kidney International,* **16,** 204–212

KASS, E.H. (1983). Should bacteriuria be treated? An interpretative essay. In *A Clinical Approach to Progress in Infectious Diseases,* edited by W. Brumfitt and J.M.T. Hamilton-Miller, pp. 78–89. Oxford; Oxford University Press

KASS, E.H., MIALL, W.E., STUART, K.L. and ROSNER, B. (1978). Epidemiologic aspects of infections of the urinary tract. In *Infections of the Urinary Tract,* pp. 1–7. Chicago; University of Chicago Press

KASS, E.H. and SCHNEIDERMAN, L.J. (1957). Entry of bacteria into the urinary tracts of patients with inlying catheters. *New England Journal of Medicine,* **256,** 556–557

KASVIKI-CHARVATI, P., DROLETTE-KEFAKIS, B., PAPANAYIOTOU, P.C. and DONTAS, A.S. (1982). Turnover of bacteriuria in old age. *Age and Ageing,* **11,** 169–174

KAYE, D. (1972). Important definitions and classification of urinary tract infection. In *Urinary Tract Infection and Its Management,* edited by D. Kaye, pp. 1–5. St. Louis; Mosby

KOZINN, P.J., TASCHDJIAN, C.L., GOLDBERG, P.K. *et al.* (1978). Advances in the diagnosis of renal candidiasis. *Journal of Urology,* **119,** 184–197

KRAFT, J.K. and STAMEY, T.A. (1977). The natural history of symptomatic recurrent bacteriuria in women. *Medicine,* **56,** 55–60

KUNIN, C.M. (1975). Long-term therapy of urinary tract infections. *Annals of Internal Medicine,* **83,** 273–274

KUNIN, C.M. (1979a). Guide to examination of the urine. In *Detection, Prevention and Management of Urinary Tract Infections,* 3rd edn, pp. 57–90. Philadelphia; Lea and Febiger

KUNIN, C.M. (1979b). Principles of urinary bacteriology and immunology. In *Detection, Prevention and Management of Urinary Tract Infections,* 3rd edn, pp. 91–151. Philadelphia; Lea and Febiger

KUNIN, C.M. (1979c). Management of urinary tract infection. In *Detection, Prevention and Management of Urinary Tract Infections,* 3rd edn, pp. 227–320. Philadelphia; Lea and Febiger

KUNIN, C.M. (1982). Urinary tract infection and new information concerning pathogenesis and management. *Journal of Urology,* **128,** 1233

KUNIN, C.M., CRAIG, W.A. and UEHLING, D.T. (1978). Trimethoprim therapy for urinary tract infection: long term prophylaxis in a uremic patient. *Journal of the American Medical Association,* **239,** 2588–2590

LAPIDES, J., COSTELLO, R.T. Jr., ZIERDT, D.K. *et al.* (1968). Primary cause and treatment of recurrent urinary infection in women: preliminary report. *Journal of Urology,* **100,** 552–555

LEVINSEN, M.E. and KAYE, D. (1972). Management of urinary tract infection. In *Urinary Tract Infection and Its Management,* edited by D. Kaye, pp. 188–226. St. Louis; Mosby

LEWIS, J.F., BRAKE, S.R., ANDERSON, D.J. and VREDEVELD, G.D. (1982). Urinary tract infection due to coagulase-negative staphylococcus. *American Journal of Clinical Pathology,* **77,** 736–739

LITTLE, P.J. (1964). A comparison of the urinary white cell concentration and the white cell excretion rate. *British Journal of Urology,* **36,** 360–363

LORENTZ, W.B. Jr. and RESNICK, M.I. (1979). Comparison of urinary lactic dehydrogenase with antibody-coated bacteria in the urine sediment as means of localizing the site of urinary tract infection. *Paediatrics,* **64,** 672–677

LOURIA, D.B. and FINKEL, G. (1965). Candida pyelonephritis. In *Progress in Pyelonephritis,* edited by E.H. Kass, pp. 179–184. Philadelphia; Davis

McALLISTER, T.A., PERCIVAL, A., ALEXANDER, J.G., BOYCE, J.M.H., DULAKE, C. and WORMALD, P.J. (1971). Multicentric study of sensitivities of urinary tract pathogens: a survey. *Postgraduate Medical Journal,* **47,** Suppl. on Clinical and Bacteriological Aspects of Urinary Tract Infection, 7–14

McCABE, W.R. and JACKSON, G.G. (1960). Treatment of chronic pyelonephritis III. Comparison of several drugs combined and one member of the combination, colistin. *American Journal of Medical Science,* **240,** 754–763

McGEACHIE, J. (1966). Recurrent infection of the urinary tract: reinfection or recrudescence? *British Medical Journal,* **1,** 952–954

McGEACHIE, J. and KENNEDY, A.C. (1963). Simplified quantitative methods of bacteriuria and pyuria. *Journal of Clinical Pathology,* **16,** 32–38

MACKEY, J.P. and SANDYS, G.H. (1965). Laboratory diagnosis of infections of the urinary tract in general practice by means of dip-inoculum transport medium. *British Medical Journal,* **2,** 1286–1288

McMILLAN, S.A. (1972). Bacteriuria of elderly women in hospital: occurrence and drug resistance. *The Lancet,* **ii,** 452–455

MANN, P.G. and SANDYS, G.H. (1978). The pros and cons of dip-inoculation. In *The Bacteriological Examination of Urine: Report of a Workshop on Needs and Methods,* edited by P.D. Meers, Public Health Laboratory Service. Monograph Series 10. London; HMSO

MARIER, R., FONG, E., JANSEN, M. *et al.* (1978). Antibody to Tamm–Horsfall protein in patients with urinary tract obstruction and vesico-ureteral reflex. *Journal of Infectious Diseases,* **138,** 781–790

MARKETOS, S.G., DONTAS, A.S., PAPANAYIOTOU, P. and ECONOMOU, P. (1970). Bacteriuria and arterial hypertension in old age. *Geriatrics,* **25,** 136–146

MARKETOS, S., PAPANAYIOTOU, P. and DONTAS, A.S. (1969). Bacteriuria and non-obstructive renovascular disease in old age. *Journal of Gerontology,* **24,** 33–36

MARRIE, T.J., KWAN, C., NOBLE, M.A., WEST, W.A. and DUFFIELD, L. (1982). *Staphylococcus saprophyticus* as a cause of urinary tract infections. *Journal of Clinical Microbiology,* **16,** 427–431

MASKELL, R. (1980). Microbiology of urinary tract infection. In *The Management of Urinary Tract Infection: an International Symposium,* edited by A.W. Asscher, pp. 41–50. Oxford; Medicine Publishing Foundation

MASKELL, R., PEAD, L. and ALLEN, J. (1979). The puzzle of 'urethral syndrome': a possible answer? *The Lancet,* **1,** 1058–1059

MASKELL, R., PEAD, L. and HALLETT, R.J. (1975). Urinary pathogens in males. *British Journal of Urology,* **47,** 691–694

MEARES, E.M. Jr. (1974). Infection stones of prostatic gland. Laboratory diagnosis and clinical management. *Urology,* **4,** 560–566

MEARES, E.M. (1975). Long term therapy of chronic bacterial prostatitis with trimethoprim-sulfamethoxazole. *Canadian Medical Association Journal,* **112** (Suppl.), 22–25

MEARES, E.M. and STAMEY, T.A. (1968). Bacteriologic localization patterns in bacterial prostatitis and urethritis. *Investigative Urology,* **5,** 492–518

MEIJER-SEVERS, G.J., AARNOUDSE, J.G., MENSINK, W.F.A. and DANKERT, J. (1979). The presence of antibody-coated anaerobic bacteria in asymptomatic bacteriuria during pregnancy. *Journal of Infectious Diseases,* **140,** 653–658

MINKOWITZ, S. *et al.* (1968). Acute glomerulonephritis associated with varicella infection. *American Journal of Medicine,* **44,** 489–492

MONTGOMERIE, J.Z., TAYLOR, D.E.M., DOAK, P.B., NORTH, J.D.K. and MARTIN, W.J. (1970). *Klebsiella* in faecal flora of renal transplant patients. *The Lancet,* **ii,** 787–791

MOORE-SMITH, B. (1971). Suprapubic aspiration in the diagnosis of urinary infection in the elderly. *Modern Geriatrics,* **1,** 124–129

MOTZKIN, D. (1972). The bacteriological diagnosis and treatment of urinary tract infection. *Journal of Urology,* **107,** 454–457

MUNDT, K.A. and POLK, B.F. (1979). Identification of site of urinary-tract infections by antibody-coated bacteria assay. *The Lancet,* **ii,** 1172–1175

MUSHER, D.M., THROSTEINSSON, S.B. and AIROLA, V.M. II (1976). Quantitative urinalysis: diagnosing urinary tract infection in men. *Journal of the American Medical Association,* **236,** 2069–2072

NANRA, R., FRIEDMAN, A., O'KEEFE, C. *et al.* (1970). Response to treatment of renal and bladder infections. In *Renal Infection and Renal Scarring,* 2nd edn, pp. 175–179, Proceedings of an International Symposium on pyelonephritis, vesico-ureteric reflux and renal papillary necrosis held at Royal Melbourne Hospital, 1970, edited by P. Kincaid-Smith and K.F. Fairley. Melbourne; Mercedes

NAUMANN, P. (1978). The value of antibiotic levels in tissue and in urine in the treatment of urinary tract infections. *Journal of Antimicrobial Chemotherapy,* **4,** 9–17

NICHOLSON, D.P. and KOEPKE, K.A. (1979). Automicrobic system for urines. *Journal of Clinical Microbiology,* **10,** 823–833

PAPANAYIOTOU, P. and DONTAS, A.S. (1972). Water-loading test in bacteriuria. *New England Journal of Medicine,* **287,** 531–534

PARSONS, C.L. and SCHMIDT, J.D. (1982). Control of recurrent lower urinary tract infection in the postmenopausal woman. *Journal of Urology,* **128,** 1224–1226

PEAD, L., CRUMP, J. and MASKELL, R. (1977). Staphylococci as urinary pathogens. *Journal of Clinical Pathology,* **30,** 427–431

PETERSDORF, R.G. (1966). Asymptomatic bacteriuria: a therapeutic enigma. In *Controversy in Internal Medicine,* edited by F.J. Ingelfinger, A.S. Relman and M. Finland, pp. 302–312. Philadelphia; Saunders

PLATT, R., POLK, B.F., MURDOCK, B. and ROSNER, B. (1983). Reduction of mortality associated with nosocomial urinary tract infection. *The Lancet,* **i,** 893–897

PORTER, I.A. and BRODIE, J. (1969). Boric acid preservation of urine samples. *British Medical Journal,* **2,** 353–355

PRÁT, V., BOHUSALAV, M., HATALA, M. *et al.* (1977). Unsere Erfahrungen mit klinischen Methoden für die Lokalisierung von Harnwegsinfekten. *Zeitschrift für Urologie und Nephrologie,* **70,** 25–31

REEVES, D.S., ROWE, R.C.G., SNELL, M.E. and THOMAS, P.B.W. (1973). Further studies on the situation of antibiotics in the prostatic fluid of the dog. In *Urinary Tract Infection,* edited by W. Brumfitt and A.W. Asscher, pp. 197–205. London; Oxford University Press

ROBERTS, A.P., ROBINSON, R.E. and BEARD, R.W. (1967). Some factors affecting bacterial colony counts in urinary infection. *British Medical Journal,* **1,** 400–403

ROCHA, H. (1972). Epidemiology of urinary tract infection in adults. In *Urinary Tract Infection and its Management,* edited by D. Kaye, pp. 142–155. St. Louis; Mosby

RONALD, A.R., BOUTROS, P. and MOURTADA, H. (1976). Bacteriuria localization and response to single dose therapy in women. *Journal of the American Medical Association,* **235,** 1854–1856

RONALD, A.R., CUTLER, R.E. and TURCK, M. (1969). Effect of bacteriuria on renal concentrating mechanisms. *Annals of Internal Medicine,* **70,** 723–733

RONALD, A.R., SILVERBLATT, F., CLARK, H. *et al.* (1971). Failure of urinary betaglucuronidase activity to localise the site of urinary tract infection. *Applied Microbiology,* **21,** 990–995

ROSALKI, B.S. and WILKINSON, H.G. (1959). Urinary lactic dehydrogenase in renal disease. *The Lancet,* **ii,** 327–328

RUBIN, R.H., FANG, L.S.T., JONES, S.R. *et al.* (1980). Single dose amoxicillin therapy for urinary tract infection: multicentric trial using antibody coated bacteria localization technique. *Journal of the American Medical Association,* **244,** 561–564

RUMANS, L.W. and VOSTI, K.L. (1978). The relationship of antibody-coated bacteria to clinical syndromes: as found in unselected populations with bacteriuria. *Archives of Internal Medicine,* **138,** 1077–1081

SANFORD, B.A., THOMAS, V.L., FORLAND, M. *et al.* (1978). Immune response in urinary tract infection determined by radio immunoassay and immunofluorescence: serum antibody levels against infecting bacterium and enterobacteriaceae common antigen. *Journal of Clinical Microbiology,* **8,** 575–579

SCARPELLI, P.T., LAMANNA, S., BIGIOLI, F. *et al.* (1979). The antibody response in chronic pyelonephritis. *Clinical Nephrology,* **12,** 7–13

SCHARDIJN, G., STATIUS VAN EPS, L.W., SWAAK, A.J.G., KAGER, J.C.G.M. and PERSIJN, P.J. (1979). Urinary β-2-microglobulin in upper and lower urinary infections. *The Lancet,* **i,** 805–807

SELLIN, M., COOKE, D.I., GILLESPIE, W.A., SYLVESTER, D.G.H. and ANDERSON, J.D. (1975). Micro-coccal urinary tract infections in young women. *The Lancet,* **2,** 570–572

SHARP, J.R., ISHAK, K.G. and ZIMMERMAN, H.J. (1980). Chronic active hepatitis and severe hepatic necrosis associated with nitrofurantoin. *Annals of Internal Medicine,* **92,** 14–19

SHARPESTONE, P. (1969). The renal handling of trimethoprim and sulphamethoxazole in man. *Postgraduate Medical Journal,* **45,** Supplement on the synergy of trimethoprim and sulphonamides: Proceedings of a Conference held at the Royal College of Physicians, London, pp. 38–42

SIROKY, M.B., MOYLAN, R.A., AUSTEN, G. Jr. *et al.* (1976). Metastatic infection secondary to genitourinary tract sepsis. *American Journal of Medicine,* **61,** 351–360

SMITH, J.W., JONES, S.R. and KAIJSER, B. (1977). Significance of antibody-coated bacteria in urinary sediment in experimental pyelonephritis. *Journal of Infectious Diseases,* **135,** 577–581

SOURANDER, L.B. (1966). Urinary tract infection in the aged: an epidemiological study. *Annales Medicinae Internae Fennae, Helsinki,* **55,** Suppl. 45

SOURANDER, L.B. and KASANEN, A. (1972). A five year follow-up of bacteriuria in the aged. *Gerontologia Clinica,* **14,** 274–281

SOURANDER, L.B., RUIKKA, I. and GRONROOS, M. (1965). Correlation between urinary tract infection, prolapse condition and function of the bladder in aged female hospital patients. *Gerontologia Clinica,* **7,** 179–184

STAMEY, T. (1967). Office bacteriology. *Journal of Urology,* **97,** 926–934

STAMEY, T.A., CONDY, M. and MIHARA, G. (1977). Prophylactic efficacy of nitrofurantoin macrocrystals and trimethoprim-sulfamethoxazol in urinary infections. Biologic effects on the vaginal and rectal flora. *New England Journal of Medicine,* **296,** 780–783

STAMEY, T.A., GOVAN, D.E. and PALMER, J. (1965). The localization and treatment of the urinary tract infections: the role of bactericidal urine levels as opposed to serum levels. *Medicine,* **44,** 1–36

STAMEY, T.A. and PFAU, A. (1963). Some functional, pathologic, bacteriologic and chemotherapeutic characteristics of unilateral pyelonephritis in man. *Investigative Urology,* **1,** 162–172

STAMEY, T.A., WEHNER, N., MIHARA, G. *et al.* (1978). The immunologic basis of recurrent bacteriuria: role of cervico-vaginal antibody in enterobacterial colonization of the introital mucosa. *Medicine,* **57,** 47–56

STAMM, W.E., WAGNER, K.F., AMSEL, R. *et al.* (1980). Causes of the acute urethral syndrome in women. *New England Journal of Medicine,* **303,** 409–415

STANSFIELD, J.M. and WEBB, J.K.G. (1953). Observation on pyuria in children. *Archives of Disease in Childhood,* **28,** 386–391

SUSSMAN, M., ASSCHER, A.W., WATERS, W.E., EVANS, J.A.S., CAMPBELL, H., EVANS, K.T. and WILLIAMS, J.E. (1969). Asymptomatic bacteriuria in the non-pregnant woman. 1 Description of population. *British Medical Journal,* **1,** 799–803

THOMAS, V., SHELOKOV, A. and FORLAND, M. (1974). Antibody-coated bacteria in the urine and the site of urinary tract infection. *New England Journal of Medicine,* **290,** 588–590

THORLEY, J.D., JONES, S.R. and SANFORD, J.P. (1974). Perinephric abscess. *Medicine,* **53,** 441–451

THROM, R., SPECTER, S., STRAUSS, R. *et al.* (1977). Detection of bacteriuria by automated electrical impedance monitoring in a clinical microbiology laboratory. *Journal of Clinical Microbiology,* **6,** 271–273

THRONTON, G.F., LYTTON, B. and ANDRIOLE, V.T. (1966). Bacteriuria during indwelling catheter drainage. *Journal of the American Medical Association,* **195,** 179–183

TURCK, M. (1972). Therapeutic principles in the treatment of urinary tract infections and pyelonephritis. *Advances in Internal Medicine,* **18,** 141–152

TURCK, M. (1975). Localization of the site of recurrent urinary tract infections in women. *Urological Clinics of North America,* **2,** 433–441

TURCK, M., RONALD, A.R. and PETERSDORF, R.G. (1968). Relapse and reinfection in chronic bacteriuria, II. The correlation between site of infection and pattern of recurrence in chronic bacteriuria. *New England Journal of Medicine,* **278,** 422–427

WACKER, W. and DORFMAN, L. (1962). Urinary lactic dehydrogenase activity. *Journal of the American Medical Association,* **181,** 972–974

WALKEY, F.A., JUDGE, T.G., THOMPSON, J. and SAKARI, N.B.S. (1967). Incidence of urinary tract infection in the elderly. *Scottish Medical Journal,* **12,** 411–414

WALLMARK, G., ARREMACK, I. and TELANDER, B. (1978). *Staphylococcus saprophyticus:* a frequent cause of acute urinary tract infection among female outpatients. *Journal of Infectious Diseases,* **138,** 791–797

WATANAKUNAKORN, C. (1979). Are wall defective microbial variants important in clinical infectious disease? *Journal of Antimicrobial Chemotherapy,* **5,** 239–247

WEISS, S. and PARKER, F. (1939). Pyelonephritis: its relation to vascular lesions and to arterial hypertension. *Medicine,* **18,** 221–315

WHITWORTH, J.A., FAIRLEY, K.F., McIVOR, M.A. *et al.* (1973). Urinary fibrin-degradation products and the site of urinary infection. *The Lancet,* **1,** 234–235

WHITWORTH, J.A., FAIRLEY, K.F., O'KEEFE, C.M. *et al.* (1974). The site of renal infection, pyelitis or pyelonephritis? *Clinical Nephrology,* **2,** 9–12

WINNINGHAM, D.G., NEMOY, N.J. and STAMEY, T.A. (1968). Diffusion of antibiotics from plasma into prostatic fluid. *Nature,* **219,** 139–143

WINNINGHAM, D.G. and STAMEY, T.A. (1970). Diffusion of sulphonamides from plasma into prostatic fluid. *Journal of Urology,* **104,** 559–563

Chapter 14

Interstitial nephropathies and pyelonephritis in the aged

Anastasius S. Dontas and Vassilios D. Tzias

Terminology, pathology and pathophysiology

Interstitial nephropathies are disorders characterized by lymphocytic and plasma cell infiltration of the medullary interstitium, increased interstitial collagen and thickening of tubular basement membranes. Subsequent changes include atrophy or loss of tubular epithelium and appearance of colloid casts within dilated tubules. Infiltration by neutrophils and eosinophils or fibrotic tissue depends on the stage of the reaction, with acute reactions evidencing the former and chronic reactions the latter. Involvement of the cortex is secondary to obstruction of medullary structures. Finally, infection when present is usually a secondary phenomenon (Heptinstall, 1976).

Functional repercussions of these changes include: (a) an inability to conserve sodium; (b) polyuria related to (a); (c) distal renal tubular acidosis and hyperkalaemia, also related to (a); (d) relatively preserved glomerular filtration rate (GFR) and proximal tubular functions (i.e. T_m PAH). In chronic, advanced stages of this process, as such cases come to the attention of the clinician, glomerular damage has become more prominent (proteinuria, hypertension) so that renal functions appear globally impaired. Thus, although in early phases distal-collecting tubule dysfunction may dominate the functional pattern, in later stages glomerular and overall tubular functions are equally damaged and such kidneys are designed as end-stage kidneys. By some mechanism increasing the sensitivity of the residual units, the latter magnify several-fold their contribution to the maintenance of stability of the body fluids in volume and composition (Bricker *et al.*, 1978).

Several causes can lead to the development of interstitial nephropathy (Freedman, 1979); (a) congenital lesions; (b) bacterial infections of the kidney, i.e. pyelonephritis; (c) disorders associated with papillary damage, including obstructions; (d) immunologic reactions, associated or not with drug sensitivity; and finally, (e) miscellaneous causes, such as systemic infections, disseminated intravascular coagulation, etc. All of these result in the common interstitial reaction irrespective of the provoking factor. We will limit this overview to the commonest aetiologies in old age, i.e. bacterial infections and drug-induced interstitial nephropathies, some of which operate through immunological mechanisms, and finally some metabolic and miscellaneous disorders. The distinction between acute and chronic forms will not be used, as most provoking factors may result in either form, both of which represent a uniform tissue reaction of differing rapidity.

A particular type of interstitial nephropathy is that associated with analgesic intake: this type is commonly associated with renal papillary necrosis, so that clinical or radiological evidence of such an injury strongly suggests analgesic aetiology, although other causes common in the elderly, i.e. diabetes, obstructions and macroglobulinaemias, may also provoke this particular pattern.

In old age, interstitial inflammation will be superimposed on the background of sclerotic renovascular disease; this involvement of vascular structures will be accompanied by earlier and more advanced glomerular damage, so that azotaemia will appear more frequently than in younger subjects.

Further, in the absence of renal infection proximal tubular functions in old age are reduced proportionally with GFR, whereas distal tubular functions are relatively more depressed. In addition, medullary functions involving several mechanisms (i.e. concentrating ability) are more impaired than are simple functions of the distal-collecting tubules (i.e. diluting ability, C_{H_2O}). Finally, there are definite sex differences: elderly men exhibit larger glomerular and proximal tubular deficits than do women, whereas distal tubular function is significantly depressed in both sexes (Dontas *et al.*, 1972).

Intrarenal infection in elderly men seriously impairs the function of all nephronal segments, whereas in women it affects only more distal segments (concentration–dilution; Dontas *et al.*, 1972). On the other hand, the clinical course of non-bacterial interstitial nephropathy will be accelerated and accentuated by the superimposition of bacterial infection, so that an advanced but covert interstitial nephropathy may reveal clinical symptoms and diagnostic laboratory findings only when complicated by bacterial infection (Freedman, 1979).

Obstructive uropathies associated with interstitial renal inflammation are dealt with in Chapter 19.

Bacterial infections

Most physicians would probably accept the term 'chronic pyelonephritis' as the entity encompassing all interstitial renal inflammatory disorders, which are aetiologically associated with bacterial infection. The diagnosis is usually *radiological,* by the finding of coarse scars, but there is frequently also evidence of functional renal disease as well as that of clinical infection. In contrast, 'acute pyelonephritis' is always associated with clinical signs of urinary tract infection (Freedman, 1979), and only occasionally is there evidence of anatomic or functional renal damage. It is, therefore, obvious that the presence of bacteria in the urine is of paramount importance in either establishing the diagnosis of acute pyelonephritis or confirming that of chronic pyelonephritis. The latter applies especially to old people, because they are more likely to have any other form of interstitial renal inflammatory disorder, as well as bacteriuria.

The changes in renal morphology and function with advancing age are discussed earlier in this book, but for our purposes these may be considered as belonging to two groups: those due to systemic factors, i.e. hypertension, diabetes, etc., and those due to local ones, i.e. drugs, instrumentation, obstructions, etc., all of which may also cause interstitial renal inflammation. Further, the increased prevalence of covert bacterial infections in old age (Brocklehurst *et al.*, 1968; Sourander, Ruikka and Kasanen, 1970; Kasviki-Charvati *et al.*, 1982) makes Freedman's question whether bacterial infection of the urinary tract produces serious renal disease 'only when it is associated with other conditions that are by themselves damaging to the kidney and that act to increase the susceptibility of the kidney to infection' more relevant.

Chronic pyelonephritis

From the definition, one might expect chronic pyelonephritis to be primarily a female disease since urinary tract infection predominantly affects women (Kunin, Deutscher and Pagquin, 1964; Raaschou, 1965; Kass *et al.*, 1978). Autopsy studies, however, indicate no differences in sex distribution (Freedman, 1979), so that in older people the finding of coarse kidney scarring (Asscher, 1980a) is all the more difficult to interpret.

Most of the patients are labelled with the diagnosis during the investigation of renal function, following a chance of finding of high blood urea during a check-up as a routine preoperative investigation. Symptoms are difficult to elicit and include the non-specific ones of urinary incontinence (Brocklehurst, 1984), dysuria, urine retention, polyuria, nocturia, etc.; only a few patients will present with back pain, vague abdominal pain and fever indicating perhaps renal infection. Finally, one has to mention the rare presentation with renal colic and the cases having only hypertension. When present, symptoms relate to the pathophysiology and pathology of pyelonephritis, the main points being as follows:

1. Impaired ability to concentrate urine with fairly well-preserved GFR. Bacterial multiplication starts in the medulla, causing extensive inflammatory reaction and eventually scarring, distortion of the tubular architecture and consequently interference with the medullary transport mechanism. That could easily account for some polyurias, nocturias, overt nephrogenic diabetes insipidus and electrolytic disturbances.
2. Overall reduction in renal mass due to spread of the inflammatory process to the cortical areas and extensive scarring resulting in the already mentioned coarsely scarred kidney. The obvious result is renal failure with all its complications, haematologic, endocrine and skeletal.
3. Hypertension; although this is a clinical finding it is mentioned here because it has aroused over the years much discussion as to its relationship with pyelonephritis and provoked many, as yet unanswered, questions. Starting with the view that inflammation of the renal medulla causes narrowing of vessels, which in turn results in hypertension (Weiss and Parker, 1939), one goes through the ischaemic tubular atrophy parenchymal change (Kincaid-Smith, 1955), which apparently correlates better with hypertension but is also found in many renal diseases, to the experimental data suggesting that vascular obstruction can cause pyelonephritis-like lesions in the kidneys (Freedman, 1966). There is also evidence of an hereditary factor in the development of high blood pressure in chronic pyelonephritis, and although the development of hypertension in younger age groups is widely accepted (Kass *et al.*, 1978; Wallace, Rothwell and Williams, 1978), this is more difficult to prove in older people.

Laboratory findings

A low Hb might indicate renal failure or blood loss because of haematuria. The white blood count will only help in the presence of active infection. Blood urea and creatinine will be a first step in assessing renal function and so will be the serum electrolytes in determining tubular function, although electrolytic changes might be due to concominant drug therapy, i.e. diuretics. Serum Ca and P are helpful in cases of advanced renal failure and renal osteomalacia (Berlyne, 1974). Blood glucose is mandatory since diabetes is always a possible background of pyelonephritis. The same applies to blood cultures even in the absence of clinical signs of sepsis, because bacteriuria is always a possibility (Asscher, 1980a).

Culture of the urine provides obviously the main hope of establishing an aetiological connection of pyelonephritis and presence of bacteria in the urine. Sterile urine is not an infrequent finding (Freedman, 1979; Asscher, 1980a) even among subjects known to excrete bacteria, and there is a growing awareness of the magnitude of the positive–negative turnover rate in elderly bacteriuric subjects with or without treatment (Kasviki-Charvati *et al.,* 1982; Nicolle *et al.,* 1983). The problem is further complicated by the fact that many non-bacterial causes can result into 'pyelonephritic insterstitial changes', and that bacteriuria and pyuria can often be provoked in otherwise negative urines by the use of special tests (Little and DeWardener, 1962; Dontas and Kasviki-Charvati, 1976). On the other hand, the spot prevalence of bacteriuria in old age ranges from 10 to 50 per cent, depending on the group examined (Dontas, 1984), without always a clear-cut association to an underlying interstitial renal inflammation (Angell, Relman and Robbins, 1968). The presence of antibody-coated bacteria in the urine will confirm the renal origin of the bacteria (Thomas, Shelokov and Forland, 1974).

The most common aerobic organism isolated is *Escherichia coli,* accounting for 80 per cent of the total in community cases, followed by *Klebsiella–Enterobacter, Proteus, Pseudomonas, Staph. aureus* and group D *Streptococcus.* Anaerobes, although common inhabitants of the genital area, fungi, salmonellae and tubercle bacilli are found less frequently. Numbers of colony-forming units in excess of 10^5/ml should be considered significant, but in special circumstances common in the elderly, i.e. presence of antimicrobial agents in the urine, indwelling catheter and high frequency of micturition, counts much lower than the above might be also regarded as significant (Brumfitt and Hamilton-Miller, 1984; Stark and Maki, 1984).

Routine urinalysis will be helpful. Pyuria is common but not specific and the same applies to red blood cells. Sterile pyuria should raise the suspicion of tuberculosis or analgesic nephropathy. Proteinuria up to 3 g/day is not unusual and larger amounts indicate glomerular damage, congestive heart failure or malignant hypertension. A positive intravenous pyelogram is still the evidence one always wants to have, although difficulties may arise in proving that the coarse scarring of the kidney in association with retraction of the corresponding papillae, dilatation of the calyces and reduced dye concentration locally (Hodson, 1967) is really due to the bacteria identified in the urine (Angell, Relman and Robbins, 1968; Asscher, 1980b). This is more so in old age, since the typical radiological features have been described in much younger age groups (Hodson, 1967), and such clinical combinations as drug-induced interstitial nephropathy and bladder bacteriuria are not uncommon in elderly women. Of course, pyelography is invaluable in showing anatomic defects or vesico-ureteric reflux, which may point out to the pathogenesis of the condition or lead to urological intervention.

A galaxy of methods have been used for the localization of the infection (Dontas, 1984), but have not been established in routine outpatient or inpatient use. Computed tomography, ultrasound, immunological studies and renal biopsy offer significant help in selected cases only.

Treatment

A radical approach to the management of these patients depends on the answers to three basic questions: (a) is there significant bacteriuria; (b) how impaired is the renal function; (c) is there room for surgical intervention? Detailed discussions on the last two subjects are to be found in Chapters 1, 5, 6, 9, 17 and 19. The management of bacteriuria will be discussed below, under acute pyelonephritis.

Acute pyelonephritis

This indicates that renal tissue is acutely infected (Berlyne, 1974); clinical urinary tract infection and positive urine cultures are always present, in contrast to chronic pyelonephritis. Fever, chills, back pain, costovertebral angle tenderness on the affected side, frequent and burning micturition, but also non-specific abdominal pain, nausea and vomiting and finally evidence of bacteraemia in the occasional patient, may all be present. Persistence of symptoms for more than 5 days and evidence of pleural effusion might indicate formation of a perinephric abscess (Cotran and Pennington, 1981). Any symptom combination is possible, as is complete lack of them in older confused and wasted patients 'going down hill' (Freedman, 1984).

In the case of acute pyelonephritis, the most important therapeutic priorities are the identification of the causative organism and the detection of possible local or systemic factors interfering with the body's defences, such as obstacles within the outflow tract, neoplasias, etc.

For the first priority, urine and blood cultures are essential. Collection of urine from old, confused and/or incontinent patients may necessitate catheterization or suprapubic aspiration. The interpretation of the urine culture follows the same guidelines as for chronic pyelonephritis; recent evidence indicates that very low microbial counts in the dysuric, symptomatic or catheterized patient should not be disregarded (Stamm *et al.*, 1982; Stark and Maki, 1984). Special care should be taken that the urine specimen is cultured immediately, because bacteria multiply easily at room temperature. Obviously, previous use of antibiotics might also give false negative results, as does the presence of antibacterial agents in the urine following cleansing of the peri-urethral area and non-effective rinsing. Urinalysis will usually show polymorphonuclears and red cells, and great numbers of bacteria particularly obvious under dark field microscopy. A polymorphonuclear leukocytosis is often present, but the usual tests of renal function are within normal limits, unless there is obstruction or the acute infection is superimposed on established renal pathology.

Macroscopically, the kidneys are enlarged and the pelvic mucosa is congested containing blood-stained or purulent urine (Berlyne, 1974). Microscopy reveals abscess formation and polymorphonuclear infiltration around and within the tubules. Abscesses radiate from the pelvis, forming the classical wedge-shaped abscess, eventually causing more destruction in the cortex than in the medulla (Freedman, 1979). Bacteria can sometimes be demonstrated in infectious foci. Areas of renal parenchyma between these abscesses can be spared as are glomeruli. Finally, there is evidence that vascular spasm is present in the early stages (Heptinstall, 1974) and that might be a factor in the pathogenesis of the pyelonephritic scar (Berlyne, 1974).

Treatment

Any elderly patient with bacteriuria *and* symptomatic urinary infection should be treated (Bendall, 1984). This statement is supported by accumulating evidence of increased mortality of bacteriuric subjects belonging to various age groups, particularly the elderly (Sourander, Ruikka and Kasanen, 1970; Dontas *et al.*, 1981; Evans *et al.*, 1982). Bearing in mind that the natural course of the disease is such that symptoms may subside even without therapy (Freedman, 1979; Cotran and Pennington, 1981) and that bacteraemia and shock may develop even in asymptomatic patients (Setia, Serventi and Lorenz, 1984), one should start treatment soon after a urine culture is obtained. Until the sensitivity tests are known one should probably give an aminoglycoside plus broad-spectrum penicillin for the seriously ill, bearing in mind the nephrotoxicity of the aminoglycosides, whereas sulphonamides, cephalosporins, penicillins or nalidixic acid derivatives will suffice in all others.

Treatment usually lasts for 7–10 days. It is always desirable to start intravenously and then switch to oral treatment. This regimen is usually successful but does not provide an answer as to what sort of follow-up the patient should have. Most authorities, in case of reinfection or persistence of symptoms, will try some form of long-term antimicrobial therapy, like short-acting sulphonamide, nitrofurantoin, nalidixic acid or newer quinoline derivatives such as norfloxacin. Others will prefer mandelamine which acts in the urine only. Unfortunately, none of the above has proved successful in the long run. Relapses, i.e. reappearance of the original organism, occur earlier than reinfections and require full investigation of possible causes, usually outflow obstructions, but also systemic disease, perinephric abscess, insufficient penetration of the drug into renal tissue or even laboratory error.

Finally, the answer to the question as to whether lots of fluids should be given or not is probably yes, particularly in feverish and dehydrated patients. Whether by doing so bacteria are washed out or the body's defences are improved is still an open question (Freedman, 1979). Nevertheless, the recent demonstration of reduced thirst and fluid intake in healthy elderly men, along with blunted renal response to higher levels of osmoregulated vasopressin (Editorial, 1984) would justify administration of excess fluids in order to prevent infection-induced and/or drug-induced hyperosmolar states.

Analgesic nephropathy

It is estimated that about 23 per cent of all consultations in the UK are made for 'rheumatic problems' (Nuki, 1983), and analgesic/anti-inflammatory drugs are prescribed for many of these patients; in the USA, 40 million persons or 1 in every 7, have symptoms for which such drugs might be prescribed (Clive and Stoff, 1984). This does not include subjects who use these agents for acute problems or who buy various analgesics over the counter for a variety of complaints, thus short-circuiting official channels and blocking possibilities of control in their use. Thus, we have witnessed an explosion in the development and marketing of analgesic/anti-inflammatory agents in the past 30 years: in 1978, more than 50 anti-rheumatic compounds were under investigation (Abruzzo, 1978). Since none of these agents is ideal for all rheumatic disorders, and most patients are unlikely to cope with moderate joint or muscle discomfort, proliferation of these agents will continue until radical new approaches to the control of inflammation are materialized.

In old age the ubiquitous osteoarthritis and other chronic bone and joint disorders provide the ground for a still larger proportion of users than in younger age groups; for example, an estimated 50 per cent of patients with rheumatoid arthritis are more than 50 years old (Kolodny and Klipper, 1976). As several organ systems are compromised in exactly those subjects who need and use these substances most, the search for evidence of clinical toxicity is well justified.

Habitual phenacetin intake has long been recognized as a cause of tubulo-interstitial inflammation, papillary damage and renal failure; further, uro-epithelial neoplasms and increased mortality from renal or cardiovascular causes are also well known (Spühler and Zollinger, 1950; Shelley, 1967; Bell *et al.*, 1969; Gault, Blennerhassett and Muehrcke, 1971; Dubach *et al.*, 1975; Bengtsson, Johannson and Angervall, 1978; Editorial, 1981; Dubach *et al.*, 1983). These adverse effects have not been limited to users of phenacetin combinations with aspirin and caffeine. As newer non-steroidal analgesic anti-inflammatory and antipyretic drugs (NSAIDs) have proliferated so have publications about their side effects from the gastrointestinal tract, and other dire consequences, allergic, haematologic, neuropathic, hepatic, etc. (Simon and Mills, 1980). The 'analgesic syndrome' includes anaemia, gastrointestinal symptoms, and ulceration, hypertension and psychoneurotic personality.

The nephropathy related to chronic analgesic intake is said to account for 10–15 per cent of all cases of chronic renal failure in reviews from Nottingham, UK (Dombey, Sagar and Knapp, 1975; Cove-Smith and Knapp, 1978), and in 15–20 per cent of patients entering maintenance dialysis and transplant programmes in Australia (Stewart, 1978). There seem to be large geographical differences in prevalence, however, both between countries and within each country, which differences are not easily accounted for on the basis of varying diagnostic habits; for example whereas one-third of fatal renal failure cases in Australia are related to analgesic intake (Ferguson, 1974), in Switzerland where analgesic nephropathy was first described these do not exceed 1.5 per cent of autopsies (Gloor, 1960), and in Liverpool, among 18 866 necropsies between 1961 and 1967, only 0.16 per cent could be so ascribed (Davies, Kennedy and Roberts, 1970).

Further, within Australia the yearly rate of end-stage renal failure due to papillary necrosis from analgesics varies between 0 and 8.4 per million, and regular analgesic consumption between 3 and 16 per cent of the population. In general, higher rates are found in areas with higher consumption, and warmer Australian areas have higher rates than more temperate ones. Further factors which have to be considered are the patterns of use and differences in the compounds absorbed (Kincaid-Smith, 1970).

Analgesic nephropathy is probably more frequent in old age than it appears from the above overall rates. Greater difficulties are met in obtaining an accurate history of prolonged analgesic intake from poor informants, and frequent acute urinary tract infections with more obvious clinical features complicate the picture. Thus, treatment may be directed against the secondary infection while disregarding the primary disease. More than 70 per cent of the published cases of analgesic nephropathy after 1980 concern subjects aged 60 and above, and in the detailed review by Cove-Smith and Knapp (1978), 27 of the 55 cases were older than 60 years.

Non-steroidal anti-inflammatory agents

All major classes of NSAIDs have been documented as able to induce adverse renal effects (Clive and Stoff, 1984). Drugs implicated include salicylates, phenacetin, phenylpropionic acid derivatives (fenoprofen, ibuprofen, naproxen, benoxaprofen), indoleacetic acid derivatives (indomethacin, sulindac), phenylacetic acid derivatives (diclofenac, phenclofenac), pyrrolacetic acid derivatives (tolmetin, zomepirac), anthranilic acid derivatives (meclofenamate, mefenamic acid), pyrazolone derivatives (phenylbutazone, oxyphenbutazone) (Morales and Steyn, 1971) and oxicams (piroxicam). The type of renal dysfunction, however, and the conditions under which adverse effects may occur, are only recently beginning to become clear.

The anti-inflammatory properties of NSAIDs appear to be related to their common ability to inhibit cyclo-oxygenase, a major enzyme in the biosynthesis of all prostaglandins from arachidonic acid (Vane, 1971). NSAIDs also inhibit 11- and 15-lipoxygenase which lead to leukotriene formation, additional metabolic products of arachidonic acid (Randall *et al.*, 1980). Finally, they interfere with leukocyte migration and function (Goodwin, 1984).

Renal release of prostaglandins is among the chief mechanisms which the body employs to prevent renal ischaemia under such adverse conditions as hypovolaemia, salt depletion, congestive heart failure, and other states associated with high adrenergic activity. In all these states, and in several animal experiments mimicking these common clinical conditions, intrarenal prostaglandin release helps maintain effective levels of renal blood flow and GFR, thus preventing pre-renal azotaemia. Inhibition of this protective mechanism by NSAIDs can reduce renal plasma flow and GFR, thus leading to an acute renal failure when superimposed on a background of borderline renal efficiency.

Under normal haemodynamic conditions the role of prostaglandins in renal autoregulation appears to be minimal: healthy, unstressed humans receiving aspirin acutely (Berg, 1977b) or for prolonged periods (Muther and Bennett, 1980) evidence no changes in GFR or renal plasma flow. After severe sodium restriction in young volunteers, only moderate decreases in GFR (12–15 per cent) have been observed (Muther, Potter and Bennett, 1981). In patients with uncomplicated rheumatoid arthritis, chronic ingestion of aspirin (5–27 kg over 4–40 years) appears not to have influenced GFR but to have provoked small but significant losses of concentrating capacity (Burry *et al.*, 1976; Akyol, Thompson and Kerr, 1982). In patients, however, with diminished GFR and renal plasma flow, severe reductions of GFR and azotaemia may result (Berg, 1977a; Kimberly and Plotz, 1977; Clive and Stoff, 1984). Thus, the intrarenal activity of the renin–angiotensin system, local prostaglandin E and sodium balance appear to be decisive factors in the haemodynamic response to aspirin.

In contrast to the above chronic reductions in GFR, severe acute oliguric renal failure with hyperkalaemia has been frequently reported in recent years following indomethacin administration in gout (Walshe and Venuto, 1979; Findling *et al.*, 1980; Galler, Folkert and Schlondorff, 1981; McCarthy *et al.*, 1982; Blackshear, Davidman and Stillman, 1983), and with other NSAIDs as well (Torres, 1982; Frais, Burgess and Mitchell, 1983). This type of acute ischaemic failure is not accompanied by either proteinuria or significant tubular dysfunction and is attributed to sudden GFR decreases in volume-contracted subjects with moderate baseline renal insufficiency. The severe hyperkalaemia and azotaemia may require haemodialysis.

An ischaemic lesion which differs from that related to prostaglandin inhibition occurs with phenacetin, whose major metabolite, *N*-acetaminophen (NAPAP, paracetamol) accumulates in the renal medulla. Such deposits lead to oxidative damage to the medullary vasa recta (wall thickening) of the loops of Henle with secondary fibrosis throughout the papilla. Another metabolite, paraphenetidin, leads to methaemoglobin and sulphhaemoglobin formation, and subsequently to haemolysis and intratubular accumulation of haemosiderin (Murray and Goldberg, 1976). The combined intratubular and peritubular ischaemic insults result in papillary necrosis (Kincaid-Smith *et al.*, 1968; Gloor, 1978).

A third, much rarer type of NSAID-related nephropathy is an acute allergic interstitial reaction with eosinophilia and renal failure (Venning, Dixon and Oliver, 1980; Katz *et al.*, 1981; Woods and Michael, 1981). Finally, a fourth type, seen with almost all NSAIDs, is that of interstitial nephropathy with renal failure and heavy proteinuria (Curt *et al.*, 1980; Gary, Dodelson and Eisinger, 1980; Wendland, Wagoner and Holley, 1980; Miller, Schorr and Lacher, 1983; Bender *et al.*, 1984; Clive and Stoff, 1984). This last pattern has a delayed onset after weeks or months of therapy and tends to improve gradually after the offending agent is discontinued. It has recently been suggested that these four types represent different points on a continuum (Bender *et al.*, 1984).

'Women comprise some 60 to 85% of terminal renal failure due to analgesics, a distinctly higher proportion than might be expected from the sex ratio of analgesic abuse in Australia' (Stewart, 1978). Further, among cases of reversible nephropathy related to NSAIDs and published since 1980, the ratio of women to men remains at 2:1, with about 71 per cent of the cases being subjects over 60. Stewart reasons that this predilection of women is related to the higher consumption of more potent 'powders' compared to tablets by Australian women, the higher fluid intake by men (beer), and the higher rates of bacteriuria in women at all ages. Bacteriuria in old age, however, is only barely more prevalent in women than in men, the ratio being about 1.2:1.0 in various groups (Dontas, 1984).

To the present authors, more important factors than higher prevalence of bacteriuria in women are (a) the heavier load of analgesic metabolites reaching the distal nephron in women, and (b) possible auto-immune reaction initiated by damaged proximal tubular cells. GFR is reduced in old age more importantly in men than in women, and the presence of infection further accentuates this trend; thus, filtered load of any substance will be heavier in the more intact female kidney with resulting higher amounts of NSAID glucuronates reaching the medulla (Gloor, 1978). If urine flow does not remain at a satisfactory level, the concentration of toxic metabolic products will affect those subjects with more intact proximal nephronal function, i.e. women. This view presupposes a lesser fluid intake among women which may be true in certain countries, e.g. Australia (Stewart, 1978). The sensation of thirst is reduced in old age (Phillips *et al.*, 1984), but we know of no data indicating systematic sex differences in drinking habits. Similarly, the more marked toxicity from gentamicin in women (Kourilsky *et al.*, 1982; Moore *et al.*, 1984) indicates gender-related differences in auto-immune or chemotactic reaction to substances released by damaged proximal tubular cells.

Treatment and evolution

If diagnosed before far advanced renal damage has occurred, analgesic nephropathy is always treatable, provided the offending agent is withdrawn (Burry, 1967). Beyond a level of serum creatinine of 300–400 μmol/l, however, renal failure of whatever aetiology inexorably progresses to total kidney failure (Rutherford *et al.*, 1977). Of course, all potentially damaging medications must be stopped and no analgesic whatsoever should be substituted for the implicated agent (Kincaid-Smith, 1970). Occasional reports where renal function has improved following discontinuation of one drug (mefenamic acid) while retaining another (indomethacin; Woods and Michael, 1981) should not become guidelines for the practitioner.

Since bacterial infection is a common complication of late stages of analgesic nephropathy, chemotherapy with non-nephrotoxic agents will remove an important factor accelerating the underlying renovascular disease, even though immediate improvement of GFR post-chemotherapy has not been documented so far. Immediate effects on blood urea among elderly dehydrated subjects can be observed following rehydration, since fluid loss is an early feature of analgesic nephropathy. Anti-hypertensive therapy, and such experimental efforts as prostaglandin E infusions (Niwa *et al.*, 1982), might also improve the renovascular status of occasional patients: the most important measure for the practitioner, however, is to keep in mind this aetiologic possibility for the many elderly subjects presenting with concentration defects, variable azotaemia and negative urine cultures.

The recent success of measures taken in Scandinavia and Canada, where phenacetin has been removed from most analgesic mixtures, proves that this serious nephropathy can be conquered. Those dealing with elderly patients should ensure that phenacetin nephropathy is not replaced by nephropathy from newer NSAIDs.

Other drug-induced interstitial nephropathies

Many drugs have been implicated in the development of interstitial nephropathies through a hypersensitivity reaction. Most cases appear *acutely* and are accompanied by renal insufficiency in subjects without known history of renal disease. Offending agents include antibiotics, particularly penicillin derivatives, sulphonamides, anticoagulants, diuretics, anticonvulsants, allopurinol, azathioprine, and various metals (Heptinstall, 1976). By far the majority of cases, however, have followed treatment with one of six drugs: methicillin, penicillin G, ampicillin, rifampicin, phenindione and lithium. It must be stressed that various offending factors are operating in patients receiving these agents, usually infections, and that non-pyelonephritic interstitial nephropathy was known before the above drugs were in use. Thus, the cause-and-effect relation of these drugs with suddenly appearing renal dysfunction in an elderly patient is difficult to prove and most reported cases have been diagnosed through renal biopsies.

The disease occurs about 2 weeks after initiation of therapy with the penicillins; it appears later with the last three agents. It is characterized by recurrence of fever after the defervescence from the infection for which the antibiotic was given. Methicillin nephropathy occurs commonly in male patients, with a slight predilection for older subjects: 32 per cent of the 72 cases reviewed by Ditlove *et al.* (1977) were 60 years or older. Younger patients exhibit this reaction in a milder form, rates of renal failure being 60 and 13 per cent, respectively, for age groups above and below 16. Further features include haematuria, proteinuria and hypertension as evidence of glomerular damage; skin rashes and blood eosinophilia; and acidosis, natriuresis and hyperkalaemia as specific signs of the tubular malfunction. As with NSAIDs, if azotaemia is absent recovery occurs within days of the discontinuation of methicillin therapy; azotaemic patients will recover usually within a few weeks, a period which can be greatly shortened by prednisone treatment (Galpin *et al.*, 1978).

There are few data as to the relative risk of methicillin nephropathy in patients receiving this antibiotic. In published cases, both the daily dose and the total amounts given have been within the recommended range. Patients receiving methicillin for prolonged periods, however, do so for severe staphylococcal osteomyelitis, endocarditis or bacteraemia. Newer penicillins and cephalosporins appear less prone to induce such reactions, but it is wise for the practitioner employing these agents to keep in mind this possible side effect (Knollen and Abernathy, 1977).

Among *chronic* interstitial nephropathies, the one due to lithium occupies a prominent place because of the popularity which this highly efficacious agent enjoys in the treatment and prevention of recurrence of manic-depressive illness. Schou (1981) estimates that 1 person out of every 1000 of the population in North Europe and USA is on lithium treatment. An early effect of ingestion of lithium salts is the inability of the collecting ducts to respond to vasopressin. Thus, a decreased concentrating ability with preserved dilution capacity and GFR are expected findings in short-term treatment. Since lithium therapy is by necessity a long-term procedure, its ulterior effects have been carefully scrutinized.

In patients treated for an average of 6 years, Hansen *et al.* (1979) found the expected impairment in concentration in over one-quarter of them, and a typical picture of chronic interstitial nephropathy with cysts in 40 per cent of obtained biopsies. Occasionally, frank diabetes insipidus persisting long after withdrawal of lithium has been reported (Simon, Garber and Arieff, 1977). Important glomerular damage and azotaemia, yet, rarely occur even when lithium is given for many years, according to various Scandinavian reports (Hansen *et al.*, 1979; Vestergaard *et al.*, 1979). Concentration defects are present anyway in depressed subjects untreated by lithium (Ellis, Coppen and Glen, 1971), but are more prominent in subjects receiving both lithium and neuroleptics (Bucht *et al.*, 1980).

As in many similar cases in the elderly, it is difficult to assess the relative importance of baseline pathology and of additional drugs in the development of lithium nephropathy. The majority of lithium-treated patients start at a young age but remain under therapy for the rest of their lives, commonly with additional neuroleptics, so that nephrotoxicity may become clinically significant. Other side effects, e.g. memory deterioration and electro-encephalographic abnormalities, are also important in old age (Christodoulou *et al.*, 1981) and may necessitate withdrawal of lithium and replacing it with alternative methods of prophylaxis, such as carbamazepine or sleep deprivation (Christodoulou *et al.*, 1978). It is important to note that no fatalities have been reported from lithium nephropathy, whereas suicides are frequent after sudden interruption of this agent.

Balkan nephropathy

This rare disorder, which is exclusively seen in the Danube basin, is still a mystery as far as its aetiology is concerned. It affects the 30–60 age group, so that it infrequently presents a diagnostic problem in older age. Patients are usually well and symptoms are insidious apart from those of progressing interstitial nephropathy. Progression to terminal renal failure is rapid, however, and 50 per cent survival after diagnosis is only 2 years. Tubular proteinuria is the first functional defect, most of the protein being of low molecular weight (e.g. β_2-microglobulin). Macroscopically, the kidneys are very small, while microscopy shows tubular atrophy and fibrosis without much cell infiltration. Recent evidence reviewed by Cotran (1981) points to a slow viral infection as a possible aetiological factor, although long-term sporadic influence of mycotoxins from fungal contamination of food has also been implicated. Increased incidence of transitional papilloma and carcinoma of pelvis and ureters has been found in these people. The combination of interstitial nephropathy, papillary necrosis and carcinoma is similar to that seen in analgesic nephropathy. Treatment is supportive only and most patients not on dialysis inevitably succumb to their disease.

Miscellaneous

Uric acid nephropathy

Uric acid crystal deposition can cause two types of renal damage. The first one is due to acute tubular obstruction by the crystals and results in acute renal failure. The most common cause is chemotherapy of different neoplastic diseases and the subsequent release of large amounts of uric acid. Oliguria, crystalluria and haematuria are usually present and diagnostic confirmation is possible if a uric acid : creatinine ratio of >1 is found in a random urine sample. Treatment includes increased water intake, alkalinization of urine, decrease of uric acid formation, and dialysis if necessary. Renal failure is usually reversible.

The second one is due to a prolonged hyperuricaemia and correlates well with uric acid serum levels. Crystals are detected in both the tubules and interstitium, surrounded by inflammatory cells and fibrosis. Blood vessels are also affected, but the nephrosclerotic changes that are found are probably due to coexistent diseases (hypertension, diabetes). Renal function is impaired in the usual fashion (mild proteinuria, loss of concentrating ability with normal GFR), ending in frank renal failure with time.

A third syndrome due to uric acid stones is discussed in Chapter 18.

Myeloma

Precipitation of paraprotein (light-chain) in the distal tubules and the collecting system causes obstruction and initiates interstitial inflammation resulting in renal failure (myeloma kidney). Amyloidosis, hypercalcaemia and recurrent infection are other factors that can cause chronic renal failure in myeloma patients. Not so frequent but more dangerous can be the acute failure as a result of dehydration, intravenous pyelography and the above-mentioned hyperuricaemia following chemotherapy. Treatment is supportive and prognosis depends largely on the nature of the main disease. Fifty per cent of myeloma patients presenting with blood urea >80 mg/100 ml will die in the next 10 weeks (DeWardener, 1973), unless dialysis is instituted; survival on long-term dialysis is poor.

Immune complex associated interstitial inflammation

This is frequently seen in autoimmune disorders, although glomerular damage is the rule. In systemic lupus erythematosus, extraglomerular involvement has been reported in different series up to 69 per cent (Tu and Shearn, 1967; Lehman, Wilson and Dixon, 1975). This is more evident in Sjögren's syndrome where interstitial infiltration by lymphocytes and plasma cells similar to the infiltration that occurs in a number of exocrine glands (Sicca syndrome) causes progressive renal functional impairment, the main features of which are inability to concentrate and acidify the urine. The renal insufficiency is rather mild and rarely uraemia is the cause of death.

Heavy metals

The role of heavy metals in inducing interstitial nephritis is not clearly defined, but may be much more common than is assumed. *Lead* in particular is capable of inducing severe chronic tubulointerstitial damage which may be progressive even after exposure has stopped (Wedeen and Batuman, 1984).

Despite their common occurrence, interstitial nephropathies are still under-recognized in old age compared to glomerular diseases. This may reflect their relative sparing of glomerular function and the really few clinically striking symptoms apart from polyuria in the chronic forms. The well-known reduction of GFR with advancing age and the numerous extrarenal factors which may additionally induce azotaemic episodes, act to focus the attention of the physician to proximal nephron pathology. Finally, the ubiquitous urinary tract infections with their eye-catching evidences of pyuria and bacteriuria draw the attention of the geriatrician chiefly to the infectious component of interstitial nephropathies which may be just grafted upon previous serious pathology. The purpose of this chapter has been to alert physicians to the strong possibilities of interstitial nephropathies being present in elderly subjects from causes other than infection and renovascular sclerosis.

References

ABRUZZO, J.L. (1978). Newer anti-rheumatic drugs. *Annals of Internal Medicine,* **89,** 132–133

AKYOL, S.M., THOMPSON, M. and KERR, D.N.S. (1982). Renal function after prolonged consumption of aspirin. *British Medical Journal,* **i,** 631–632

ANGELL, M.E., RELMAN, A.S. and ROBBINS, S.L. (1968). 'Active' chronic pyelonephritis without evidence of bacterial infection. *New England Journal of Medicine,* **278,** 1303–1305

ASSCHER, A.W. (1980a). *The Challenge of Urinary Tract Infections.* London; Academic Press

ASSCHER, A. (1980b). Urinary tract infection. *Journal of the Royal College of Physicians of London,* **15,** 232–238

BELL, D., KERR, D.N.S., SWINNEY, J. and YEATES, W.K. (1969). Analgesic nephropathy: clinical course after withdrawal of phenacetin. *British Medical Journal,* **iii,** 378–382

BENDALL, M.I. (1984). A review of urinary tract infection in the elderly. *Journal of Antimicrobial Chemotherapy,* **13,** Suppl. B, 69–78

BENDER, W.L., WHELTON, A., BESHORNER, W.E., DARWISH, M.O., HALL-CRAGGS, M. and SOLEZ, K. (1984). Interstitial nephritis, proteinuria and renal failure caused by nonsteroidal anti-inflammatory drugs. *American Journal of Medicine,* **76,** 1006–1012

BENGTSSON, U., JOHANNSON, S. and ANGERVALL, L. (1978). Malignancies of the urinary tract and their relation to analgesic abuse. *Kidney International,* **13,** 107–113

BERG, K.Z. (1977a). Acute effects of acetylsalicylic acid in patients with chronic renal insufficiency. *European Journal of Clinical Pharmacology,* **11,** 111–116

BERG, K.Z. (1977b). Acute effects of acetylsalicylic acid on renal function in normal man. *European Journal of Clinical Pharmacology,* **11,** 117–123

BERLYNE, G.M. (1974). *A Course in Renal Disease.* Oxford; Blackwell

BLACKSHEAR, J.L., DAVIDMAN, M. and STILLMAN, M.T. (1983). Identification of risk for renal insufficiency from nonsteroidal anti-inflammatory drugs. *Archives of Internal Medicine,* **143,** 1130–1134

BRICKER, N.S., FINE, L.G., KAPLAN, M., EPSTEIN, M., BOURGOIGNIE, J.J. and LIGHT, A. (1978). 'Magnification phenomenon' in chronic renal disease. *New England Journal of Medicine,* **299,** 1287–1293

BROCKLEHURST, J.C. (1984). Ageing, bladder function and incontinence. In *Urology in the Elderly,* edited by J.C. Brocklehurst, pp. 1–18. Edinburgh; Churchill Livingstone

BROCKLEHURST, J.C., DILLANE, J.B., GRIFFITHS, L. and FRY, J. (1968). The prevalence and symptomatology of urinary tract infection in an aged population. *Gerontologia Clinica,* **10,** 242–253

BRUMFITT, W. and HAMILTON-MILLER, J.M.T. (1984). A review of the problem of urinary tract infection management and the evaluation of a potential new antibiotic. *Journal of Antimicrobial Chemotherapy,* **13,** Suppl. B, 121–133

BUCHT, G., WAHLIN, A., WENTZEL, T. and WINBLAD, B. (1980). Renal function and morphology in long-term lithium and combined lithium–neuroleptic treatment. *Acta Medica Scandinavica,* **208,** 381–385

BURRY, A.F. (1967). The evolution of analgesic nephropathy. *Nephron,* **5,** 185–190

BURRY, H.C., DIEPPE, P.A., BRESNIHAN, F.B. and BROWN, C. (1976). Salicylates and renal function in rheumatoid arthritis. *British Medical Journal,* **1,** 613–615

CHRISTODOULOU, G.N., KOKKEVI, A., LYKOURAS, E.P., STEFANIS, C.N. and PAPADIMITRIOU, G.N. (1981). Effects of lithium on memory. *American Journal of Psychiatry,* **138,** 847–848

CHRISTODOULOU, G.N., MALLIARAS, D.F., LYKOURAS, E.P., PAPADIMITRIOU, G.N. and STEFANIS, C.N. (1978). Possible prophylactic effect of sleep deprivation. *American Journal of Psychiatry,* **135,** 375–376

CLIVE, D.M. and STOFF, J.S. (1984). Renal syndromes associated with nonsteroidal anti-inflammatory drugs. *New England Journal of Medicine,* **310,** 563–572

COTRAN, R.S., RUBIN, R.H. and TOLKOFF-RUBIN, N. (1986). Tubulointerstitial diseases. In *The Kidney,* 3rd edn, edited by B.M. Brenner and F.C. Rector, pp. 1143–1174. Philadelphia; Saunders

COVE-SMITH, J.R. and KNAPP, M.S. (1978). Analgesic nephropathy: an important cause of chronic renal failure. *Quarterly Journal of Medicine,* **47,** 49–69

CURT, G.A., KALDANY, A., WHITLEY, L.G., CROSSON, A.W., ROLLA, A., MERINO, M. *et al.* (1980). Reversible rapidly progressive renal failure with nephrotic syndrome due to fenoprofen calcium. *Annals of Internal Medicine,* **92,** 72–73

DAVIES, D.J., KENNEDY, A. and ROBERTS, C. (1970). The aetiology of renal medullary necrosis: a survey of adult cases in Liverpool. *Journal of Pathology,* **100,** 257–268

DE WARDENER, H.E. (1973). *The Kidney.* London; Churchill

DITLOVE, J., WEIDMANN, P., BERNSTEIN, M. and MASSRY, S.G. (1977). Methicillin nephritis. *Medicine,* **56,** 483–491

DOMBEY, S.L., SAGAR, D. and KNAPP, M.S. (1975). Chronic renal failure in Nottingham and requirements for dialysis and transplant facilities. *British Medical Journal,* **ii,** 484–485

DONTAS, A.S. (1984). Urinary tract infections and their implications. In *Urology in the Elderly,* edited by J.C. Brocklehurst, pp. 162–192. Edinburgh; Churchill Livingstone

DONTAS, A.S. and KASVIKI-CHARVATI, P. (1976). Significance of diuresis-provoked bacteriuria. *Journal of Infectious Diseases,* **134,** 174–180

DONTAS, A.S., KASVIKI-CHARVATI, P., PAPANAYIOTOU, P.C. and MARKETOS, S.G. (1981). Bacteriuria and survival in old age. *New England Journal of Medicine,* **304,** 939–943

DONTAS, A.S., MARKETOS, S.G. and PAPANAYIOTOU, P. (1972). Mechanisms of renal tubular defects in old age. *Postgraduate Medical Journal,* **48,** 295–303

DUBACH, U.C., LEVY, P.S., ROSNER, B., BAUMELER, H.R., MÜLLER, A., PEIER, A. *et al.* (1975). Relation between regular intake of phenacetin-containing analgesics and laboratory evidence for urorenal disorders in a working female population of Switzerland. *Lancet,* **i,** 539–543

DUBACH, U.C., ROSNER, B. and PFISTER, E. (1983). Epidemiologic study of abuse of analgesics containing phenacetin. *New England Journal of Medicine,* **308,** 357–362

EDITORIAL (1981). Analgesic nephropathy. *British Medical Journal,* **i,** 339–340

EDITORIAL (1984). Thirst and osmoregulation in the elderly. *Lancet,* **ii,** 1017–1018

ELLIS, C.G., COPPEN, A. and GLEN, A.I.M. (1971). Urine concentration in depressive illness. *Journal of Neurology, Neurosurgery and Psychiatry,* **34,** 30–31

EVANS, D.A., KASS, E.H., HENNEKENS, C.H., ROSNER, B., MIAO, L., KENDRICK, M.I. *et al.* (1982). Bacteriuria and subsequent mortality in women. *Lancet,* **i,** 156–158

FERGUSON, I. (1974). How safe are analgesics? The Queensland experience. *Australian and New Zealand Journal of Medicine,* **2,** 603

FINDLING, G.W., BECKSTROM, D., RAWSTHORNE, L., KOZIN, F. and ITSKOVITA, H. (1980). Indomethacin induced hyperkalemia in three patients with gouty arthritis. *Journal of the American Medical Association,* **244,** 1127–1128

FRAIS, M.A., BURGESS, E.D. and MITCHELL, L.B. (1983). Piroxicam-induced renal failure and hyperkalaemia. *Annals of Internal Medicine,* **99,** 129–130

FREEDMAN, L.R. (1966). Experimental pyelonephritis. XII, Changes mimicking chronic pyelonephritis as a consequence of renal vascular occlusion in the rat. *Yale Journal of Biology and Medicine,* **39,** 113–117

FREEDMAN, L.R. (1979). Interstitial renal inflammation, including pyelonephritis and urinary tract infection. In *Strauss and Welt's Diseases of the Kidney,* **2,** 817–876. Boston; Little, Brown

FREEDMAN, L.R. (1984). Urinary tract infection in the elderly. *New England Journal of Medicine,* **309,** 1451–1452

GALLER, M., FOLKERT, V.W. and SCHLONDORFF, D. (1981). Reversible acute renal insufficiency and hyperkalemia following indomethacin therapy. *Journal of the American Medical Association,* **246,** 154–155

GALPIN, J.E., SHINABERGER, J.H., STANLEY, T.M., BLUMENKRANTZ, M.J., BAYER, A.S., FRIEDMAN, G.S. *et al.* (1978). Acute interstitial nephritis due to methicillin. *The American Journal of Medicine,* **65,** 756–765

GARY, N.S., DODELSON, R. and EISINGER, R.P. (1980). Indomethacin associated acute renal failure. *The American Journal of Medicine,* **65,** 135–136

GAULT, M.H., BLENNERHASSETT, J. and MUEHRCKE, R.C. (1971). Analgesic nephropathy: a clinicopathologic study using electron microscopy. *The American Journal of Medicine,* **51,** 740–756

GLOOR, F. (1960). Über verschiedene Formen der Papillennekrosen der Nieren. *Pathologie und Microbiologie,* **23,** 263–271

GLOOR, F.G. (1978). Changing concepts in pathogenesis and morphology of analgesic nephropathy as seen in Europe. *Kidney Internationa1,* **132,** 27–33

GOODWIN, J.S. (1984). Mechanism of action of nonsteroidal anti-inflammatory agents. *The American Journal of Medicine,* **77**(1A), 57–64

HANSEN, H.E., HESTBECH, J., SØRENSEN, J.L., NØRGAARD, K., HEILSKOV, J. and AMDISEN, A. (1979). Chronic interstitial nephropathy in patients on long-term lithium treatment. *Quarterly Journal of Medicine,* **NS 48,** 577–591

HEPTINSTALL, R.H. (1974). *Pathology of the Kidney.* Boston; Little, Brown

HEPTINSTALL, R.H. (1976). Interstitial nephritis: a review. *American Journal of Pathology,* **83,** 214–236

HODSON, G.L. (1967). The radiological contribution toward the diagnosis of chronic pyelonephritis. *Radiology,* **88,** 857–866

KASS, E.H. (1978). Horatio at the orifice. The significance of bacteriuria. *Journal of Infectious Diseases,* **138,** 546–557

KASS, E.H., MIALL, W.E., STUART, K.L. and ROSNER, B. (1978). Epidemiologic aspects of infections of the urinary tract. In *Infections of the Urinary Tract,* edited by E.H. Kass and W. Brumfitt, pp. 1–7. Chicago; The University of Chicago Press

KASVIKI-CHARVATI, P., DROLETTE-KEFAKIS, B., PAPANAYIOTOU, P.C. and DONTAS, A.S. (1982). Turnover of bacteriuria in old age. *Age and Ageing,* **11,** 169–174

KATZ, S.M., CAPALDO, R., EVERTS, E.A. and DiGREGORIO, J.G. (1981). Tolmetin; association with reversible renal failure and acute interstitial nephritis. *The Journal of the American Medical Association,* **246,** 243–245

KIMBERLY, R.P. and PLOTZ, P.H. (1977). Aspirin-induced depression of renal function. *New England Journal of Medicine,* **296,** 418–424

KINCAID-SMITH, P. (1955). Vascular obstruction in chronic pyelonephritic kidneys and its relation to hypertension. *Lancet,* **ii,** 1263–1265

KINCAID-SMITH, P. (1970). Analgesic nephropathy. *British Medical Journal,* **ii,** 618

KINCAID-SMITH, P., SAKER, B.M., McKENZIE, I.F.C. and MURIDEN, K.D. (1968). Lesions in the blood supply of the papilla in experimental analgesic nephropathy. *Medical Journal of Australia,* **1,** 203–206

KNOLLEN, C.E. and ABERNATHY, R. (1977). Nephropathy associated with methicillin therapy. *Archives of Internal Medicine,* **137,** 997–1000

KOLODNY, A.L. and KLIPPER, A.R. (1976). Bone and joint diseases in the elderly. *Hospital Practice,* **11,** 91–101

KOURISLSKY, O., SOLEZ, K., MOREL-MAROGER, L., WHELTON, A., DUHOUX, P. and SRAER, J.D. (1982). The pathology of acute renal failure due to interstitial nephritis in man with comments on the role of interstitial inflammation and sex in gentamicin nephrotoxicity. *Medicine,* **61,** 258–268

KUNIN, C.M., DEUTSCHER, R. and PAGQUIN, A.J. (1964). Urinary tract infection in school children: an epidemiologic clinical and laboratory study. *Medicine,* **43,** 91–130

LEHMAN, D.H., WILSON, C.B. and DIXON, F.J. (1975). Extraglomerular immunoglobin deposits in human nephritis. *The American Journal of Medicine,* **58,** 765–786

LITTLE, P.J. and DE WARDENER, H.E. (1962). The use of prednisolone phosphate in the diagnosis of pyelonephritis in man. *Lancet,* **i,** 1145–1146

McCARTHY, J.T., TORRES, V., ROMERO, J.C., WOCHOS, D.N. and VELOSA, J.A. (1982). Acute intrinsic renal failure induced by indomethacin. *Mayo Clinic Proceedings,* **57,** 289–296

MILLER, F.C., SCHORR, W.J. and LACHER, J.W. (1983). Zomepirac-induced renal failure. *Archives of Internal Medicine,* **143,** 1171–1173

MOORE, R.D., SMITH, C.R., LIPSKY, J.J., MELLITS, E.D. and LIETMAN, P.S. (1984). Risk factors for nephrotoxicity in patients treated with aminoglycosides. *Annals of Internal Medicine,* **100,** 352–357

MORALES, A. and STEYN, L. (1971). Papillary necrosis following phenyl-butazone ingestion. *Archives of Surgery,* **103,** 420–422

MURRAY, T. and GOLDBERG, M. (1976). Analgesic abuse and renal disease. *Annual Review of Medicine,* **26,** 537–550

MUTHER, R.S. and BENNETT, W.M. (1980). Effects of aspirin on glomerular filtration rate in normal humans. *Annals of Internal Medicine,* **92,** 386–387

MUTHER, R.S., POTTER, D.M. and BENNETT, W.M. (1981). Aspirin-induced depression of glomerular filtration rate in normal humans: role of sodium balance. *Annals of Internal Medicine,* **94,** 317–321

NICOLLE, L.E., BJORNSON, J., HARDING, G.K.M. and MACDONNELL, J.A. (1983). Bacteriuria in elderly institutionalized men. *New England Journal of Medicine,* **309,** 1420–1424

NIWA, T., MAEDA, K., NAOTSUKA, Y., ASADA, H., KOBAYASHI, S., YOKOHANA, M. *et al.* (1982). Improvement of renal function with prostaglandin E_1 infusion in patients with chronic renal disease. *Lancet,* **i,** 687

NUKI, G. (1983). Non-steroidal analgesic and anti-inflammatory agents. *British Medical Journal,* **287,** 39–43

PHILLIPS, P.A., ROLLS, B.J., LEDINGHAM, J.G.G., FORSLING, M.L., MORTON, J.J., CROWE, M.J. *et al.* (1984). Reduced thirst after water deprivation in healthy elderly men. *New England Journal of Medicine,* **311,** 753–759

RAASCHOU, F. (1965). Definition of chronic pyelonephritis. In *Progress in Pyelonephritis,* edited by E.H. Kass, pp. 373–375. Philadelphia; Davis

RANDALL, R.W., EAKINS, K.E., HIGGS, G.A., SALMON, J.A. and TATESON, J.E. (1980). Inhibition of arachidonic acid cyclo-oxygenase and lipoxygenase activities of leukocytes by indomethacin and compound BW755C. *Agents Actions,* **10,** 553–555

RUBIN, R.H., TOLKOFF-RUBIN, N.E. and COTRAN, R.S. (1986). Urinary tract infection, pyelonephritis and reflux nephropathy. In *The Kidney,* 3rd edn, edited by B.M. Brenner and F.C. Rector, pp. 1085–1142. Philadelphia; Saunders

RUTHERFORD, W.E., BLONDIN, J., MILLER, J.P., GREENWALT, A.S. and VAVRA, J.D. (1977). Chronic progressive renal disease: rate of change of serum creatinine concentration. *Kidney International,* **11,** 62–70

SCHOU, M. (1981). Problems of lithium prophylaxis: efficacy, serum lithium, selection of patients. In *Aspects of Preventive Psychiatry,* edited by G.N. Christodoulou; *Bibliotheca Psychiatrica,* Vol. 160, pp. 30–37. Basel; Karger

SETIA, U., SERVENTI, I. and LORENZ, P. (1984). Bacteremia in a long-term care facility; spectrum and mortality. *Archives of Internal Medicine,* **144,** 1633–1635

SHELLEY, J.H. (1967). Phenacetin: through the looking glass. *Clinical Pharmacology and Therapeutics,* **8,** 427–429

SIMON, N.M., GARBER, E. and ARIEFF, A.J. (1977). Persistent nephrogenic diabetes insipidus after lithium carbonate. *Annals of Internal Medicine,* **86,** 446–447

SIMON, L.S. and MILLS, J.A. (1980). Nonsteroidal anti-inflammatory drugs. *New England Journal of Medicine,* **302,** 1179–1185, 1237–1243

SOURANDER, L.B., RUIKKA, I. and KASANEN, A. (1970). A health survey on the aged with a five-year follow-up. *Acta Socio-Medica Scandinavica,* Suppl. 3, 5–40

SPÜHLER, O. and ZOLLINGER, H.W. (1950). Die chronische interstitielle Nephritis. *Helvetica Medica Acta,* **17,** 564–567

STAMM, W.E., COUNTS, G.W., RUNNING, K.R., FIHN, S., TÜRCK, M. and HOLMES, K.K. (1982). Diagnosis of coliform infection in acutely dysuric women. *New England Journal of Medicine,* **307,** 463–468

STARK, R.P. and MAKI, D.G. (1984). Bacteriuria in the catheterized patient. *New England Journal of Medicine,* **311,** 560–564

STEWART, J.H. (1978). Analgesic abuse and renal failure in Australasia. *Kidney International,* **13,** 72–78

THOMAS, V., SHELOKOV, A. and FORLAND, M. (1974). Antibody-coated bacteria in the urine and the site of urinary tract infection. *New England Journal of Medicine,* **290,** 588–590

TORRES, V.E. (1982). Present and future of the nonsteroidal anti-inflammatory drugs in nephrology. *Mayo Clinic Proceedings,* **57,** 389–393

TU, W.H. and SHEARN, M.A. (1967). Systemic lupus erythematosus and latent tubular dysfunction. *Annals of Internal Medicine,* **67,** 100–103

VANE, U.R. (1971). Inhibition of prostaglandin synthesis as a mechanism of action for aspirin-like drugs. *Nature (New Biology),* **234,** 231–238

VENNING, V., DIXON, A.J. and OLIVER, D.O. (1980). Mefenamic acid nephropathy. *Lancet,* **ii,** 745–746

VESTERGAARD. P., AMDISEN, A., HANSEN, H.E. and SCHOU, M. (1979). Lithium treatment and kidney function: a survey of 237 patients in long-term treatment. *Acta Psychiatrica Scandinavica,* **60,** 504–520

WALLACE, D.M.A., ROTHWELL, D.L. and WILLIAMS, D.I. (1978). The long-term follow-up of surgically treated vesico-ureteric reflux. *British Journal of Urology,* **50,** 479–482

WALSHE, J.J. and VENUTO, R.C. (1979). Acute oliguric renal failure induced by indomethacin: possible mechanism. *Annals of Internal Medicine,* **91,** 47–49

WEDEEN, R.P. and BATUMAN, V. (1984). Tubulo-interstitial nephritis induced by heavy metals and metabolic disturbances. In *Tubulointerstitial Nephropathies,* edited by R.S. Cotran, pp. 211–241. New York; Churchill Livingstone

WEISS, S. and PARKER, F.J. (1939). Pyelonephritis. Its relation to vascular lesions and to arterial hypertension. *Medicine,* **18,** 221–315

WENDLAND, M.L., WAGONER, R.D. and HOLLEY, K.E. (1980). Renal failure associated with fenoprofen. *Mayo Clinic Proceedings,* **55,** 103–107

WOODS, K.L. and MICHAEL, J. (1981). Mefenamic acid nephropathy. *British Medical Journal,* **282,** 1471

Chapter 15

Glomerular disease in the aged

Brian M. Murray and Leopoldo Raij

Introduction

Glomerulonephritis has classically been considered as a disease of children and the middle-aged and to be rare in the elderly. As a result there is a paucity of published studies in this area and few systematic attempts to examine the incidence, presentation and prognosis of the various glomerular diseases have been made (Abrass, 1985). Consequently, the true incidence of glomerulonephritis in the elderly remains unknown. In this chapter, we review the general picture of glomerulonephritis and its varied presentation in the elderly, with particular emphasis on presentation, prognosis and management. The pathogenesis of glomerulonephritis will not be discussed, as it has been extensively reviewed elsewhere (Raij and Michael, 1980; Cameron, 1982).

In studies performed during the 1960s (Nesson and Robbins, 1960; Samiy, Field and Merrill, 1961; Lee, Stirling and Sharpstone, 1966; Sapir, Yardley and Walker, 1968), the predominant impression was that glomerulonephritis in the elderly was a rare disease with atypical clinical presentations and a high mortality rate. Most of the cases of acute glomerulonephritis were felt to be post-streptococcal. With the more frequent use of ante-mortem renal biopsy and the diagnostic techniques of immunofluorescence and electron microscopy, it has become clear that the disease is more common than at first thought, the aetiology essentially as diverse as in other age groups, and the prognosis not as unfavourable as previously believed.

One of the most systematic and comprehensive reviews of glomerular disease in the elderly is that of Moorthy and Zimmerman (1977), who performed a clinicopathologic analysis of 115 patients, 60 years of age or older, who presented with renal disease. Only patients in whom the nature of the renal disease was confirmed by renal biopsy were included. Since the study was retrospective, obvious systemic diseases, such as diabetes or amyloidosis, in which the diagnosis could have been established without a renal biopsy, may be under-represented. Of the 115 cases, 78 were attributed to a primary glomerular disease, 27 were secondary to a systemic disorder, usually a vasculitis or amyloidosis, and 10 were due to miscellaneous causes such as interstitial nephritis or acute tubular necrosis. The most common diagnoses were rapidly progressive glomerulonephritis (19 cases), glomerulonephritis of unknown aetiology (16 cases) and membranous nephropathy (15 cases).

Nephrotic syndrome

The spectrum of diseases causing the nephrotic syndrome tends to vary with age, with minimal lesion disease being most common in children and membranous nephropathy in adults. Three studies (Moorthy and Zimmerman, 1977; Zech *et al.*, 1982; Bolton, 1984a; see also Chapter 21) have recently looked at the causes of this disease in the elderly and have come to essentially similar conclusions. Membranous nephropathy was the commonest cause, accounting for approximately one-third of all cases, followed by minimal lesion disease and various other forms of glomerular disease (*Table 15.1*). All studies found a high incidence of amyloidosis (9–14 per cent).

Table 15.1 Causes of the nephrotic syndrome in the elderly

Type	*Moorthy and Zimmerman (1977)*	*Zech* et al. *(1982)*	*Bolton (1984b)*	*Total* (%)
Membranous GN	13	31	21	65 (38%)
Minimal lesion GN	9	19	13	41 (24%)
Proliferative GN	2	10	6	18 (10%)
Focal sclerosis	2	3	10	15 (9%)
Amyloidosis	3	10	9	22 (13%)
Others	4	3	4	11 (6%)
Total:	33	76	63	172

In general, it is not possible to differentiate between the different causes of the nephrotic syndrome on a clinical basis and a renal biopsy is generally required for diagnosis. While most nephrologists would agree with this approach, it has been challenged in a recent study (Kassirer, 1983) which provided suggestive evidence that treatment with steroids and observation of the response was at least as good if not better than biopsy-directed management. However, this is probably more a reflection of the fact that the therapies available are neither very good nor very harmful, rather than an indictment of the use of biopsy *per se*. We will now consider the various causes of the nephrotic syndrome individually.

Membranous glomerulonephritis

In elderly patients presenting with the nephrotic syndrome, the most commonly encountered diagnosis is membranous nephropathy. The extensive review of Noel *et al.* (1979) showed two peaks of incidence of membranous nephropathy, the larger one in the 16–20 age group and the smaller one in the 61–70 age group (*Figure 15.1*). Seventy to 80 per cent of patients with membranous glomerulonephritis present with the nephrotic syndrome, while the remainder have non-nephrotic proteinuria (Row *et al.*, 1975). Gross haematuria is rare, but microscopic haematuria is seen in between 40 and 60 per cent and hypertension in from 25 to 40 per cent (Gluck *et al.*, 1973; Row *et al.*, 1975; Noel *et al.*, 1979). Histological changes vary with the stage of the disease (Glassock *et al.*, 1981), but the characteristic finding is that of a thickened basement membrane on light microscopy. Electron microscopy reveals subepithelial deposition of electron-dense material, thought to be immune complexes, which stain for IgG and C_3 and

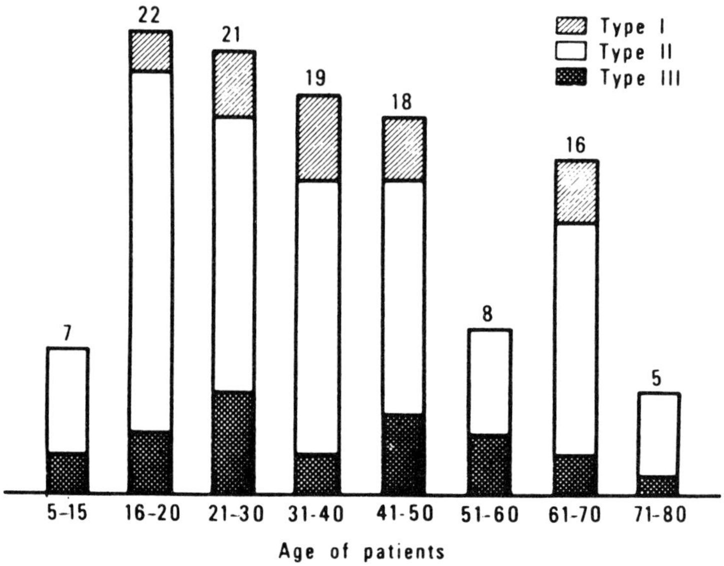

Figure 15.1 Distribution of the age of patients presenting with membranous nephrophathy (From Noel *et al.*, 1979, reproduced with permission)

occasionally IgA and IgM on immunofluorescence microscopy. Early in the disease, glomeruli may appear normal by light microscopy and the diagnosis can only be made by either electron or immunofluorescence microscopy.

Analysis of three recent series (Gluck *et al.*, 1973; Row *et al.*, 1975; Noel *et al.*, 1979) of patients with membranous nephropathy shows that about 16 per cent of all cases present after age 60. From the data available in the foregoing studies, it is not possible to conclude whether the presentation in the elderly was different from the mainstream. Moorthy and Zimmerman (1977), in their series, found that clinical features were similar in elderly patients to those seen in other adults, with 87 per cent presenting as a nephrotic syndrome.

Membranous nephropathy tends to have a variable course and Cameron (1979) has summarized the long-term outlook. As many as 25 per cent of patients will undergo spontaneous remission of proteinuria and a further 20–25 per cent a partial remission (protein excretion >200 mg/day but <2 g/day). The remainder will have a persistent nephrotic syndrome and as many as half of these may progress to end-stage renal failure in from 3 to 15 years. Patients presenting with nephrotic syndrome tended to have a poor prognosis, as did adults when compared with children. Erwin *et al.* (1973) found that 42 per cent of patients developed renal insufficiency an average of 40 months after onset, whereas in the series of Noel *et al.* (1979) only 19 per cent developed renal insufficiency and half of these progressed to end-stage renal disease between 2 months and 6 years after the development of renal insufficiency. There is no firm evidence that the prognosis of the nephrotic syndrome is worse in the elderly. However, in the study of Noel *et al.* (1979), patients over 60 did have a higher incidence of elevated creatinine at presentation and a greater proportion progressed to end-stage renal failure.

The variable and indolent course of membranous nephropathy with its tendency to spontaneous clinical remission makes evaluation of potential treatments difficult and extrapolation from short-term uncontrolled studies treacherous. An early controlled study (Black, Rose and Brewer, 1970) showed no evidence of benefit from steroid therapy, but numbers were small and the period of follow-up short. In contrast, the report of the Collaborative Study of the Adult Idiopathic Nephrotic Syndrome (1979) showed evidence of a beneficial effect of high dose steroids (120 mg on alternate days for 2 months) both in terms of a higher number of remissions of the nephrotic syndrome and a slower rate of decline in renal function. The study was prospective, randomized and double blind. The principal concern about the results obtained by this study was the unusually severe course of the disease in the placebo group and the surprise that such a short course of steroids would have such long-term effects.

Recently, Ponticelli *et al.* (1984) reported in a randomized prospective multicentre study on the efficacy of a 6-month course of methylprednisolone alternating with chlorambucil and found a higher rate of complete remission in the treated group. In addition, only the control group showed a significant decrease in renal function over a 2-year follow-up period. How then do we treat the elderly patient presenting with membranous nephropathy? The upper age limit in the collaborative study was 65, so that its general applicability to the geriatric population is uncertain. However, on the basis that (a) the clinical manifestations and course of the disease seem no different in the elderly and (b) given the relatively non-toxic nature of the steroid regimen proposed, it seems reasonable to follow the advice of Glassock *et al.* (1981). He proposes a course of alternate day steroid therapy to patients with proven membranous nephropathy, provided that renal function is well preserved and no specific contraindications to such therapy exist. The recommended dose is 1.5–2 mg/kg on alternate days for 2 months, then tapered over 4 weeks. The addition of more toxic cytotoxic agents to the steroid regimen cannot be advocated until controlled trials show a greater efficacy over steroids alone.

Minimal change disease

Minimal change disease is characterized by the presence of the nephrotic syndrome in patients with normal glomerular histology by light microscopy and diffuse epithelial foot process fusion by electron microscopy. Immunofluorescence microscopy is usually negative, but may reveal the presence of focal deposits of IgM or C3 (Prasad, Zimmerman and Burkholder, 1977) in the mesangium. It has been proposed by some (Tejani and Nicastri, 1983) that those patients showing IgM deposition may represent a separate entity. However, the vast majority of cases reported have been in young adults and 'IgM nephropathy' has not been recognized as a significant cause of glomerular disease in the aged. While minimal change disease is characteristically associated with the nephrotic syndrome of childhood, it is also a frequent cause of the nephrotic syndrome in the elderly, constituting roughly 25 per cent of all cases (see *Table 15.2*). The effectiveness of steroid therapy in inducing remission of the nephrotic syndrome in children is well recognized, although recurrent relapses can be a difficult management problem and even require treatment with cyclophosphamide (Glassock *et al.*, 1981).

There have been several studies of minimal change disease in adults (Pollak *et al.*, 1968; Sharpstone, Ogg and Cameron, 1969; Hopper *et al.*, 1970; Hayslett *et al.*, 1973; Lim, Sibley and Spargo, 1974), but few have included many elderly patients. Cameron *et al.* (1974) studied 49 adult patients with minimal change disease. They noted that at onset, compared with children, adults with the disease were more likely

Table 15.2 Clinical features of presentation in adult patients with minimal change disease (Data from Cameron *et al.*, 1974)

	>60 years old	*<60 years old*
Number of patients	12	38
Proteinuria >3 g/day	100%	100%
Hypertension (diastolic BP >90 mmHg)	58%	45%
Haematuria (>5 rbc/hpf)	17%	36%
Serum creatinine (>130 μmol/l)	70%	58%

to exhibit hypertension (31 per cent), diminished renal function (70 per cent) and non-selective proteinuria (51 per cent). However, despite these features, generally associated with a poor prognosis, the outlook was good. Eighty per cent responded to prednisone therapy with early loss of proteinuria, although relapses were frequent. Of 17 patients treated with cytotoxic drugs (5 for steroid resistance and 12 for steroid intolerance), 14 responded and 11 remained in remission. This study included 12 patients aged 60 years and over. As can be seen (*Table 15.2*), clinical features at onset were similar to those of the adult group in general. As regards clinical course, of the 10 patients for whom adequate data is available, 2 underwent spontaneous remission, 6 responded to steroid therapy, 1 to azathioprine and only 1 patient was resistant to therapy and died of renal failure.

Table 15.3 Prognosis of minimal change disease in adults patients (Data from Pollak *et al.*, 1968; Sharpstone, Ogg and Cameron, 1969; Hopper *et al.*, 1970; Hayslett *et al.*, 1973; Lim, Sibley and Spargo, 1974; Cameron *et al.*, 1974)

	>60 years old	*<60 years old*
Number of cases	26	104
Spontaneous remissions	5	8
Steroid remissions	15	71
Cytotoxic remissions	2	8
Resistant	4 (16%)	17 (17%)

Combining the data from all studies (*Table 15.3*) and comparing it with the corresponding data from younger adults in the same series, it can be seen that the prognosis in the elderly is similar, with between 80 and 90 per cent being steroid responsive and only the occasional patients progressing to renal failure.

Focal glomerulosclerosis

This entity was first described by Rich (1957) as characterized by focal and segmental involvement of glomeruli by an acellular sclerosis which initially involves deep glomeruli. Immunofluorescence microscopy is negative or shows staining with IgM and C3. First recognized in the context of 'steroid resistant lipoid nephrosis', its significance and aetiology have remained a matter of controversy. It has been claimed by several authors that there are two forms of the disease (Brown *et al.*, 1978; Tejani *et al.*, 1983) representing distinct nosologic entities: (a) an 'early' malignant form, where the lesion is present at or near the onset of profuse proteinuria, and in which patients tend to be resistant to steroids and alkylating agents and progress rapidly to renal failure; and (b) a 'late' form, in which the lesion is not initially present but the patient follows a relapsing, steroid-responsive syndrome and focal sclerosis does not develop until the disease has been present for several years. In general, the lesion is unresponsive to steroid or cytotoxic therapy.

While it has been estimated that focal glomerulosclerosis accounts for some 10–15 per cent of cases of the nephrotic syndrome in both adults and children, it is considered an uncommon disease in the elderly. A review of 12 series from the literature in 1978 (Bolton, Westervelt and Sturgill, 1978) revealed only 6 cases over the age of 60, out of a total of 260 adult cases. Bolton *et al.* (1978) reported cases of focal glomerulosclerosis in 4 elderly patients, including 3 septuagenarians. All had steroid-resistant nephrotic syndrome.

Acute renal failure complicating the nephrotic syndrome

The occurrence of renal failure in patients with minimal change nephrotic syndrome was first reported by Chamberlain, Pringle and Wrong (1968) and Connolly, Wrong and Jones (1968). In their cases, renal failure was reversible and they proposed that hypovolaemia leading to acute tubular necrosis might be the cause. Lowenstein *et al.* (1981) reported data on 15 patients with minimal change disease. All presented with anasarca, massive proteinuria despite oliguria and markedly depressed serum albumin (0.4–2.4 g/dl). Serum creatinines ranged from 200 to 850 μmol/l. Renal biopsy did not reveal any structural basis for the decreased renal function, as most cases showed only changes consistent with minimal change disease and occasional mesangial hypercellularity. Significant glomerular sclerosis was seen in only 1 patient. This group found that glomerular filtration rate improved with the induction of a diuresis in 13 of 15 patients, whether or not proteinuria resolved. Large doses of frusemide were generally required and some patients were also given salt-poor albumin. Measurements of inulin and PAH clearance revealed extremely low filtration fractions. They postulated that increased hydrostatic pressure in the proximal tubules and in Bowman's space, consequent to renal interstitial oedema, may be responsible for the renal insufficiency. Two of their patients did not respond to diuretics or steroid therapy and progressed to dialysis. At autopsy, the kidneys from these two patients still showed only 'minimal change' and did not differ in appearance from the earlier biopsy.

This is not unlike our own experience (Raij *et al.*, 1976) with 5 elderly patients who developed irreversible renal failure coincident with the nephrotic syndrome. Light microscopy revealed the changes of focal sclerosis in 2, and focal and segmental mesangial hypercellularity in the other 3 patients. Again, all patients showed massive proteinuria, despite oliguria, indicating a marked increase in glomerular permeability to these molecules. The mechanism of this irreversible renal failure remains to be explained.

Nephrotic syndrome associated with non-steroidal anti-inflammatory agents

The occurrence of renal insufficiency accompanied by heavy proteinuria in association with the use of the non-steroidal anti-inflammatory agent, fenoprofen, was first reported in 1979 (Brezin *et al.*, 1979). Since then, numerous reports have appeared confirming the initial findings and implicating several other of these agents. The subject has been recently reviewed (Garella and Matarese, 1984).

The average age of patients who developed the syndrome was 62. Onset of the syndrome was on the average 5 months after initiation of the offending agent, with a range from 1 month to 2 years. Oedema was the most frequent presenting symptom and the vast majority of patients had nephrotic range proteinuria. Peripheral or urinary eosinophilia was rare. One feature was the high incidence of renal insufficiency and as many as 40 per cent of patients required dialysis. Renal biopsy usually revealed an acute interstitial nephritis. While glomeruli appeared normal by light microscopy, electron microscopy showed fusion of the foot processes. Nearly 60 per cent of cases have been associated with fenoprofen use. Of interest is that indomethacin, the most commonly prescribed non-steroidal anti-inflammatory drug, has been rarely implicated as a cause of the syndrome. In general, improvement in renal function and disappearance of proteinuria follow discontinuation of the drugs. Occasionally, prednisone therapy has been given (Finkelstein *et al.*, 1982).

Glomerulopathies of neoplasia

We cannot leave the subject of nephrotic syndrome in the elderly without mentioning its occasional association with neoplasia. This subject has been extensively reviewed by Eagen and Lewis (1977). The first description of the nephrotic syndrome in association with cancer is attributed to Volhard (see Revol *et al.*, 1966). The subject received little attention until the report of Lee, Yamauchi and Hopper (1966), who found that in 11 per cent of nephrotic patients, the syndrome was associated with a neoplasia. The glomerulopathies of neoplasia have been classified into those occurring in association with (1) carcinomas, (2) Hodgkin's disease and other lymphoproliferative disorders, and (3) miscellaneous benign and malignant neoplasms.

In the case of carcinomas, 70 per cent of cases of the nephrotic syndrome are due to membranous nephropathy and are felt to represent an example of immune complex disease. Several antigen antibody systems have been postulated as causing the disease including tumour-associated antigens (Couser *et al.*, 1974), re-expressed fetal antigens (Costanza *et al.*, 1973), viral antigens (Oldstone *et al.*, 1974), and antibodies either to renal (Ozawa *et al.*, 1975) or non-renal tissue. Numerous types of carcinoma have been associated with the nephrotic syndrome, most commonly lung, colorectal and stomach carcinoma. In up to half of the cases, the tumour is occult at the time of development of the nephrotic syndrome. One feature is the poor prognosis of such patients, with a median survival of only 3 months after discovery of the tumour (Eagen and Lewis, 1977). In those cases where the tumour is amenable to therapy, surgical resection of the tumour often leads to disappearance of the renal disease.

On the other hand, in patients with Hodgkin's disease, the most common diagnosis is minimal change disease (Potter *et al.*, 1978). Again, the renal disease may antedate the clinical appearance of the tumour and frequently remits if the Hodgkin's disease is treated, whether by radiation alone or chemotherapy. Patients with Hodgkin's disease and the nephrotic syndrome do not seem to have a poorer prognosis than other patients with this neoplasia.

The above-described studies raise the question whether in elderly patients, presenting with the nephrotic syndrome, a systematic search for a neoplasm should be undertaken. As mentioned earlier, the incidence of associated neoplasia has been estimated by several authors (Eagen and Lewis, 1977; Cameron, 1979) to be about 10 per cent. In only half of the patients will the nephrotic syndrome precede clinical evidence of a tumour. Thus, a systematic tumour work-up cannot be advocated routinely. However, it would be prudent to check all the patients for abnormal weight loss, unexplained anaemia, guaiac positive stools and chest X-ray.

Rapidly progressive renal failure

This may be defined as progressive renal insufficiency of less than 2 months duration and covers a wide range of renal diseases. The glomerular diseases which can present in this way include those which present classically as *an acute nephritic syndrome.* This is characterized by a sudden onset of oliguria with dark or frankly bloody urine, hypertension, oedema and rising creatinine. The disease often follows an infection, most commonly with the β-haemolytic streptococcus, and is frequently accompanied by a low serum complement. A number of systemic diseases, including systemic lupus erythematosus, Henoch–Schönlein purpura, infectious endocarditis or shunt nephritis can have a similar presentation and a careful physical examination must be performed to exclude these. In addition, two other primary glomerular diseases can occasionally give rise to this clinical picture, membranoproliferative glomerulonephritis and idiopathic IgA nephropathy. While a typical history and appropriate serology can often suggest the diagnosis, recourse to a renal biopsy is often necessary.

Another glomerular disease which can present as insidiously progressive renal failure is *rapidly progressive glomerulonephritis* (RPGN). The hallmark of this disease is the presence of extensive extracapillary proliferation (crescents) in the glomeruli. It is a heterogeneous disease often representing severe forms of more common glomerulonephritides, e.g. post-streptococcal GN, SLE, Henoch–Schönlein purpura, vasculitis or Berger's disease, but in many cases no multisystem disease or infectious cause can be found. The patients usually present with the insidious onset of the clinical features of uraemia. Blood pressure may be normal or mildly elevated and oligo-anuria may also be present. The urine sediment is usually 'active', but the degree of haematuria and/or proteinuria variable. Serum assay for circulating anti-GBM antibody may be helpful (see below) but when negative, a renal biopsy is required for diagnosis and institution of therapy as quickly as possible.

Finally, one needs to consider a number of non-glomerular causes of progressive renal insufficiency. *Acute interstitial nephritis* should always be considered. Skin rash and blood eosinophilia may help in diagnosis but are not invariably present. Of particular interest is the occurrence of interstitial nephritis in association with nephrotic proteinuria following the use of non-steroidal agents (see above). Severe atherosclerotic disease of the renal vessels may result in *bilateral renal artery obstruction.* Migration of *cholesterol emboli* to the kidney can also result in sudden deterioration of renal function. Severe *malignant hypertension* is another potential cause of reversible acute renal insufficiency and the rare systemic diseases *haemolytic uraemic syndrome* and *thrombotic thrombocytopenic purpura* can usually be recognized from their other manifestations.

Moorthy and Zimmerman (1977) identified 32 cases of acute renal failure due to glomerular disease among their series of 115 cases. Seventeen were due to RPGN and a further 7 to vasculitides (including Wegener's granulomatosis). Other causes of this syndrome were rare. In particular, acute nephritic syndrome seems to have been a relatively rare clinical presentation of glomerular disease in the elderly, with only 5 cases out of 115, 4 due to post-infectious glomerulonephritis and 1 to IgA nephropathy.

Post-infectious glomerulonephritis

A number of infections, most commonly streptococcal pharyngitis or pyoderma, can lead to a diffuse proliferative glomerulonephritis. In classic post-streptococcal glomerulonephritis (PSGN), after a latent period of 7–21 days the patient typically presents with the acute onset of microscopic haematuria, oliguria, pedal and periorbital oedema. Flank pain, hypertension, congestive cardiac failure and even encephalopathy may be present. While severe renal failure requiring dialysis may occur, most patients show only mild elevations in serum creatinine. Serum complement is decreased in nearly 90 per cent of cases (Glassock *et al.*, 1981). Most patients recover from the acute episode and in children there seems to be no major long-term sequelae. This is particularly true of the epidemic form of the disease as illustrated by the study of Potter *et al.* (1978) in Trinidad, where follow-up of 760 cases showed persistent urinary abnormalities in only 1.8 per cent, hypertension in 1.4 per cent and azotaemia in only a single patient, 2–6 years after the acute episode. It has always been suspected that the disease in adults may be less benign. Baldwin *et al.* (1976) have claimed that 'more than half' of all patients with PSGN may show evidence of irreversible damage. Moreover, the disappearance of proteinuria or haematuria did not necessarily imply an inactive nephritis. In many cases urinary abnormalities and hypertension returned after many years of seemingly good renal function. These conclusions have, however, been challenged (Editorial, 1977; Kurtzman, 1978), mainly on the basis that only a small proportion of the patients with sporadic PSGN were available for follow-up and that the studies involved mostly hospitalized patients who would tend to have more severe forms of the disease. A more recent review studied 57 cases of the sporadic form of the disease in adults (Lien, Meadows and Mathew, 1979). In this series, only 15 per cent of patients who were alive at follow-up (mean 7 years) had abnormalities in the form of hypertension, microscopic haematuria, proteinuria or an elevated serum creatinine.

Post-streptococcal glomerulonephritis was initially felt to be rare in the elderly, but during the 1960s a number of studies appeared which suggested that the disease was not uncommon but difficult to diagnose ante mortem. Nesson and Robins (1960), in a retrospective study of autopsy data, reported that 46 per cent of deaths due to acute glomerulonephritis occurred after the age of 60. Lee, Stirling and Sharpstone (1966) reported 7 patients with acute fatal glomerulonephritis between the ages of 53 and 70; 2 almost certainly represented cases of idiopathic RPGN and only 2 had true post-infectious disease clinically, with a history of sore throat and elevated ASO titre. Finally, Sapir, Yardley and Walker (1968), in a review of 52 cases of acute glomerulonephritis seen in adults, noted a greater tendency of older patients to present with exertional dyspnoea and pulmonary oedema than as an acute nephritic syndrome. Nine of the 52 patients were over 60 years of age, and 7 of these patients died, giving a mortality rate of nearly 80 per cent in this group. However, the diagnosis of post-infectious glomerulonephritis was not strictly applied and many cases, especially in the elderly group, may have represented cases of RPGN. Most of these studies were done in the predialysis era. More recent studies have challenged their findings (Moorthy and Zimmerman, 1977; Lien *et al.*, 1979; Montoliu *et al.*, 1981).

Analysis of the 5 cases of acute PSGN occurring in patients over 60 in the study of Lien *et al.* (1979) revealed only 1 death which was probably unrelated to renal causes. The other 4 patients were alive 6–11 years after the initial attack and, while 1 had hypertension and an elevated creatinine with evidence of glomerulosclerosis on biopsy, the other 3 had normal renal function with no urinary abnormalities. The series of Moorthy and Zimmerman (1977) included 5 patients with diffuse proliferative glomerulonephritis. All had discernible urinary abnormalities, 3 had elevated ASO titres and only 1 patient progressed to end-stage renal failure requiring dialysis.

Finally, Montoliu *et al.* (1981) reported on 7 cases of well-documented post-infectious glomerulonephritis in patients over 60. The clinical picture was invariably one of acute renal failure and oliguria in all cases, hypertension in 5 and peripheral oedema in 4. Haematuria was constant and gross in 5 of the patients. Hypocomplementaemia was found in 5 of the 7 patients. Despite the fact that 4 of the 7 patients required haemodialysis during the acute phase, prognosis was generally good with only 1 fatality due to sepsis. The other 6 patients all recovered with return of renal function in the 3 patients who required dialysis. At follow-up, 3 patients were free of any evidence of persistent renal disease, while the other 3 patients showed evidence of mild persistent renal abnormalities with creatinines between 100 and 170 mol/l. Two had persistent microscopic haematuria, 1 of which also had persistent proteinuria. None was hypertensive. Thus, these recent studies indicate that PSGN in the elderly tends to present in a similar fashion to other age groups and is a more benign disease than was initially thought. Most of the data reviewed here concerns PSGN. While it is our impression that non-streptococcal post-infectious glomerulonephritis also occurs in the elderly, its true incidence in this age group is difficult to document. For a more extensive review of the subject of post-infectious glomerulonephritis, although not necessarily in the elderly, we refer the reader to the review by Kim and Michael (1978).

Rapidly progressive glomerulonephritis (RPGN)

The idiopathic form of this disease refers to an entity characterized by extensive (over 50 per cent) involvement of glomeruli with extracapillary proliferation in the form of crescents. While RPGN may occur in association with infectious diseases, e.g. post-streptococcal glomerulonephritis and infective endocarditis, or multisystem diseases, e.g. SLE, Henoch–Schönlein purpura, more than 70 per cent of cases are idiopathic or occur in the setting of 'Goodpasture's syndrome'. The idiopathic forms of RPGN can be divided into three groups, principally on the basis of the findings on immunofluorescence microscopy (Couser, 1982).

Type I. Anti-GBM mediated RPGN

This is characterized by deposition of anti-GBM antibody in a linear fashion along glomerular capillary walls. The antibody often can also be detected in the serum. Many of these patients have pulmonary haemorrhage, the classic 'Goodpasture's syndrome', but as many as 10–30 per cent do not. Patients tend to be young adult males.

Type II. RPGN associated with granular immune deposits

This is characterized by glomerular deposits principally of IgG and C3 in a 'granular' pattern. More than 75 per cent of such cases are associated with some well-defined clinical disorder, e.g. SLE or mesangiocapillary GN, but the remaining 25 per cent seem to have a primary renal disease. Patients tend to be middle-aged or older.

Type III. RPGN without glomerular immune deposits

Here, the kidney is either totally negative by immunofluorescence microscopy or shows a non-specific pattern of trace to 1+ focal deposits of IgM and/or C3. Patients tend to be middle-aged to elderly males. Some consider this to be an exclusively glomerular manifestation of vasculitis (see Chapter 16).

While the onset of RPGN may be rapid with oliguria, microscopic haematuria and oedema, more commonly it presents insidiously with circulatory overload or symptoms of uraemia. Renal biopsy reveals the characteristic crescentic glomerulonephritis. The natural history of untreated RPGN is impossible to determine, as most reported cases have received some form of therapy. It is generally felt that, untreated, the disease progresses to end-stage renal failure over a period of days to months, although spontaneous recovery of the disease has been described. Maxwell *et al.* (1979) described three such cases, all in elderly patients with type III disease. They initially required dialysis, but were given no specific treatment and all recovered sufficient renal function to be able to discontinue dialysis 4–14 months later. In general, however, the prognosis of RPGN is poor. Couser (1982), reviewing the literature prior to the introduction of either pulse methylprednisolone or plasmaphaeresis found that some 73 per cent of patients either died or progressed to dialysis within 2 years. In general, it has been felt that types II and III disease carry a better prognosis than disease associated with the anti-GBM antibody. Beirne *et al.* (1977) found that in their patients with either 'Goodpasture's syndrome' or anti-GBM nephritis without pulmonary haemorrhage, the mortality rate was 58 per cent and only 16 per cent of patients were alive and off dialysis. In contrast, in patients with either granular or negative immunofluorescence, the mortality rate was only 27 per cent and 56 per cent retained adequate renal function.

In the series of Moorthy and Zimmerman (1977), RPGN was the most common cause of renal insufficiency in the elderly, accounting for over 50 per cent of all cases of acute renal failure biopsied. *Table 15.4* summarizes the incidence of the various

Table 15.4 Frequency of different subtypes of rapidly progressive glomerulonephritis in patients over 60

	Type I (anti-GBM disease)	*Type II (granular deposits)*	*Type III (NID disease)*
Morrin *et al.* (1978)	2	1	7
Beirne *et al.* (1977)	4	3	3
Moorthy and Zimmerman (1977)	2	9	6
Total:	8 (22%)	13 (35%)	16 (43%)

subtypes of RPGN in three series from the literature (Moorthy and Zimmerman, 1977; Beirne *et al.*, 1977; Morrin *et al.*, 1978). It confirms the fact that anti-GBM disease is not a common cause of RPGN in the elderly. The majority of cases are due to disease characterized by either granular Ig deposits or negative immunofluorescence. The particularly high incidence of type III disease in the elderly is also reflected in the fact that 12 of the 16 patients with this disease described in the review of Stilmant *et al.* (1974) were over the age of 55.

The prognosis of RPGN in the elderly appears to be poor. Analysis of 10 cases in Morrin's study (Morrin *et al.*, 1978) shows a 60 per cent mortality rate with only 1 patient surviving off dialysis. In another study (Moorthy and Zimmerman, 1977) patients fared no better, with 63 per cent dying during the period of observation and only 3 of 17 patients not requiring dialysis. The outcome was even more disappointing in the 7 cases reported by Montoliu *et al.* (1981): all presented with an advanced degree of renal dysfunction and none was treated with plasmaphaeresis, steroids or immunosuppression. In 6 of the 7 dialysis was required as the initial therapy and no patient regained renal function. Four patients died and the other 3 required chronic maintenance dialysis. This high mortality in the elderly occurred despite the fact that the subgroups of disease predominating (types II and III) are generally considered to be more benign (Beirne *et al.*, 1977). This may reflect the fact that the elderly as a group are more susceptible to the complications both of the disease and treatment.

There is general consensus that the renal prognosis of RPGN without treatment is dismal, but there is considerable controversy about the optimal form of treatment (Couser, 1982; Bolton, 1984b; Kincaid-Smith and Walker, 1984). At various times dramatic responses have been claimed for a number of agents including oral steroids, cytotoxic drugs, antilymphocyte globulin and anticoagulants, but, unfortunately, none has been substantiated in controlled trials. Furthermore, it seems unlikely that any such trial will ever be performed both because of the rarity of the disease and because it is felt by some that withholding treatment may be unethical (Stilmant *et al.*, 1974).

Bolton and Couser (1979) reported a new approach to the treatment of RPGN by the use of high dose methylprednisolone (50 mg/kg lean body weight) followed by oral prednisone (60 mg/day) and subsequent tapering. Bolton (1984b) has recently summarized his experience with 30 patients, 14 with granular type II, and 16 with no immune deposits, type III disease. Of 14 patients with type II, half were treated with pulse therapy and 6 showed improvement. Only 2 of the 7 treated with conventional doses of oral prednisone improved. However, the latter may have had more advanced disease, since a higher percentage initially required dialysis. Of 16 patients with type III disease, 14 received pulse therapy and 12 showed improvement. Seven of 9 patients in this group were able to discontinue dialysis. However, the 2 patients who were treated conventionally also showed considerable improvement. When the results obtained with pulse therapy are compared with those of conventional or no therapy (Couser, 1982), pulse methylprednisolone does indeed seem to lead to an improved outcome.

On the other hand, there is suggestive evidence that pulse methylprednisolone is not as effective in anti-GBM mediated RPGN (type I disease), with only 17 per cent of patients showing improvement (Lockwood *et al.*, 1976; Kincaid-Smith and Walker, 1984). However, these authors reported beneficial effects of a regimen of intensive plasma-exchange, cytotoxic drugs and corticosteroids in patients with 'Goodpasture's syndrome'. Since these initial reports, plasmaphaeresis has been used widely in 'Goodpasture's syndrome' and stabilization of renal function reported in over 50 per cent of treated patients. Although controlled studies have not been done and the effect of increased availability of dialysis and earlier recognition of the disease is difficult to estimate, many feel it is the treatment of choice for RPGN mediated by anti-GBM antibody (Kincaid-Smith and Walker, 1984). In a recent review by Lockwood and Peters (1980) of 35 patients with RPGN due to anti-GBM disease, they found that recovery of renal function seemed to depend on the level of renal function existing at the time when plasmaphaeresis was instituted. Thus, in 18 patients with creatinine $>$600 mol/l only 2 survived without long-term dialysis, whereas in 17 patients with acutely deteriorating renal failure but creatinine $<$600 mol/l, 15 responded with improvement in renal function. Pulmonary haemorrhage was controlled in all but 1 of 32 patients. Eleven patients died within 1 year of follow-up, 2 of pulmonary haemorrhage, 5 of infections, and 4 of cardiovascular causes.

These authors claimed similar results with the use of this type of therapy in the treatment of RPGN not mediated by anti-GBM antibody (Lockwood and Peters, 1980; Hind *et al.*, 1983). The results obtained were comparable to those achieved by Bolton's group (Bolton, 1984b) with pulse steroid, but with a higher incidence of complications. In particular, Wing *et al.* (1980) found 5 episodes of serious 'life-threatening infections' in 8 patients treated with plasmaphaeresis for RPGN.

The following guidelines would seem reasonable for patients with RPGN:

A. *Non anti-GBM RPGN (types II and III)*

Mild cases without oliguria and a creatinine <450 mol/l may be treated with traditional doses of prednisone (60 mg daily or 120 mg altern.d.). Addition of immunosuppressives, cyclophosphamide or azathioprine, while they may increase the number of responses, are also likely to increase potential complications.

In more advanced (>450 mol/l) and oliguric disease, many would favour the use of pulse methylprednisolone initially, as outlined by Bolton and Couser (1979). There is no evidence to suggest that plasma exchange offers any further advantage. On the other hand, the occurrence of coincident pulmonary haemorrhage would be an indication for high dose steroids and, if no response, plasma-exchange, regardless of the level of renal function.

B. *Anti-GBM RPGN (type I)*

It appears that in anti-GBM mediated RPGN there is potential for improvement of renal function if plasma-exchange and immunosuppression are used, but the benefit seems to be confined largely to those patients with non-oliguric disease and with a creatinine less than 600 mol/l (Lockwood and Peters, 1980). Response to pulse methylprednisolone has been disappointing in this disease.

Membranoproliferative glomerulonephritis

This is a histopathologic entity which may present under a number of clinical guises including a classical nephrotic syndrome (50 per cent), asymptomatic proteinuria (30 per cent), with or without haematuria, or an acute nephritic syndrome (20–30 per cent) (Cameron *et al.*, 1983). The disease may be idiopathic or secondary to a number of associated diseases such as SLE, congenital complement deficiencies or sickle cell anaemia (Glassock *et al.*, 1981). Two types are classically described: type I, or subendothelial deposit disease with electron-dense material situated mainly subendothelially in the glomerular capillaries, and type II dense linear deposit disease, in which a refractile electron-dense material almost completely replaces the lamina densa of the glomerular capillary basement membranes. The disease is frequently associated with a low serum complement, and 'C3 nephritic factor' is often detectable in the serum (Glassock *et al.*, 1981). Most cases present over the age of 5 and under the age of 30 and the disease is rare in the elderly. In a recent series (Cameron *et al.*, 1983), only 4 of the 104 patients were over the age of 60 and all had type I disease. Moorthy and Zimmerman (1977), in their review, found only 2 cases of membranoproliferative glomerulonephritis among 78 cases of primary glomerular disease in the elderly. Both presented with the nephrotic syndrome and exhibited progressive renal failure. This remains a rare cause of glomerular disease in the elderly.

Recently, 2 reports have provided evidence that antiplatelet agents may be useful in slowing the progression of renal insufficiency in this disease. Zimmerman *et al.* (1983), in a small prospective trial involving 22 patients, showed that treatment with dipyridamole and warfarin was associated with stabilization of renal function and decreased urinary protein excretion. More recently, Donadio *et al.* (1984), in a larger randomized double-blind controlled trial, showed that combined treatment with dipyridamole (75 mg t.i.d.) and aspirin (325 mg t.i.d.) resulted in better maintenance of the glomerular filtration rate and a lesser progression to end-stage renal disease. This is particularly encouraging because of the low toxicity of this regimen, with only 3 of 40 patients having to stop treatment because of bleeding complications.

Idiopathic IgA nephropathy

This pathologic entity was first described by Berger and Hinglais (1968), who noted a focal glomerulitis with predominant IgA deposition in a group of paediatric patients with idiopathic haematuria. While episodes of haematuria frequently related to a viral infection is the commonest mode of presentation, the syndrome may also present as non-nephrotic proteinuria, but only rarely as acute nephritic or full-blown nephrotic syndrome. In general, the outlook for patients with IgA nephropathy is considered good, although as many as 25 per cent of patients ultimately developed renal insufficiency usually within 6 years of diagnosis (Droz, 1976). Features which made such deterioration more likely include a decreased glomerular filtration rate at initial presentation, persistent nephrotic range proteinuria, moderate hypertension, and the presence of diffuse proliferation or focal sclerotic changes on biopsy. The disorder may be found at any age, but is uncommon before the age of 10 or over the age of 50. We reviewed several published reports of this disease in adults, totalling 168 cases, and found only 8 in patients over the age of 60. In the series of Moorthy and Zimmerman (1977) there were 5 cases of focal proliferative glomerulonephritis which presented as benign recurrent haematuria with associated IgA deposits in 4.

In another study (Clarkson *et al.*, 1977), of the 4 patients over 60 with IgA deposits on biopsy, 1 presented with haematuria, 1 with proteinuria and 2 with acute nephritic syndrome; all 4 patients had elevated creatinines at presentation (140–>410 μmol/l). Although long-term follow-up on an individual basis was not available, the authors noted a general tendency for a decrease in renal function and an excess of hypertension with age. In contrast, the patients reported by Moorthy and Zimmerman (1977) exhibited stable renal function, although the length of follow-up was not stated. In summary then, IgA nephropathy seems to be a rare disease in the elderly. When presenting as benign recurrent haematuria it seems to carry a good prognosis, but may follow an indolent progressive course especially in patients exhibiting significant proteinuria. No therapy has been found to alter the clinical expression of the disease, although rigorous control of hypertension (Raij *et al.*, 1984) may slow down its progression, as shown in experimental models.

Glomerular involvement in systemic disease

Diabetes

The kidney is one of the major targets of the microvascular complications of diabetes and over the past decade much has been learned about the aetiology and natural history of the disease (Mauer *et al.*, 1981).

Nephropathy complicates roughly 50 per cent (Mauer *et al.*, 1981) of cases of juvenile-onset diabetes (type 1) in children and is a major cause of morbidity and mortality in this group (Knowles, 1976). Most of what we understand about this disease has been obtained from studies of juvenile onset diabetes. Typically, the disease is initially silent with a negative urinalysis and normal or even slightly elevated creatinine clearance. The first clinical finding of disease is the occurrence of fixed proteinuria. Proteinuria is rare before the 10th year of disease, but, once present, is steadily progressive usually reaching the nephrotic range and associated with a progressive and inexorable fall in creatinine clearance. End-stage renal failure is reached, on average, 20 years after initial diagnosis.

Nephropathy also complicates adult-onset non-ketotic (type 2) diabetes (Bell, 1953), but has been much less intensively studied in this group, probably because in this population the morbidity of renal disease is overshadowed by that of large vessel disease (Knowles, 1976). Whereas in the series reported by the Joslin clinic, renal failure was considered the cause of death in 42 per cent of patients below age 20 at the onset of diabetes, it accounted for only 0.8 per cent of deaths in those who presented after the age of 60 (Balodimos, 1971). Nevertheless, type 2 diabetes mellitus is the most prevalent form of diabetes, since 80 per cent of all diabetic patients present initially after age 40, and is by far the commonest form of diabetes in the elderly (Kilvert *et al.*, 1984).

A considerable amount of information on the incidence and course of nephropathy in this form of diabetes has been obtained from studies of the Pima Indians. This tribe of southwestern American Indians is characterized by the highest recorded prevalence of diabetes in the world, since over 40 per cent of those above age 35 develop type 2 diabetes. A study of 105 autopsies revealed nodular glomerulosclerosis, compatible with diabetic nephropathy in 56 per cent of cases (Kamenetzky *et al.*, 1976). Furthermore, dipstick-positive proteinuria was seen in 22 per cent of all cases of diabetes, including almost 50 per cent of those with diabetes for 15 years or longer. Of interest, proteinuria was present in 17 per cent of newly diagnosed diabetics and this was particularly so in patients presenting after age 65. This tendency for proteinuria to develop soon after diagnosis in the elderly diabetic is in contrast to juvenile onset diabetes where fixed proteinuria is rare before 10 years. While this might reflect an increased susceptibility of older diabetics to the microvascular complications of diabetes, this difference is more likely to be due to the difficulty of determining the precise time of onset of carbohydrate intolerance in adult-onset disease where glucose intolerance may precede symptomatic diabetes for many years. Another interesting feature of this study was the low incidence of uraemia, with only 4–7 per cent of diabetic patients exhibiting an elevated serum creatinine. Even in those patients with diabetes for more than 15 years duration, only 13.8 per cent had serum creatinines >1.5 mg/dl, suggesting that diabetic nephropathy may be less likely to progress in adult-onset patients compared to their younger counterparts.

Finally, Fabre *et al.* (1982) have recently reported the findings of a cross-sectional study of 510 patients with maturity onset diabetes mellitus. They confirmed the finding that abnormal protein excretion (>150 mg/d) was common, occurring in 48 per cent of patients and usually appearing sooner in the course of the disease. However, the nephrotic syndrome was rare, being present in only 2 per cent as compared to 45 per cent of juvenile-onset diabetics 20–50 years old at death (Bell, 1953). Again, most patients with maturity onset diabetes maintained an adequate GFR; the GFR was considered normal in 83 per cent of patients without proteinuria and in 65 per cent of those with elevated urinary protein excretion. Only 1 patient died of renal insufficiency. Thus, while the occurrence of diabetic nephropathy in elderly diabetic patients appears to be just as frequent as in the juvenile form, the prognosis of such renal involvement appears to be considerably better. Since hypertension accelerates the glomerulopathy of type I diabetes, it would be sensible to pay careful attention to the control of blood pressure in patients with adult-onset diabetes. In addition, although there is as yet no conclusive evidence that tight control slows the progression of clinical diabetic nephropathy, it still seems reasonable to strive for the lowest blood glucose levels compatible with the avoidance of hypoglycaemia.

Rheumatic diseases

Renal involvement is common in systemic lupus erythematosus (SLE) and is occasionally seen in mixed connective tissue disease. However, lupus nephritis is an uncommon problem in the elderly because this disease tends to present at a younger age. A review of five major series from the literature (Pollack *et al.*, 1964; Kellum and Maserick, 1966; Estes and Christian, 1971; Harvey *et al.*, 1975; Lee *et al.*, 1977) revealed that only 4 per cent of cases of SLE presented after the age of 60. Details of the types of nephritis and their clinical course in these elderly patients were not available.

It is still unclear whether rheumatoid arthritis can cause a glomerulopathy *per se*. Claims have been made for the occurrence of both a membranous nephropathy (Samuels *et al.*, 1978) and a proliferative glomerulonephritis (Davis *et al.*, 1979). However, the issue is obscured by the fact that such involvement is rare and that many of the drugs used in this disease such as penicillamine and gold can cause glomerulopathies in their own right. One review of renal involvement in 5232 hospitalized patients with rheumatoid arthritis found only 11 cases of glomerular disease (Davis *et al.*, 1979). Five were attributed to gold nephropathy, 2 to amyloidosis, 3 to post-infectious glomerulonephritis and 1 to concurrent diabetes. No specific information is available in elderly patients with rheumatoid arthritis.

Amyloidosis

This refers to a spectrum of disease processes characterized by the tissue deposition of protein fibrils, in a β-pleated conformation. A considerable amount has been learned in recent years concerning the aetiology of this disease, and an extensive classification derived for clinical purposes by Kyle and Bayrd (1975) is probably sufficient. Over 80 per cent of cases fall into this category of primary amyloidosis or amyloidosis associated with myeloma. It is now clear that both probably represent different aspects of the same disease since, in both, amyloid deposition is associated with abnormal plasma cell function and the production of monoclonal paraprotein. The distinction is made only on the basis that, in primary amyloidosis, the criteria for diagnosis of a plasma cell dyscrasia are not satisfied. The common origin of these two entities is also reflected in their similar clinical features. Both are common in males and usually present in the sixth or seventh decades with over 50 per cent of cases occurring after the age of 60. From the renal point of view, proteinuria, frequently nephrotic in range, is the commonest presenting feature, being present in over 90 per cent of patients. As we saw earlier, amyloidosis accounts for up to 10 per cent of cases of the nephrotic syndrome seen in the elderly. Also, renal insufficiency is quite common; about 50 per cent of patients have elevated serum creatinine concentrations at presentation. Other clinical features which may suggest the diagnosis include peripheral and autonomic neuropathy, restrictive cardiomyopathy, hepatosplenomegaly, pinch purpura and a non-inflammatory polyarthropathy (Kyle and Bayrd, 1975).

About 8 per cent of cases of amyloidosis occur in association with some chronic inflammatory or infectious process, most often rheumatoid arthritis, but also tuberculosis, the paraplegic state, and many others (Kyle and Bayrd, 1975). Such a reactive amyloidosis usually presents as the nephrotic syndrome or hepatosplenomegaly. The diagnosis of amyloidosis is usually made by the detection of the characteristic eosinophilic deposits in biopsies of affected organs which stain with Congo red. Unfortunately, no clearly effective therapy exists for amyloidosis and the prognosis is poor, with death usually occurring within 2 years of diagnosis (Glenner, 1980).

Plasma cell dyscrasias

Renal disease is a frequent and usually ominous complication of multiple myeloma, occurring in over half of patients at some time during their course. As plasma cell dyscrasias occur mainly in the older age groups, this accounts for a small but definite cause of renal disease in the elderly. The usual manifestation is that of a tubulo-interstitial disease with tubular obstruction, atrophy and interstitial inflammation, the so-called 'myeloma kidney' (DeFronzo *et al.*, 1978). Light chains are primarily responsible for this type of renal impairment. Other potential causes of renal impairment in myeloma include hypercalcaemia which is often reversible and, rarely nowadays, hyperuricaemia (Bernstein and Humes, 1978). Initially, no glomerular lesions were identified (Levi *et al.*, 1968), but in recent years it has become increasingly recogized that glomerular disease may occur from deposition of light chains and be manifest in one of two forms, amyloidosis or light-chain disease.

Amyloidosis we have already considered. The other glomerular manifestation of plasma cell dyscrasias has come to be known as *light-chain nephropathy*. While cases of nodular glomerulosclerosis complicating myeloma may be found in the older literature, the first description of this entity which implicated the deposition of light chains is attributed to Randall *et al.* (1976), who described 2 patients with a lobular glomerulonephritis and deposition of kappa light chains. One had myeloma but, in the second, no evidence of myeloma was found. Both died of advanced renal failure. In a recent review of the literature, Ganeval *et al.* (1984) found that kappa-chain deposits occurred more frequently than lambda chains with a ratio of 4:1. Onset was usually in the sixth decade and about 25 per cent of the patients were over 60. The clinical presentation was generally one of renal insufficiency and proteinuria, occasionally nephrotic in range.

The most characteristic finding by light microscopy is thought to be multifocal nodular accumulation of eosinophilic material in the mesangium which is PAS positive but negative on Congo red stain. However, this is not an invariable finding and was present in only 5 of 14 patients at the Necker Hospital. Seven of the remainder showed thickening of the basement membrane only and, in 2, light microscopy was normal (Ganeval *et al.*, 1984). Tubular atrophy, rather than ectasia, was present and conventional immunofluorescence was usually negative. Use of specific anti-light-chain sera usually revealed deposition of kappa chains in a linear fashion along the glomerular (GBM) and tubular basement membranes (TBM), with coarse granular deposits in the mesangium.

Lambda light-chain nephropathy showed similar glomerular staining, but lacked TBM deposits (Ganeval *et al.*, 1984). Electron microscopy usually revealed dark granular material at the site of the Ig deposits. The disease may be associated with clinically overt myeloma or Waldenstrom's macroglobulinaemia at presentation, but in up to one-third of cases no monoclonal component was detectable in either urine or serum. In one case myeloma did not become evident for 8 months after development of renal disease and, in another, followed for up to 4 years, no sign of myeloma had appeared at last report (Ganeval *et al.*, 1984).

In general, the course of the nephropathy has been one of rapidly progressive deterioration in renal function with end-stage renal failure supervening within 1 year. In the series of Tubbs *et al.* (1981), 6 of 11 patients required dialysis, but detailed follow-up data on the other 5 patients are not available.

Ganeval *et al.* (1984) have argued that because of its close association with lymphoplasmacytic dyscrasias and the seemingly causal effect of light-chain deposition, it would seem logical to treat these patients with chemotherapy as in myeloma. Preud'homme *et al.* (1980) have described one patient who presented with a creatinine of 310 mol/l and whose renal function improved on chemotherapy. In addition, Ganeval *et al.* (1984) noted a slower degree of progression to dialysis in their patients given chemotherapy, as compared with those treated conservatively. However, the latter tended to be seen initially at a more advanced stage of the disease and stronger evidence will be required before such therapy can be advocated, especially in view of its poor record in amyloidosis. Finally, it is of interest to note that in the one patient reported who was transplanted, there was marked recurrence of the disease in the transplanted kidney (Case Records of the Massachusetts General Hospital, 1981).

Mixed essential cryoglobulinaemia

Cryoglobulins were first defined as cold precipitating or gelling plasma proteins. Most proteins involved in cryoprecipitation proved to be immunoglobulins and have been divided into three types (Brouet *et al.*, 1974):

Type I. Isolated monoclonal Igs or Bence-Jones proteins.
Type II. Mixed cryoglobulins with a monoclonal component usually an antibody against polyclonal Igs.
Type III. A mixture of polyclonal Igs.

The presence of cryoglobulins has been associated with a large number of infections, collagen-vascular and lymphoproliferative diseases (Brouet *et al.*, 1974), but in as many as 30–40 per cent of patients no underlying disease is clinically obvious and the condition is termed 'essential cryoglobulinaemia'. The first description of 'essential mixed cryoglobulinaemia', with its typical triad of purpura, arthralgia and renal involvement, is attributed to Lerner and Watson (1947). Melzer *et al.* (1966) described 9 cases with a similar syndrome, 4 of whom had severe renal disease consisting of a diffuse proliferative nephritis. Until recently, most descriptions of cryoglobulinaemic nephropathy have consisted of anecdotal case reports with scanty follow-up data, but recently two major series have been published. Unfortunately, in neither of these studies can the data for the elderly patients be separately analysed.

Table 15.5 Clinical presentation of renal disease in mixed essential cryoglobulinaemia in 44 patients (Data from Gorevic *et al.*, 1980)

	No. of cases (%)
Microscopic haematuria:	
−/proteinuria	10 (23%)
+/proteinuria	12 (27%)
Isolated proteinuria	6 (14%)
Acute nephritic syndrome	6 (14%)
Nephrotic syndrome	8 (18%)
Acute renal failure	2 (4%)

Gorevic *et al.* (1980) described the clinical course of 40 patients with significant quantities of mixed cryoglobulins (*Table 15.5*). Prominent clinical symptoms included recurrent palpable purpura (100 per cent), polyarthralgias (72.5 per cent) and renal disease (55 per cent). Hepatic involvement with hepatomegaly and elevated alkaline phosphatase was frequent (70 per cent) and other common symptoms included leg ulcers (30 per cent), Raynaud's phenomenon (25 per cent), intermittent abdominal pains (20 per cent) and lymphadenopathy (17.5 per cent). Over two-thirds of the patients were women, with a mean age of 51 years. 22.5 per cent of patients were over 60 years of age. In these patients, a high incidence of HB_s-Ag was found in cryoglobulins. Renal involvement implied a worse prognosis, with a 70 per cent mortality compared with 30 per cent in patients without renal involvement after an average follow-up of 7.6 years.

Renal involvement in this syndrome has been looked at in more detail by Tarantino *et al.* (1981), who reviewed 44 patients with mixed cryoglobulinaemia. The mode of presentation was variable, with a combination of proteinuria and/or microscopic haematuria accounting for over 60 per cent of cases. Renal disease rarely predated the appearance of purpura; it appeared simultaneously with purpura in 29 per cent and in the remainder developed 2 months to 7 years later. Renal biopsy revealed membrano-proliferative glomerulonephritis in 22 of 35 cases; the remainder showed a mesangial proliferative pattern, with 16 cases showing prominent intraluminal thrombi in the glomerular capillaries. Crescents were rare. Granular deposits of IgG, IgM and C3 were almost invariable on immunofluorescence microscopy and occurred in three different patterns: (1) intraluminal thrombi, alone or in association with scanty parietal deposits, (2) peripheral subendothelial deposits, and (3) mesangial deposits only. Electron microscopy revealed characteristic crystalloid deposits consisting of straight or slightly curved pairs of cylinders with a faint cross-striation, appearing as annular bodies on cross-section.

Two patients died during an initial bout of acute renal failure, and follow-up (mean 53.8 months) was available on 39 patients: 10 patients had a complete prolonged and undisturbed remission; 16 patients maintained normal renal function despite persistent urinary abnormalities; the remaining 13 patients experienced further exacerbations either in the form of acute renal failure with acute nephritic and/or nephrotic syndrome. Two of these patients died during acute renal disease and 3 progressed to chronic renal failure. This does not, however, represent the natural course of the disease, as most of these patients at some point were treated with either steroids or cytotoxic agents in a haphazard fashion. This was also true of the series of Gorevic *et al.* (1980) and is almost inevitable in such a rare disease in which it takes so long to accumulate a sizeable number of cases. Conclusions are made even more difficult by the waxing and waning nature of the disease. Whereas

Gorevic *et al.* (1980) favoured intervening as little as possible, Tarantino *et al.* (1981) generally felt that immunosuppressive therapy was effective and in particular stressed the effectiveness of high dose methylprednisolone in acutely controlling systemic symptoms such as fever, purpura and arthralgias. In addition, 8 out of 15 patients with renal manifestations showed clinical improvement after this therapy.

This group has recently reported more extensively (DeVecchi *et al.* 1983) on their experience in treating 15 patients with essential mixed cryoglobulinaemia with pulse methylprednisolone followed by immunosuppressive drugs. Treatment was instituted either for an increase in plasma creatinine of more than 30 per cent of baseline, a plasma creatinine >250 mol/l at presentation, or an increase of more than 40 per cent in protein excretion. Creatinine improved promptly in 10 of 13 episodes treated with a mean fall in serum creatinine from 330 to 190 mol/l 1 month later. Geltner *et al.* (1981) recently reported 4 patients who had an improvement in renal function and healing of vasculitic ulcers with the use of plasmaphaeresis combined with prednisone and chloramhucil. Such aggressive therapy may be indicated in patients with severe progressive systemic manifestations of vasculitis, particularly with deterioration in renal function (see Chapter 16).

References

ABRASS, C. (1985). Glomerulonephritis in the elderly. *American Journal of Kidney Disease,* **4,** 409–418

BALDWIN, D.S., GLUCK, M.C., SCHACHT, R.G. and GALLO, G. (1976). The long term course of poststreptococcal glomerulonephritis. *Annals of Internal Medicine,* **80,** 342–358

BALODIMOS, M.D. (1971). Diabetic nephropathy. In *Joslin's Diabetes Mellitus,* 11th edn, edited by A. Marble, P. White, R.F. Bradley and L.P. Krall, pp. 526–561. Philadelphia; Lea and Febiger

BEIRNE, G.J., WAGNILD, J.P., ZIMMERMAN, S.W. *et al.* (1977). Idiopathic crescentic glomerulonephritis. *Medicine,* **56,** 369–381

BELL, E.T. (1953). Renal vascular disease in diabetes mellitus. *Diabetes,* **2,** 376–389

BERGER, J. and HINGLAIS, N. (1968). Les depots intercapillaries d'IgA–IgG. *Journal de Urologie et de Nephrologie,* **74,** 694–695

BERNSTEIN, S.P. and HUMES, H.D. (1978). Reversible renal insufficiency in multiple myeloma. *Archives of Internal Medicine,* **142,** 2083–2086

BLACK, D.A.K., ROSE, G. and BREWER, D.R. (1970). Controlled trial of prednisone in adult patients with the nephrotic syndrome. *British Medical Journal,* **3,** 421–426

BOLTON, W.K. (1984a). Nephrotic syndrome in the aged. In *Proceedings of the Ninth International Congress of Nephrology,* **72A.**

BOLTON, W.K. (1984b). The case for aggressive use (of high-dose steroids). In *Controversies in Nephrology and Hypertension,* edited by R.G. Narins, pp. 421–459. New York; Churchill Livingstone

BOLTON, W.K. and COUSER, W.G. (1979). Intravenous pulse methylprednisolone therapy of crescentic rapidly progressive glomerulonephritis. *American Journal of Medicine,* **66,** 496–502

BOLTON, W.K., WESTERVELT, F.B. and STURGILL, B.C. (1978). Nephrotic syndrome and focal glomerulosclerosis in aging man. *Nephron,* **20,** 307–315

BREZIN, J.P., KATZ, S.M. *et al.* (1979). Reversible renal failure associated with nonsteroidal anti-inflammatory agents. *New England Journal of Medicine,* **301,** 1271–1273

BROUET, J.C., CLAUVEL, J.P., DANON, F. *et al.* (1974). Biologic and clinical significance of cryoglobulins. *American Journal of Medicine,* **57,** 775–788

BROWN, C.R., CAMERON, J.S., TURNER, D.R. *et al.* (1978). Focal segmental glomerulosclerosis with rapid decline in renal function ('malignant FSGS'). *Clinical Nephrology,* **10,** 51–61

CAMERON, J.S. (1979). Pathogenesis and treatment of membranous nephropathy. *Kidney International,* **15,** 88–103

CAMERON, J.S. (1982). Glomerulonephritis: current problems and understanding. *Journal of Laboratory and Clinical Medicine,* **99,** 755–787

CAMERON, J.S., TURNER, D.R., HEATON, J. *et al.* (1983). Idiopathic mesangiocapillary glomerulonephritis. Comparison of Types I and II in children and adults and long-term prognosis. *American Journal of Medicine,* **79,** 175–192

CAMERON, J.S., TURNER, D.R., OGG, C.S. *et al.* (1974). The nephrotic syndrome in adults with 'minimal change' glomerular lesions. *Quarterly Journal of Medicine,* **43,** 461–488

CASE RECORDS OF THE MASSACHUSETTS GENERAL HOSPITAL (Case 1—1981). *New England Journal of Medicine,* **309,** 53–63

CHAMBERLAIN, M.J., PRINGLE, A. and WRONG, O.M. (1968). Oliguric renal failure in the nephrotic syndrome. *Quarterly Journal of Medicine,* **35,** 215–235

CLARKSON, A.R., SEYMOUR, A.E., THOMPSON, A.J. *et al.* (1977). IgA nephropathy: a syndrome of uniform morphology, diverse clinical features and uncertain prognosis. *Clinical Nephrology,* **8,** 459–471

COLLABORATIVE STUDY OF THE ADULT IDIOPATHIC NEPHROTIC SYNDROME (1979). A controlled study of short-term prednisone treatment in adults with membranous nephropathy. *New England Journal of Medicine,* **301,** 1301–1306

CONNOLLY, N.E., WRONG, O.M. and JONES, N.F. (1968). Reversible renal failure in idiopathic nephrotic syndrome with minimal glomerular changes. *The Lancet,* **1,** 665–668

CONSTANZA, M.E., PINN, V., SCHWARTZ, R.S. and NATHANSON, L. (1973). Carcinoembryonic antigen-antibody complexes in a patient with colonic carcinoma and nephrotic syndrome. *New England Journal of Medicine,* **289,** 520–522

COUSER, W.G. (1982). Idiopathic rapidly progressive glomerulonephritis. *American Journal of Nephrology,* **2,** 57–69

COUSER, W.G., WAGONFIELD, J.B., SPARGO, B.H. and LEWIS, E.J. (1974). Glomerular deposition of tumor antigen in membranous nephropathy associated with colonic carcinoma. *American Journal of Medicine,* **57,** 962–970

DAVIS, J.A., COHEN, A.H., WEISBART, R. and PAULUS, H.E. (1979). Glomerulonephritis in rheumatoid arthritis. *Arthritis and Rheumatism,* **22,** 1018–1023

DEFRONZO, R.A., COOKE, C.R., WRIGHT, J.R. and HUMPHREY, R.L. (1978). Renal function in patients with multiple myeloma. *Medicine,* **57,** 151–166

DEVECCHI, A., MONTAGNINO, G., POZZI, C. *et al.* (1983). Intravenous methylprednisolone pulse therapy in essential mixed cryoglobulinemia therapy. *Clinical Nephrology,* **19,** 221–227

DONADIO, J.V., ANDERSON, C.F., MITCHELL, J.C. *et al.* (1984). Membranoproliferative glomerulonephritis. A prospective clinical trial of platelet-inhibitor therapy. *New England Journal of Medicine,* **310,** 1421–1427

DROZ, D. (1976). Natural history of primary glomerulonephritis with mesangial deposits of IgA. *Contributions to Nephrology,* **2,** 150–157

EAGEN, J.W. and LEWIS, E.J. (1977). Glomerulopathies of neoplasia. *Kidney International,* **11,** 297–306

EDITORIAL (1977). Is poststreptococcal glomerulonephritis progressive? *British Medical Journal,* **2,** 775–776

ERWIN, D.T., DONADIO, J.V., Jr. and HOLLEY, K.E. (1973). The clinical course of idiopathic membranous nephropathy. *Mayo Clinic Proceedings,* **48,** 697–712

ESTES, D. and CHRISTIAN, C.L. (1971). The natural history of systemic lupus erythematosus by prospective analysis. *Medicine,* **33,** 291–437

FABRE, J., BALANT, L.P., DAYER, P.G., FOX, H.M. and VERNET, A.T. (1982). The kidney in maturity onset diabetes mellitus: a clinical study of 510 patients. *Kidney International,* **21,** 730–738

FINKELSTEIN, A., FRALEY, D.S., STACHURA, I. *et al.* (1982). Fenoprofen nephropathy: lipoid nephrosis and interstitial nephritis. *American Journal of Medicine,* **72,** 81–87

GANEVAL, D., NOEL, L.H., PREUD'HOMME, J.L. *et al.* (1984). Light-chain deposition disease: its relation with AL-type amyloidosis. *Kidney International,* **26,** 1–9

GARELLA, S. and MATARESE, R.A. (1984). Renal effects of prostaglandins and clinical adverse effects of nonsteroidal anti-inflammatory agents. *Medicine,* **63,** 165–181

GELTNER, K., KOHN, R.W., GOREVIC, P. and FRANKLIN, E.C. (1981). The effect of combination therapy (steroids, immunosuppressives and plasmapheresis) on 5 mixed cryoglobulinemia patients with renal, neurologic and vascular involvement. *Arthritis and Rheumatism,* **24,** 1121–1127

GLASSOCK, R., COHEN, A., ADLER, S. and WARD, H. (1986). Primary glomerular diseases. In *The Kidney,* 3rd edn, edited by B.M. Brenner and F.C. Rector, pp. 929–1013. Philadelphia; Saunders

GLENNER, G.G. (1980). Amyloid deposits and amyloidosis. *New England Journal of Medicine,* **302,** 1283–1292, 1333–1343

GLUCK, M.C., GALLO, G., LOWENSTEIN, J.L. and BALDWIN, D.S. (1973). Membranous glomerulonephritis. *Annals of Internal Medicine,* **78,** 1–12

GOREVIC, P.D., KASSAB, H.J., LEVO, Y. *et al.* (1980). Mixed cryoglobulinemia: clinical aspects and long-term follow-up of 40 patients. *American Journal of Medicine,* **69,** 287–308

HARVEY, A.M., SHULMAN, L.E., TUMULTY, A., CONLEY, C.L. and MUEHRCKE, R.C. (1975). Systemic lupus erythematosus: review of the literature and clinical analysis of 138 cases. *Medicine,* **33,** 291–437

HAYSLETT, J.P., KASHGARIAN, M., SPARGO, B. *et al.* (1973). Clinicopathological correlations in the nephrotic syndrome due to primary renal disease. *Medicine,* **52,** 93–100

HIND, C.R.K., LOCKWOOD, C.M., PETERS, D.K. *et al.* (1983). Prognosis after immunosuppression of patients with crescentic nephritis requiring dialysis. *Lancet,* **1,** 263–265

HOPPER, J. Jr., RYAN, P., LEE, J.C. and ROSENAD, W. (1970). Lipoid nephrosis in 37 adult patients. *Medicine,* **49,** 321–341

KAMENETZKY, S.A., BENNETT, P.H., DIPPE, S.E., MILLER, M. and LECOMPTE, P.M. (1976). A clinical and histologic study of diabetic nephropathy in Pima Indians. *Diabetes,* **23,** 61–68

KASSIRER, J.P. (1983). Is renal biopsy necessary for optimal management of the idiopathic nephrotic syndrome? *Kidney International,* **24,** 561–575

KELLUM, R.E. and HASERICK, J.R. (1966). Systemic lupus erythematosus. *Archives of Internal Medicine,* **113,** 200–207

KILVERT, A., FITZGERALD, M.G., WRIGHT, A.D. and NATTRASS, M. (1984). Newly diagnosed, insulin-dependent diabetes mellitus in elderly patients. *Diabetes Medicine,* **1,** 115–118

KIM, Y. and MICHAEL, A.F. (1978). Infection and nephritis. In *Pediatric Kidney Disease,* 1st edn, edited by C.M. Edelmann Jr., pp. 828–837. Boston; Little, Brown

KINCAID-SMITH, P. and WALKER, R.G. (1984). The case for plasmapheresis. In *Controversies in Nephrology and Hypertension,* edited by R.G. Narins, pp. 463–493. New York; Churchill Livingstone

KNOWLES, H.C. Jr. (1976). Magnitude of the renal failure problem in diabetic patients. *Kidney International,* **2** (Suppl. 2), 52–57

KURTZMAN, N.A. (1978). Does acute poststreptococcal glomerulonephritis lead to chronic renal disease? *New England Journal of Medicine,* **298,** 796

KYLE, R.A. and BAYRD, E.D. (1975). Amyloidosis. Review of 236 cases. *Medicine,* **54,** 271–299

LEE, H.A., STIRLING, G. and SHARPSTONE, P. (1966). Acute glomerulonephritis in middle-aged and elderly patients. *British Medical Journal,* **2,** 1361–1363

LEE, J.C., YAMAUCHI, H. and HOPPER, J. Jr. (1966). The association of cancer and the nephrotic syndrome. *Annals of Internal Medicine,* **69,** 41–51

LEE, P., UROWITZ, M.B., BOOKMAN, A.M., KOEHLER, B.E., SMYTHE, H.A., GORDON, D.A. and OGRYZLO, M.A. (1977). Systemic lupus erythematosis. A review of 110 cases with reference to nephritis, the nervous system, infections, aseptic necrosis and prognosis. *Quarterly Journal of Medicine,* **46,** 1–32

LERNER, A.B. and WATSON, C.J. (1947). Studies of cryoglobulins I: Unusual purpura associated with rheumatoid factor activity. *American Journal of the Medical Sciences,* **214,** 416–421

LEVI, D.F., WILLIAMS, R.C. and LINSTROM, R.D. (1968). Immunofluorescent studies of the myeloma kidney with special reference to light chain disease. *American Journal of Medicine,* **44,** 922–933

LIEN, J.M.S., MATHEW, T.M. and MEADOWS, R. (1979). Acute poststreptococcal glomerulonephritis in adults: a long-term study. *Quarterly Journal of Medicine,* **48,** 99–111

LIM, V.S., SIBLEY, R. and SPARGO, B. (1974). Adult lipoid nephrosis: clinicopathological correlations. *Annals of Internal Medicine,* **81,** 314–320

LOCKWOOD, C. and PETERS, D. (1980). Plasma exchange in glomerulonephritis and related vasculitides. *Annual Review of Medicine,* **31,** 167–179

LOCKWOOD, C.M., PINCHING, A.J., SWENY, P. *et al.* (1977). Plasma exchange and immunosuppression in the treatment of fulminating immune-complex crescentic nephritis. *Lancet,* **1,** 63–67

LOCKWOOD, C.M., REES, A.J., PEARSON, T.A. *et al.* (1976). Immunosuppression and plasma exchange in the treatment of Goodpasture's syndrome. *Lancet,* **1,** 711–715

LOWENSTEIN, J., SCHACHT, R.G. and BALDWIN, D.S. (1981). Renal failure in minimal change nephrotic syndrome. *American Journal of Medicine,* **70,** 227–233

MAUER, S.M., STEFFES, M.W. and BROWN, D.M. (1981). The kidney in diabetes. *American Journal of Medicine,* **70,** 603–612

MAXWELL, D.R., OZAWA, T., NIELSEN, R.L. and LUFT, F.C. (1979). Spontaneous recovery from rapidly progressive glomerulonephritis. *British Medical Journal,* **3,** 643

MELTZER, M., FRANKLIN, E.C., ELIAS, K. *et al.* (1966). Cryoglobulinemia. A clinical and laboratory study. II cryoglobulins with rheumatoid factor activity. *American Journal of Medicine,* **40,** 837–856

MONTOLIU, J., DANNELL, A., TORRAS, A. and REVERT, L. (1981). Acute and rapidly progessive forms of glomerulonephritis in the elderly. *Journal of the American Geriatrics Society,* **29,** 108–116

MOORTHY, A.V. and ZIMMERMAN, S.W. (1977). Renal disease in the elderly: clinicopathologic analysis of renal disease in 115 elderly patients. *Clinical Nephrology,* **14,** 223–229

MORRIN, P., HINGALIS, N., NABARRA, B. and KREIS, H. (1978). Rapidly progressive glomerulonephritis — a clinical and pathologic study. *American Journal of Medicine,* **65,** 446–460

NESSON, H.R. and ROBBINS, S.L. (1960). Glomerulonephritis in older age groups. *Archives of Internal Medicine,* **105,** 23–32

NOEL, L.H., ZANETTI, M., DROZ, D. and BARBANEL, C. (1979). Long-term prognosis of idiopathic membranous glomerulonephritis. *American Journal of Medicine,* **6**, 82–89

OLDSTONE, M.B.A., THEOFILOPOULOS, A.N., GUNVEN, P. and KLEIN, G. (1974). Immune complexes associated with neoplasia: presence of Epstein–Barr virus antigen–antibody complexes in Burkett's lymphoma. *Intervirology,* **4**, 292–302

OZAWA, T., PLASS, R., LARCHER, J. *et al.* (1975). Endogenous immune complex nephropathy associated with malignancy I. Studies on the nature and immunopathogenic significance of glomerular bound antigen and antibody, isolation and characterization of tumor specific antigen and antibody and circulating immune complexes. *Quarterly Journal of Medicine,* **49**, 523–541

POLLAK, V.E., PIRANI, C.L. and SCHWARTZ, F.D. (1964). The natural history of the renal manifestations of systemic lupus erythematosus. *Journal of Laboratory and Clinical Medicine,* **63**, 537–550

POLLAK, V.E., ROSEN, S., PIRANI, C.L. *et al.* (1968). Natural history of lipoid nephrosis and of membranous glomerulonephritis. *Annals of Internal Medicine,* **69**, 1171–1196

PONTICELLI, L., ZUCCHELLI, P., IMBASCIATI, E. *et al.* (1984). Controlled trial of methylprednisolone and chlorambucil in idiopathic membranous nephropathy. *New England Journal of Medicine,* **310**, 946–950

POTTER, E.V., ABIDH, S., SHARRETT, A.R. *et al.* (1978). Clinical healing two to six years after poststreptococcal glomerulonephritis in Trinidad. *New England Journal of Medicine,* **298.**, 767–772

PRASAD, D.R., ZIMMERMAN, S.W. and BURKHOLDER, P.M. (1977). Immunohistologic features of minimal-change nephrotic syndrome. *Archives of Pathology and Laboratory Medicine,* **101**, 345–349

PREUD'HOMME, J.L., MOREL-MAROGER, R.L., BROUET, J.C. *et al.* (1980). Synthesis of abnormal immunoglobulins in lymphoplasmacytic disorders with visceral light-chain deposition. *American Journal of Medicine,* **69**, 703–710

RAIJ, L., KEANE, W.F., LEONARD, A. and SHAPIRO, F.L. (1976). Irreversible acute renal failure in idiopathic nephrotic syndrome. *American Journal of Medicine,* **61**, 207–214

RAIJ, J. and MICHAEL, A.F. (1980). Immunologic aspects of kidney disease. In *Clinical Immunology,* edited by C.W. Parker, pp. 1009–1050. Philadelphia; Saunders

RAIJ, L., AZAR, S. and KEANE, W. (1984). Mesangial immune injury, hypertension and progressive glomerular damage in Dahl rats. *Kidney International,* **26**, 137–143

RANDALL, R.E., WILLIAMSON, W.C. Jr., MULLINAX, F. *et al.* (1976). Manifestations of systemic light chain deposition. *American Journal of Medicine,* **60**, 293–299

REVOL, L., VIOLA, J.J., REVILLAUD, J.P. and MANUEL, Y. (1966). Proteinurie associée à des manifestations paraneoplastiques au cours d'un cancer bronchogenie. *Lyon Medical,* **212**, 907–916

RICH, A.R. (1957). A hitherto undescribed vulnerability of the juxtamedullary glomeruli in lipoid nephrosis. *Bulletin of Johns Hopkins Hospital,* **100**, 174–175

ROW, P.G., CAMERON, J.S., TURNER, D.R. *et al.* (1975). Membranous nephropathy. Long term follow-up and association with neoplasia. *Quarterly Journal of Medicine,* **44**, 207–239

SAMIY, A.M., FIELD, R.A. and MERRILL, J.P. (1961). Acute glomerulonephritis in elderly patients. *Annals of Internal Medicine,* **54**, 603–609

SAMUELS, B., LEE, J.C., ENGLEMAN, E.P. and HOPPER, J. Jr. (1978). Membranous nephropathy in patients with rheumatoid arthritis. *Medicine,* **57**, 319–327

SAPIR, D.G., YARDLEY, J.H. and WALKER, W.G. (1968). Acute glomerulonephritis in older patients. *Johns Hopkins Medical Journal,* **32**, 145–152

SHARPSTONE, P., OGG, C.S. and CAMERON, J.S. (1969). Nephrotic syndrome due to primary renal disease in adults. *British Medical Journal,* **2**, 533–539

STILMANT, M., BOLTON, W.K., STURGILL, B. *et al.* (1974). Crescentic glomerulonephritis without immune deposits. Clinicopathologic features. *Kidney International,* **15**, 189–195

TARANTINO, A., DEVECCHI, A., MONTAGNINO, G. *et al.* (1981). Renal disease in essential mixed cryoglobulinemia. *Quarterly Journal of Medicine,* **50**, 1–30

TEJANI, A. and NICASTRI, A.D. (1983). Mesangial IgM nephropathy. *Nephron,* **35**, 1–5

TEJANI, A., NICASTRI, A.D., SEN, N. *et al.* (1983). Long-term evaluation of children with nephrotic syndrome and focal segmental glomerulosclerosis. *Nephron,* **35**, 225–231

TUBBS, R.R., GEPHARDT, G.N., MACMAHON, J.T. *et al.* (1981). Light-chain nephropathy. *American Journal of Medicine,* **71**, 263–269

WING, W.J., BURNS, F.J., FRALEY, D.S. *et al.* (1980). Infectious complications with plasmapheresis in rapidly progressive glomerulonephritis. *Journal of the American Medical Association,* **244**, 2423–2426

ZECH, P., COLON, S., POINTET, P. *et al.* (1982). The nephrotic syndrome in adults aged over 60: etiology, evolution and treatment of 76 cases. *Clinical Nephrology,* **18**, 232–236

ZIMMERMAN, S.W., MOORTHY, A.W., DREHER, W.H. *et al.* (1983). Prospective trial of warfarin and dipyramidole in patients with membranoproliferative glomerulonephritis. *American Journal of Medicine,* **75**, 920–927

Chapter 16

Renal vasculitis in the aged

Assumpta Serra-Cardús and J. Stewart Cameron

Introduction

Several questions need to be answered when approaching the subject of renal vasculitis in the elderly: (a) its incidence above 60 years of age; (b) the clinical features of the vasculitides in the elderly compared with those of patients under 60 years of age; (c) identification of the types of vasculitis that are specially prevalent in this period of life; and conversely, which forms are seldom seen in this population.

Data mainly extracted from our own series of patients with renal vasculitis are provided, in an attempt to answer these questions. Conclusions and comments of the present review only apply to patients with severe renal involvement, and not to patients with vasculitis in whom nephrologic involvement is of minor relevance or is absent.

In the elderly, the signs and symptoms of renal disease and vasculitis tend to be non-specific and atypical, and clinical detection not infrequently poses a problem. The difficulty in the diagnosis of other types of disease in the elderly (appendicitis, endocarditis, etc.) also extends to vasculitis. Patients may present with progressive renal failure of unknown aetiology, non-specific single organ involvement (respiratory, gastrointestinal) or with general symptoms (fever, abdominal pain), and only careful search of clinical signs of vasculitis may unmask the underlying disease or prompt a diagnostic biopsy. Conversely, other diseases in the elderly can mimic vasculitis (e.g. cholesterol embolism). The clinical importance of a precise diagnosis stems from the fact that patients with vasculitis and progressive renal involvement may benefit from treatment.

Vasculitis is seen nowadays in the elderly more often than in the past. The reasons for this phenomenon are twofold: first, the mean age of death of the population has increased, and secondly, the awareness of these diseases in the medical community is greater. In addition, prompt diagnosis and successful treatment has resulted in the survivors of vasculitis increasingly attending outpatients clinics.

The following description of renal vasculitis will be divided into two basic sections; in the first, problems in the definition, nomenclature and the pathology and pathogenesis are dealt with. In the second, a clinical description of the vasculitides in a nephrologic context is made, with emphasis on the impact of the disease on the elderly. Comparison is made between the data of patients older and younger than 60 years of age. Prognosis and treatment are dealt with in a final section.

I. Definition, nomenclature, pathology and pathogenesis

Definition and nomenclature

What constitutes a renal vasculitis? Problems in the classification of renal vasculitis

The problem of 'microscopic polyarteritis' and idiopathic 'segmental necrotizing glomerulitis'

Necrosis and cellular infiltration of the vessel wall are taken as the histological features of vasculitis. In the kidney, every artery can be involved, from the main renal artery to the capillaries of the glomerular tuft. It is the latter involvement which produces glomerular changes that are identified as a type of 'glomerulonephritis'. Traditionally, the presence of arterial involvement has been a precondition of the diagnosis of vasculitis. Wainwright and Davson first suggested, in 1950, that necrotizing glomerular lesions alone might be the only evidence of vasculitis within the kidney. This glomerular appearance is referred to as 'microscopic polyarteritis' (Davson, Ball and Platt, 1948), although 'segmental necrotizing glomerulitis' is probably a more accurate descriptive term. A recent study from our unit, including more than 50 patients, has recently presented evidence that this approach is probably valid (Serra *et al.*, 1984).

In addition, some patients do not have a clear clinical picture of vasculitis or evidence of vasculitis (arteritis, arteriolitis) histologically, but present with a pattern of 'idiopathic' segmental necrotizing glomerulitis, often with severe crescent formation and negative findings for immunoglobulins on immunofluorescence (Sonsino *et al.*, 1972; Stilmant *et al.*, 1979; Moorthy and Zimmerman, 1980; Neild *et al.*, 1983). In some of these cases the only manifestation of vasculitis could be glomerular capillaries, other vascular lesions being absent or not evident clinically or in the small biopsy specimen. In some cases who come to post mortem, this has been proven, but remains undecided in those patients who survive or those who are not subjected to careful post-mortem examination of many tissues. At present, there is no satisfactory answer as to how these patients should be regarded or treated. On balance, they should probably be regarded (and treated) as having vasculitis affecting only the glomeruli (see Chapter 15).

Definition of Wegener's granulomatosis

The definition of Wegener's granulomatosis constitutes another problem in the classification of the vasculitides, as it may present identical clinical and histological features to 'microscopic polyarteritis', thus raising the question as to which cases with evident clinical vasculitis should be included under the diagnosis of Wegener's granulomatosis. Different authors have used different criteria. A strict view would include only those patients with *histological* evidence of a necrotizing granulomatous vasculitis in biopsies of the upper respiratory tract, nose or ear. Separation of patients with Wegener's granulomatosis from those with 'microscopic polyarteritis' and respiratory involvement, but no identifiable granulomas, may be important in view of the very successful results achieved with cyclophosphamide and plasmaphaeresis in Wegener's granulomatosis.

In practice, this distinction is difficult, and even when there are evident upper respiratory lesions, biopsies often show nothing but non-specific necrosis, even when the base of the lesion is included in the biopsy. Bronchial and even open lung biopsy are not necessarily more useful, and an unacceptable delay of several days may occur before the material can be taken and processed. This has led some authors, reasonably, to accept a *clinical* diagnosis of Wegener's granulomatosis when there is prominent involvement of lung, sinuses, ears or upper respiratory tract with what appear clinically to be vasculitic lesions (Haworth, 1983; Pinching *et al.*, 1983). Unfortunately, this is also fraught with difficulties: in ill, infected patients with vasculitis, the chest X-ray may show diffuse changes unrelated to vasculitis, or vasculitis which is not granulomatous. Finally, in cases coming to post mortem after intensive treatment and in whom no granuloma are found despite a clinical picture suggestive of Wegener's granulomatosis, the effects of treatment in the suppression of the granulomas should be considered.

Vasculitis with known aetiology

Difficulties in classification of the vasculitides also arise because, in a minority of patients, specific circumstances can be identified which seem to play a part in the pathogenesis of the disease. Infections, drugs and neoplastic disease, plus a number of more or less well-defined immunological disorders, are sometimes associated with vasculitis. Clinical classifications, or the ones based upon the size of vessel, the type of inflammatory lesions seen (granulomatous or non-granulomatous), on the supposed aetiology or specific organ involvement are not entirely satisfactory in defining clear-cut entities; in addition, one must take into account the pattern of glomerular injury: besides the common pattern of segmental necrotizing glomerulitis with or without crescent formation, endocapillary glomerulonephritis or a collapsed glomerular tuft without obvious pathology may be seen. Probably no available classification describes renal vasculitis comprehensively; *Table 16.1* attempts to define each case at various levels (e.g. between hepatitis B antigenaemia and involvement of medium-sized vessels with classical polyarteritis nodosa, and not with necrotizing glomerulitis); there are no absolute one-to-one correspondences.

Henoch–Schönlein purpura

Another serious area of confusion lies in the diagnosis of Henoch–Schönlein purpura in the adult. Henoch–Schönlein purpura shows a typical leukocytoclastic vasculitis affecting principally skin, joints, guts and kidneys, but has a striking age distribution (5–15 years) and a strong association with IgA (Habib and Cameron, 1982), which is found in deposits within the skin, gut and renal lesions. The condition is rare over the age of 20. Many patients diagnosed in middle and old age as having Henoch–Schönlein purpura are probably suffering from other forms of vasculitis. Unless there is evidence of IgA deposition in isolation or as the predominant immunoglobulin in the glomeruli, the diagnosis should be viewed with extreme suspicion in any adult. However, typical cases of Henoch–Schönlein purpura can be seen in the elderly, even in the eighth or ninth decade of life (Ballard, Eisinger and Gallo, 1970; Brun *et al.*, 1971; Fillastre, Morel-Maroger and Richet, 1971; Bar-On and Rosenmann, 1972; Kalowski and Kincaid-Smith, 1973; Case Records of the Massachusetts General Hospital, 1974; Kauffmann and Houwert, 1981; Habib and Cameron, 1982).

Table 16.1 Specific circumstances, vessel involvement, type of glomerular injury and clinical course in renal vasculitis (From Serra and Cameron, 1985, reproduced with permission)

Precipitating events or associated diseases	*Size of vessel involved*	*Glomerular pathology*	*Course*
Infections: hepatitis B beta-haemolytic streptococci otitis media	—Large (aorta) (renal branches)	Ischaemic only	'One shot'
Drugs: sulphonamides penicillin iodide thiourea alclofenac etc.	—Medium arteries (lobular, arcuate)	—Focal necrotizing glomerulitis ('microscopic polyarteritis')	
Neoplasms: chronic lymphocytic leukaemia lymphoma myeloma	± Granuloma formation —Small (arterioles)	—Crescentic glomerulonephritis ± Glomerular lesions	—Continuing disease
Identifiable systemic diseases: systemic lupus erythematosus Henoch–Schönlein purpura rheumatoid arthritis mixed cryoglobulinaemia subacute bacterial endocarditis polychondritis Behçet's disease serum sickness complement deficiencies anti-GBM dermatomyositis etc.	± —Venules —Capillary	—Endocapillary proliferative glomerulonephritis —Others	

Pathology of renal vasculitis

The pathologic findings of patients with predominant renal vasculitis differ from those found in unselected series in two aspects (Serra and Cameron, 1985):

(1) The organ distribution of vasculitic lesions is different; cardiac, hepatic, gastrointestinal, testicular and central and peripheral nervous system vessel vasculitis is significantly higher in the unselected series; contrarily, purpura, pulmonary and splenic involvement are more often seen in the renal series.
(2) Glomerulonephritis is mainly seen in the renal series; three main types of glomerular changes are seen in those patients who come to a renal unit:segmental necrotizing glomerulitis 'microscopic polyarteritis' and/or crescentic glomerulonephritis (83 per cent), diffuse endocapillary proliferative glomerulonephritis (9 per cent), and normal or ischaemic glomeruli (8 per cent) (Serra *et al.*, 1984; Serra and Cameron, 1985, unpublished). Other types of glomerular changes have also been described (Habib *et al.*, 1973; Montes *et al.*, 1975; Duffy *et al.*, 1976; Michalak, 1978; Spargo, Seymour and Ordoñez, 1980).

Pathologic findings in the elderly patients are similar to those under 60 years of age: in our series, 19 of 63 patients were more than 60 years old. The proportion of vasculitic lesions in the kidney or elsewhere was greater in the elderly than in the younger: 14/19 (74 per cent) versus 26/44 (59 per cent), although not significantly so. The type and prevalence of glomerular lesions was also similar: in the elderly 17/19 (89 per cent) had segmental necrotizing glomerulitis and 2/19 (11 per cent) had diffuse endocapillary proliferative glomerulonephritis. We did not find any patient above 60 years with normal or only ischaemic glomeruli.

Renal structures potentially involved in the vasculitic process are vessels, glomeruli, interstitium and tubules.

Vessel involvement in the vasculitides (Novak, Christiansen and Sorensen, 1982; Heptinstall, 1983)

Acute necrotizing vasculitis is characterized by fibrinoid necrosis of the vessel wall with infiltration by polymorphonuclear leukocytes, eosinophils, and mononuclear cells within and around the vessel wall; thrombosis can be seen occasionally. Fibrinoid necrosis may be limited to the intimal area of the vessel in the acute renal lesions of some patients with Wegener's granulomatosis, and very little polymorphonuclear reaction is also noted within the vessel wall of these patients (Novak, Christiansen and Sorensen, 1982). The infiltrating cells in Wegener's granulomatosis are mainly T-lymphocytes (both helper and suppressor) and monocytes (Gerhardt, Ahmad and Tubbs, 1983). Healed lesions can be recognized by the presence of mural fibrosis, rupture of the elastic laminae and irregular intimal thickening; aneurysms can be seen at this stage. In some cases acute and healed lesions can be seen in combination, while in others, lesions are at the same stage. Arteries of different calibre are involved. Arcuate or interlobular arteries are the most commonly affected in the classic or 'macroscopic' polyarteritis nodosa of Kussmaul and Maier (Zeek's periarteritis nodosa), while interlobular arteries, arterioles and the glomerular capillary tuft are mainly involved in the 'microscopic' form of polyarteritis (Zeek's hypersensitivity angiitis); overlap between both 'macroscopic' and 'microscopic' types of lesions occurs (Davson, Ball and Platt, 1948; Ralston and Kvale, 1949; Knowles, Zeek and Blankenhorn, 1953; de Shazo *et al.*, 1977; Ronco *et al.*, 1983).

In our series of patients with predominant renal vasculitis the renal vessels involved are, when consideration is given to the biopsy findings, arterioles (47 per cent), small arteries (63 per cent) and less commonly medium sized arteries (10 per cent) (Serra, 1983). In post-mortem studies, these percentages are somewhat different: 29 per cent, 86 per cent and 29 per cent, respectively. The proportion of arterioles—lower in necropsy than in biopsy findings—can be underestimated if careful post-mortem study of many tissues is not performed. It should be noted that when medium sized arterial vasculitis is seen at post mortem, it is in our experience invariably associated with arteriole or small artery vasculitis. There is no difference between the elderly and patients under 60 years, regarding the type of vessel involved.

Glomerular involvement (glomerulonephritis, glomerulitis)

In classic polyarteritis nodosa, the glomeruli show mainly non-specific ischaemic shrinkage of the capillary tuft. In other forms of vasculitis characterized by small vessel involvement (hypersensitivity vasculitis, Wegener's granulomatosis, allergic angiitis and granulomatosis, and other vasculitis), there is glomerulonephritis. This may take the form of segmental necrotizing glomerulitis ('microscopic polyarteritis'), crescentic and other types of glomerulonephritis.

(a) Segmental necrotizing glomerulitis (microscopic polyarteritis) (Figure 16.1)

The glomerular lesions consist of areas of glomerular fibrinoid necrosis, usually focal and segmental, which are frequently seen together with minimal endocapillary proliferation, crescent formation and capillary thrombosis. Fresh damage and variable degrees of glomerular scarring and organization may coexist in the same glomerulus (Richet and Habib, 1959; Spargo, Seymour and Ordoñez, 1980). When crescents are conspicuous, pathologic differentiation from rapidly progressive crescentic glomerulonephritis is difficult (Meadows, 1973; Spargo, Seymour and Ordoñez, 1980; Heptinstall, 1983).

(b) Crescentic glomerulonephritis

The possibility of vasculitis exists whenever segmental crescentic glomerulonephritis is encountered (Spargo, Seymour and Ordoñez, 1980). Idiopathic crescentic glomerulonephritis without glomerular proliferation and negative immunofluorescence, commonly seen in the elderly (Stilmant *et al.*, 1979; Samiy, 1983), poses a special diagnostic challenge, as it can be the only apparent pathological manifestation of vasculitis. Confusion with primary glomerular disease should be avoided by careful search for vascular lesions. Some authors suggest that vasculitis cannot be ruled out, even in the cases where typical vascular lesions are absent outside the glomeruli (Spargo, Seymour and Ordoñez, 1980; Novak, Christiansen and Sorensen, 1982).

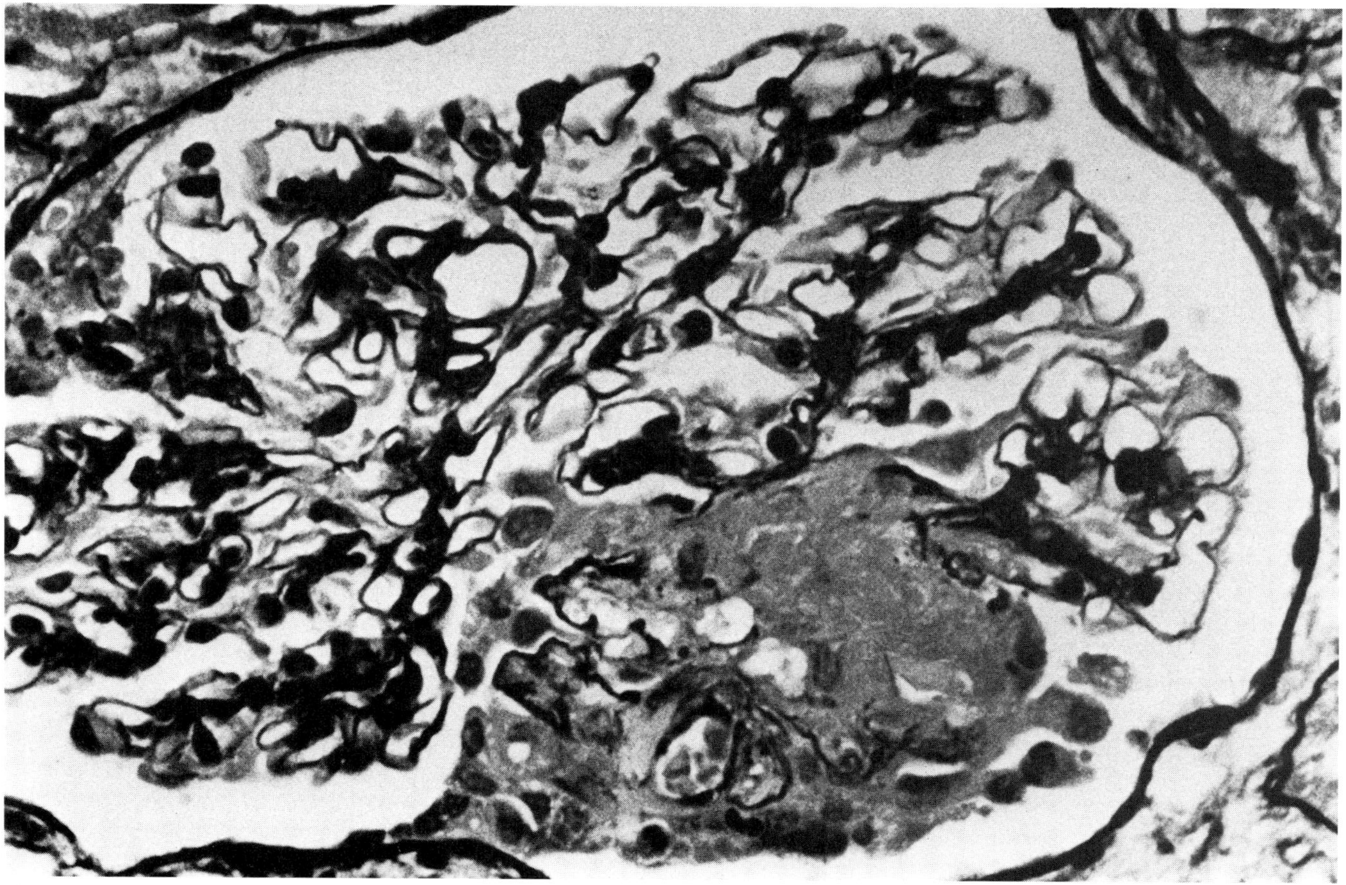

Figure 16.1 Segmental necrotizing glomerulitis, 'microscopic polyarteritis'. Part of the glomerular tuft shows necrosis, the rest of the glomerulus being completely normal. There is some suggestion of crescent formation (left of the glomerulus). The immunofluorescence showed heavy segmental deposition of fibrin and little IgG, IgM and C3 in the areas of necrosis (PASM stain, ×400) (From Serra et al., 1984, reproduced with permission)

(c) Other glomerulonephritis

Mesangial proliferative, membranous, mesangiocapillary and endo-extracapillary glomerulonephritis have been reported in patients with positive hepatitis B surface antigen associated with classic polyarteritis nodosa (Duffy *et al.*, 1976; Michalak, 1978). Mesangiocapillary glomerulonephritis has been associated occasionally with polyarteritis nodosa in patients with negative hepatitis B surface antigen and in children (Habib *et al.*, 1973; Montes *et al.*, 1975). Mesangial and endothelial proliferation has been associated with the urticarial form of hypocomplementemic cutaneous vasculitis (Spargo, Seymour and Ordoñez, 1980). In our experience of 63 patients with vasculitis and predominant renal involvement, 8 had diffuse endocapillary proliferative glomerulonephritis and 5 had normal or mild mesangial proliferation in the glomeruli (Serra *et al.*, 1984; Serra and Cameron, 1985, unpublished).

(d) Henoch–Schönlein purpura and glomerulonephritis (Habib and Cameron, 1982)

The histological features of the glomerulonephritis in adults with Henoch–Schönlein purpura (HSP) do not differ from those in children (Ballard, Eisinger and Gallo, 1970; Brun *et al.*, 1971; Fillastre, Morel-Maroger and Richet, 1971; Bar-On and Rosenmann, 1972; Case Records of the Massachusetts General Hospital, 1974; Heptinstall, 1974; Kauffmann and Houwert, 1981). Several patterns have been described: some present glomeruli which appear basically normal but with superimposed focal and segmental lesions, usually proliferative and occasionally with necrosis; crescents, which in HSP are usually small, frequently overlie the affected segment of the glomerulus. In others, there is a constant expansion and hypercellularity of the mesangial areas, sometimes severe. Superimposed on this basic mesangial proliferative pattern are glomerular focal and segmental lesions. In this proliferative variety of glomerular involvement, the segments affected and the crescents tend to be larger. In a minority, the lesions are much more severe and most of the glomeruli are affected by extensive crescent formation and glomerular proliferation. Occasionally, glomerular involvement in HSP may mimic a mesangiocapillary glomerulonephritis.

Immunofluorescence and electron microscopy findings

Reported *immunofluorescence* studies of the *vasculitic vessel lesions* have been variable (Serra and Cameron, 1985); different patterns of immunoglobulins, albumin, complement and other antigens have been found by different authors (Mellors and Ortega, 1956; Paronetto and Strauss, 1962; Michalak, 1978; Droz *et al.*, 1979; Pirani and Silva, 1979; Ronco *et al.*, 1983; Serra, 1983), while only fibrinogen has been demonstrated by others (Burkholder, 1968; Berger, Yaneva and Hinglais, 1971).

Electron microscopy of the *vasculitic lesions* in small blood vessels are singularly lacking. Renal studies of 2 patients with small vessel vasculitis were reported to show fibrin, poorly defined electron-dense deposits, polymorphonuclear leukocyte infiltration and degeneration with free lysosomal structures among the smooth muscle cells of the vascular renal lesions (Pirani and Silva, 1979). A recent study of the vascular lesions of patients with Wegener's granulomatosis involving mainly interlobular renal arteries, emphasized the presence of platelets intermixed with fibrin in the early vasculitic lesions and the presence of accentuated endothelial cell alterations occurring along with the intimal infiltrate (Novak, Christiansen and Sorensen, 1982).

Immunofluorescent studies of the *glomerular lesions* in vasculitis are different in relation to the type of glomerular involvement.

(1) In segmental necrotizing glomerulitis ('microscopic polyarteritis') or crescentic glomerulonephritis (Serra and Cameron, 1985), immunofluorescence was negative or weakly positive (except for fibrin) in a segmental fashion in 73 patients from our own and Ronco's series (Ronco *et al.*, 1983; Serra *et al.*, 1984; Serra and Cameron, 1985, unpublished), and in other renal studies (Mellors and Ortega, 1956; Paronetto and Strauss, 1962; Berger, Yaneva and Hinglais, 1971; Kincaid-Smith, 1975; Kanfer *et al.*, 1976; Droz *et al.*, 1979); only one of our patients with segmental necrotizing glomerulitis associated with chronic lymphatic leukaemia and diabetes presented with diffuse subepithelial deposits of immune globulins and complement (Serra *et al.*, 1984). When segmental necrotizing glomerulitis or crescentic glomerulonephritis are seen associated with Wegener's granulomatosis, either negative immunofluorescence (Hyman *et al.*, 1973; Droz *et al.*, 1979; Pinching *et al.*, 1983) or deposition of IgG or C3 and less frequently IgM or IgA in the basement membrane have been reported (Fauci and Wolff, 1973; Wolff *et al.*, 1974; Berlyne, 1979; Droz *et al.*, 1979). The presence of diffuse deposits is rare in the previously mentioned glomerular pattern of renal vasculitis, although a report from Cohen *et al.* (1981) including a small number of patients with rapidly progressive crescentic glomerulonephritis showed that all of them, including a few with vasculitis, presented definite glomerular diffuse deposition of immune globulins and complement.

(2) Immunofluorescence of other types of glomerulonephritis: mesangial proliferative, membranous, mesangiocapillary and endo-extracapillary glomerulonephritis in patients with hepatitis B surface antigen associated with vasculitis are variable; deposition of IgG, IgM, C3, Clq, fibrinogen and hepatitis B surface antigen (HB_sAg) have been reported (Duffy *et al.*, 1976; Michalak, 1978). Granular immunofluorescent reactions for IgG, IgM, IgA, Clq and C3 have been reported in the urticarial form of hypocomplementemic cutaneous vasculitis (Spargo, Seymour and Ordoñez, 1980). In our experience, only 1 from 8 patients with diffuse endocapillary proliferative glomerulonephritis showed diffuse deposits of C3, IgG, IgM and IgA. Immunofluorescent studies were always negative in our patients who presented normal glomeruli or minimal mesangial proliferation (Serra *et al.*, 1984; Serra and Cameron, 1985, unpublished).

Immunofluorescent studies are crucial in distinguishing other forms of necrotizing glomerular lesions that can be associated with vasculitis, such as Henoch–Schönlein purpura (IgA, fibrin, C3) (Habib and Cameron, 1982), antiglomerular basement membrane glomerulonephritis (linear IgG) (Wu Ming-Jiang *et al.*, 1980) or systemic lupus erythematosus (IgG, IgA, IgM, C3, C4, Clq) (Adu and Cameron, 1982).

Electron microscopic studies of the glomerular lesions

(1) Electron microcopy in 28 patients with segmental necrotizing glomerulitis ('microscopic polyarteritis') with or without crescent formation (Serra *et al.*, 1984) showed extensive abnormalities of the endothelial and mesangial cells (degeneration, swelling, expansion and hypertrophy), and in some cases the presence of cytoplasmic mesangial processes extending into the peripheral

glomerular capillary loops between the endothelial cells and the glomerular basement membrane. Non-specific findings included deposits of fibrin, presence of extraglomerular cells (leukocytes, platelets) and products of cellular degeneration in the affected glomerular segments. Massive fibrin deposits are also present in the capsular space, in the walls of the intertubular blood vessels and very massively in the interstitium. Abnormalities of the glomerular basement membrane such as collapse, rupture and very abnormal epithelial cells with frequent severe segmental or diffuse crescent formation are frequently seen. Severe obsolescence of glomerular capillary loops are commonly found (Mandache and Nicolescu, 1970; Bohman, Olsen and Peterson, 1974; Jenis and Lowenthal, 1977; Serra *et al.*, 1984).

Similar findings have been reported in patients with Wegener's granulomatosis (Zollinger and Mihatsch, 1978). In most cases lesions of segmental necrotizing glomerulitis are associated with crescents; study of fresh crescents has shown them to consist of fibrin, proliferating capsular or visceral epithelial cells and monocytes; in later stages, basement membrane-like material and collagen fibres can be seen in Bowman's space (Min *et al.*, 1974). A variable number of subendothelial, intramembranous, subepithelial and mesangial electron-dense deposits have been reported in some cases with probable segmental necrotizing glomerulitis and crescentic glomerular lesions (Min *et al.*, 1974; Dunnill, 1976; Jenis and Lowenthal, 1977; Pirani and Silva, 1979), while we believe that electron-dense deposits are rare in segmental necrotizing glomerulitis ('microscopic polyarteritis') (Serra *et al.*, 1984). Localized subepithelial deposits, both 'hump'-like and small ones surrounded by 'spike'-like basement membrane material, have been described in the segmental necrotizing glomerulitis associated with Wegener's granulomatosis (Wolff *et al.*, 1974); however, 2 patients from our study (Serra *et al.*, 1984) showed negative immunofluorescence.

(2) Electron microscopy of our patients with proliferative glomerulonephritis associated with vasculitis showed the invariable presence of electron-dense deposits (Serra *et al.*, 1984). Other studies including a small number of these patients have shown similar results (Mandache and Nicolescu, 1970; Bohman, Olsen and Peterson, 1974; Jenis and Lowenthal, 1977; Pirani and Silva, 1979).

In summary, electron microscopy has been useful in defining the ultrastructural morphology of the glomerular lesions; however, there is no specific electron microscopic feature in vasculitis with renal involvement which could be more useful in the diagnosis and clinical management of these patients in relation to the ones provided by optic microscopy in immunohistochemical studies.

Tubular involvement in the vasculitides (Heptinstall, 1983)

The tubules show no characteristic lesions. Acute tubular damage with necrosis of the epithelium is a common finding (Droz *et al.*, 1979). Dilatation and atrophy of the convoluted tubules can be seen in association with renal ischaemia (Patalano and Sommers, 1961). Tubular atrophy is seen associated with healed lesions of vasculitis.

Interstitial tissue involvement in the vasculitides (Heptinstall, 1983)

Variable degrees of cellular infiltration are commonly associated with renal vasculitis. These infiltrates are mainly composed of plasma cells and lymphocytes; eosinophils, polymorphonuclears and histiocytes can be found in some cases.

Eosinophils are particularly numerous when vasculitis is associated with allergic angiitis and granulomatosis. A periglomerular distribution of the infiltrates is a common finding when glomerular lesions consist of segmental necrotizing glomerulitis ('microscopic polyarteritis'). Interstitial lesions are one of the main lesions in some vasculitis. Necrotizing granulomata can be found in Wegener's granulomatosis and allergic angiitis and granulomatosis. Papillary necrosis associated with calyceal arteritis has been described (Heaton and Bourke, 1976), as well as ureteric lesions (Melin *et al.*, 1982; Ronco *et al.*, 1982).

Is renal biopsy useful in renal vasculitis?

Renal biopsy seemed, for some time, to be contraindicated in patients suspected as having vasculitis. The basis for such fear appeared to be the potential rupture of arterial aneurysms. In predominant renal vasculitis of the microscopic type, however, arterial aneurysms are infrequently seen, and an increased incidence of complications has not been reported in this group of patients; in only 1 of 63 patients did a haemorrhage occur, in the context of a haemorrhagic diathesis (Serra *et al.*, 1984; Serra and Cameron, 1985, unpublished). Therefore, renal biopsy is safe in predominant renal vasculitis; but is it useful? The diagnostic yield in detecting vasculitis depends on the clinical status of the patient; it appears to be more useful as the severity of the vasculitis increases (*Figure 16.2*). This is probably due to the more widespread vasculitic lesions seen in ill patients who subsequently die at the acute stage. Despite the fact that extraglomerular vasculitis is infrequently seen in patients who survive, glomerular lesions of vasculitis ('segmental necrotizing glomerulitis') identify the vasculitis in 64 per cent of the patients, and thus make renal biopsy a very

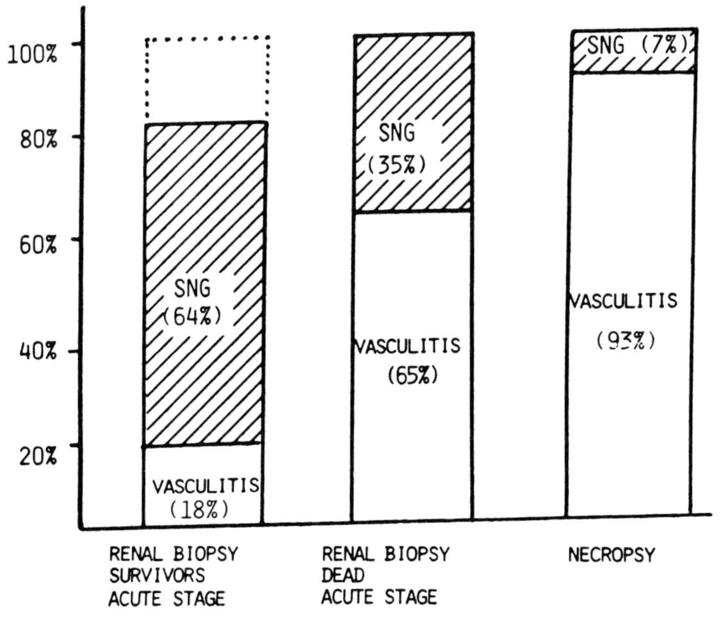

Figure 16.2 Relative contribution of the detection of extraglomerular vasculitis and SNG (segmental necrotizing glomerulitis, 'microscopic polyarteritis') to the diagnosis of vasculitis affecting the kidney (From Serra and Cameron, 1985, reproduced with permission)

useful diagnostic tool in the context of vasculitis with predominant renal involvement.

Renal biopsy also provides valuable prognostic and therapeutic guidelines: visualization of major crescents in most of the glomeruli calls for a more aggressive treatment; furthermore, tubular atrophy, presence of sclerotic lesions, or lesions of acute tubular necrosis, are associated with increased mortality, but scarcely influenced by treatment. In some patients, acute tubular necrosis may be a reversible cause of oliguria clinically attributable to severe glomerular involvement and may need different clinical and therapeutic considerations.

Pathogenesis of the glomerular lesions in renal vasculitis

It seems that immune complexes, alone or in combination with cell-mediated reactions (granulomatous vasculitis), could be responsible, as accepted in systemic vasculitis, for the renal vascular lesions. A description of the pathogenesis of the extraglomerular vasculitis is not dealt with in this chapter, and a comprehensive description of these lesions can be found elsewhere (Unanue and Dixon, 1967; Cupps and Fauci, 1981; Ito, Matsuo and Andres, 1983). The glomerulus, as a differentiated vascular structure, can share common mechanisms with the remaining vascular lesions, and some glomerular changes seen in association with certain vasculitides (necrotizing lesions) are explained on the basis of the vascular nature of the glomerulus.

The pathogenesis of the glomerular lesions in vasculitis has specific mechanisms, most of which have been described in experimental animal observation.

(1) *Immune complex deposition* and glomerular inflammation, as in extraglomerular (vessel) vasculitis, would result from activation of humoral mediator systems; vasculitis and glomerulonephritis occurring in 'single shot' acute serum sickness provide a model for this mechanism (Unanue and Dixon, 1967; Christian and Sergent, 1976). The size of immune complexes, the ratio between antigen and antibody, platelet-induced release of vasoactive amines (histamine–serotonin) and complement activation and subsequent attraction of polymorphonuclear leukocytes secondary to immune complex deposition are thought to play a role in the pathogenesis of both vascular or glomerular lesions (Kniker and Cochrane, 1965; Henson and Cochrane, 1971; Cochrane, 1979). However, immune complexes have not been consistently demonstrated in human vasculitis and associated glomerulonephritis, and when present, their pathogenetic role has been questioned (Dunnill, 1976; Meadows, 1978). Other mechanisms have been proposed that do not necessarily involve the mediation by immune complexes, i.e. coagulation mechanisms, such as fibrin-related pathways, and cell-mediated reactions.

(2) *Fibrin deposition* may be important in the production of glomerulonephritis and crescent formation, and is found in the glomerular and vascular lesions of patients with vasculitis. Deposition of fibrin, intracapillary proliferation and crescent formation are demonstrated experimentally (Vasalli and McCluskey, 1964), and defibrination with Ancrod or anticoagulation with large doses of heparin or dicumarol have been shown to reduce or prevent both glomerular fibrin deposition and crescent formation (Vasalli and McCluskey, 1964; Halpern *et al.*, 1965).

(3) *Cell-mediated mechanisms:* identification of macrophages and monocytes in the glomerulus by new techniques suggests the participation of cell-mediated immunity in the production of glomerulonephritis. The experimental demonstration that accumulation of monocytes and macrophages is responsible for the glomerular hypercellularity supports the cell-mediated hypothesis (Hunsicker *et al.*, 1979; Holdsworth, Neale and Wilson, 1980). Further experimental evidence indicates that segmental necrotizing glomerulitis lesions (often seen in renal vasculitis) may be cell mediated, and can be produced by the interaction between sensitized T-lymphocytes and antigens present in the immune complexes within the mesangial regions. Similarities between this model and the delayed type of cell-mediated immunity (type IV) have been suggested (Bhan *et al.*, 1978, 1979).

Morphological similarities between vasculitis and glomerulonephritis in humans and in animal models suggest common mechanisms in the production of vasculitis and glomerulonephritis. However, so far, they have only been clinically demonstrated in patients with vasculitis associated with hepatitis B virus which involves immune complexes (Michalak, 1978). There has been no direct evidence that cell-mediated immunity accounts for any form of human glomerulonephritis, although indirect evidence has been obtained in some patients with antiglomerular basement membrane disease, and has been suggested in idiopathic crescentic glomerulonephritis with negative deposits and in Wegener's granulomatosis (McCluskey and Bhan, 1982). Recently we have shown, using monoclonal antibodies, an excess of monocytic cells and T-lymphocytes in the glomeruli of patients with vasculitis (Nolasco *et al.*, 1985).

Aetiology and pathogenesis of Henoch–Schönlein purpura (Cupps and Fauci, 1981)

Different agents (infections, drugs, vaccines, food) have been implicated and deposition of immune complexes has been the presumptive mechanisms of the disease. IgA and C3 have been demonstrated in the blood vessels from both normal and involved skin. Increased numbers of IgA-bearing lymphocytes and IgA-containing circulating immune complexes in the peripheral circulation are observed, suggesting an IgA immune complex-mediated disease. Deposition of IgA has also been demonstrated in the renal biopsy of patients with Henoch–Schönlein purpura. Reports of the disease occurring in patients with congenital absence of C2 suggests that the disease can occur in the absence of the early components of the classic complement pathway. One possible mechanism of disease would be the deposition of IgA immune complexes in blood vessels and glomeruli, with activation of the alternative complement pathway and subsequent generation of chemotactic factors with influx of polymorphonuclear leukocytes.

II. Clinical aspects of the vasculitides in a renal unit with special reference to the elderly

Introduction

The clinical manifestations of the vasculitides depend on the context in which the vasculitis is seen. It is now clear that the dermatological, rheumatological, or renal clinical manifestations, and even nomenclature, greatly differ in published series. Therefore, when dealing with descriptions and prognosis of the vasculitides it is important to bear in mind that what may be true in a certain context is not necessarily applicable to another.

Unselected series and series from renal units differ in relation to the type of vasculitis seen, presentation, clinical aspects and outcome (Serra and Cameron, 1985). A description of the various clinical aspects of renal vasculitis is made in this section, with emphasis in the differences found between patients who are 59 years or younger, and elderly patients. It should be noted that these data refer *only* to those patients with vasculitis who are seen in renal units, and extrapolation to other patients with vasculitis, whether young or elderly, is not justified. Interestingly, the nature of the vasculitides included in the renal series is often unclear, the prevalent histopathology being a segmental necrotizing glomerulitis ('microscopic polyarteritis') in most cases, associated with crescent formation (Serra and Cameron, 1985). Vasculitis which may affect the elderly in other unselected series is rarely seen in a nephrologic context: giant cell temporal arteritis is one such example (Paulley and Hughes, 1960; Lie, 1978; Goodman, 1979). In the present report, some vasculitides are deliberately not included: essential mixed cryoglobulinaemia, systemic lupus erythematosus (rare in the elderly), Takayasu's arteritis and lymphomatoid granulomatosis.

Age of onset, prodromes, precipitating events and associated diseases

Most patients with renal vasculitis are Caucasian (Serra *et al.*, 1984), in contrast to other forms of renal disease. Vasculitis with predominant renal involvement can be seen above 60 years of age, the prevalence in our series being 30 per cent of the patients with vasculitis (19 of 63 patients), most of them with segmental necrotizing glomerulitis ('microscopic polyarteritis') (Serra *et al.*, 1984; Serra and Cameron, 1985, unpublished). The prevalence of patients with Wegener's granulomatosis and predominant renal involvement older than 60 years is 35 per cent (8 of 23) (Novak, Christiansen and Sorensen, 1982; Pinching *et al.*, 1983).

Prodromes and possible *precipitating events* are found in as many as 24 per cent of the patients from the renal series, including a previous history of sore throat or flu-like illness (16 per cent) and a drug intake (anti-rheumatic drugs, cotrimoxazole, penicillamine, etc.) in 8 per cent of the patients (Serra *et al.*, 1984; Serra and Cameron, 1985, unpublished). No difference is found between patients over 60 years compared with younger individuals in relation to the history of previous infections (11 per cent versus 18 per cent) or drug intake (16 per cent versus 27 per cent), respectively. A mild course for the vasculitis has been described when hypersensitivity to a known antigen (e.g. a drug) is detected (Fauci, Haynes and Katz, 1978); however, when the kidney is predominantly involved, the prognosis does not seem to be so benign (Serra *et al.*, 1984). In our series, association of vasculitis with an *identified underlying disease* was present in 7 of 63 patients (11 per cent): 2 lymphomas, 1 chronic lymphatic leukaemia, 1 breast carcinoma, 2 relapsing polychondritis and 1 rheumatoid arthritis. Only 2 patients, both with neoplasia (leukaemia and breast carcinoma), were above 60 years of age.

Mode of presentation

Only one-third of patients who will develop renal vasculitis initially present with evidence of renal disease; isolated renal involvement is rarely seen at presentation; the only 3 patients who presented to our unit in such a way were over 60 years of age (Serra *et al.*, 1984; Serra and Cameron, 1985, unpublished). An extrarenal presentation was observed in two-thirds of the renal patients (Friedman and Kincaid-Smith, 1972; Serra *et al.*, 1984), including a multisystemic involvement in half of these cases, and in a similar proportion an isolated involvement of many organ/systems. Skin and lung are the organs more frequently involved; no significant differences are observed between elderly and younger patients.

Table 16.2 Presentation of renal disease in patients with renal vasculitis

	>60 years ($n = 19$)	*<60 years* ($n = 44$)
Urinary findings:		
Isolated microscopic haematuria	0 (0%)	2 (5%)
Proteinuria <2.5 g/24 h	3 (16%)	9 (20%)
Microscopic haematuria and proteinuria	14 (74%)	27 (61%)
Nephrotic syndrome	1 (5%)	5 (11%)
Not performed	1 (5%)	1 (3%)
Renal function:		
Normal	1 (5%)	22 (50%)*
Reduced	5 (26%)	4 (9%)
Rapid impairment	13 (69%)	18 (41%)†
without oliguria	10 (53%)	12 (27%)
with oliguria	3 (16%)	6 (14%)

* $P<0.001$.
† $P<0.05$.

Renal presentation (*Table 16.2*) invariably includes proteinuria and haematuria, and in more than half of the cases it is associated with impaired renal function. Oliguria is the renal presentation in a minority (14 per cent) (Droz *et al.*, 1979; Serra *et al.*, 1984). It should be noted that the greatest difference between patients under 60 years of age and elderly patients is in relation to renal function at the time of presentation. Normal renal function at the time of presentation was found in only 5 per cent of the elderly, versus 50 per cent in patients under 60 years ($P<0.001$). In addition, progressive deterioration of renal function is more frequent in the elderly (69 per cent versus 41 per cent) ($P<0.05$) (*Table 16.2*). As a form of renal presentation, oliguria is equally prevalent between both age groups. The explanation for these differences can be found in the paucity of clinical signs of vasculitis in the elderly patients compared with the younger (see below; *Table 16.3*). A nephrotic syndrome can be occasionally seen (Friedman and Kincaid-Smith, 1972; Kanfer *et al.*, 1976; Droz *et al.*, 1979; Serra *et al.*, 1984).

However, other diseases associated with vasculitis must be ruled out before the diagnosis of primary vasculitis associated with nephrotic syndrome is made: essential mixed cryoglobulinaemia (Tarantino *et al.*, 1981), Henoch–Schönlein purpura (Habib and Cameron, 1982), lymphomas and leukaemias (Durante, Lum and McIntosh, 1977), systemic lupus erythematosus (Adu and Cameron, 1982), or the presence of HBsAg or intravascular coagulation. In our series, 6 patients had vasculitis and a nephrotic syndrome: 2 had a lymphoproliferative disease, and in a third patient, intraglomerular hyaline thrombi suggested the presence of associated

Table 16.3 Clinical features of renal vasculitis in the aged (Data from Kanfer *et al.*, 1976; Droz *et al.*, 1979; Serra *et al.*, 1984; Serra and Cameron, 1985, unpublished)

	>60 years	*<60 years*	*P**
Fever	13/24 (54%)	45/56 (80%)	($P<0.01$)
General symptoms	18/21 (86%)	39/53 (74%)	NS
Skin	8/21 (38%)	34/53 (64%)	($P<0.05$)
Purpura	8/21†	21/53	
ENT	6/19 (32%)	16/44 (36%)	NS
Ocular	3/19 (16%)	16/44 (36%)	NS
Musculoskeletal	12/24 (50%)	44/56 (79%)	($P<0.02$)
GI, pancreas, liver	8/21 (38%)	27/53 (51%)	NS
Respiratory	11/23 (48%)	34/56 (61%)	NS
CNS	1/21 (5%)	10/53 (19%)	NS
PNS	2/21 (10%)	15/53 (28%)	NS
Heart	2/19 (11%)	6/44 (14%)	NS
Hypertension	7/24 (29%)	22/56 (39%)	NS

*Chi-square
†The only skin lesion seen in elderly patients was purpura.
CNS, central nervous system; ENT, ear, nose and throat; GI, gastrointestinal; NS, not significant; PNS, peripheral nervous system.

intravascular coagulation (Serra *et al.*, 1984; Serra and Cameron, 1985, unpublished).

General clinical features (Serra *et al.*, 1984; Serra and Cameron 1985) (*Table 16.3*)

Clinical signs and symptoms in vasculitis are often non-specific, and patients who present with vasculitis at a renal unit are no exception. Fever, general symptoms (weakness, weight loss), skin lesions, musculoskeletal disease and diverse organ involvement are often seen (Davson, Ball and Platt, 1948; Wainwright and Davson, 1950; Friedman and Kincaid-Smith, 1972; Kanfer *et al.*, 1976; Droz *et al.*, 1979; Serra *et al.*, 1984). The clinical difficulty of attaining a correct diagnosis in these patients is well known. Sometimes, only a careful search for subtle signs (dermatological lesions, ocular involvement) is the clue to the clinical suspicion, and a skin or renal biopsy leads to the diagnosis. Such difficulty is more obvious in the elderly; fever is seen in only half of these patients compared to the younger population (80 per cent) ($P<0.01$); the skin lesions, which provide a very useful hint in two-thirds of patients under 60, are seen in only one-third of the elderly population ($P<0.05$), and in every one of the 8 patients over 60, it took the form of purpuric lesions. Musculoskeletal involvement is less often seen in the elderly (*Table 16.3*).

It is not surprising, therefore, that elderly patients are more difficult to recognize as harbouring a vasculitis, and the diagnosis is made in a late stage of the disease, often when the renal function is severely damaged. Ear, nose and throat (ENT), ocular, gastrointestinal, pancreas, liver, respiratory, central nervous system (CNS), peripheral nervous system (PNS) and cardiac involvement are found with similar frequency in both age groups (*Table 16.3*). Patients with Wegener's granulomatosis with severe renal involvement have similar clinical features to the patients with segmental necrotizing glomerulitis, but present predominant upper and lower respiratory tract involvement; however, gastrointestinal involvement is rare in these patients, but abnormal liver function tests are commonly found (Camilleri *et al.*, 1983; Pinching *et al.*, 1983).

Hypertension is seen in less than one-third of patients with vasculitis (elderly, and under 60 years), but it does not represent a problem of clinical management. Accelerated hypertension is seldom seen.

Renal involvement at the time of renal biopsy (*Table 16.4*)

The renal differences between young and elderly patients at the time of renal presentation have been previously described: renal function is normal in only 5 per cent of the elderly patients and in 50 per cent of those under 60; however, the latter figure drops to 14 per cent by the time these patients come to renal biopsy. Elderly patients also develop more severe renal involvement after presentation: at the time of renal biopsy, oliguria is seen more often in the elderly (42 per cent) than in the young (27 per cent). Development of severe renal failure is rapid: the mean interval between renal presentation and biopsy is 2 months, and less than 1 month in two-thirds of the patients. Oliguria and rapid impairment of renal function are clearly associated with increased mortality: half of the patients in whom these were present were dead at the end of the observation period, most of them (75 per cent) in the acute stage of the disease. The finding that the presence of severe renal involvement is the main factor that determines prognosis in the acute stage indicates the need for urgent nephrological assessment in vasculitis when renal involvement is first noted (Serra *et al.*, 1984).

Table 16.4 Renal involvement at the time of renal biopsy

	>60 years ($n = 19$)	*<60 years* ($n = 44$)
Creatinine <120 μmol/l	1/19 (5%)	6/44 (14%)
Creatinine 120–200 μmol/l	3/19 (17%)	9/44 (21%)
Creatinine 200–499 μmol/l	5/19 (25%)	12/44 (27%)
Creatinine 500–1000 μmol/l	2/19 (11%)	5/44 (11%)
Oliguria	8/19 (42%)	12/44 (27%)

P = not significant

Laboratory investigations at referral (*Table 16.5*)

Constant laboratory features in patients with predominant renal disease are elevated erythrocyte sedimentation rate (ESR), anaemia, leukocytosis with increased polymorphonuclear cells and hypoalbuminaemia; moderate eosinophilia is seen in a number of patients, most of them with a history of asthma, lung involvement or drug-related vasculitis (Friedman and Kincaid-Smith, 1972; Kanfer *et al.*, 1976; Droz *et al.*, 1979; Serra *et al.*, 1984). No differences are seen between the group of patients under 60 years of age and elderly patients except for eosinophilia (*Table 16.5*).

Circulating immune complexes detected by different methods are found to be present in most patients with renal vasculitis (Ronco *et al.*, 1983; Serra *et al.*, 1984).

Positive results are found in most patients using the platelet aggregating titre (PAT), the Clq-binding test, or other methods (Ronco *et al.*, 1983; Serra *et al.*, 1984).

Low levels of complement components are rare in patients with predominant renal vasculitis, and have found to be normal or high in most reports of patients with vasculitis and predominant renal involvement (Kanfer *et al.*, 1976; Droz *et al.*, 1979; Ronco *et al.*, 1983; Serra *et al.*, 1984).

Table 16.5 Laboratory features of renal vasculitis in the aged (Data from Droz *et al.*, 1979; Serra *et al.*, 1984; Serra and Cameron, 1985, unpublished)

	>60 years	*<60 years*	*P**
Anaemia	19/21 (90%)	43/53 (81%)	NS
Leukocytosis	13/21 (62%)	36/53 (68%)	NS
Eosinophilia	2/16 (13%)	35/53 (66%)	($P<0.001$)
Increased ESR	17/18 (94%)	37/41 (90%)	NS
Decreased complement	0/14 (0%)	1/36 (3%)	NS
Rheumatoid factor	3/9 (33%)	9/23 (39%)	NS
ANA	2/13 (15%)	3/41 (7%)	NS
Clq-binding	0/3 (0%)	2/8 (25%)	—
PAT	3/4 (75%)	6/7 (86%)	—
Cryoglobulins	1/1 (100%)	0/3 (0%)	—

*Chi-square.
ANA, antinuclear antibodies; ESR, erythrocyte sedimentation rate; NS, not significant; PAT, platelet aggregation test.

HLA-DR2 and HLA-B8 are found with increased frequency in patients with Wegener's granulomatosis (Katz *et al.*, 1979; Elkon *et al.*, 1983). No HLA typing studies have been published in patients with segmental necrotizing glomerulitis ('microscopic polyarteritis') unrelated to Wegener's granulomatosis.

It has been suggested (Bron, Strott and Shapiro, 1965) that *radiology* is an important aid in the diagnosis of vasculitis, especially in revealing lesions in patients without other clinical signs of diffuse vessel involvement. The splanchnic arteriogram does appear to show micro-aneurysms in a high proportion of patients with polyarteritis nodosa of the 'classic' type, but the technique is of much less use in microscopic polyarteritis or Wegener's granuloma. We found micro-aneurysms in only 1 of 7 patients with proven microscopic polyarteritis in the kidney (Serra *et al.*, 1984), and Camilleri *et al.* (1983) in none of 8.

Hepatitis B surface antigen (HBsAg) has been found in the serum of 6–40 per cent of patients with classic polyarteritis (Sack, Cassidy and Bole, 1975; Conn *et al.*, 1976; Fauci *et al.*, 1979; Leib, Restivo and Paulus, 1979; Cohen, Conn and Ilstrup, 1980; Scott *et al.*, 1982), demonstrated in the vascular and glomerular lesions in some patients (Michalak, 1978), and found to be associated with essential mixed cryoglobulinaemia (Levo *et al.*, 1977; Tarantino *et al.*, 1981); however, it seems to be infrequent in renal vasculitis. No explanation is readily available for this difference, although the proportion of positive cases will vary with the local carriage rate. In some patients, an elevated antistreptolysin titre accompanied by the presence of some of the clinical features of acute glomerulonephritis suggested the diagnosis of severe post-infectious glomerulonephritis (Inglefinger *et al.*, 1977; Serra *et al.*, 1984).

Clinical involvement in adults with Henoch–Schönlein purpura

It is well documented that Henoch–Schönlein purpura may occur up to the ninth decade of life. However, only a few cases of Henoch–Schönlein purpura in patients over 60 years have been reported (Ballard, Eisinger and Gallo, 1970; Bar-On and Rosenmann, 1972; Kalowski and Kincaid-Smith, 1973; Case Records of the Massachusetts General Hospital, 1974; Kauffmann and Houwert, 1981), and we have seen only 3 cases, the oldest being 72 years of age (Serra and Cameron, 1985, unpublished). The clinical manifestations in adults with Henoch–Schönlein purpura are similar to the children, although there is some suggestion that prior drug treatment and severe arthralgia are more common (80 per cent of cases), and abdominal symptoms and signs less common (35 per cent of cases) (Habib and Cameron, 1982). The clinical manifestations of the nephritis in adults are similar to those in childhood: isolated macroscopic or microscopic haematuria or proteinuria, haematuria and proteinuria with or without hypertension, nephrotic syndrome, and nephritic–nephrotic syndrome. Mild uraemia is common; rarely, there is a rapid onset with severe progressive uraemia which requires dialysis.

Information collected from the literature on a total of 14 patients with Henoch–Schönlein purpura more than 60 years old, showed that only 4 had important renal failure early in the follow-up; in the remaining, renal involvement was not present or it was manifested as urinary sediment abnormalities, mild deterioration of the renal function or nephrotic syndrome (Ballard, Eisinger and Gallo, 1970; Bar-On and Rosenmann, 1972; Kalowski and Kincaid-Smith, 1973; Serra and Cameron, 1985, unpublished).

Prognosis and treatment

Prognosis

The prognosis of patients with vasculitis as a whole varies according to whether non-renal (unselected) series (Frohnert and Sheps, 1967; Cohen, Conn and Illstrup, 1980) or series which come from renal units are considered (Friedman and Kincaid-Smith, 1972; Kanfer *et al.*, 1976; Droz *et al.*, 1979; Serra *et al.*, 1984). The prognosis is worse in the latter, the chance of survival being 59, 54, 42 and 39 per cent at 1, 2, 5 and 10 years in our own data of predominantly patients with microscopic polyarteritis (Serra *et al.*, 1984; Serra and Cameron, 1985, unpublished). In the predominantly renal series it is not surprising that there is one subgroup which fares worse: the elderly. *Figure 16.3* shows the 1-, 2-, 5- and 10-year survival curves of 42, 36, 25 and 25 per cent in the elderly versus 68, 64, 52 and 48 per cent in the patients under 60 ($P<0.05$). The difference is mainly due to the greatly increased mortality in the elderly during the acute stage. Renal failure and vasculitis are the main causes of death in the acute stage in both groups of patients, and no differences in the immediate causes of death can be found between these two age groups.

Wegener's granulomatosis has been treated as a separate entity: the prognosis in Wegener's granulomatosis has greatly improved since the introduction of corticosteroids and cyclophosphamide treatment. However, this improvement has been reported in patients who, although they frequently had renal disease (85 per cent), had only mild involvement: in Fauci's series (1983), only 9 of the 75 patients reported had renal failure. The mortality in Wegener's granulomatosis with severe

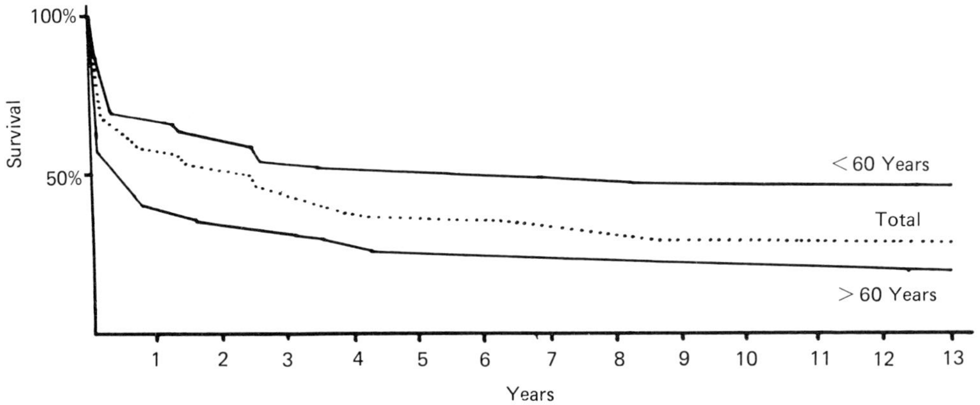

Figure 16.3 Actuarial survival curve of patients with predominantly renal vasculitis. Total figures are shown as dotted line. The survival curves of patients younger than 60 years (top) and older than 60 years (bottom) are also shown

nephritis and/or oliguria remains unacceptably high (Pinching *et al.*, 1983), although death may be postponed in many cases to a later phase of the disease, and relates more to treatment than to the underlying pathology. It is unclear if elderly patients with Wegener's granulomatosis have different prognosis than younger patients. A recently published study distinguishes the outcome of patients over 60 years: 4 of 6 elderly patients died, but the proportion was similar in the younger group (7 of 12) (Pinching *et al.*, 1983).

The long-term follow-up of adults with *Henoch–Schönlein purpura* suggests that the prognosis is not very different from that in children, with only 10 per cent of the patients being dead or in renal failure about 5 years from onset. Most patients were by then totally asymptomatic (50 per cent), or have only some evidence of renal involvement (Ballard, Eisinger and Gallo, 1970; Fillastre, Morel-Maroger and Richet, 1971; Bar-On and Rosenmann, 1972; Kalowski and Kincaid-Smith, 1973; Cameron, 1979). Patients above 60 years seem to have a worse prognosis than younger patients when severe renal failure is present, although one elderly patient who needed haemodialysis recovered renal function treated with plasmaphaeresis (Kauffmann and Houwert, 1981). From 16 patients, including 3 from our own unit, more than 60 years old, at least 5 patients died, 4 early in the follow-up, of renal failure, and the fifth late in the follow-up of myocardial infarction (Ballard, Eisinger and Gallo, 1970; Bar-On and Rosenmann, 1972; Kalowski and Kincaid-Smith, 1973; Case Records of the Massachusetts General Hospital, 1974; Kauffmann and Houwert, 1981; Serra and Cameron, 1985, unpublished).

We have recently presented data of the short- and long-term outcome of a large group of patients with predominant renal vasculitis which revealed that two distinct phases in the vasculitis can be observed: (a) a great percentage of patients die during the first weeks of hospital admission; (b) those who survive follow two clinical courses—some pursue a stable clinical course, and others have continuing symptoms. The prognosis in either case is different. Interestingly, very few patients have a 'recurrent' course of their vasculitis (Serra *et al.*, 1984). Although no firm guidelines for treatment can be outlined, the need and type of treatment should probably be separately considered for each of the described stages of renal vasculitis: acute and long-term.

Treatment

Treatment in the acute stage

Although in several patients clinical manifestations of the vasculitis are present before the first hospital admission, renal involvement is associated with a severe bout of vasculitis, and an 'acute' stage is often observed. A large proportion of these patients with predominant renal vasculitis die shortly after admission to the renal unit. In our series of 63 patients seen from 1965 to 1984, 20 died in the acute stage. Causes of death were renal failure or complications of the vasculitis (Serra *et al.*, 1984; Serra and Cameron, 1985, unpublished).

Treatment in the acute stage of renal vasculitis has been variable: drugs such as *corticosteroids, immunosuppressive agents* (azathioprine and cyclophosphamide mainly), *quadruple chemotherapy* (combination of corticosteroids, immunosuppressive agents, heparin and dipyridamole) and pulses of *intravenous methylprednisolone* have been used irregularly in these patients usually with little success (Droz *et al.*, 1979; Hind *et al.*, 1983; Pinching *et al.*, 1983; Serra *et al.*, 1984). In our series, 8 patients were treated only with corticosteroids, 33 with corticosteroids and immunosuppressive agents, mainly azathioprine, and 12 received quadruple treatment; in 17 patients, intravenous pulses of 1 g of methylprednisolone were added to the other treatments. No correlation between the drug regimen used and the outcome was observed in our series of 63 patients (*Figure 16.3*), the mortality being considerable in the acute stage: 20 of 63 (32 per cent). However, this figure might underestimate the true value of treatment: patients admitted to a renal unit for vasculitis and renal failure are often very ill, and survival may be a matter of days; the diagnosis of vasculitis is not always made soon after admission, and a considerable delay in the beginning of treatment is not infrequently recorded in these circumstances; aggressive treatment is chosen either when the diagnosis is clear or the patient is very ill, perhaps too late for the drugs to be effective. Patients with vasculitis might be untreated because the diagnosis is unclear, the patient severely ill, or fear of using immunosuppressive drugs. In our series, the decision not to treat affected the elderly more than the young: 31 per cent versus 9 per cent ($P<0.05$).

Despite this gloomy panorama, recently published series indicate that *plasmaphaeresis* seems to have a favourable effect in the improvement of both survival and renal function in the acute stage of the disease (Hind *et al.*, 1983; Pinching *et al.*, 1983). In our series of 63 patients, only 5 received plasmaphaeresis: 2 were able to stop haemodialysis, and the 3 others showed improvement of their renal function (Serra and Cameron, 1985, unpublished). These later results offer some hope to patients with vasculitis and severe renal involvement. A controlled trial is in progress in London to see if such observations can be confirmed.

Oliguria as a clinical factor affecting the outcome in the acute stage

The status of renal function strongly influences the outcome of the patients in the acute stage of the disease. Treatment mainly benefits patients without oliguria, and it should be seriously considered in these subgroups (Friedman and Kincaid-Smith, 1972; Droz *et al.*, 1979; Serra *et al.*, 1984). In our series (*Table 16.6*), including mainly patients with microscopic polyarteritis, 38 non-oliguric patients were treated, and improvement in 30 (80 per cent) was noted. Renal function also improved in 28 (74 per cent). The quick clinical response seen, favoured treatment

Table 16.6 Survival in the acute stage of vasculitis: relation to oliguria

		<60 years ($n=44$)		*>60 years* ($n=19$)		
Oliguric ($n=12$)	Treated ($n=12$)	7 (58%)	**Death**	3 (100%)	Treated ($n=3$)	Oliguric ($n=8$)
		5 (42%)	**Improved**	0 (0%)		
	Untreated ($n=0$)	—	**Death**	5 (100%)	Untreated ($n=5$)	
		—	**Improved**	0 (0%)		
Non-oliguric ($n=32$)	Treated ($n=28$)	4 (14%)	**Death**	0 (0%)	Treated ($n=10$)	Non-oliguric ($n=11$)
		22 (79%)	**Improved**	8 (80%)		
		2 (7%)	**Unchanged**	2 (20%)		
	Untreated ($n=4$)	1 (25%)	**Death**	0 (0%)	Untreated ($n=1$)	
		3 (75%)	**Improved**	1 (100%)		

n = number of patients.

as the cause of clinical improvement, although spontaneous remission in some patients cannot be ruled out. Contrarily, the effects of treatment when oliguria is present are far less clear, and although some patients seem to benefit from treatment, the majority die at this stage (Friedman and Kincaid-Smith, 1972; Kanfer *et al.*, 1976; Droz *et al.*, 1979). In our series, 15 of 20 oliguric patients were treated: all untreated died; and only 5 (33 per cent) of the 15 treated improved, and in 3 of them it was paralleled by an improvement in renal function. Other series of patients with microscopic polyarteritis treated with cyclophosphamide or azathioprine and corticosteroids in addition to plasmaphaeresis show better results in the short term, although a late considerable increase of mortality, mainly from infection, is found (Hind *et al.*, 1983).

Age may influence the outcome of vasculitis in the acute stage; elderly patients often die when oliguric: in our series, none of the 8 elderly oliguric patients survived. The decision not to treat, which affected 5 oliguric elderly patients, might have been responsible for such a poor outcome (*Table 16.6*).

Long-term follow-up, treatment and outcome

Observations of patients who survive the acute stage of the disease reveal that two distinctive clinical courses are depicted: some patients lead a 'stable' clinical course of their vasculitis, with no symptoms, normalization of the erythrocyte sedimentation rate (ESR) and biological data, and a high expectancy for survival; contrarily, a residual activity of the vasculitis is present in a group of survivors of the acute stage, the ESR is high, and various clinical markers indicate a continuing activity of the vasculitis. The term 'smouldering' vasculitis has been used to refer to these patients, and the clinical course is associated with a low expectancy of survival (Serra *et al.*, 1984). In our series, 43 of 63 (72 per cent) patients survived the acute stage, and the follow-up extends up to 19 years. A 'stable' clinical course was seen in 18 (42 per cent) and a 'smouldering' course in 20 (47 per cent). Recurrent vasculitis was observed in 2, and 3 patients were lost to follow-up. No difference was found between those patients under 60 years of age or those above 60 in relation to the proportion of the two main subgroups identified in the long-term follow-up.

Few reports in the literature deal with the outcome of the renal function in patients with predominant renal vasculitis. It has previously been mentioned that the renal status strongly influences survival in the acute stage. However, this is not the case once the patient has overcome this very critical period of the vasculitis. In our recently published series, those who were clinically stable always showed lack of progression of the deterioration of their renal function through the years; in the subgroup of patients with persistent ('smouldering') activity of their vasculitis renal function either remained stable (25 per cent), improved (50 per cent) or deteriorated (25 per cent) (Serra *et al.*, 1984; Serra and Cameron, 1985, unpublished). In a few patients, hypertension can develop in the long-term course of renal vasculitis; conversely, hypertension in the acute stage can disappear during the long-term follow-up. No difference is apparent between young and elderly patients related to either long-term renal outcome or hypertension.

The 'stable' and 'smouldering' clinical subgroups have different outcomes: 3 of 18 (17 per cent) stable patients versus 12 of 20 (60 per cent) of the patients with 'smouldering' activity of the vasculitis died in the long term; therefore, treatment must be separately analysed for each of them. The treatments used in this later period of the disease are essentially similar to that employed in the acute phase. However, there is a tendency to reduction or withdrawal of the drugs.

In relation to the usefulness of treatment in the 'stable' group of patients, it is uncertain if control of symptoms or increase in survival is achieved with drugs. The fear of the clinician of withdrawing corticosteroids or immunosuppressive drugs after the patient has overcome a severe episode of vasculitis, even in 'stable' conditions, is understandable. That long-term treatment is probably not needed, however, is suggested by the fact that the majority of 'stable' patients in our previously published study were off treatment at the first year of follow-up (Serra *et al.*, 1984). Unfortunately, there is no single laboratory determination or combination of laboratory tests that absolutely measures the state of disease activity; serial studies of immune complexes in patients with vasculitis have not been done to prove their usefulness in this respect. Recently, an anti-leucocyte antibody which appears specific for vasculitis has been described (van der Woude *et al.*, 1985) which may be useful not only in diagnosis but also in assessment of disease activity; subsequent studies have shown it to be present in microscopic polyarteritis as well as Wegener's granuloma.

Use of corticosteroids and immunosuppressive agents in the 'smouldering' group is probably warranted; despite the evidence that drugs have not been demonstrated as useful in prolonged survival, the symptomatic improvement of the signs such as pulmonary infiltrates, skin rash, episodes of asthma, severe arthromyalgias, etc., favours a therapeutic attitude towards this subgroup.

Summary

Vasculitis with renal involvement is common in the middle aged and elderly, and is probably underdiagnosed in the old because of its non-specific presentation. Isolated segmental necrotizing glomerulitis associated in most cases with crescents, again common in the elderly, probably represents vasculitis apparently affecting only the glomerular capillaries. The only clinical differences in our series were that elderly patients were less often febrile, purpuric, eosinophilic or had musculoskeletal involvement; their renal disease, however, was more severe than the middle-aged patients, and the elderly were more often oligo-anuric. Survival of those aged over 60 is poorer than younger patients, partly because of less aggressive treatment. Immunosuppressive agents have improved on the results obtained with corticosteroids, and plasma exchange seems likely to improve these still further. Even so, up to half of the patients with renal vasculitis die, the majority within the first year.

References

ADU, D. and CAMERON, J.S. (1982). Lupus nephritis. In *Clinics in Rheumatic Disease,* edited by G.R.V. Hughes, pp. 153–182. Baltimore; Williams and Wilkins

BALLARD, H.S., EISINGER, R.P. and GALLO, G. (1970). Renal manifestations of the Henoch–Schönlein syndrome in adults. *The American Journal of Medicine,* **49,** 328–335

BAR-ON, H. and ROSENMANN, E. (1972). Schönlein Henoch syndrome in adults. A clinical and histological study of renal involvement. *Israel Journal of Medical Science,* **8,** 1702–1715

BERGER, J., YANEVA, H. and HINGLAIS, N. (1971). Immunohistochemistry of glomerulonephritis. In *Advances in Nephrology,* edited by J. Hamburger, J. Crosnier and M.H. Maxwell, pp. 11–30. Chicago; Year Book

BERLYNE, G.M. (1979). Renal involvement in the collagen diseases. In *Renal Diseases,* edited by D. Black and N.F. Jones, pp. 653–686. Oxford; Blackwell

BHAN, A.K., COLLINS, A.B., SCHNEEBERGER, E.E. and McCLUSKEY, R.T. (1979). A cell-mediated reaction against glomerular-bound immune complexes. *Journal of Experimental Medicine,* **150,** 1410–1420

BHAN, A.K., SCHNEEBERGER, E.E., COLLINS, A.B. and McCLUSKEY, R.T. (1978). Evidence for a pathogenic role of a cell-mediated immune mechanism in experimental glomerulonephritis. *Journal of Experimental Medicine,* **148,** 246–260

BOHMAN, S.O., OLSEN, S. and PETERSON, V.P. (1974). Glomerular ultrastructure in extracapillary glomerulonephritis. *Acta Pathologica et Microbiologica Scandinavia,* Sect. A, Suppl. 249, **82,** 29–54

BRON, K.M., STROTT, C.A. and SHAPIRO, A.P. (1965). The diagnostic value of angiographic observations in polyarteritis nodosa. *Archives of Internal Medicine,* **116,** 450–454

BRUN, C., BRYLD, C., FENGER, L. and JORGENSEN, F. (1971). Glomerular lesions in adults with the Schönlein Henoch syndrome. *Acta Pathologica et Microbiologica Scandinavia,* Sect. A, **79,** 559–583

BURKHOLDER, P.M. (1968). Immunology and immunohistopathology of renal diseases. In *Structural Basis of Renal Disease,* edited by E.L. Becker, pp. 197–237. New York; Hoeber Medical Division/Harper and Row

CAMERON, J.S. (1979). The nephritis of Schönlein Henoch purpura: current problems. In *Progress in Glomerulonephritis,* edited by P. Kincaid-Smith, A.J.F. Apice and R.C. Atkins, pp. 283–309. New York; Wiley

CAMILLERI, M., PUSEY, C.D., CHADWICK, V.S. and REES, A.J. (1983). Gastrointestinal manifestations of systemic vasculitis. *Quarterly Journal of Medicine,* **LII:** 141–149

CASE RECORDS OF THE MASSACHUSETTS GENERAL HOSPITAL (1974). Case 23–1974. *New England Journal of Medicine,* **290,** 1365–1372

CHRISTIAN, C.L. and SERGENT, J.S. (1976). Vasculitis syndromes: clinical and experimental models. *The American Journal of Medicine,* **61,** 385–392

COCHRANE, C.G. (1979). Immune complex mediated tissue injury. In *Mechanisms of Immunopathology,* edited by S. Cohen, P.A. Ward and R.T. McCluskey, pp. 29–48. New York; Wiley

COHEN, A.H., BORDER, W.A., SHANKEL, E. and GLASSOCK, R.J. (1981). Crescentic glomerulonephritis: immune versus non immune mechanisms. *The American Journal of Nephrology,* **1,** 78–83

COHEN, R.D., CONN, D.L. and ILSTRUP, D.M. (1980). Clinical features, prognosis and response to treatment in polyarteritis. *Proceedings of the Staff Meetings of the Mayo Clinic,* **55,** 146–155

CONN, D.L., McDUFFIE, F.C., HOLLEY, K.E. and SCHROETER, A.L. (1976). Immunologic mechanisms in systemic vasculitis. *Proceedings of the Staff Meetings of the Mayo Clinic,* **51,** 511–518

CUPPS, T.R. and FAUCI, A.S. (1981). Pathophysiology of vasculitis. In *The Vasculitides,* edited by T.R. Cupps and A.S. Fauci. Philadelphia; Saunders

DAVSON, J., BALL, J. and PLATT, R. (1948). The kidney in periarteritis nodosa. *Quarterly Journal of Medicine,* **17,** 175–202

DROZ, D., NOEL, L.H., LEIBOWITCH, M. and BARBANEL, C. (1979). Glomerulonephritis and necrotizing angiitis. In *Advances in Nephrology,* edited by J. Hamburger, J. Crosnier and M.H. Maxwell, pp. 343–363. Chicago; Year Book

DUFFY, J., LIDSKY, M.D., SHARP, J.T., DAVIS, J.S., PERSON, D.A., BLAINE HOLLINGER, F. *et al.* (1976). Polyarthritis, polyarteritis and hepatitis B. *Medicine (Baltimore),* **55,** 19–37

DUNNILL, M.S. (1976). Polyarteritis nodosa and Wegener's granulomatosis. In *Pathological Basis of Renal Disease,* pp. 177–193. London; Saunders

DURANTE, D., LUM, G. and McINTOSH, R.M. (1977). The kidney in leukemia and lymphoma. In *Kidney Disease. Hematological and Vascular Problems,* edited by R.M. McIntosh, J. Guggenheim and R.W. Schrier, pp. 163–172. New York; Wiley

ELKON, K.B., SUTHERLAND, D.C., REES, A.J., HUGHES, G.R.V. and BATCHELOR, J.R. (1983). HLA antigen frequencies in systemic vasculitis: increase in HLA-DR2 in Wegener's granulomatosis. *Arthritis and Rheumatism,* **26,** 102–105

FAUCI, A.S. (moderator), HAYNES, B.P. and KATZ, P. (discussants) (1978). The spectrum of vasculitis. Clinical, pathologic, immunologic and therapeutic considerations. *Annals of Internal Medicine,* **89,** 660–676

FAUCI, A.S., HAYNES, B.F., KATZ, P. and WOLFF, S.M. (1983). Wegener's granulomatosis: prospective clinical and therapeutic experience with 85 patients for 21 years. *Annals of Internal Medicine,* **98,** 76–85

FAUCI, A.S., KATZ, P., HAYNES, B.F. and WOLFF, S.M. (1979). Cyclophosphamide therapy of severe systemic necrotizing vasculitis. *New England Journal of Medicine,* **301,** 235–238

FAUCI, A.S. and WOLFF, S.M. (1973). Wegener's granulomatosis: studies in eighteen patients and a review of the literature. *Medicine (Baltimore),* **52,** 535–561

FILLASTRE, J.P., MOREL-MAROGER, L. and RICHET, G. (1971). Schönlein Henoch purpura in adults. *The Lancet,* **1,** 1243–1244

FRIEDMAN, A. and KINCAID-SMITH, P. (1972). Arteritis with impaired renal function. In *Glomerulonephritis,* part II, edited by P. Kincaid-Smith, T.H. Mathew and E.L. Becker, pp. 1047–1056. New York; Wiley

FROHNERT, P.P. and SHEPS, S.G. (1967). Long term follow-up study of periarteritis nodosa. *The American Journal of Medicine,* **43,** 8–14

GERHARDT, G.M., AHMAD, M. and TUBBS, R.R. (1983). Pulmonary vasculitis (Wegener's granulomatosis). Immunohistochemical study of T and B cell markers. *The American Journal of Medicine,* **74,** 700–704

GOODMAN, B.W. (1979). Temporal arteritis. *The American Journal of Medicine,* **67,** 839–854

HABIB, R. and CAMERON, J.S. (1982). Schönlein Henoch purpura. In *The Kidney and Rheumatic Diseases,* edited by P.A. Bacon and N.M. Hadler, pp. 178–201. London; Butterworths

HABIB, R., KLEINKNECHT, C., GUBLER, M.C. and LEVY, M. (1973). Idiopathic membranoproliferative glomerulonephritis in children. Report of 105 cases. *Clinical Nephrology,* **1,** 194–214

HALPERN, B., MILLIEZ, P., LAGRUE, G., FRAY, A. and MORARD, J.C. (1965). Protective effect of heparin in experimental immune nephritis. *Nature,* **205,** 257–259

HAWORTH, S.J. (1983). Renal involvement in Wegener's granulomatosis. The Hammersmith experience. In *Nephrology '83,* edited by G. D'Amico and G. Colasanti, pp. 33–43. Milan; Wichtig Editore

HEATON, J.M. and BOURKE, E. (1976). Papillary necrosis with calyceal arteritis. *Nephron,* **16,** 57–63

HENSON, P.M. and COCHRANE, C.G. (1971). Acute immune complex disease in rabbits. The role of complement and of leukocyte-dependent release of vasoactive amines from platelets. *Journal of Experimental Medicine,* **133,** 554–571

HEPTINSTALL, R.H. (1974). Schönlein Henoch syndrome; lung hemorrhage and glomerulonephritis or Goodpasture's syndrome. In *Pathology of the Kidney,* Vol. II, pp. 563–599. Boston; Little, Brown

HEPTINSTALL, R.H. (1983). Polyarteritis (periarteritis) nodosa, other forms of vasculitis and rheumatoid arthritis. In *Pathology of the Kidney,* Vol. II, pp. 793–838. Boston; Little, Brown

HIND, C.R.K., LOCKWOOD, C.M., EVANS, D.J. and REES, A.J. (1983). Prognosis after immunosuppression of patients with crescentic nephritis requiring dialysis. *The Lancet,* **1,** 263–265

HOLDSWORTH, S.R., NEALE, T.J. and WILSON, C.B. (1980). The participation of macrophages and monocytes in experimental immune complex glomerulonephritis. *Clinical Immunology and Immunopathology,* **15,** 510–524

HUNSICKER, L.G., SHEARER, T.P., PLATTNER, S.B. and WEISENBURGER, D. (1979). The role of monocytes in serum sickness nephritis. *Journal of Experimental Medicine,* **150,** 413–425

HYMAN, L.R., WAGNILD, J.P., BEIRNE, G.J. and BURKHOLDER, P.M. (1973). Immunoglobulin A distribution in glomerular disease: analysis of immunofluorescence localizations and pathogenetic significance. *Kidney International,* **3,** 397–408

INGELFINGER, J.R., McCLUSKEY, R.T., SCHNEEBERGER, E.E. and GRUPE, W.E. (1977). Necrotizing arteritis in acute poststreptococcal glomerulonephritis. *Journal of Pediatrics,* **91,** 228–232

ITO, S., MATSUO, S. and ANDRES, G. (1983). Pathogenesis of systemic angiitis. In *Nephrology '83,* edited by G. D'Amico and G. Colasanti, pp. 5–11. Milan; Wichtig Editore

JENIS, E.H. and LOWENTHAL, D.T. (1977). Polyarteritis nodosa. In *Kidney Biopsy Interpretation,* pp. 179–192. Philadelphia; Davis

KALOWSKI, S. and KINCAID-SMITH, P. (1973). Glomerulonephritis in Henoch Schönlein syndrome. In *Glomerulonephritis: Morphology, Natural History and Treatment,* edited by P. Kincaid-Smith, T. Mathew and E.L. Becker. pp. 1123–1132. New York; Wiley

KANFER, A., SRAER, J.D., FEINTUCH, M.J., MOREL-MAROGER, L., BEAUFILS, Ph. and RICHET, G. (1976). Insuffisance rénale aiguë au cours de la périartérite noueuse. *Nouvelle Press Médicale,* **5**, 1883–1888

KATZ, P., ALLING, D.W., HAYNES, B.F. and FAUCI, A.S. (1979). Association of Wegener's granulomatosis with HLA-B8. *Clinical Immunology and Immunopathology,* **14**, 268–270

KAUFFMANN, R.H. and HOUWERT, D.A. (1981). Plasmapheresis in rapidly progressive Henoch Schönlein glomerulonephritis and the effect on circulating IgA immune complexes. *Clinical Nephrology,* **16**, 155–160

KINCAID-SMITH, P. (1975). Polyarteritis nodosa and other forms of arteritis. In *The Kidney, a Clinicopathological Study,* pp. 295–301. Oxford; Blackwell

KNIKER, W.T. and COCHRANE, C.G. (1965). Pathogenetic factors in vascular lesions of experimental serum sickness. *Journal of Experimental Medicine,* **122**, 83–98

KNOWLES, H.C., ZEEK, P.M. and BLANKENHORN, M.A. (1953). Studies on necrotizing angiitis. IV. Periarteritis nodosa and hypersensitivity angiitis. *Archives of Internal Medicine,* **92**, 789–805

LEIB, E.S., RESTIVO, C. and PAULUS, H.E. (1979). Immunosuppressive and cortiocosteroid therapy of polyarteritis nodosa. *The American Journal of Medicine,* **67**, 941–947

LEVO, Y., GOREVIC, P.D., KASSAB, H.J., ZUCKER-FRANKLIN, D. and FRANKLIN, E.C. (1977). Association between hepatitis B virus and essential mixed cryoglobulinemia. *New England Journal of Medicine,* **296**, 1501–1504

LIE, J.T. (1978). Disseminated visceral giant cell arteritis (histopathologic description and differentiation from other granulomatosis vasculitides). *The American Journal of Clinical Pathology,* **69**, 299–305

McCLUSKEY, R.T. and BHAN, A.K. (1982). Cell mediated mechanism in renal diseases. *Kidney International,* **21**, s–6, s–12

MANDACHE, E. and NICOLESCU, P. (1970). Electron microscopy observations on the participation of blood leukocytes in the production of some renal glomerular lesions. *Virchows Archiv Abteilung (A) Pathologie Anatomie,* **351**, 306–315

MEADOWS, R. (1973). The collagen disease. In *Renal Histopathology. A Light Microscopy Study of the Renal Disease,* pp. 259–276. London; Oxford University Press

MEADOWS, R. (1978). The collagen disease. In *Renal Histopathology. A Light, and Immunofluorescent Microscopy Study of Renal Disease,* pp. 393–421. Oxford; Oxford University Press

MELIN, J.P., LEMAIRE, P., BIREMBAUF, P., AUBERT, L. and CHANARD, J. (1982). Polyarteritis nodosa with bilateral ureteric involvement. *Nephron,* **32**, 87–89

MELLORS, R.C. and ORTEGA, L.G. (1956). Analytical pathology. III. New observations on the pathogenesis of glomerulonephritis, lipid nephrosis, periarteritis nodosa and secondary amyloidosis in man. *The American Journal of Pathology,* **32**, 455–499

MICHALAK, T. (1978). Immune complexes of hepatitis B surface antigen in the pathogenesis of polyarteritis nodosa. A study of seven necropsy cases. *The American Journal of Pathology,* **90**, 619–632

MIN, K.W., GYORKEY, P., YIUM, J.J. and EKNOYAN, G. (1974). The morphogenesis of glomerular crescents in rapidly progressive glomerulonephritis. *Kidney International,* **5**, 47–56

MONTES, M., ANDRES, G., ELWOOD, C.M., SEPULVEDA, M.R. and DECOTEAU, W.E. (1975). Membranoproliferative glomerulonephritis with polyarteritis: a case report. *Human Pathology,* **6**, 391–397

MOORTHY, A.V. and ZIMMERMAN, S.W. (1980). Renal disease in the elderly: clinicopathologic analysis of renal disease in 115 elderly patients. *Clinical Nephrology,* **14**, 223–229

NEILD, G.H., CAMERON, J.S., TURNER, D.R., WILLIAMS, D.G., CHANTLER, C. *et al.* (1983). Rapidly progressive glomerulonephritis with extensive glomerular crescent formation. *Quarterly Journal of Medicine,* **52**, 395–406

NOLASCO, F., CAMERON, J.S. and HARTLEY, B. (1985). T lymphocyte and macrophage involvement in the glomerular lesions of microscopic polyarteritis. *Proceedings of the EDTA-European Renal Association,* **22**, 752–758

NOVAK, R.F., CHRISTIANSEN, R.G. and SORENSEN, E.T. (1982). The acute vasculitis of Wegener's granulomatosis in renal biopsies. *The American Journal of Clinical Pathology,* **78**, 367–371

PARONETTO, F. and STRAUSS, L. (1962). Immunocytochemical observations in periarteritis nodosa. *Annals of Internal Medicine,* **56**, 289–296

PATALANO, V.J. and SOMMERS, S.C. (1961). Biopsy diagnosis of periarteritis nodosa. *Archives of Pathology,* **72**, 1–7

PAULLEY, J.W. and HUGHES, J.P. (1960). Giant cell arteritis of the aged. *British Medical Journal,* **2,** 1562–1567

PINCHING, A.J., LOCKWOOD, C.M., PUSSELL, B.A., REES, A.J., SWENY, P., EVANS, D.J. *et al.* (1983). Wegener's granulomatosis: observations on 18 patients with severe renal disease. *Quarterly Journal of Medicine,* **52,** 435–460

PIRANI, C.L. and SILVA, F.G. (1979). The kidneys in systemic lupus erythematosus and other collagen diseases: recent progress. In *Kidney Diseases: Present Status,* edited by J. Churg, B.H. Spargo, F.K. Mostofi and M.R. Abell, pp. 98–139. Baltimore; Williams and Wilkins

RALSTON, D.E. and KVALE, W.F. (1949). The renal lesions of periarteritis nodosa. *Proceedings of the Staff Meetings of the Mayo Clinic,* **24,** 18–27

RICHET, G. and HABIB, R. (1959). Les localisations rénales de la péri-artérite noueuse. *Journal d'Urologie,* **65,** 77–82

RONCO, P., MIGNON, F., LANOE, Y., ROLAND, J., MOREL-MAROGER, L. and GATTEGNO, B. (1982). Ureteral stenosis in Wegener's granulomatosis. Report of a case. *Nephron,* **30,** 201–204

RONCO, P., VERROUST, P., MIGNON, F., KOURILSKY, O., VANHILLE, Ph., MEYRIER, A. *et al.* (1983). Immunopathological studies of polyarteritis nodosa and Wegener's granulomatosis: a report of 43 patients with 51 renal biopsies. *Quarterly Journal of Medicine,* **52,** 212–223

SACK, M., CASSIDY, J.T. and BOLE, G.G. (1975). Pronostic factors in polyarteritis. *Journal of Rheumatology,* **2,** 411–420

SAMIY, A.H. (1983). Renal disease in the elderly. In *The Medical Clinics of North America,* edited by A.H. Samiy, pp. 463–480. Philadelphia; Saunders

SCOTT, D.G.I., BACON, P.A., ELIOT, P.J., TRIBE, C.R. and WALLINGTON, T.B. (1982). Systemic vasculitis in a District General 1972–1980: clinical and laboratory features, classification and prognosis in 80 cases. *Quarterly Journal of Medicine,* **51,** 292–311

SERRA, A. (1983). Natural history of the renal vasculitides. *Doctoral thesis.* Universidad Autónoma de Barcelona, Spain

SERRA, A. and CAMERON, J.S. (1985). Clinical and pathological aspects of renal vasculitis. *Seminars in Nephrology,* **5,** 15–33

SERRA, A., CAMERON, J.S., TURNER, D.R., HARTLEY, B., OGG, C.S., NEILD, G.H. *et al.* (1984). Vasculitis affecting the kidney: presentation, histopathology and long-term outcome. *Quarterly Journal of Medicine,* **53,** 181–208

SHAZO, R.D., LEVINSON, A.I., LAWLESS, O.J. and WEISBAUM, G. (1977). Systemic vasculitis with coexistent large and small vessel involvement. A classification dilema. *Journal of the American Medical Association,* **238,** 1940–1942

SONSINO, E., NABARRA, B., KAZATCHKINE, M., HINGLAIS, N. and KREIS, H. (1972). Extracapillary proliferative glomerulonephritis so called malignant glomerulonephritis. In *Advances in Nephrology,* edited by J. Hamburger, J. Crosnier and M.H. Maxwell, pp. 121–163. Chicago; Year Book

SPARGO, B.H., SEYMOUR, A.E. and ORDOÑEZ, N.G. (1980). Vasculitis. In *Renal Biopsy Pathology with Diagnostic and Therapeutic Implications,* pp. 205–218. New York; Wiley

STILMANT, H.M., BOLTON, W.K., STURGILL, B.C., SCHMITT, G.W. and COUSER, W.G. (1979). Crescentic glomerulonephritis without immune deposits: clinicopathologic features. *Kidney International,* **15,** 184–195

TARANTINO, A., DE VECCHI, A., MONTAGNINO, G., IMBASCIATI, E., MIHATSCH, M.J., ZOLLINGER, H.U. *et al.* (1981). Renal disease in essential mixed cryoglobulinemia. *Quarterly Journal of Medicine,* **50,** 1–30

UNANUE, E.R. and DIXON, F.J. (1967). Experimental glomerulonephritis: immunological events and pathogenetic mechanisms. *Advances in Immunology,* **6,** 1–90

VAN DER WOUDE, F.J., RASMUSSEN, N., LOBATTO, S., WIIK, A., PERMIN, H., VAN ES, L.A. *et al.* (1985). Autoantibodies against neutrophils and monocytes: tool for diagnosis and marker of disease activity in Wegener's granulomatosis. *Lancet,* **i,** 425–429

VASALLI, P. and McCLUSKEY, R.T. (1964). The pathogenic role of the coagulation process in rabbit Masugi nephritis. *The American Journal of Pathology,* **45,** 653–677

WAINWRIGHT, J. and DAVSON, J. (1950). The renal appearances in the microscopic form of periarteritis nodosa. *Journal of Pathology and Bacteriology,* **62,** 189–196

WOLFF, S.M., FAUCI, A.S., HORN, R.G. and CALE, D.C. (1974). Wegener's granulomatosis. *Annals of Internal Medicine,* **81,** 513–525

WU MING-JIANG, RAJARM, R., SHELP, D., BEIRNE, G. and BURKHOLDER, P.M. (1980). Vasculitis in Goodpasture's syndrome. *Archives of Pathology and Laboratory Medicine,* **104,** 300–302

ZOLLINGER, H.U. and MIHATSCH, M.J. (1978). Special forms of glomerulonephritis. In *Renal Pathology in Biopsy (Light, Electron and Immunofluorescent Microscopy and Clinical Aspects),* pp. 317–366. Berlin; Springer

Chapter 17

Renal cystic disease in the elderly

V.E. Torres, K.E. Holley, G.W. Hartman and C. Garcia Iglesias

Introduction

Cystic diseases of the kidney are a very heterogeneous group of disorders which have in common the presence of renal cysts (from the Greek *kystis,* bladder), that is, sac-like structures containing fluid or semi-solid material. The pathogenesis of these diseases is incompletely understood and no specific defect that might be responsible for the development of the cysts during fetal or post-natal life has been identified at a biochemical level. Some cysts develop during embryogenesis, others late in life; some cysts arise from a genetic abnormality and are regarded as hereditary, others are not (Bernstein, 1976). Since individually most cysts look alike, classifications of renal cystic disorders have usually been based on the number and distribution of the cysts, microdissection characteristics, and genetic and clinical patterns (Spence and Singleton, 1972; Bernstein, 1976; Steg, 1978). These are provisional classifications to clarify and organize the current knowledge, but they will eventually become obsolete when more is learned of the aetiology and pathogenesis of these disorders. It is likely that diseases now viewed as homogeneous disorders will turn out to be a group of related disorders with different underlying metabolic abnormalities.

A classification of the renal cystic diseases that can be seen in elderly patients is shown in *Table 17.1.* Some renal cystic diseases are excluded from this classification because they are not compatible with a normal life expectancy and are seen exclusively in neonates, infants, children or young adults. Bilateral multicystic dysplasia, infantile polycystic kidney disease, phakomatosis, and renal cystic disorders in syndromes of multiple malformations will not be further discussed in this chapter.

Table 17.1 Classification of renal cystic disorders in the elderly

Unilateral multicystic kidney
Multilocular cyst
Simple cysts
Autosomal dominant polycystic kidney disease
Acquired cystic disease of the kidneys
Adult medullary cystic disease
Medullary sponge kidney
Cystic disease of the renal sinus
Pelvicaliceal diverticula
Neoplastic cysts
Inflammatory cysts

Unilateral multicystic kidneys

Unilateral multicystic kidneys are a rare form of renal dysplasia that needs to be considered in the differential diagnosis of a non-visualized kidney in the adult (Spence, 1955; Becker and Robinson, 1970; Greene, Feinzaig and Dahlin, 1971; Kyaw and Newman, 1971; Lang and Gershanik, 1978; Walker *et al.,* 1978).

Pathology

These kidneys consist of a grape-like cluster of cysts held together by connective tissue and have lost the typical reniform outline (*Figure 17.1*). The composition of cystic fluid resembles plasma in regards to sodium, potassium, creatinine, urea and sugar. The ureter is characteristically absent, rudimentary or atretic.

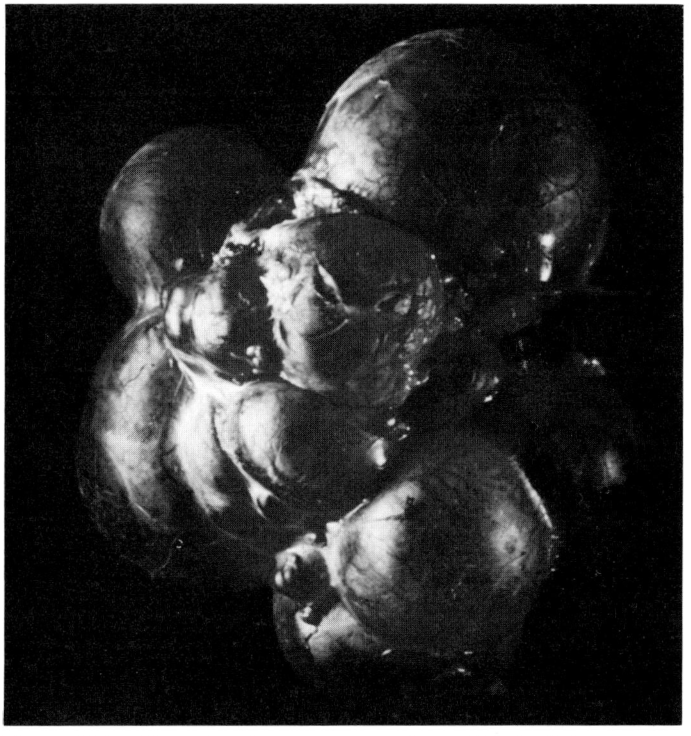

Figure 17.1 Characteristic appearance of a multicystic kidney; grape-like cluster of cysts held together by connective tissue

Pathogenesis

The cause of multicystic renal dysplasia is uncertain, but a primary defect in the ureteric development is strongly suspected. Experimentally, a typical multicystic kidney can be produced by transient ureteric obstruction during renal development.

Clinical manifestations

Multicystic dysplastic kidneys are the most common cause of an abnormal mass in the newborn and, when bilateral, are incompatible with life. Unilateral multicystic kidneys, however, may not be detected until adult age or may go completely undetected during life and be discovered at autopsy. Multicystic kidneys are most commonly found in the adult as an incidental finding during the evaluation of hypertension, nephrolithiasis or urinary tract infection. Occasionally, however, the diagnosis of multicystic kidney will be associated with the presence of abdominal or flank discomfort due to the mass effect of the lesion.

Imaging

The diagnosis of this condition requires lack of visualization of the kidney by excretory urogram and the inability to obtain a retrograde pyelogram because of partial or complete absence or obliteration of the ureter. Very frequently, calcified cysts are shown on X-ray by the presence of varying size ring-like calcifications (*Figure 17.2*).

Treatment

Nephrectomy is not necessary except in those few patients who have abdominal or flank discomfort.

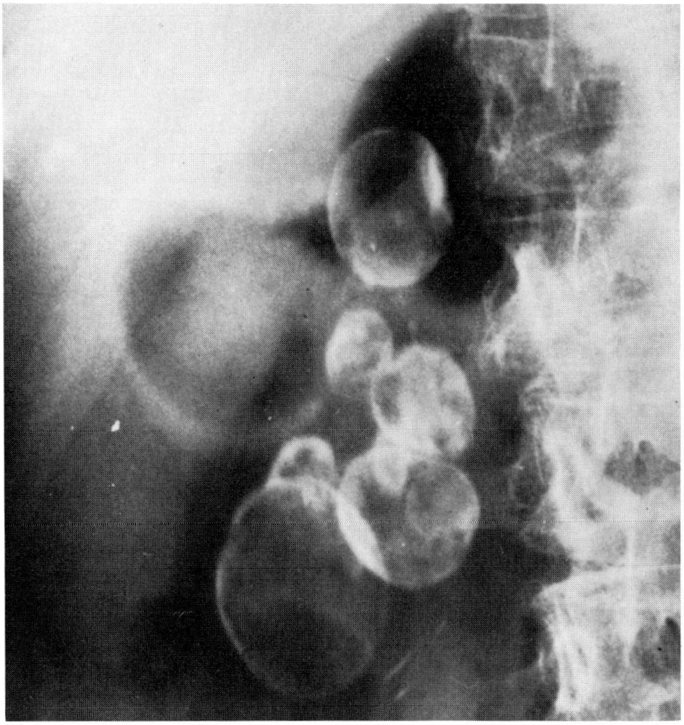

Figure 17.2 Ring-like calcifications in a multicystic kidney

Multilocular renal cysts

Multilocular renal cysts constitute a well-defined entity (Meland and Braasch, 1933; Baldauf and Schulz, 1975; Epstein *et al.*, 1978; Sadlowski *et al.*, 1979; Akhtar and Qadeer, 1980; Banner *et al.*, 1981; Taxy and Marshall, 1983) consisting of a well-circumscribed, encapsulated renal mass composed of multiple non-communicating cysts of varying size (*Figure 17.3*).

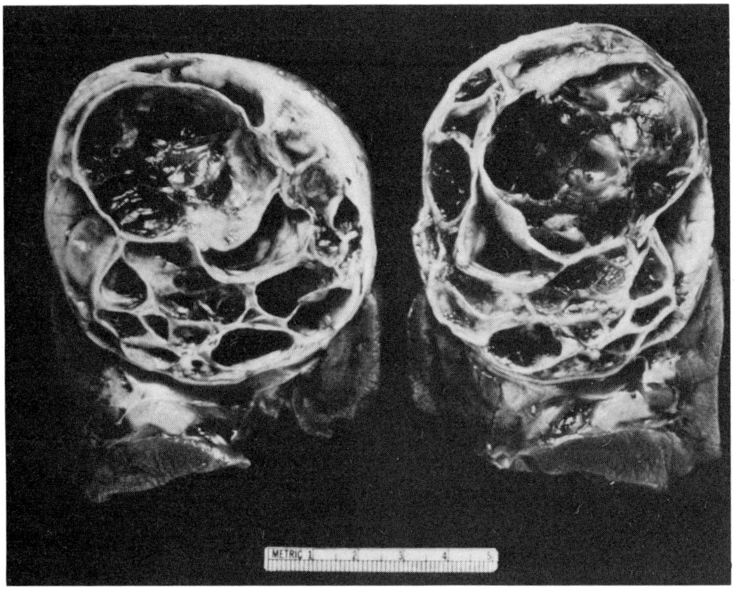

Figure 17.3 Multilocular cyst. Well-circumscribed, encapsulated renal mass composed of multiple non-communicating cysts

Pathology

Histologically, two types of multilocular cysts have been described. In both types, no fully developed nephrons or segments of nephrons can be found in the septa of the cysts, while the remaining kidney tissue outside the cyst is normal. The first type of multilocular cysts is most frequently found in adults; the septa in this type are composed of fibrous tissue. The second type of multilocular cysts is found in infants and young children only and is considered by some authors to be a benign equivalent of a nephroblastoma; the septa in this type contain variable amounts of embryonic tissue composed of clusters of small cells with varying degrees of differentiation into structures such as tubules, glomeruli and mesenchymal tissues, including smooth and striated muscle. The locules of the cysts are lined with flattened or plump, cytologically atypical but reactive type, epithelial cells. In some cases, proliferation of these cells has been interpreted as evidence of their neoplastic nature and occasionally histologic evidence of renal adenocarcinoma has been found. The biologic course of these tumours, however, has been consistently benign. No metastasis or local recurrence has ever been described following nephrectomy for a multilocular cyst which contains a renal cell carcinoma.

Pathogenesis

The pathogenesis of multilocular cysts is unknown. Recent reviews suggest that multilocular cysts are neoplasms, usually benign but occasionally harbouring histologic malignancy. A few cases have been reported where development of a multilocular cyst has occurred in a kidney previously normal by excretory urography. There is also evidence that these lesions increase in size, resulting in compression and damage of the surrounding normal renal parenchyma. It is possible, however, that not all multilocular cysts have a singular pathogenesis and some multilocular cysts, especially in children, may be congenital and dysplastic.

Clinical manifestations

Multilocular cysts are less rare than initially suspected. Approximately half of the cases reported have occurred in children and half in adults. The ages of the adult patients at diagnosis have ranged from 18 to 72 years old, with a peak incidence in the sixth decade. Multilocular cysts are typically solitary and unilateral. Bilateral multilocular renal cysts are very rare and have been described only in children. The presenting symptoms are usually an abdominal mass, pain or haematuria.

Imaging and differential diagnosis

Multilocular cysts are usually first detected on excretory urography. The urographic evidence of multilocular cysts is usually indistinguishable from other renal masses. Central and peripheral calcification occurs more commonly than initially reported. By ultrasonography, multilocular cysts are complex masses with well-defined cysts mixed with highly echogenic stroma. The role of computed tomography in the diagnosis of these lesions has not been well evaluated. On angiography, these lesions are generally avascular or sparsely vascular, rarely being moderately vascular or

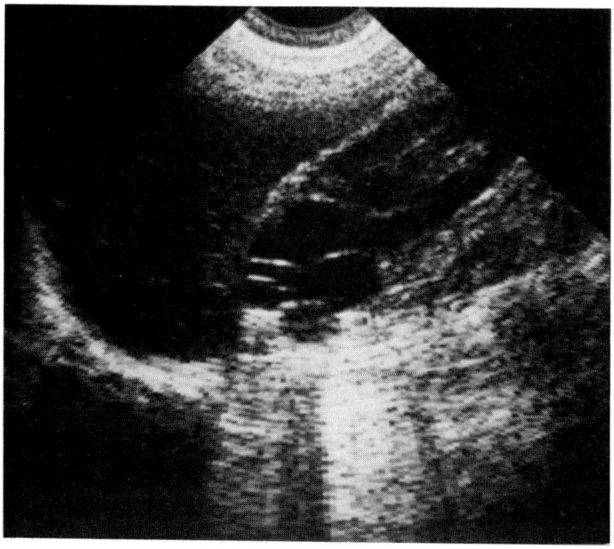

Figure 17.4 Surgically proven multilocular cyst in the upper pole of the right kidney demonstrated by ultrasonography

hypervascular. The angiographic appearance is, therefore, insufficient to rule out a renal cell carcinoma. Cyst puncture reveals clear fluid with benign cytology. Only one or a few cysts are filled with contrast media if this is instilled, while the bulk of the multilocular cyst remains unopacified (*Figure 17.4*).

Treatment

If technically possible, partial nephrectomy is the treatment of choice for multilocular cysts. The occurrence of renal cell carcinoma in multilocular cysts is not frequent enough to justify routine nephrectomy in these cases. However, thorough tissue sampling for histologic studies and use of frozen sections should be done at the time of surgery to rule out the presence of a renal adenocarcinoma which would necessitate complete nephrectomy. A preoperative diagnosis of multilocular cysts free of renal adenocarcinoma is difficult to establish. On the other hand, atypical hyperplasias in multilocular cysts may on occasion be erroneously interpreted as low grade adenocarcinomas. In any case, the biological course of multilocular cysts is usually benign, even in those cases with associated renal cell carcinoma with no reports of local or metastatic recurrence following nephrectomy for a multilocular cyst with adenocarcinoma.

Simple cysts

Simple cysts are the most common renal disorder, and they are especially frequent in elderly patients. Over 50 per cent of people over 50 years old have at least one cyst on post-mortem examination. Our own experience of 100 post-mortem examinations over the age of 90 indicated that one or more cysts are present in almost 100 per cent of the cases. Twenty-four per cent of patients over the age of 40 have cysts detectable by computed tomography of the abdomen obtained for reasons unrelated to the kidney (Laucks and MacLachlan, 1981). They can be single or multiple, are usually asymptomatic, and rarely lead to complications. Their clinical significance resides in the fact that they need to be differentiated from hypernephroma and, when very numerous, polycystic kidney disease.

Pathology

Simple renal cysts are usually lined by a single layer of epithelial cells and filled with a clear, serous fluid (Kissane, 1983). They are usually small and grow slowly, but huge cysts up to 30 cm in diameter have been described. The inner surface of these cysts is glistening and usually smooth, but some cysts may be trabeculated by partial septa that divide the cavity into broadly interconnecting locules (*Figure 17.5*). These septate simple cysts should not be confused with multilocular cysts.

Pathogenesis

Many clinical and pathologic studies suggest that most, if not all, simple renal cysts are acquired. Several hypotheses have been proposed to explain their pathogenesis. Early experimental animal studies suggested that tubular obstruction and ischaemia might play a role (Heppler, 1930). Interstitial fibrosis in the medulla and papilla increases with age and tubular obstruction secondary to this interstitial

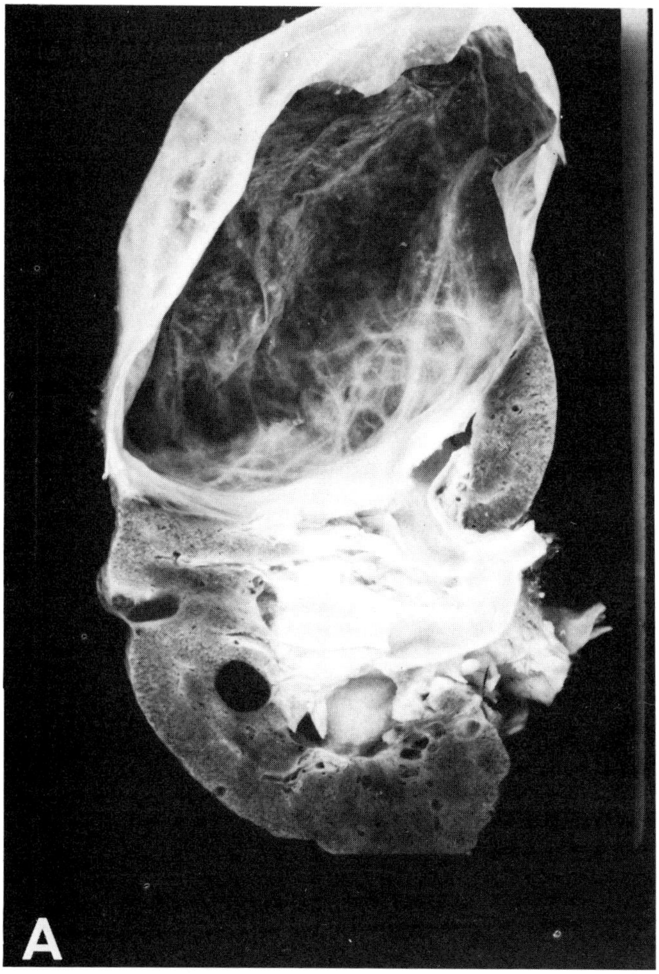

Figure 17.5 See caption opposite

fibrosis might contribute to the development of the cysts (Keresztury and Megyeri, 1962; Darmady, Offer and Woodhouse, 1973). Support for the obstructive theory has also been sought in the higher frequency of simple cysts in patients evaluated for prostatism, as compared to an unselected urologic population (Steg, 1976a; Baert and Steg, 1977). It has not been proven, however, that patients with prostatism have a higher prevalence of simple renal cysts than age-matched controls. Therefore, a contributory role of obstruction to the formation of simple renal cysts is likely, but not proven.

Microdissection studies suggest that they may originate from localized defects in the tubular wall with formation of a diverticulum that progresses to a simple cyst (Steg, 1976a; Baert and Steg, 1977). Using microdissection techniques, diverticula in the distal convoluted tubules are frequently found after the age of 20 and numerically increase with age (*Figure 17.6*). Alterations of the tubular basement membrane also occur with aging. These alterations may be the result of changes in maturation and cross-linking of collagen that also occur with age and may lead to

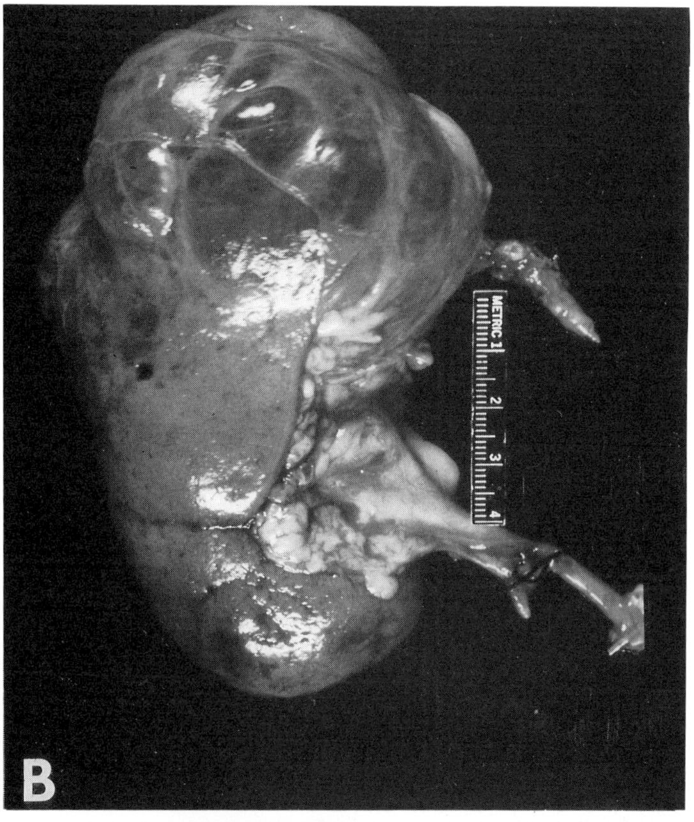

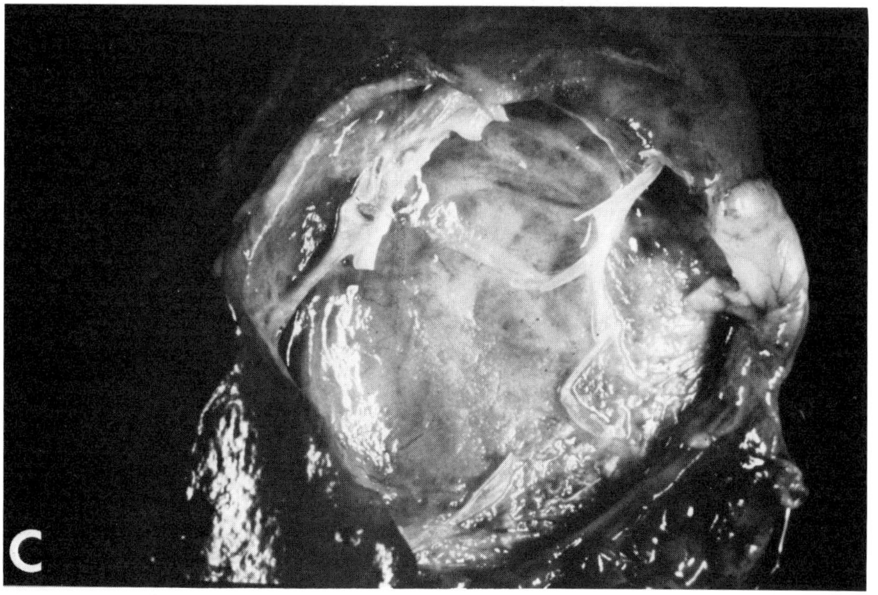

Figure 17.5 (A) Kidney of a 97-year-old patient containing multiple benign simple cysts of variable sizes; (B) kidney with large septated cyst in a 74-year-old patient; (C) same as (B) after opening the cyst

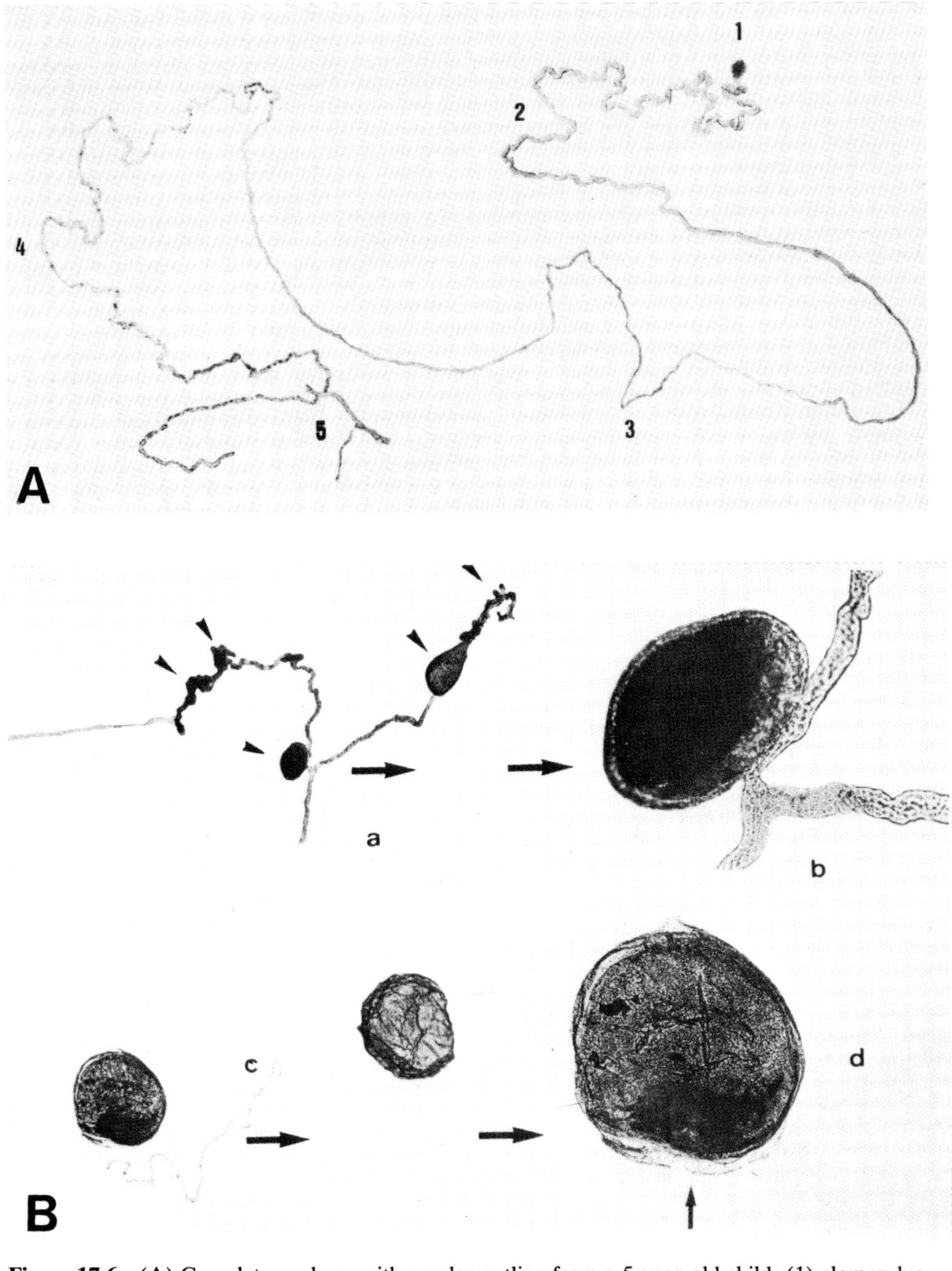

Figure 17.6 (A) Complete nephron with regular outline from a 5-year-old child: (1) glomerulus, (2) proximal convoluted tubule, (3) loop of Henle, (4) distal convoluted tubule, (5) collecting tubule. (B) Distal convoluted tubules from a normal kidney of a 70-year-old man. Note diverticula, ectasia and cyst formation (From Baert and Steg, 1977, reproduced with permission)

weakening of the basement membrane, formation of tubular diverticula and development of simple cysts. If this hypothesis is proved to be correct, the development of renal simple cysts would then be determined not only by genetic factors controlling the metabolism of connective tissue but also by environmental factors such as exposure to drugs that might alter metabolism of collagen.

As opposed to the cysts in autosomal dominant polycystic kidney disease, the composition of cystic fluid in renal simple cysts usually resembles that of interstitial fluid (Bricker and Patton, 1955; Clarke, Hurwitz and Dubinsky, 1956; Steg, 1976b). Another difference is that small molecular tracers, such as inulin, para-aminohippuric acid, sodium *o*-iodohippurate and sodium pertechnetate, are not found in the cystic fluid aspirated from patients to whom these drugs have been administered intravenously. Therefore, renal simple cysts do not appear to be in communication with the tubular lumina. The information provided by the microdissection and by the chemical studies are not necessarily contradictory. It is possible that renal simple cysts result from progressive dilatation of saccular tubular diverticula with increasingly narrow necks which are eventually completely cut off from the tubule.

Clinical manifestations

Simple renal cysts occur equally in both kidneys and are found more frequently in the lower pole, followed by the upper pole and then the mid-section of the kidney (Braasch and Hendrick, 1944; Hale and Morgan, 1969; Steg, 1976c). Both slight male and female predominance have been reported. Most frequently, the cysts are asymptomatic, but they may be discovered at the time of a nephro-urologic evaluation for some unrelated problem. It is, therefore, important that the presence of these cysts does not distract from the diagnosis of other more important intrarenal or extrarenal lesions. Large renal cysts may cause abdominal or flank discomfort, usually described as a sensation of weight or a dull ache. More frequently, however, this pain can be explained by another coincident lesion such as nephrolithiasis Simple cysts in the upper pole of the right kidney can produce pain in the right upper abdominal quadrant, under the costal margin and in the right side of the back and should be considered in the differential diagnosis of right upper quadrant abdominal pain (Quinby and Bright, 1977).

Rare cases of gross haematuria due to vascular erosion by an enlarging cyst have been well documented (Smith, Rich and Barnes, 1977; Brown, 1978), but another cause of macrohaematuria or microhaematuria is usually found in the great majority of patients with simple renal cysts who have haematuria.

When the simple cysts lie at or near the hilus, a urographic pattern of caliceal obstruction or hydronephrosis is frequently found (Reid, 1966; Evans and Coughlin, 1970; Hinman, 1978). In most but not all cases, these apparent obstructive changes seen on the excretory urogram are of no functional significance. A dynamic hippuran/DTPA radioactive renal scan before and after administration of frusemide is helpful to assess the degree of functional obstruction (Roth and Roberts, 1980).

Rare cases of renin-dependent hypertension caused by solitary intrarenal simple cysts have been described (Babka, Cohen and Sode, 1974; Rockson, Stone and Gunnells, 1974; Churchill *et al.*, 1975; Hoard and O'Brien, 1976; Rose and Pruitt, 1976; Johnson and Radwin, 1976; Kala *et al.*, 1976; Mang *et al.*, 1978). The proposed mechanism is arterial compression by the cyst, causing segmental renal ischaemia. These cases have been well documented by renal vein renin studies and cure of the hypertension following surgical or percutaneous drainage of the cyst.

A rare but dramatic complication is that of infection of a renal cyst (Limjoco and Strauch, 1966; Deliveliotis, Zorzos and Varkarakis, 1967; Altemus, Salazar and Rotherham, 1968; Stables and Jackson, 1974; Mindell, 1975; Patel, Witts and Ward, 1978; Sagalowsky and Solotkin, 1980). The usual presentation is with high fever, flank pain and tenderness, and frequently a sympathatic pleural effusion. Most patients are females and the most common pathogen is *Escherichia coli*. Urine cultures are frequently negative. Ultrasonography is helpful in making the diagnosis. As opposed to uncomplicated simple cysts, infected cysts have irregular borders with internal echoes. The distinction between an infected simple cyst and a primary abscess of the kidney, however, may be difficult and depends on the recognition of a smooth contour to the inner surface of the lesion at percutaneous renal cystography.

Imaging and differential diagnosis

By far the most common diagnostic problem raised by the detection of a simple cyst is its differentiation from a renal cell carcinoma (Clayman *et al.*, 1984; Williamson *et al.*, 1985). With the advent of excretory urography in 1928 and nephrotomography in 1954, the combined use of routine tomography with excretory urograms in many institutions since the 1960s and the more recent introduction of ultrasonography, computed tomography and magnetic resonance imaging, unsuspected renal masses have been increasingly detected (Lloyd *et al.*, 1978). Excretory urography with routine tomography allows visualization of small renal masses that would otherwise be obscured by overlying bowel content and gas. Although excretory

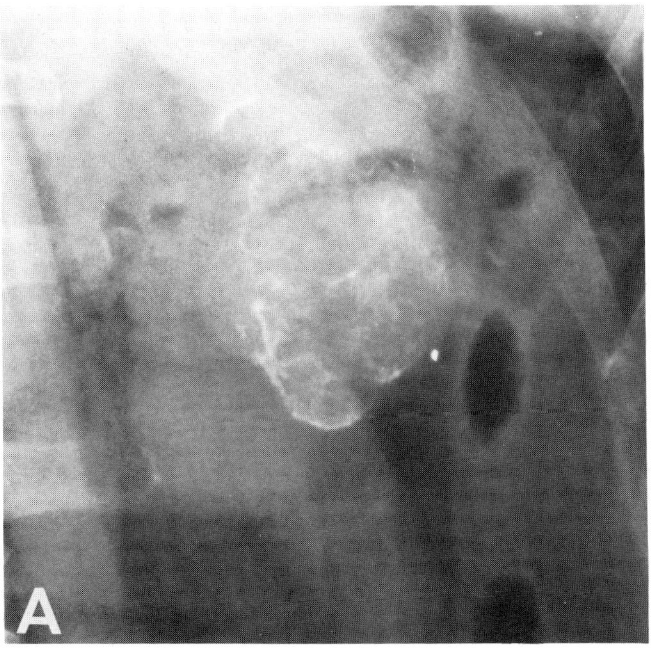

Figure 17.7 See caption opposite

urography is the basic imaging modality used in the detection of renal masses, it has limited usefulness in determining whether a lesion is benign or malignant. Calcification is detected in only 1–2 per cent of simple cysts (Daniel *et al.*, 1972). The calcification in these cases is usually peripheral. Demonstration of mottled or punctate calcium within a mass in the absence of peripheral calcification is highly indicative of a malignant lesion (*Figure 17.7*). The masses containing only

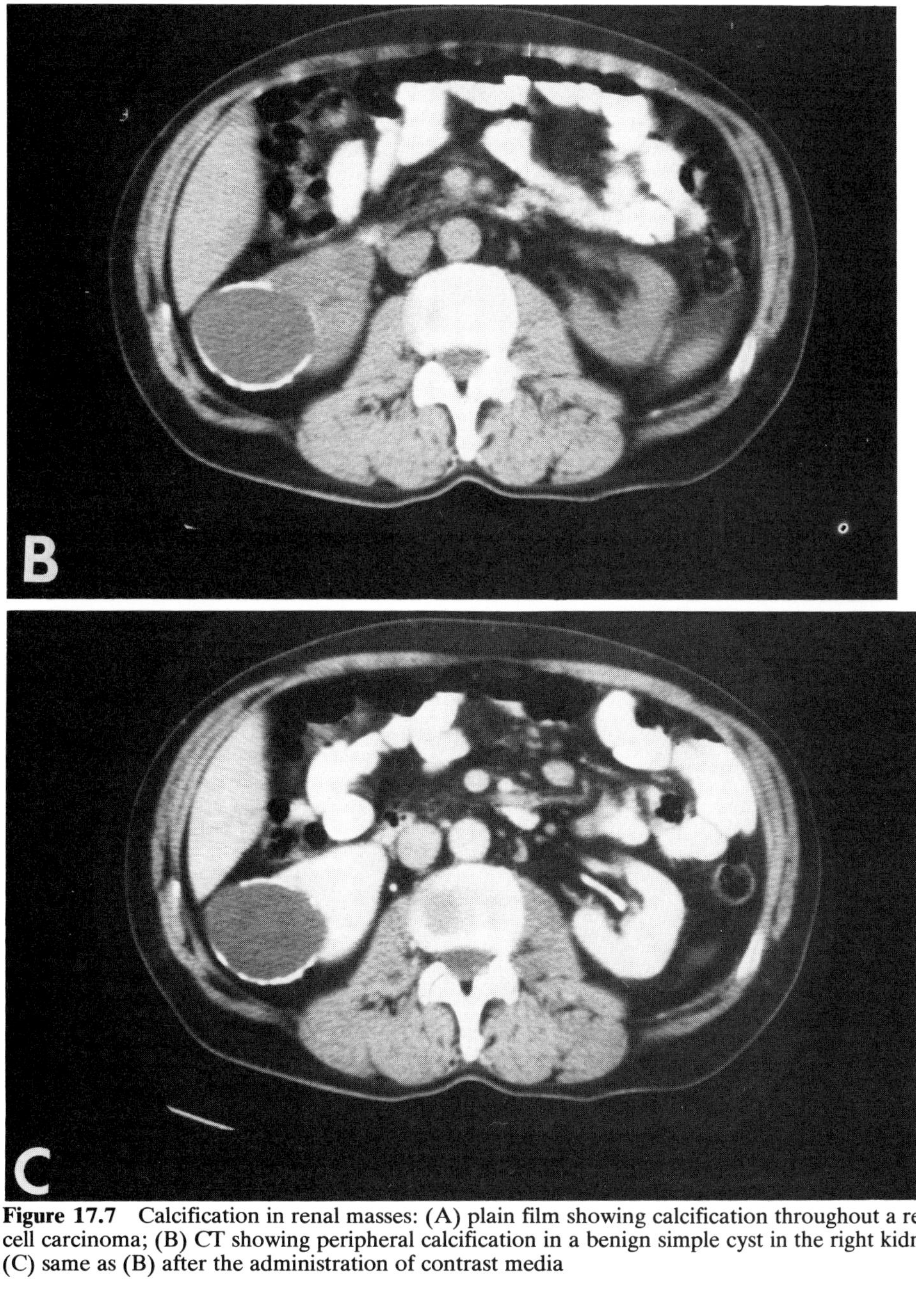

Figure 17.7 Calcification in renal masses: (A) plain film showing calcification throughout a renal cell carcinoma; (B) CT showing peripheral calcification in a benign simple cyst in the right kidney; (C) same as (B) after the administration of contrast media

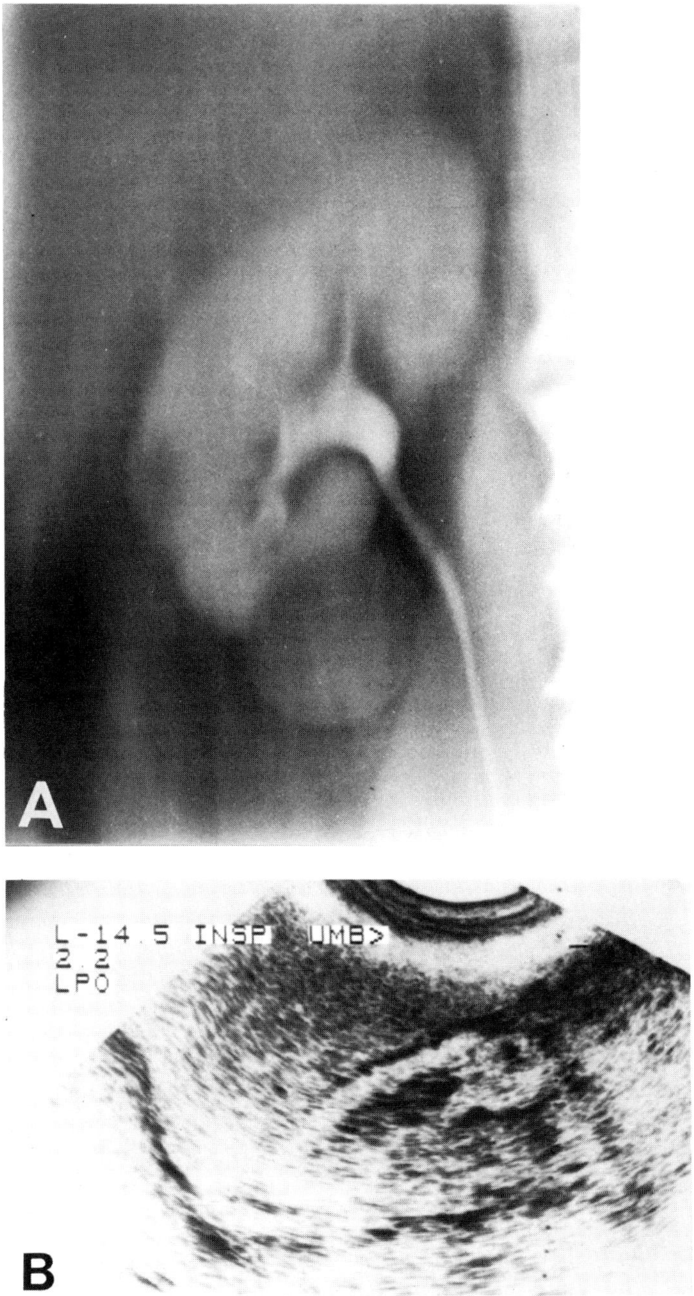

Figure 17.8 Renal cell carcinoma: (A) tomogram obtained during excretory urography demonstrates a relatively radiolucent mass, which is sharply demarcated and has a thin wall; (B) ultrasonography shows a solid echogenic mass

peripheral curvilinear (eggshell) calcification, however, also have a significant chance, at least 20 per cent, of being malignant. Other urographic findings suggestive of malignancy include invasion of the collecting system, lobulated or thickened wall of the mass, and homogenous or relatively high density of the mass.

Because the appearance of a renal mass on the excretory urogram alone almost never excludes a malignancy (*Figure 17.8*), ultrasonography, computed tomography or arteriography are commonly required to characterize the lesion. Ultrasonography is commonly used because of the lack of ionizing radiation, lack of invasiveness, limited cost and general availability. The ultrasound features which permit the diagnosis of benign simple cysts are lack of internal echoes, smooth walls and enhancement of echoes deep to the lesion (*Figure 17.9*). If all of these criteria

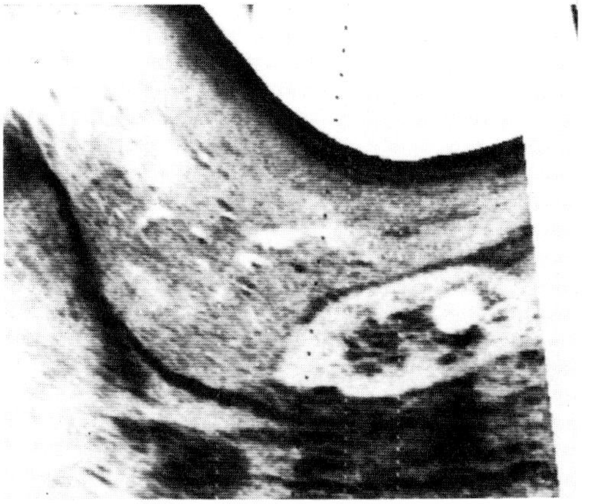

Figure 17.9 Ultrasonography of the right kidney containing a typical benign intrarenal cyst with smooth walls, enhancement of echoes deep to the cyst, and without internal echoes

are met, accuracy approaches 100 per cent and further evaluation is not necessary. The computed tomography criteria which permit the diagnosis of benign simple cysts are a density that is near that of water, thin or imperceptible wall, sharp interface with renal parenchyma, and no significant increase in density after the administration of intravenous contrast material (*Figure 17.10*). As with ultrasound, if all these criteria are met, further evaluation of the mass is not necessary.

Masses which by ultrasonography are primarily cystic but contain internal echoes such as a thick septum or nodule are often benign simple cysts, but percutaneous needle aspiration is necessary to exclude the very rare tumour within the wall of a cyst. To allow the diagnosis of a benign simple cyst, the fluid obtained from the cyst has to be clear or straw-coloured, with a protein content below 3g/dl, a low or normal concentration of lactic dehydrogenase activity, and free of malignant cells or cells containing intracellular fat.

Since the acceptance of ultrasonography and computed tomography for the differential diagnosis of renal masses, the number of angiograms performed for this purpose has declined dramatically. Angiography is still helpful, especially in patients with complex, multiple renal masses such as patients with multiple cysts and a possible solid renal mass.

Several algorithms have been proposed for the evaluation of renal masses (Clayman *et al.*, 1984). While these algorithms can be helpful as a general guide, they do not take into consideration the strength and weaknesses of various

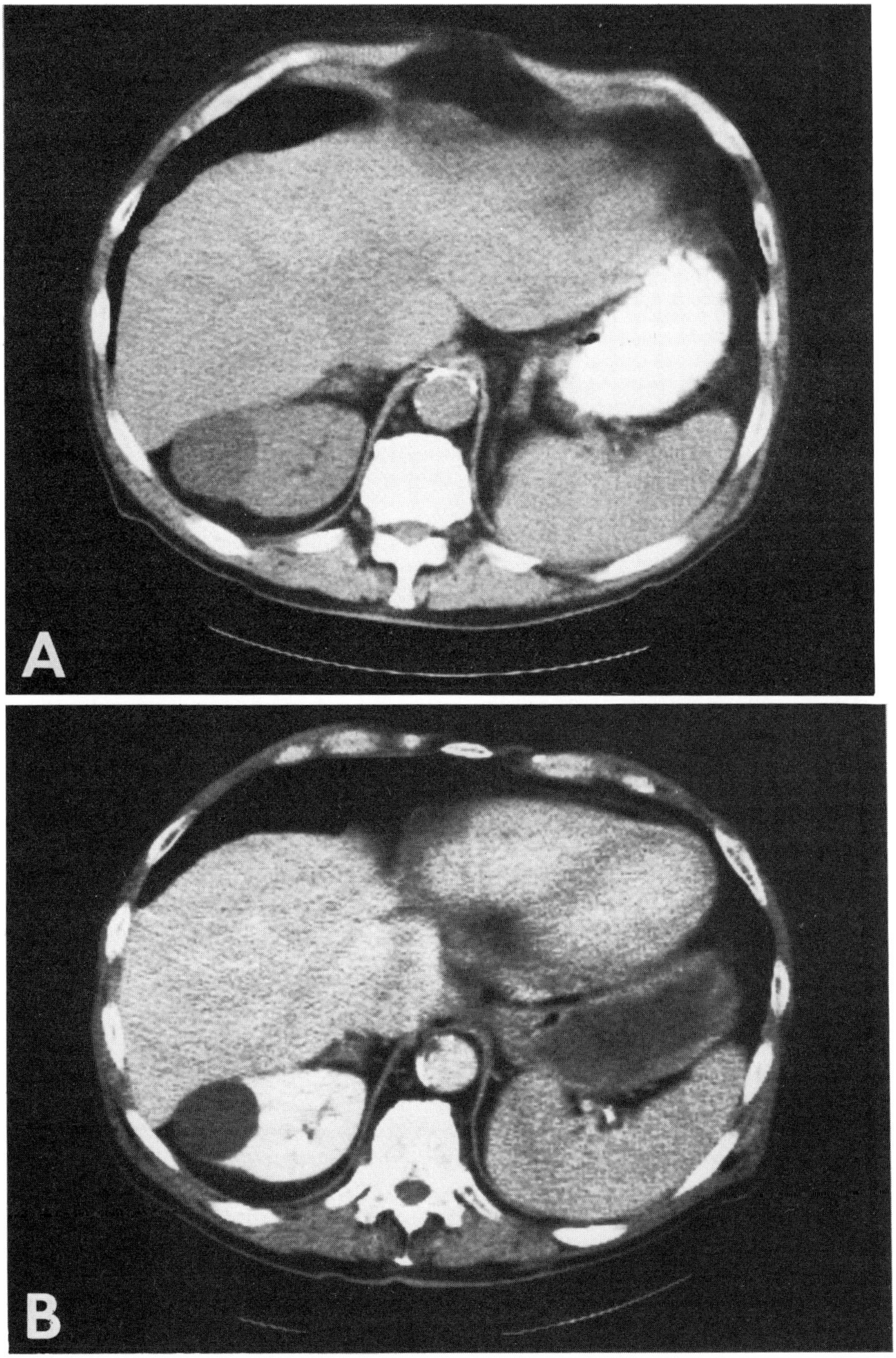

Figure 17.10 Computed tomography of a benign simple cyst in the lateral aspect of the right kidney: (A) pre-contrast media shows a water density mass with a thin wall and a sharp interface with the renal parenchyma; (B) post-contrast media shows no enhancement of the cyst

diagnostic modalities at the specific institution, the varying abilities of the different modalities in evaluating masses of varying size and location, and coexisting medical conditions which may dictate a unique pattern of diagnostic testing in a given patient.

Simple renal cysts frequently are not solitary and one or more additional cysts may be present in the same or contralateral kidney. Occasionally, however, simple cysts may be very numerous and cause parenchymal and pyelocaliceal distortion. When both kidneys are extensively and diffusely involved, differentiation from autosomal dominant polycystic kidney disease may be difficult. Because of the obvious implications, it is important that the diagnosis of autosomal dominant polycystic kidney disease is not made in this situation unless a familial history consistent with autosomal dominant transmission can be documented.

Treatment

The improvement of the diagnostic techniques during the past decade has dramatically reduced the indications for surgery in the management of benign simple cysts. At present surgery is only indicated in the rare cases where there is still doubt of the precise diagnosis after using less invasive investigations, in the rare complicated cysts that cannot be adequately treated percutaneously and in the symptomatic cysts that recur rapidly after percutaneous drainage (Steg, 1976d). Drainage of the infected simple cyst is essential. The penetration of antibiotics such as amoxicillin, minocycline and rifampicin into the cyst is poor. While surgery used to be required for cyst drainage, more recent reports indicate that percutaneous drainage might be equally successful. Percutaneous aspiration of a renal cyst is easily accomplished and should be done for a diagnostic purpose whenever the cyst might be responsible for pain, obstruction or hypertension. In some cases, there is no reaccumulation of cystic fluid after aspiration, and in these cases, cyst aspiration is also of therapeutic value. Instillation of some materials such as pantopaque has been advocated by some authors to induce an inflammatory reaction in the cyst wall that results in a decrease in the size of some renal cysts (Vestby, 1967; Raskin *et al.*, 1975).

Autosomal dominant polycystic kidney disease

While benign simple cysts are the most prevalent renal cystic disorder, autosomal dominant polycystic kidney disease (ADPKD) is undoubtedly the most important. This is also true in the geriatric population, especially with the recent recognition that survival of patients with this disease to an elderly age is not as rare as initially thought and that significant pathology may result from associated extrarenal disorders. The existence of polycystic kidneys has been known for centuries, as illustrated by the drawing published by Rayer in 1837 and reproduced in *Figure 17.11(A)*. Nevertheless, ADPKD did not become a well-defined entity, clearly separated from other renal cystic disorders, until the twentieth century. During the early part of this century, reports of large series of patients (Bunting, 1906; Cairns, 1925; Shapiro, 1929; Oppenheimer, 1934; Fergusson, 1949; Bell, 1950; Newman, 1950; Higgins, 1952; Funck-Brentano *et al.*, 1964; Ward, Draper and Lavengood, 1967), including many from our institution (Braasch, 1916; Schacht, 1931; Braasch and Schacht, 1933; Walters and Braasch, 1934; Rall and Odel, 1949; Comfort *et al.*,

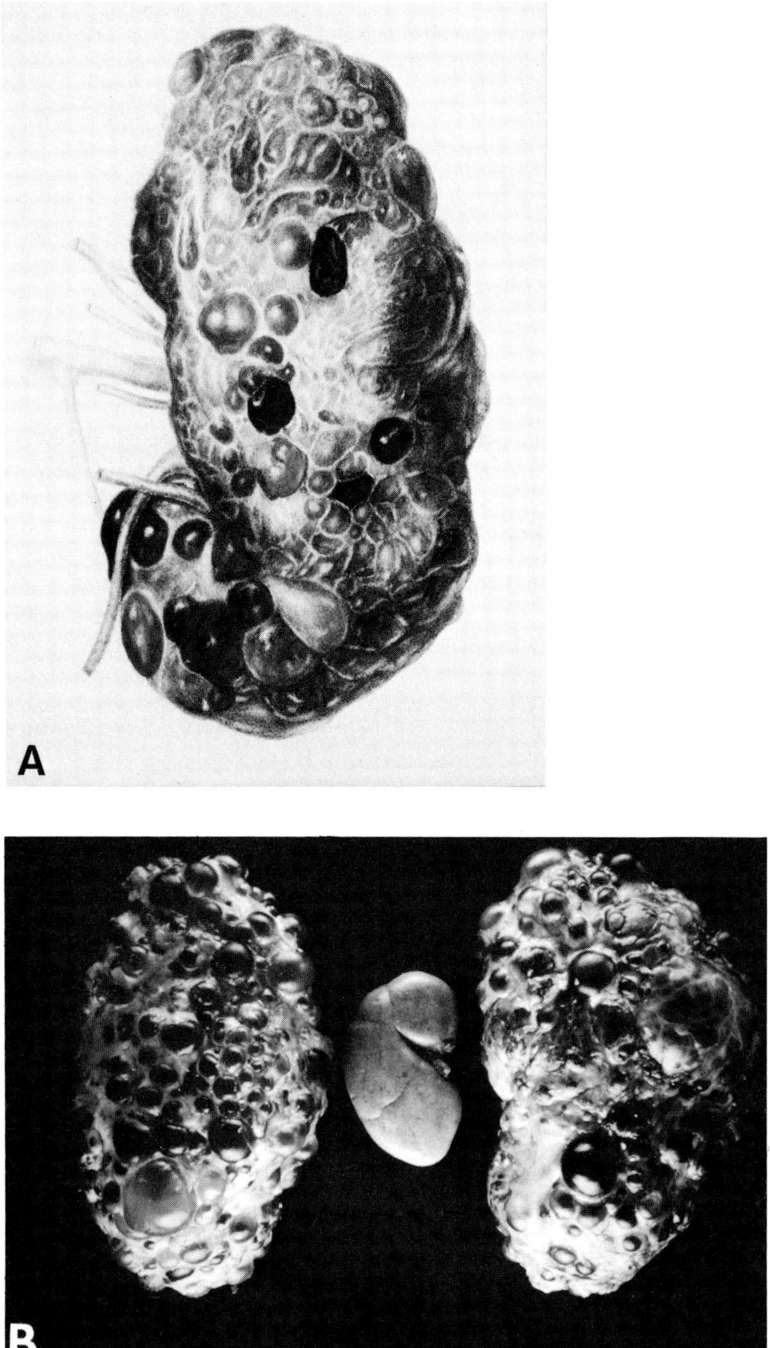

Figure 17.11 (A) Drawing of a typical polycystic kidney published by Rayer in 1837; (B) typical appearance of polycystic kidneys, compared to a normal kidney

1952; Simon and Thompson, 1955), helped to define its clinical characteristics and hereditary pattern. Among these early reports, the initial description by Lejars (1888) and the classical work by Dalgaard (1957) deserve special mention. These early studies included mostly patients with advanced disease. The prognosis of ADPKD based on these studies appeared rather dismal. More recent studies (Gabow, Iklé and Holmes, 1984; Churchill *et al.*, 1984; Delaney *et al.*, 1985) have examined populations with less advanced disease, mostly including non-azotaemic patients or patients detected by family screening. The prognosis of the disease based on these studies is considerably better.

Epidemiology

There have been two population based epidemiological studies of polycystic kidney disease in the adult. The first is a classical study by Dalgaard (1957) in Copenhagen between 1920 and 1953. The second is a more recent study by Iglesias *et al.* (1983) in Olmsted County, Minnesota, USA, between 1935 and 1980. Based on the Olmsted County data, the calculated lifetime risk of having a diagnosis of ADPKD is approximately 1 per 1000 (Torres, Holley and Offord, 1985). This is a conservative value, since it does not include the autopsy cases. Up to 50 per cent of patients with ADPKD may have escaped detection during life in the Olmsted County study. Patients with ADPKD were diagnosed earlier in life in the Olmsted County study than those patients reported in the Copenhagen study. The patients diagnosed at autopsy in Olmsted County had mild forms of the disease, with normal renal function or only mild renal insufficiency. Their age reflected the age of the general autopsy population. Comparison of these two epidemiological studies of ADPKD covering two different time periods suggests that ADPKD is becoming recognized earlier and more often during life and that milder cases are compatible with a normal life expectancy (*Figure 17.12*) (Iglesias *et al.*, 1983; Torres, Holley and Offord, 1984; Delaney *et al.*, 1985).

The survivorship of patients with ADPKD is better than initially thought and appears to be improving. The survivorship of the Olmsted County patients was considerably better than that of the Copenhagen patients (Dalgaard, 1957; Iglesias *et al.*, 1983; Torres, Holley and Offord, 1984; Delaney *et al.*, 1985). Several explanations may account for this observation. First, the expected survival of the general population between the two different time periods improved. Secondly, the diagnosis and inclusion of milder cases in the Olmsted County study would also contribute to a better survival. Thirdly, and most important, the development of therapeutic advances such as antihypertensive and antimicrobial therapies and especially the introduction of renal replacement therapies has played an important part. Approximately 50 per cent of deaths in the Copenhagen study were due to uraemia. A slightly lower proportion of deaths of patients diagnosed in Olmsted County between 1935 and 1957 was due to uraemia, whereas none of the patients diagnosed between 1957 and 1980 died of renal failure.

At a national level in the USA, 5 subjects per million per year enter the Medicare end-stage renal disease program as a result of ADPKD (Eggers, Connerton and McMullan, 1984). The prevalence of end-stage renal disease secondary to polycystic kidneys has been steadily increasing since 1974, and there is no sign of a plateau. Approximately 8 per cent of the total end-stage renal disease enrolment is due to ADPKD. The price of this improved survivorship is high. During 1983, 168 million dollars were spent to maintain 6720 polycystic kidney patients on

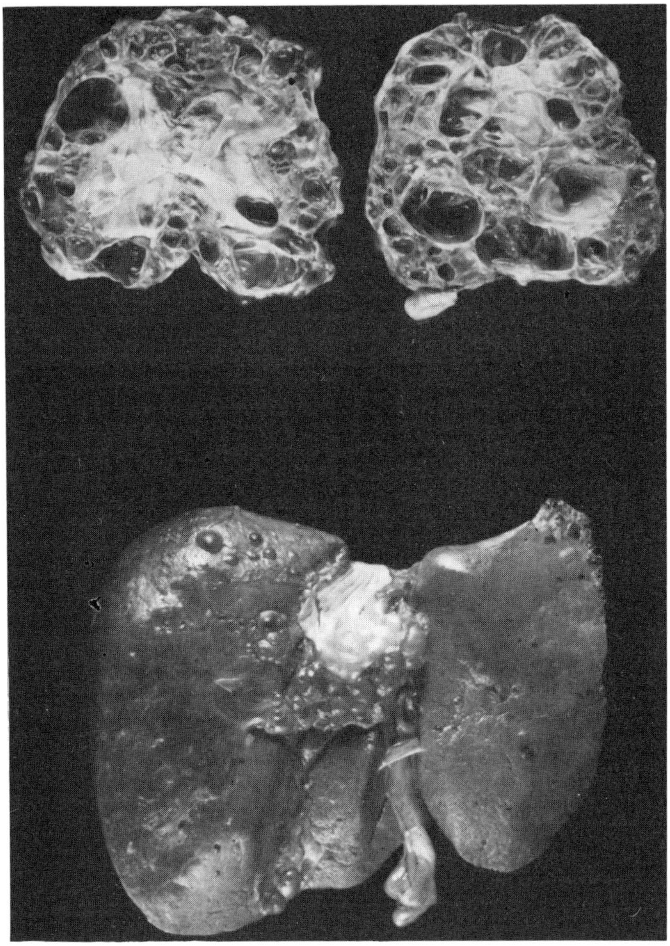

Figure 17.12 Polycystic kidneys and liver of an 85-year-old patient. Cause of death, pulmonary embolism after a hip fracture. Combined kidney weight, 885 g. Plasma urea, 22 mg/dl. Autosomal dominant polycystic kidney disease documented in members of four generations of her family

haemodialysis. Since the enrolment of end-stage renal disease patients is projected to increase steadily before it plateaus around the year 2030, it can be calculated that the cost of the end-stage renal disease program for ADPKD in the year 2030 will be nearing half a billion 1983 dollars. By itself, this should be enough reason to stimulate a research effort to study the pathogenesis of ADPKD as well as possible therapeutic approaches.

Pathology

The kidneys in ADPKD are almost always enlarged, to massive proportions in advanced cases. Characteristically, there is bilateral and diffuse involvement of the renal cortex and medulla with numerous small and larger cysts (*Figure 17.11*). Although the external surface of the kidney is distorted by innumerable cysts, the kidneys retain their characteristic reniform shape. Islands of normal renal parenchyma can be seen between the cysts. The contents of the cysts range from clear, straw-coloured fluid to dark-reddish gelatinous material (Kissane, 1983).

Pathogenesis

During the past decade, there have been some significant advances in the understanding of the pathogenesis of this disease. Until recently, ADPKD has been thought to result from an abnormal embryogenesis. Early hypothesis defended a lack of union of the metanephric nephrons with the collecting ducts of mesonephric origin or a failure to involute of primitive metanephric nephrons. Even when histological (Eggers, Connerton and McMullan, 1984), microdissection (Osathanondh and Potter, 1964) and functional studies (Bricker and Patton, 1955; Eggers, Connerton and McMullan, 1984) proved this explanation untenable, the basic idea of an abnormal embryogenesis was perpetuated by Potter's hypothesis, based on her observation of an abnormal branching of the collection ducts, that the cystic dilatation of the tubules in ADPKD resulted from an abnormal tubular development during fetal life (Osathanondh and Potter, 1964). More recently, Potter's hypothesis has been challenged. Microdissection of early polycystic kidneys has failed to confirm any abnormal branching, but has shown a great number of diverticula in all segments of the nephron which are thought to be the precursors of macroscopic cysts (Baert, 1978).

Two main hypotheses have been proposed to explain the pathogenesis of diverticula and cyst formation. According to the first hypothesis, the cysts would develop as the result of intratubular obstruction produced by a hyperplastic epithelium (Evan, Gardner and Bernstein, 1979). Indeed, the epithelium lining the cysts is frequently hyperplastic, and papillary projections into the lumen are commonly observed. It is easy to imagine how these papillary projections, conveniently located, can produce tubular obstruction. Nevertheless, at least according to one study, the epithelial hyperplasia is a late phenomenon not found in the early stages of polycystic kidneys (Milutinovic and Agodoa, 1983). In addition, direct measurements of intracystic pressures in two studies have revealed these pressures to be normal or low except in azotaemic patients (Bjerle, Lindqvist and Michaelson, 1971; Huseman *et al.*, 1980).

According to the second hypothesis, the cystic dilatation of the tubules would be the result of an increased compliance due to a weak basement membrane (Carone *et al.*, 1974; Grantham, 1983). It is supported by the finding of an abnormal basement membrane with multilayered lamina densa in early polycystic kidneys (Mulitinovic and Agodoa, 1983), by the observation of a high urinary excretion of 3-hydroxyproline, suggesting an abnormal turnover of type 4 basement membrane collagen in these patients (Chanard *et al.*, 1980), and by the association of this disorder with other conditions where an abnormal collagen metabolism has also been proposed; for example, intracranial aneurysms, aortic aneurysms and dissections, valvular abnormalities, Marfan's syndrome, colon diverticulosis, and inguinal hernia (Torres, Holley and Offord, 1985).

Histological studies of these cysts using transmission and scanning electron microscopy and functional evaluation by chemical analysis of the cystic fluid have also supported the concept that the cysts in ADPKD are dilated tubules, lined by a functional epithelium, that retain features characteristic of the nephron segment from which they arise (Cuppage *et al.*, 1980).

Recent experiments using an autosomal dominant model of polycystic kidney and liver disease with intracranial aneurysms in mice (Werder *et al.*, 1984), as well as a chemical model of polycystic kidney disease in rats using nordihydroguiaretic acid (Gardner and Evan, 1984), have clearly demonstrated that the expression of both the genetic disorder and the chemically induced disease is clearly influenced by environmental factors. When the mice with the autosomal dominant polycystic kidney disease are raised under normal laboratory conditions, nearly 100 per cent die from uraemia before reaching 1 year of age. If the mice, however, are raised in a germ-free environment, very few cysts develop and nearly 100 per cent of the animals are alive at 2 years of age. Similar observations have been made in rats used in the chemically induced model. The explanation of this phenomenon is not yet understood.

Finally, Reeders *et al.* (1986) have reported recently that there are polymorphisms closely linked with ADPKD near the α-globin locus on the short arm of chromosome 16. This is a major step towards identification of the gene responsible for ADPKD, and further progress in this direction should lead to better understanding of this disease.

Clinical manifestations

The clinical diagnosis of ADPKD may be made at any time during infancy, childhood or adulthood, but it is more frequently made during the third, fourth and fifth decades of life. The average age in the Olmsted County study was 36 years (Iglesias *et al.*, 1983). The diagnosis is usually made during the evaluation for abdominal or flank pain, haematuria or hypertension. Less frequently, the diagnosis is made during the work-up of a urinary tract infection or renal insufficiency, or because the patient has become aware of an abdominal mass. Although not necessarily the presenting complaints, many of these symptoms or manifestations are already present at the time of the initial evaluation, or they develop later on during the course of the disease. The clinical manifestations of the Olmsted County patients diagnosed between 1935 and 1980 are shown in *Table 17.2.*

Table 17.2 Characteristics of the patients with a clinical diagnosis of ADPKD in Olmsted County between 1935 and 1980

Positive family history	26/34 (76%)
Abdominal/flank pain	32/34 (94%)
Hypertension:	
diastolic > 90 mmHg	32/34 (94%)
diastolic >100 mmHg	21/34 (62%)
Gross haematuria	15/34 (44%)
Microhaematuria only	13/34 (38%)
Proteinuria	24/34 (71%)
Urinary tract infection	15/34 (44%)
Angina pectoris/myocardial infarction	5/34 (15%)
Cerebrovascular accident	3/34 (9%)
Gout	6/34 (18%)
Diaphragmatic hernia	2/15* (13%)
Diverticulosis	7/12* (58%)

*Includes only patients who had appropriate radiologic studies. Two of the patients with diverticulosis had episodes of diverticulosis with colonic perforation.

Pain, located in the abdomen, flank or back is the most common initial complaint and it is almost universally present in patients with ADPKD. The pain can be caused by enlargement of one or more cysts, bleeding, either confined inside the cyst or leading to gross haematuria with passage of clots, or a perinephric haematoma; urinary tract infection (acute pyelonephritis, infected cysts, perinephric abscess); nephrolithiasis and renal colic; rarely, a coincidental hypernephroma. In addition, patients with ADPKD may have abdominal pain related to definitely or presumably associated conditions. Dull aching and an uncomfortable sensation of heaviness may result from a large polycystic liver. Although rarely, hepatic cysts may become infected (*Figure 17.13*), especially after renal transplantation (Gesundheit *et al.*,

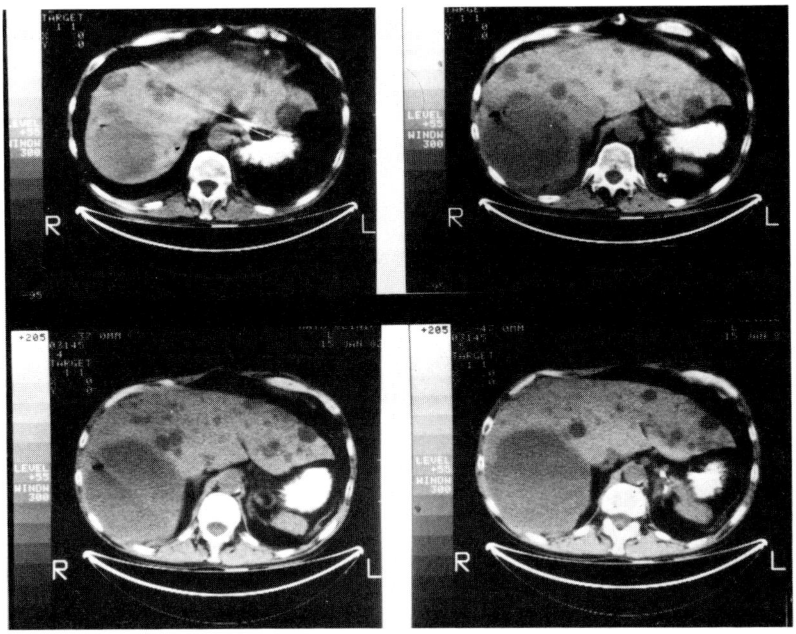

Figure 17.13 Computed tomography of a polycystic liver after renal transplantation. Note the large infected cyst, containing air, in the right lobe of the liver

1982; Bourgeois *et al.*, 1983). Abdominal pain can also result from diverticulitis which has been reported to occur with increased frequency in patients with ADPKD maintained on dialysis (Karanicolas *et al.*, 1979; Scheff *et al.*, 1980). This has also been our experience. ADPKD patients may also be at a higher risk of developing aortic abdominal aneurysms (Chapman and Hilson, 1980; Montoliu, Torras and Revert, 1980). Of course, these patients may also develop pain for reasons completely unrelated to their underlying disease. It goes without saying that abdominal pain in a patient with polycystic kidneys may be a diagnostic challenge.

Hypertension

Hypertension is one of the most common early manifestations of ADPKD (Gabow, Iklé and Holmes, 1984). Even when renal function is normal, hypertension has been found in 50–75 per cent of the patients. In fact, the clinical course of hypertension in ADPKD is very unlike that of hypertension in chronic glomerulonephritis or tubulo-interstitial nephropathies. In ADPKD, the hypertension is usually more severe early in the course of the disease and becomes less of a problem with the progression of the renal insufficiency (Calabrese *et al.*, 1982). Studies of the renin–angiotensin–aldosterone system have not convincingly demonstrated that they play an important role in its pathogenesis. The hypertension in ADPKD is accompanied by an increase in plasma volume, with normal levels of plasma renin activity and serum aldosterone (Nash, 1977). Because the plasma renin activity and serum aldosterone would have been expected to be suppressed in this situation, renin stimulation has been implied from these results. Normalization of pressure, while on a severely sodium-restricted (10 mmol sodium) diet, and the lack of effect of saralasin on the blood pressure of these patients, however, argues against a renin dependency of this hypertension (Nash, 1977; Anderson, Miller and Linas, 1979; Calabrese *et al.*, 1982). On the other hand, the way in which these patients respond to an acute saline expansion may be intimately related to this peculiar behaviour of hypertension in ADPKD.

In patients with polycystic kidneys and normal renal function, the natriuretic response to an acute saline expansion is blunted as compared to controls, whereas in patients with polycystic kidneys and renal insufficiency, the natriuretic response is exaggerated (D'Angelo *et al.*, 1975). This may explain why ADPKD patients develop hypertension early before the deterioration of renal function at which time they are sodium retainers, whereas the hypertension tends to become less severe with the development of renal insufficiency at which time they are sodium wasters. The mechanisms responsible for the blunted natriuretic response to an acutely administered sodium load in patients' ADPKD and normal renal function is not entirely understood. D'Angelo *et al.* (1975) have suggested that this blunted natriuretic response might be due to incomplete arterial vasodilatation secondary to the anatomic lesions peculiar to these patients.

Nephrolithiasis and obstruction

The incidence of nephrolithiasis appears to be increased in ADPKD. The true incidence, however, is difficult to assess since the passage of stones is frequently not documented and renal colic in these patients may also be due to passage of blood clots. In addition, cyst wall calcification may be falsely taken for opaque renal calculi. All this considered, the frequency of nephrolithiasis in some series has ranged between 18 and 34 per cent (Delaney *et al.*, 1985). The composition of the renal calculi does not appear to be different from the general stone population. Calcium oxalate, calcium phosphate and uric acid stones have been reported. No metabolic abnormalities predisposing to stone formation have been so far identified. It is possible that the high incidence of stones in these patients is accounted by the anatomic distortion with stagnation of the urine.

Ureteral obstruction is not infrequent in ADPKD. It can be caused by a calculus, clot or compression by a cyst. Because of the non-specific symptoms and the caliceal distortion present in ADPKD, the obstruction may be difficult to detect. Unilateral or bilateral renal shutdown may rarely occur as a result of intracystic bleeding, with compression and obstruction of the renal pelvis (Camey and Le Duc, 1972; Barbaric, Spataro and Segal, 1977; Tadros, 1979).

Laboratory findings

In addition to the microhaematuria and mild degrees of proteinuria, sterile pyuria is very common. Urinary doubly refractile bodies (oval fat bodies) are also observed in the urine sediment of 60 per cent of patients; the presence of these bodies in ADPKD patients does not indicate a coexistent renal disorder (Duncan, Cuppage and Grantham, 1985). Hyperuricaemia and erythrocytosis are also found with increased frequency. There is a decreased maximal urine concentrating capacity, whereas the capacity to dilute the urine is normal. Inability to acidify the urine and reduced ammonium formation has been described in some patients, but this defect may not be different from that encountered in other patients with moderate to severe renal disease (Martinez-Maldonado, 1985).

Diagnosis

Most frequently, the diagnosis of polycystic kidney disease is established by excretory urography with nephrotomography, classically demonstrating the spider deformity of the caliceal pattern and the moth-eaten appearance of the nephrogram. Ultrasonography has displaced excretory urography as the main screening test for polycystic kidney disease. It is more sensitive than excretory urography and avoids radiation exposure. It is less sensitive, however, than computed tomography. When

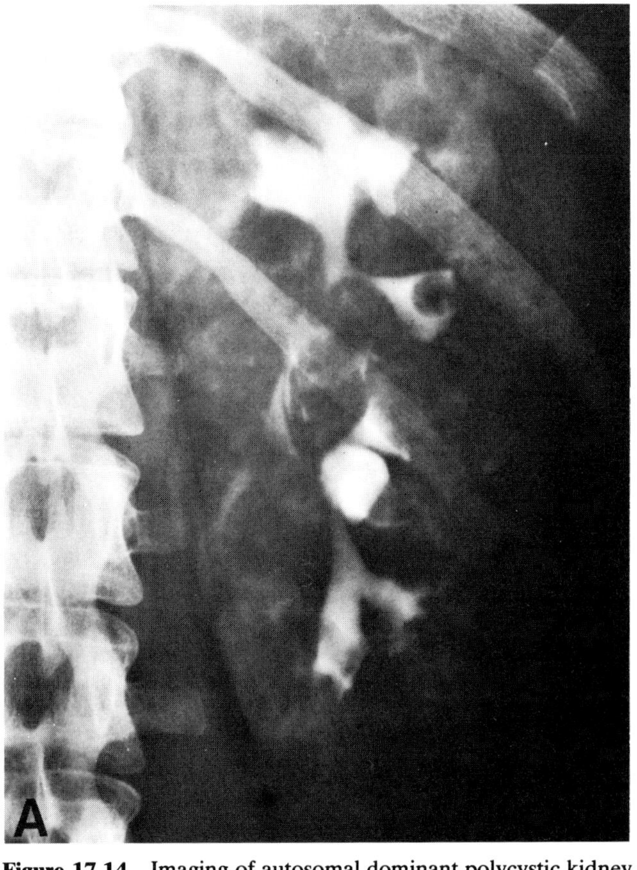

Figure 17.14 Imaging of autosomal dominant polycystic kidney disease: (A) caliceal deformity and moth-eaten appearance of the nephrogram demonstrated by excretory urography with nephrotomography; (B) polycystic liver and kidney disease demonstrated by ultrasonography; (C) computed tomography of polycystic kidney; (D) computed tomography of polycystic liver and pancreas (arrow); (E) magnetic resonance imaging of polycystic kidneys and liver

the result of ultrasonography is questionable, computed tomography should be performed to rule out an early stage of development of the disease (Levine and Grantham, 1981). Computed tomography has taken the place of renal arteriography in the early diagnosis of polycystic kidneys. Using renal arteriography, essentially 100 per cent of the patients with polycystic kidney disease may be diagnosed after age 20. Even with the use of renal arteriography, however, up to 40 per cent of patients with ADPKD are not diagnosed in the 15–19-year age group (Milutinovic *et al.*, 1980). Arteriography is still necessary when a coexisting renovascular lesion or a hypernephroma is suspected. The role of magnetic resonance imaging has not yet been established (*Figure 17.14*).

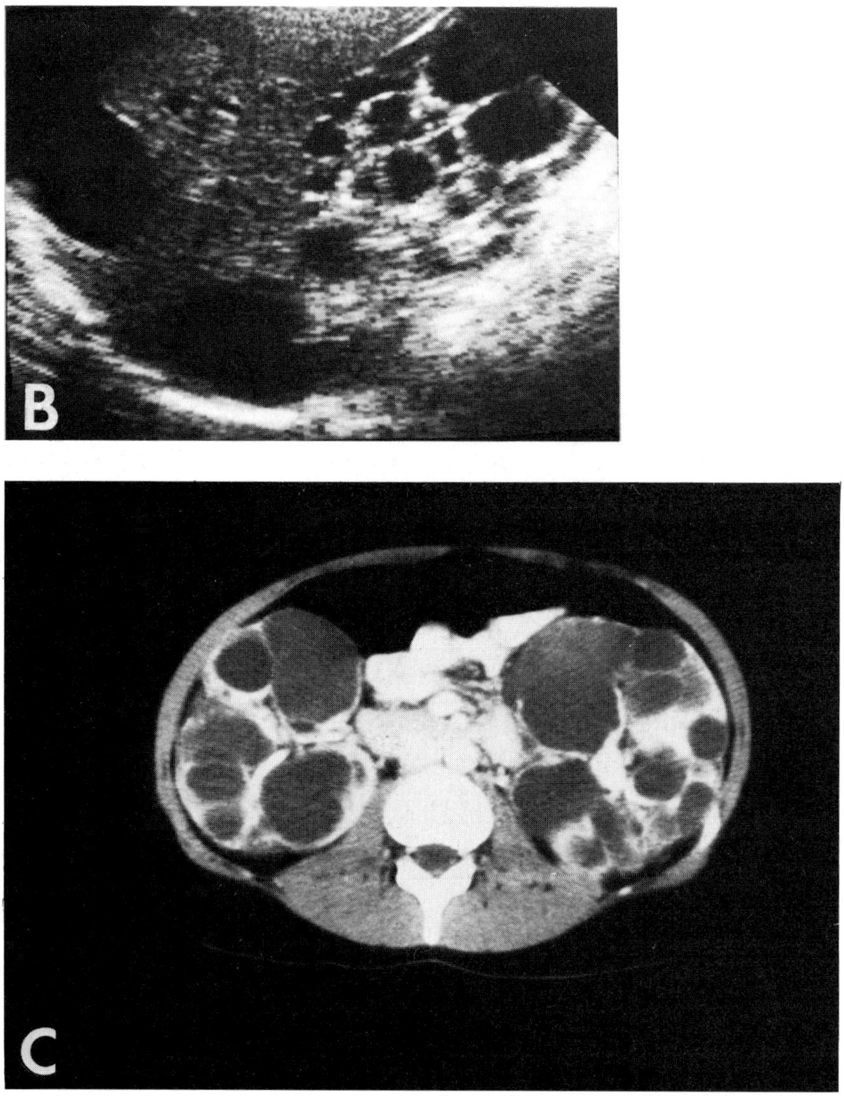

Figure 17.14 *continued*

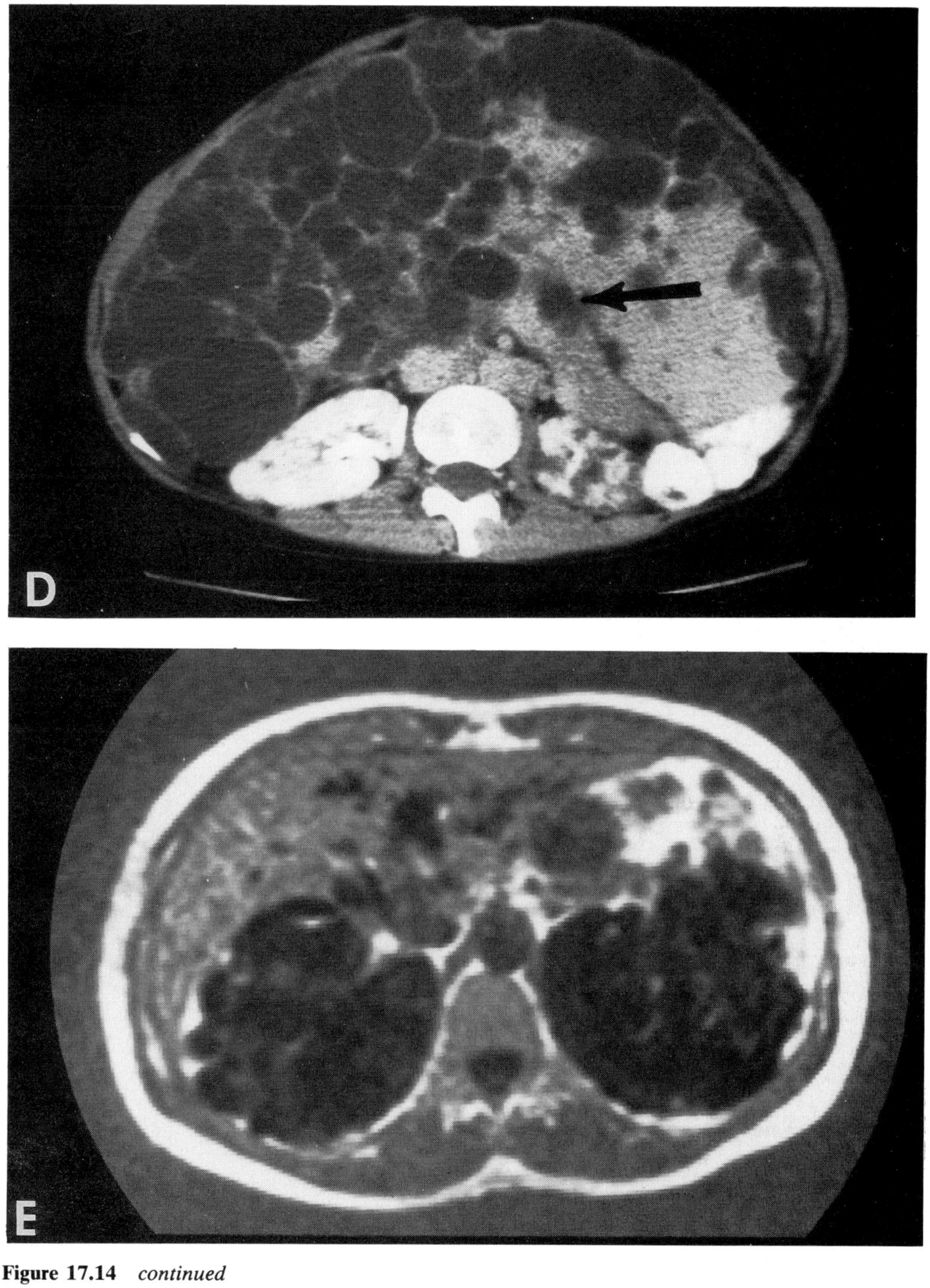

Figure 17.14 *continued*

Associated conditions

ADPKD has been associated with a variety of extrarenal disorders. As previously mentioned, patients with this disease now survive longer. Because of the improved survivorship, the morbidity and mortality related to these associated disorders is likely to become more important. Not all of these associations have been well documented and some of them, such as coexisting renal cell carcinomas, may just represent chance associations.

Hepatic cysts

The development of liver cysts correlates with the age of the patient and impairment of renal function (Milutinovic *et al.*, 1980). In some reports, cystic liver disease is more prominently severe in females than in males (Torres, Holley and Offord, 1985). In a few patients, massive hepatic cystic disease can result in portal hypertension, but hepatic insufficiency from a polycystic liver, if it occurs, is exremely rare. Less frequently, cysts can also be found in other locations, such as the pancreas, spleen, ovaries, pineal gland, testes, etc.

Intracranial aneurysms

The association of intracranial aneurysms and ADPKD has been established on the basis of large retrospective autopsy studies (Suter, 1949; Brown, 1951; Bigelow, 1953). The overall prevalence of intracranial aneurysms in the general population ranges in several large autopsy studies from 0.2 to 9.9 per cent, with the more recent studies indicating a frequency of approximately 5 per cent. The observed frequency of coexisting intracranial aneurysms and ADPKD has been significantly higher than expected by chance association alone. Approximately 20 per cent of ADPKD patients have intracranial aneurysms at autopsy. Only one small, prospective angiographic study of ADPKD patients has been published (Wakabayashi *et al.*, 1983). In this study, asymptomatic, unruptured intracranial aneurysms were found in 41 per cent of the patients (7 out of 17), suggesting that the frequency of unruptured aneurysms in ADPKD might have been underestimated in autopsy studies. In the Olmsted community study, intracranial aneurysms were found in 19 per cent of the patients, and rupture resulting in subarachnoid haemorrhage was the immediate cause of death in 7 per cent (Iglesias *et al.*, 1983).

From studies in the general population, it is known that the vast majority of intracranial aneurysms never rupture. Since cerebral angiography is not free of significant morbidity and intracranial aneurysm surgery has significant morbidity and mortality even in the best hands, accurate knowledge of the natural history of unruptured intracranil aneurysms is essential for intelligent treatment decisions. In a recent prospective study of intracranial aneurysms in the general population at the Mayo Clinic, the only variable that was found to be of unquestionable value in predicting the risk of rupture was aneurysm size (Wiebers, Whisnant and O'Fallon, 1981). None of 44 aneurysms smaller than 1 cm in diameter ruptured, whereas 8 of 29 aneurysms 1 cm or more in diameter eventually did.

There is no information on the natural history of intracranial aneurysms associated with ADPKD. Assuming that the natural history of these aneurysms was not different from the natural history of all intracranial saccular aneurysms, decision analysis has been used to assess whether or not patients with ADPKD should undergo routine cerebral angiography for intracranial aneurysms and prophylactic surgery. It was found that arteriography should not be carried out routinely, because its benefit exceeds 1 year only if the prevalence of aneurysms exceeds 30 per cent, if the surgical complication rate is 1 per cent or less, and if the patient is under 25 years of age (Levey, Pauker and Kassirer, 1983). Therefore, there appears to be little justification to screen for the presence of intracranial aneurysms in asymptomatic elderly patients.

Other cardiovascular complications

Several case reports of associations of ADPKD and cardiovascular abnormalities have appeared in the literature (diMatteo *et al.*, 1965; Chapman and Hilson, 1980; Montoliu, Torras and Revert, 1980; Selgas *et al.*, 1981). In a recent larger series, an 18 per cent frequency of cardiovascular abnormalities was found (Leier *et al.*, 1984). Dilatation of the aortic root, bicuspid aortic valve, mitral valve prolapse and coarctation of the aorta were the most frequent abnormalities. Valvular and aortic abnormalities have also been found in autopsy series at the Mayo Clinic (Torres, Holley and Offord, 1985). Aortic aneurysms or dissections, bicuspid aortic valve and aortic coarctation were observed. Of these, dissecting thoracic aortic aneurysms were the most common (*Figure 17.15*). The observed frequency of coexisting polycystic kidney disease and dissecting thoracic aortic aneurysm in these autopsy series was 7.3 times higher than expected by chance association alone.

Carcinoma in polycystic kidneys

Focal cellular hyperplasia of the tubular epithelium is a common abnormality in ADPKD, but whether this constitutes a pre-neoplastic state is still questionable. Many case reports of the association of ADPKD and renal cell carcinoma have been published, but these do not prove the existence of an association, since chance association of two relatively common disorders can be expected in a considerable number of patients. In many large series of patients, the association of renal cell carcinoma and ADPKD has not been found. Furthermore, development of renal cell carcinoma in polycystic kidney patients on haemodialysis or after renal transplantation has been reported rarely and it does not appear to be a common problem. No patient in the Olmsted County study and only one patient in the Mayo Clinic autopsy series had renal cell carcinoma (Ishikawa *et al.*, 1980; Iglesias *et al.*, 1983). The observed frequency of renal cell carcinoma and ADPKD coexisting in the same patient was not higher than expected by chance association alone (Ishikawa *et al.*, 1980). The only argument that would support the possibility that ADPKD is a pre-malignant state is the fact that the renal cell carcinoma in many of the reported cases was multicentric or bilateral (Ng and Suki, 1980). When ADPKD and renal cell carcinoma coexist in the same patient, the diagnosis is challenging (*Figure 17.16*). Pain in association with fever, weight loss, anaemia, or a striking change in the configuration of the kidney and the presence of mottled calcifications within a renal cyst should raise the suspicion of coexisting renal cell carcinoma. In this situation, renal arteriography is the most helpful diagnostic test.

Clinical course

A decline of renal function occurs in most, but not all, patients with ADPKD diagnosed during life if they are followed for sufficiently long periods of time. These

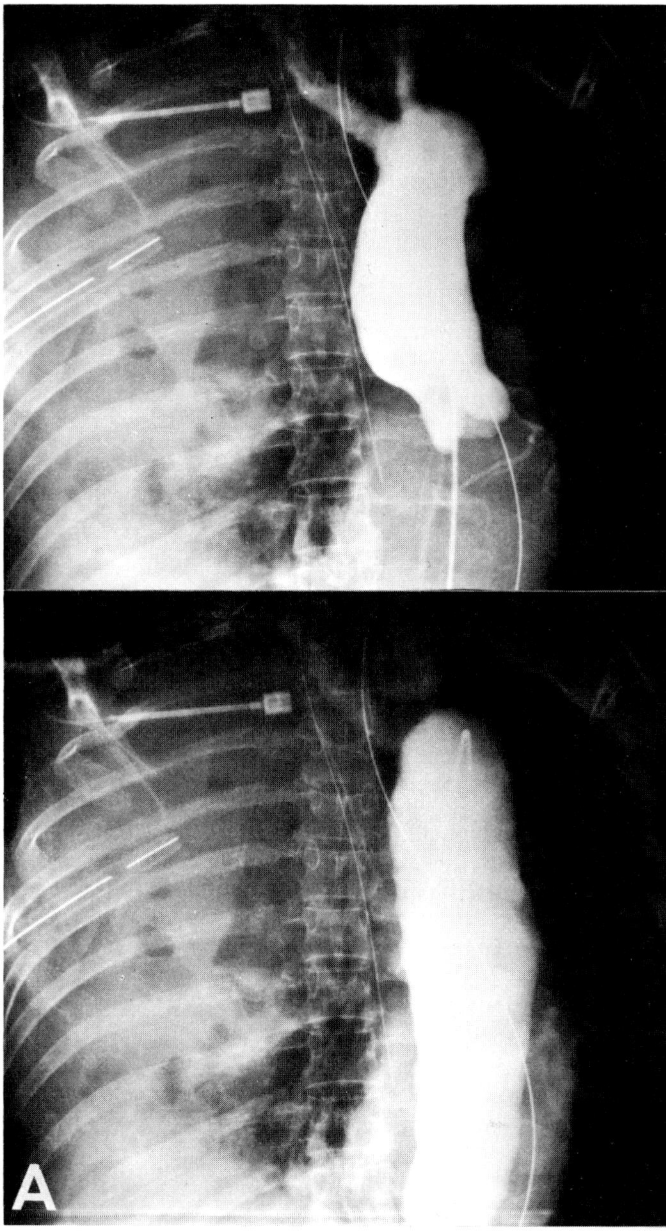

Figure 17.15
See caption opposite

patients have a prolonged period of stable renal function followed by a slow decline of renal function that is predictable from the reciprocal plot of plasma creatinine against time (Franz and Reubi, 1983; Delaney *et al.*, 1985). A diversion from the initial slope in these patients should alert the physician to the possibility of an intercurrent renal disease, a reaction to a medication or the development of obstruction. It is important to avoid undue pessimism when assessing the prognosis of ADPKD in an individual patient. In the Olmsted community study, for example, the actuarial kidney survival 15 years after the diagnosis of polycystic kidney disease

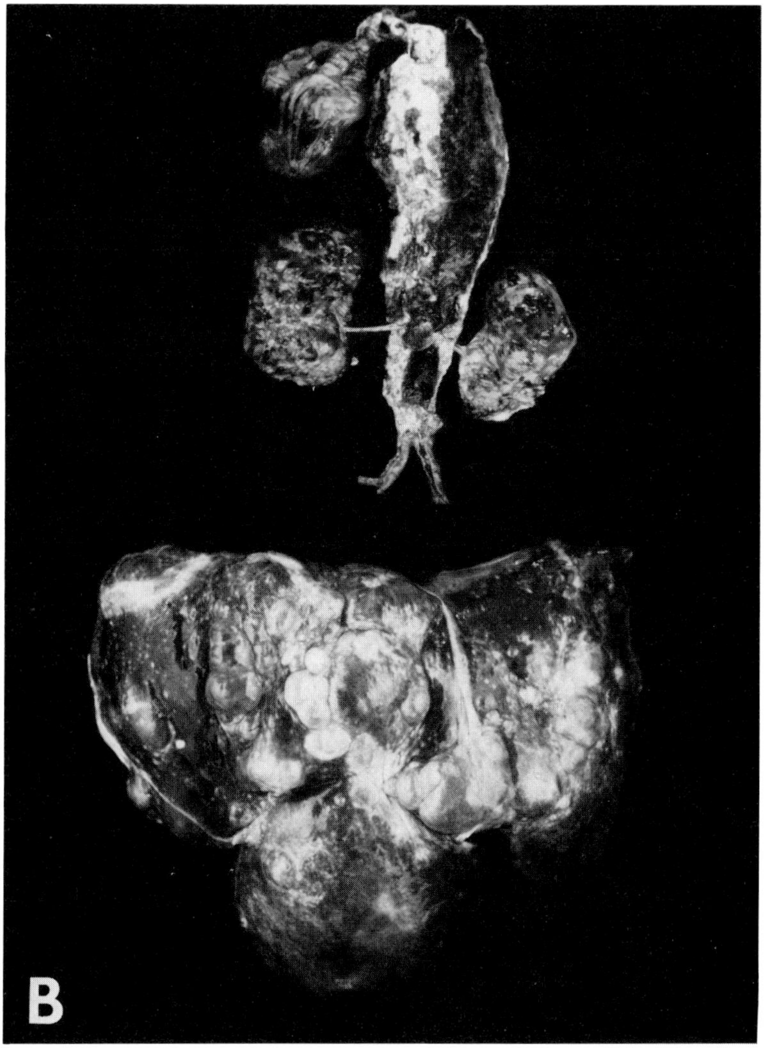

Figure 17.15 (A) Aortogram demonstrating a dissecting aortic aneurysm in a patient with autosomal dominant polycystic kidney disease; (B) heart, aorta, polycystic kidneys and polycystic liver of the same patient

in symptomatic patients was approximately 50 per cent (Iglesias *et al.*, 1983). The kidney survival was better in the patients diagnosed more recently as well as in the patients who at the time of the diagnosis were normotensive, had a normal serum creatinine or plasma urea and had no proteinuria on the urinalysis. It is, therefore, important when assessing the prognosis of polycystic kidney disease in an individual patient, to take into consideration multiple factors peculiar to this patient rather than extrapolating from large clinical series. In a series of patients presenting to a referral centre, 70 per cent had end-stage renal disease by age 65 (Mitcheson, Williams and Castro, 1977). In studies including not only symptomatic but also asymptomatic patients, however, the risk of developing end-stage renal disease by age 73 years is only 48 per cent (Churchill *et al.*, 1984).

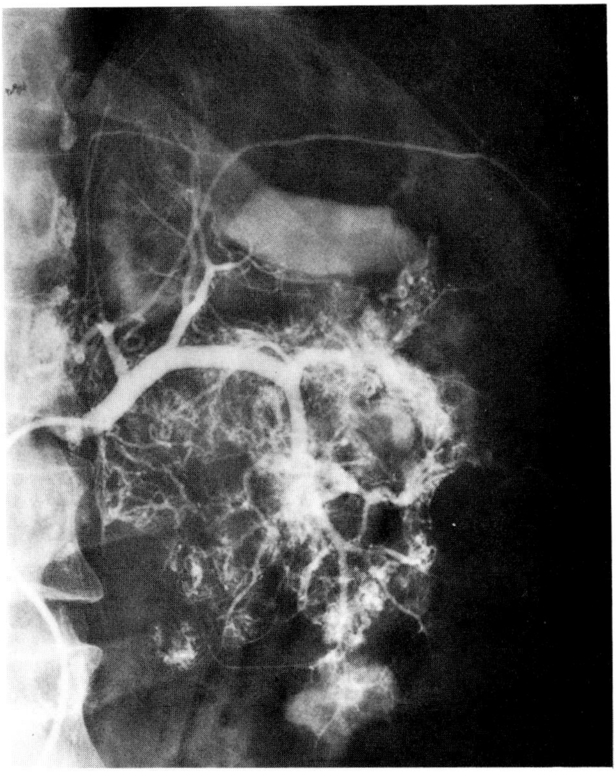

Figure 17.16 Renal cell carcinoma in a patient with autosomal dominant polycystic kidney disease. Hypervascular mass demonstrated by renal arteriography. Polycystic kidney disease had been previously diagnosed. The patient presented with anaemia and fever of unknown origin

The introduction of renal replacement therapies has eliminated uraemia as the leading cause of death in ADPKD. Cardiovascular pathology and infections account for approximately 90 per cent of the deaths of these patients treated by haemodialysis or peritoneal dialysis and after renal transplantation (Kramer *et al.*, 1982). Malignant disease has a relatively minor role in all three groups of patients, not supporting earlier reports that ADPKD patients might have a higher risk for the development of lymphoma and malignancy after renal transplantation (Hoover and Fraumeni, 1973; Advisory Committee, 1977).

Treatment

There is no specific therapy for ADPKD. The goal of treatment is to prevent complications and, if possible, slow down the rate of progression of the renal disease (Grantham and Slusher, 1984). The patients should be advised against the use of constrictive belts and the practice of contact sports, as well as caution against narcotic or analgesic abuse for frequently occurring chronic pain. Cyst decompressive procedures are of no proven value, although re-evaluation of these procedures may be justified on the basis of a recent report. Hypertension should be strictly controlled. The best antihypertensive treatment for these patients has not been established. In the presence of normal renal function and capacity to retain sodium, mild sodium restriction and the use of a beta-blocker agent are probably adequate. The use of diuretics, which may increase intratubular pressure, may be unwise. Severe sodium restriction in patients with renal insufficiency, unable to conserve sodium, should be avoided since it may lead to contraction and deterioration of renal function. Reduction of dietary protein intake may be of value to slow down the rate of progression of renal insufficiency. Unnecessary urinary tract manipulation should be avoided; when absolutely necessary, antimicrobial prophylaxis should be prescribed.

The treatment of infected renal cysts poses special problems because of the variable penetration of different antibiotics into the cysts (Muther and Bennett, 1981; Schwab *et al.*, 1983). Most antibiotics enter the proximal cyst to some extent. Lipid soluble antibiotics with an alkaline pK, such as clindamycin, enter the distal cyst well. Other lipid soluble antibiotics that may be useful in the treatment of these infected cysts are chloramphenicol, tetracycline, trimethoprim and erythromycin. Because of the reported increased risk for diverticulitis, prevention of constipation is important. In cases of unilateral or bilateral ureteral obstruction by a cyst, surgical relief of the obstruction is frequently necessary to relieve the pain and preserve renal function. Percutaneous draining of a compressing large renal cyst can be successful in rare cases. When end-stage renal disease occurs, dialysis and, in the younger patients, renal transplantation are indicated. Patients with ADPKD on maintenance haemodialysis do well compared with other types of renal disease, probably because they maintain a higher haemoglobin. Bleeding secondary to heparinization during dialysis occurs only rarely and usually these cases can be satisfactorily managed by using low or regional heparinization.

Finally, the discovery of ADPKD in an elderly patient raises the question of genetic counselling. We believe that relatives at risk, children and siblings, benefit from screening, but repercussions on insurability and employability should be considered in each individual case. The benefits from screening are early treatment and prevention of complications, choice of alternative family planning for those with ADPKD, and reassurance of those without ADPKD. Recommendations for screening include blood pressure measurements at age 10 and 15 and ultrasonography at age 20 (earlier in special circumstances, e.g. contact sports).

Acquired cystic disease of the kidneys

The terms 'acquired cystic disease of the kidneys' and 'acquired polycystic kidney disease' have been used to describe the cystic degeneration of the renal parenchyma that occurs in end-stage kidneys probably as a result of prolonged uraemia. This lesion was initially described by Dunnill *et al.* (1977) as a hazard of long-term intermittent maintenance haemodialysis and has been confirmed by many other authors (Elliott, McDougall and Buchanan, 1977; Moorthy and Beirne, 1978; Ishikawa *et al.*, 1980; Konishi, Mukawa and Kitada, 1980; Fayemi and Ali, 1980; Krempien and Ritz, 1980; Hughson, Hennigar and McManus, 1980; Feiner, Katz and Gallo, 1981; Case Records of the MGH, 1982; Mickisch *et al.*, 1984; Levine *et al.*, 1984). It appears that these cystic changes can start prior to the initiation of dialysis and that they develop regardless of the type of dialysis being used. This phenomenon is therefore likely to be related to the uraemic state, rather than a consequence of the dialysis procedures. The role of uraemia is also supported by the regression of these cystic changes that can occur after successful renal transplantation (Ishikawa *et al.*, 1983).

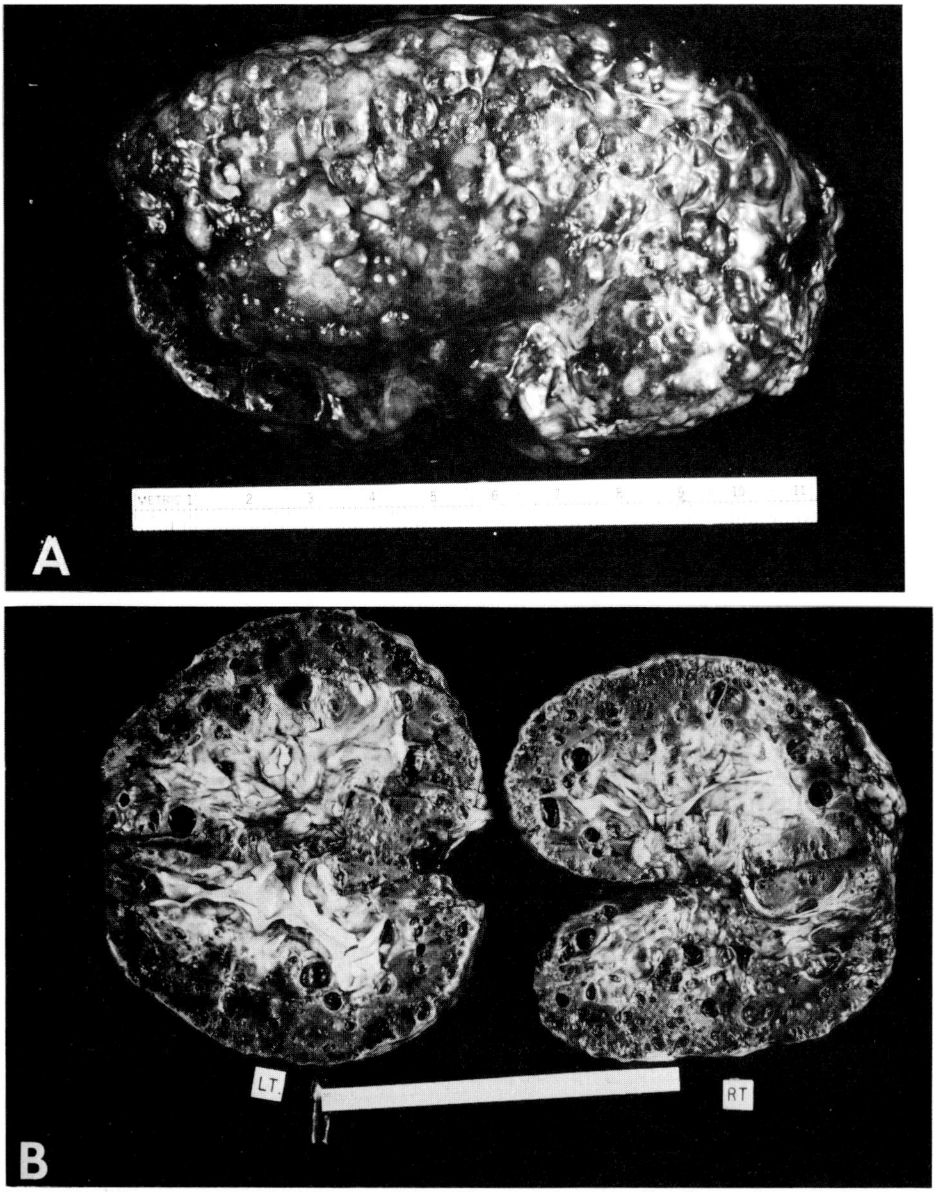

Figure 17.17 Acquired cystic disease of the kidneys: (A) external surface; (B) cut surface

Pathology

The kidneys are frequently larger than expected for an end-stage kidney, but true renal enlargement is rarely observed. The cysts, which are usually smaller than in autosomal dominant polycystic kidney disease, tend to occur in the renal cortex, but also involve the renal medulla (*Figure 17.17*). They may be lined by a simple cuboidal epithelium or by a hyperplastic multilayered epithelium with papillary projections. Two types of cysts have been distinguished on the basis of surface morphology. One type, with large numbers of microvilli, is presumably derived from proximal tubules. The second type has a smoother surface and is presumably derived from various segments of the distal nephron (Mickisch *et al.*, 1984). The continuity between the cysts and the renal tubules has been confirmed by microdissection studies (Feiner, Katz and Gallo, 1981). Deposition of oxalate crystals is frequently observed in the renal interstitium surrounding the cysts, in the walls of the cysts and in the lumen (Dunnill, Millard and Oliver, 1977).

Pathogenesis

Tubular obstruction by interstitial fibrosis or deposition of oxalate, ischaemia and accumulation of toxic metabolites have all been proposed to play a role. It is possible that biologically active substances which are retained in uraemia and not removed by dialysis, such as the mitogenic polyamines, could stimulate epithelial and smooth muscle cell proliferation and result in a variety of abnormalities in end-stage kidneys, including atypical cysts, renal cell tumours and nodular formation in the intrarenal arteries and arterioles. Nevertheless, the evidence to support these hypotheses is sparse and much more needs to be learned about pathogenesis and the biological and clinical significance of this disorder (McManus and Hughson, 1979; Gardner, 1984).

Clinical manifestations

In most patients, the cystic degeneration of the renal parenchyma that occurs on long-term dialysis is a silent process. The number of patients with cysts, as well as the number and size of the cysts, increases with duration of the dialysis. Using sensitive computed tomography techniques, multiple renal cysts were observed in approximately 80 per cent of patients who have been on haemodialysis for more than 3 years (Ishikawa *et al.*, 1980). In another study including 30 long-term dialysis patients, diffuse bilateral cysts were observed in 43.3 per cent of the patients, occasional cysts (fewer than 5 per kidney) in 16.7 per cent, and no renal cysts in 40 per cent (Levine *et al.*, 1984). With the increasing number and size of the cysts, the kidney volume also increases. Determinations of kidney volume by computed tomography suggest that the volume of the kidney decreases during the first 3 years of dialysis and then increases as the result of cyst formation (Ishikawa *et al.*, 1980). It has been reported that the cysts occur more frequently in dialysed patients who are anuric than in those who maintain some urine output, but it is unclear whether this observation could be explained by a longer duration of intermittent haemodialysis in the anuric patients (Mickisch *et al.*, 1984). Similarly, it has been reported that cysts occur less frequently in dialysed patients with underlying diabetic nephropathy, than in patients whose renal failure was secondary to a different aetiology, but this also could be explained by a shorter time on dialysis of the diabetic patients (Mickisch *et al.*, 1984). No other significant correlation between the occurrence of acquired cystic disease and patient age, gender, ethnic origin or nature of the original renal disease have been made. The frequency of these cystic changes does not appear to be influenced by the efficiency of dialysis as reflected by blood chemistry parameters (Levine *et al.*, 1984).

Complications of acquired cystic disease of the kidneys have incuded intracystic bleeding, gross haematuria, retroperitoneal haemorrhage and malignant transformation.

Intracystic bleeding can be the cause of unexplained flank or back pain in haemodialysis patients. Rarely, the bleeding has been documented by the appearance of a radiodense cyst on computed tomography (Levine *et al.*, 1984). The haemorrhagic cysts can rupture into the pelvis, giving rise to gross haematuria, or into the retroperitoneum, causing a retroperitoneal haemorrhage. Retroperitoneal haemorrhage is a life-threatening complication that usually has a dramatic presentation (Tuttle, Minielly and Fay, 1971; Vanichayakornkul *et al.*, 1974; Tsai and Shimizu, 1975; Milutinovic, Follette and Scribner, 1977; Case Records of the MGH, 1982). Heparinization during haemodialysis and the use of anticoagulants to prevent the clotting of arteriovenous fistulas may play a contributory role. The typical presentation of these patients is with severe abdominal and flank or back pain, distended abdomen, hypoactive or absent bowel sounds, and a palpable abdominal mass. In some cases, fever, femoral nerve compression and obstructive jaundice have been observed. Spontaneous retroperitoneal bleeding has been estimated to occur in 1–3 per cent of all chronic haemodialysis patients. In many of these cases, the retroperitoneal haemorrhage results from the rupture of a sclerotic artery in the wall of the cyst.

Whether acquired cystic disease of the kidneys should be regarded as a premalignant state is controversial. In their original description, Dunnill *et al.* (1977) described three types of renal tumours associated with acquired cystic disease. These were papillary tumours, tumours exhibiting tubular differentiation and solid tumours. These tumours were frequently multicentric. A major problem is how to assess their malignant potential. The distinction between renal cell adenomas and carcinomas is frequently made on the basis of size; if the renal cell tumour is less than 3 cm in diameter, the risk of metastasizing is usually small. Whether renal cell carcinomas will become a major medical problem in the long-term maintenance of the haemodialysis population is uncertain. Recently, Gardner (1984) has reviewed and summarized the published information based on 160 long-term haemodialysis patients with acquired renal cystic disease and 278 long-term haemodialysis patients without renal cysts. Renal tumours were found in 25 per cent of the 160 patients with acquired renal cystic disease, but were not reported in any of the patients with non-cystic kidneys. Seven of the 160 patients or 4.3 per cent of the total population with acquired renal cystic disease had renal carcinomas. Of these, two were metastatic.

Imaging and treatment

Only the complications of acquired cystic disease of the kidneys may require treatment. Until more information becomes available, it seems reasonable to follow small (<3 cm) renal tumours by serial computed tomography or ultrasound examinations (Levine *et al.*, 1984). Surgical intervention would be indicated for large solid tumours with invasive features or when there is evidence of progressive tumour enlargement. The treatment of retroperitoneal bleeding is usually conservative, but therapeutic embolization or nephrectomy may become necessary in some cases.

Adult medullary cystic disease

Medullary cystic disease and nephronophthisis, initially described as two different diseases, are synonymous terms that define a heterogeneous group of disorders rather than a single entity (Gardner and Evan, 1979). At least two forms are recognized on the basis of inheritance and clinical presentation—a juvenile recessive form and an adult dominant form. Sporadic cases may represent recessive cases in families with a small offspring or new dominant mutations. Only the adult dominant form of this disease is within the scope of this chapter.

Pathology

The kidneys are small, and the characteristic pathologic change is the presence of multiple cysts most commonly seen at the cortical medullary junction and along the medullary collecting ducts. Nevertheless, these cysts are not universally present and, when present, are not necessarily confined to the medulla. For this reason, some authors object to the term 'medullary cystic disease' (Steele, Lirenman and Beattie, 1980).

Pathogenesis

Little is known about the pathogenesis of this disorder. The hypothesis that a nephrotoxic substance resulting from an inborn error of metabolism might be the cause of this disease, essentially a form of chronic interstitial nephritis, is not supported by the fact that recurrence of this disease does not occur after renal transplantation.

Clinical manifestations

The adult dominant form of the disease is usually recognized during the second to fifth decades of life, has an insidious onset and progresses rapidly to end-stage renal failure. A late onset of the disease, during the seventh and eighth decades of life, has been observed in some families, and, therefore, medullary cystic disease should be considered in the differential diagnosis of chronic renal failure even in the elderly (Wrigley *et al.*, 1973; Swenson, Kempson and Friedland, 1974). In some of these elderly patients, the clinical course has been unusually prolonged. Inability to concentrate urine and wasting of sodium are usually present. The urinary sediment is characterisically benign and the proteinuria is usually mild, below 1 g per 24 h. Anaemia is a very frequent finding, but there is no evidence to support that the degree of anaemia is out of proportion to the degree of insufficiency. Hypertension may be present, but is not a prominent feature of this disease. Extrarenal disorders, such as retinitis pigmentosa, metaphyseal chondrodysplasia, cerebellar ataxia and hepatic fibrosis, which are frequently associated with the juvenile form of medullary cystic disease, are not observed in the adult form. Osteodystrophy is less frequent.

Imaging

Detection of the cysts by radiographic procedures is frequently unsuccessful, since these are usually small (1 mm to 1 cm in diameter). The value of ultrasonography or computed tomography in the detection of these cysts is still undetermined.

Treatment

The treatment of medullary cystic disease is merely supportive. Because of the tendency to salt wasting, volume contraction and renal azotaemia, unnecessary sodium restriction or use of diuretics should be avoided.

Medullary sponge kidney

Medullary sponge kidney (MSK) or precaliceal canalicular ectasia is a disorder characterized by tubular dilatation of the collecting ducts and cyst formation strictly confined to the medullary pyramids, especially to their inner, papillary portions (Lenarduzzi, 1939; Cacchi and Ricci, 1948; Ekstróm *et al.*, 1959; Kuiper, 1976).

Pathology

Precaliceal canalicular ectasia may involve one or more renal papillae in one or both kidneys. These dilated tubules may be surrounded by a normal appearing medullary interstitium or, in cases of more prominent cystic disease, inflammatory cell filtration and interstitial fibrosis. The renal size is usually normal or slightly enlarged (Ekstróm *et al.*, 1959; Kuiper, 1976).

Pathogenesis

MSK is usually regarded as a non-hereditary disease, despite rare reports of familial cases. It is more controversial whether it should be considered a congenital or acquired disorder. Although there have been cases of MSK diagnosed in childhood, others remark that the rarity of this disorder in children favours the interpretation that this is an acquired disease (Bernstein, 1976). Progression of the tubular ectasia and development of new tubular dilatation and medullary cysts have been documented in some patients. It is possible that MSK is only a structural abnormality and results from a variety of different physical, chemical or genetic factors.

Clinical manifestations

The prevalence of MSK by age, sex and race is unknown. The frequency in different clinical series has varied widely between 0.5 and 21 per cent, depending not only on the type of population being studied but also on the different diagnostic criteria used to identify MSK (Palubinskas, 1963; Mayall, 1970; Yendt, 1982). In large unselected series of excretory urographies done for different indications, the frequency of MSK is approximately 0.5 per cent. Higher frequencies, between 2.3 and 21 per cent, have been observed in patients with idiopathic calcium nephrolithiasis. Early reports suggest a male predominance, but both sexes probably are equally involved. In fact, females with idiopathic calcium nephrolithiasis have underlying MSK more frequently than males (Parks, Coe and Strauss, 1982). Most patients are diagnosed in their fourth or fifth decade, but infrequently the diagnosis is not made until the sixth, seventh or eighth decade.

Medullary sponge kidney is usually a benign disorder that may remain asymptomatic and undetected for life. Mild impairment of tubular functions, such as a mild concentration defect, a reduced capacity to lower the urine pH after administration of ammonium chloride as compared to controls (Higashihara *et al.*, 1984) and possibly a reduced maximal excretion of potassium after short-term intravenous potassium chloride loading may be common in these patients (Green *et al.*, 1984). As many as 30–40 per cent may fit the definition of incomplete distal renal tubular acidosis. The complete form of distal renal tubular acidosis with hypokalaemia occurs more rarely (Deck, 1965; Jayasinghe *et al.*, 1984). The major complication of MSK kidney is the deposition of gross or microscopic calculi in the dilated or cystic tubules, often responsible for the development of gross or microscopic haematuria and episodes of renal colic. The association between precaliceal tubular ectasia and nephrolithiasis is well documented. Patients with MSK and nephrolithiasis have a higher rate of stone formation than other patients with idiopathic nephrolithiasis (Parks, Coe and Strauss, 1982). The major factor responsible for the formation of stones in these patients is the stagnation of the urine in the dilated or cystic tubules.

Other metabolic factors, such as impaired acidification mechanisms and hypercalciuria, may also play a role. Hypercalciuria and hyperparathyroidism have been frequently reported in patients with MSK and nephrolithiasis (Maschio *et al.*, 1982). The hypothesis that these patients have renal leak hypercalciuria resulting in parathyroid overactivity and eventually autonomous hyperparathyroidism remains unproven (Dlabal, Jordan and Dorfman, 1979). In fact, absorptive hypercalciuria seems to be more common than renal leak hypercalciuria in MSK, and parathyroid adenomas rather than hyperplasia have been found in most patients with MSK who have had documented hyperparathyroidism (O'Neill, Breslau and Pak, 1981). Although in a small number of selected patients the prevalence of parathyroid hyperactivity has been remarkably higher, the frequency of hyperparathyroidism in a larger number of patients with MSK was not different from that observed in a large unselected group of patients with calcium nephrolithiasis—approximately 5 per cent (Parks, Coe and Strauss, 1982). Similarly, the frequency of hypercalciuria in patients with calcium nephrolithiasis, with or without MSK, was not different. It is, therefore, possible that the hypercalciuria frequently observed in these patients is related to the metabolic stone disease, rather than to the dilatation of the papillary collecting ducts. Patients with MSK may have a greater anatomic propensity to form stones, but the evaluation and treatment of any possible metabolic defect should not be different from other stone formers, since they have the same spectrum of metabolic abnormalities (O'Neill, Breslau and Pak, 1981). The stones are most commonly calcium oxalate or calcium phosphate. Although the diagnosis of MSK is frequently made during the evaluation of a urinary tract infection, the rate of infection is not different in calcium stone formers with or without MSK. Hypertension is not more frequent than in the general population, and the renal function remains normal, except in rare patients with chronic pyelonephritis resulting from recurrent episodes of obstruction and infection and multiple surgeries.

Imaging

The diagnosis of MSK is made by excretory urography that characteristically reveals the anterograde visualization by contrast media of dilated collecting tubules (Kuiper, 1976). Medullary sponge kidneys are commonly bilateral, but they may be unilateral in up to one-fourth of the cases. The degree of tubular dilatation is highly variable and the wide range of reported frequencies of this abnormality is in part due to the variable degrees of collecting duct dilatation that different observers have decided to consider abnormal. Degrees of tubular dilatation include papillary blush which is the mildest form of MSK, linear striations consistent with tubular dilatation, and different cystic forms which have been described like a bunch of flowers, cluster of grapes, etc. (*Figure 17.18*). Mild cases of precaliceal ectasia can easily be overlooked if the excretory urography is not of high quality, clearly outlining most caliceal fornices, or if the images are obscured by overlying bowel. A definite

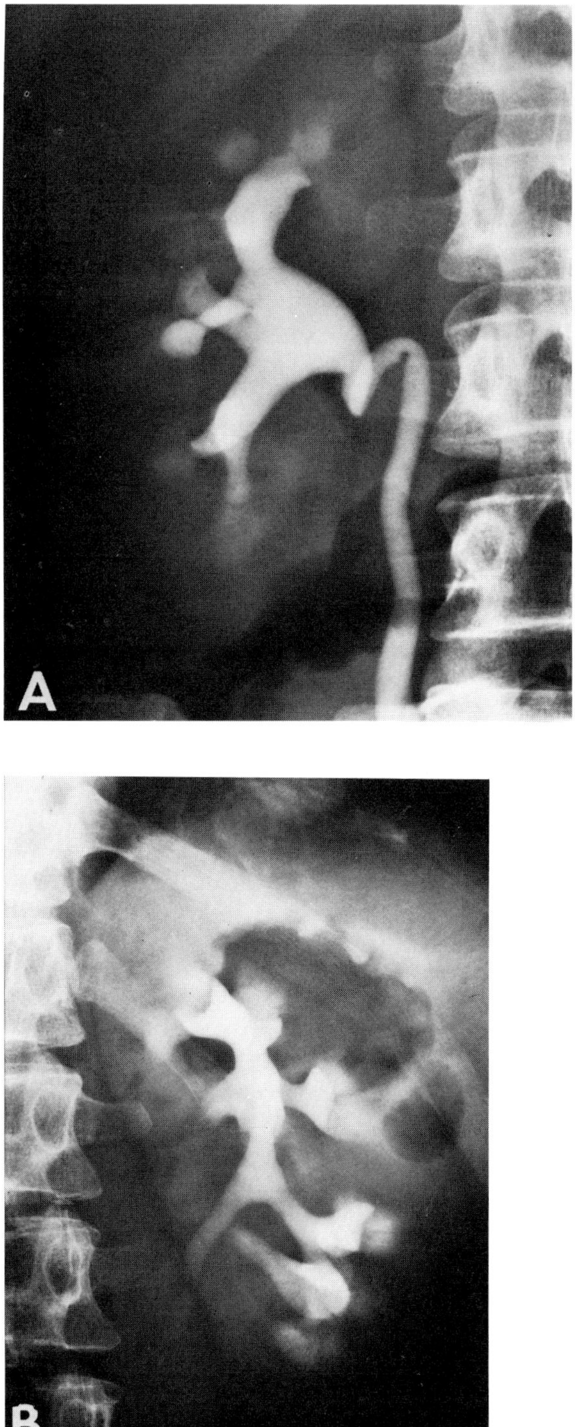

Figure 17.18 See caption opposite

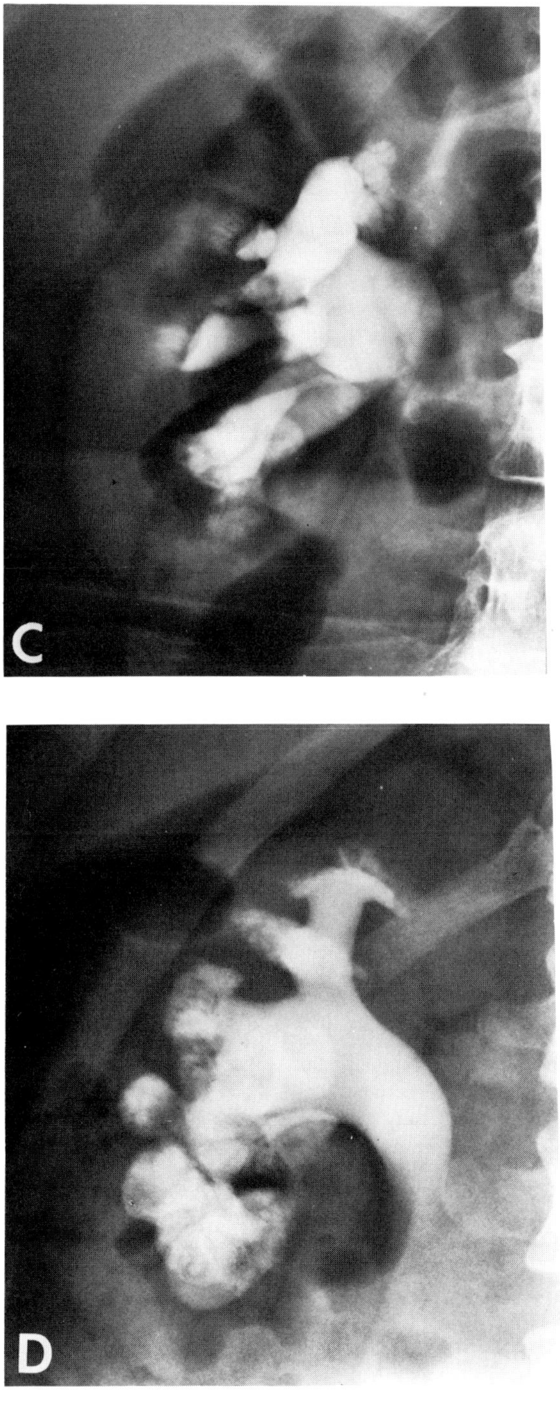

Figure 17.18 Medullary sponge kidney. Spectrum of degrees of collecting duct dilatation: (A) papillary blush; (B) linear radiation; (C), (D) marked dilatation

diagnosis of MSK can be made when the dilated collecting ducts are visualized on early and delayed films without the use of compression and in the absence of ureteral obstruction. Deposition of calcium salts within these dilated tubules may give the radiographic appearance of renal calculi or nephrocalcinosis. The distribution of the renal calculi in these patients is characteristic, in clusters fanning away from the calyx.

Although MSK can occasionally be detected by ultrasonography or computed tomography, the contribution of these techniques to the diagnosis of this condition is very limited. In rare cases, MSK can mimic the urographic appearance of ADPKD (Reed, Rutsky and Witten, 1984). In these cases, computed tomography, ultrasonography and arteriography help too distinguish these two lesions, clearly showing that the cortical layer is free of cysts, except where large medullary cysts protrude through the cortex to the surface. In rare cases, MSK and ADPKD may coexist (Nemoy and Forsberg, 1968; Abreo and Steele, 1982).

Treatment

There is no specific treatment for MSK. The treatment of nephrolithiasis and urinary tract infection, when present, is the same as it would be in the general population. Thiazides and inorganic phosphates have been found to be effective in preventing stones in these patients. Extensive or repeated unnecessary investigations for haematuria should be avoided.

Cystic disease of the renal sinus

Less is known about the cystic disorders involving the renal sinus than of those involving the renal parenchyma. The differential diagnosis of mass-occupying lesions in the area of the renal sinus is difficult and many different processes may look the same on excretory urography. Identification of different types of lesions has now become much easier with newer techniques such as computed tomography and magnetic resonance imaging. The cystic disorders of the renal sinus are benign conditions and they should not be confused with other more serious mass-occupying lesions of the renal pelvis or renal parenchyma. Two types of cystic lesions have been described in the area of the renal sinus—the hilum cysts and the parapelvic cysts.

Pathology and pathogenesis

The hilus cysts have only been described in autopsy studies and have been thought to be due to regressive changes in the fat tissue of the renal sinus, especially in kidneys with abundant fat in the renal sinus because of renal atrophy. The cysts result from fluid replacement of adipose tissue which undergoes regressive changes owing to localized vascular disease and/or atrophy due to recent wasting. The wall of these cysts is lined by a single layer of flattened mesenchymal cells and the cystic fluid is clear and contains abundant lipid droplets (Barrie, 1953; Hellweg, 1954). The parapelvic cysts are of lymphatic origin. The wall of the cyst is very thin and lined by flat endothelial cells. The composition of the cystic fluid resembles that of lymph with electrolyte concentrations similar to those of plasma and higher concentrations of albumin than globulins, as expected in the renal lymph (Deliveliotis and Kavidis, 1969; Bollack *et al.*, 1967). It seems doubtful that hilar cysts and parapelvic cysts indeed represent two different entities since the clinical characteristics of the patients with these disorders are in fact very similar. The lymphatic origin of the parapelvic cysts is not only supported by the structure of the wall of the cyst and the composition of the cystic fluid, but also by the location of the cysts and the good correspondence in many cases between the observed number of cysts and the normal number of renal hilar lymphatic channels. The mechanism responsible for the dilatation of these lymphatic channels is not known.

Recently, it has become recognized that parapelvic cysts are multiple and bilateral much more frequently than initially thought, although in clinical and surgical series only the larger cysts are recognized and the smaller cysts are overlooked (Paramo and Segura, 1972; Vela Navarrete *et al.*, 1973; Vela Navarrete and Garcia Robledo, 1982, 1983). The term 'polycystic disease of the renal sinus' has been recently proposed to describe the bilateral presentation of multiple parapelvic cysts (Vela Navarrete *et al.*, 1983). They are in direct contact with the extrarenal pelvic surface and/or extend into the renal sinus distorting the caliceal infundibuli and calices. The kidney may appear slightly enlarged, but the enlargement is exclusively due to the expansion of the renal sinus, whereas the area of the renal parenchyma *per se* remains normal. A left side predominance in occurrence, number and size has been noted. There is no communication between the different cysts or with the renal pelvis.

Clinical manifestations

The parapelvic cysts are most frequently diagnosed after the fourth decade of life, and they are usually asymptomatic. They are usually discovered in the course of evaluations for conditions such as urinary tract infections, nephrolithiasis, hypertension and prostatism. Despite considerable distortion of the calices and infundibuli, the pressure in these lymphatic cysts is low and not likely to result in significant functional obstruction. Indeed, renal function in patients with bilateral multiple parapelvic cysts is usually normal. The evidence that supports a pathogenetic role of these cysts in the hypertension or nephrolithiasis of these patients is not convincing. Nevertheless, a high prevalence of medullary sponge kidneys has been noted in patients with bilateral parapelvic cysts (Vela Navarrete and Garcia Robledo, 1982, 1983), and a higher prevalence of nephrolithiasis in patients with parapelvic cysts cannot be ruled out. Occasionally, parapelvic cysts are the only finding in the course of evaluations for otherwise unexplained lumbar or flank pain.

Imaging

Usually, the diagnosis of parapelvic cysts can be done by excretory urography with nephrotomography. The most common abnormality is the deformity caused by the elongation of the infundibuli extending into delicately lined calices. Contrary to simple renal cysts, there is no sharp interface between the contrast-laden parenchyma and the cysts on the nephrotomogram. In fact, the renal sinus fat displaced by the expanding parapelvic cyst may be detectable as a radiolucent halo which has been called the peripheral fat sign (Crummy and Madsen, 1966). As opposed to medullary cysts in medullary sponge kidney and to communicating pelvic diverticula, these cysts never become opacified by contrast media. The introduction of computed tomography and ultrasonography has facilitated the

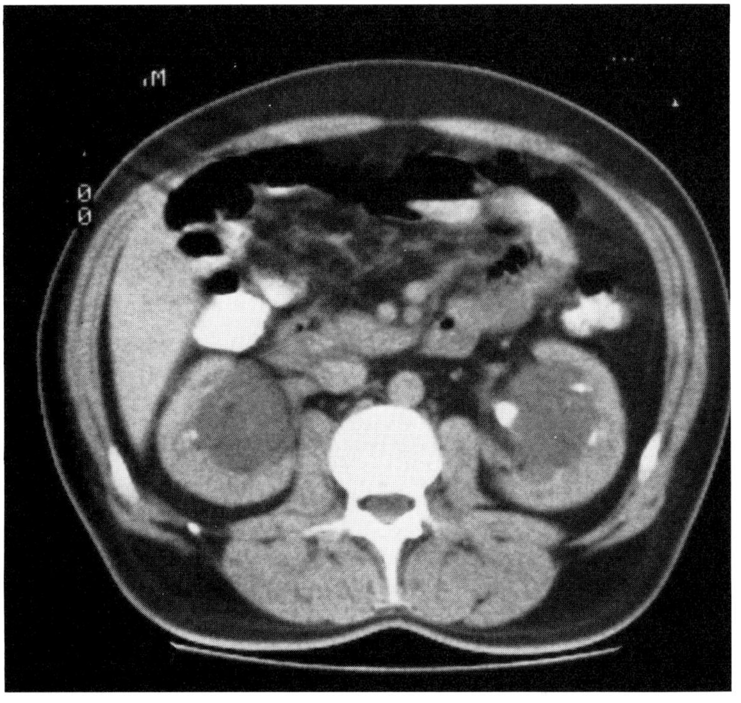

Figure 17.19 Cystic disease of the renal sinus. Demonstration by computed tomography of multiple bilateral parapelvic cysts

differentiation of parapelvic cysts from other benign conditions such as renal sinus lipomatosis (Hurwitz, Benjamin and Cooper, 1978) as well as from more serious diseases such as neoplasms of the renal pelvis and kidney or ADPKD (*Figure 17.19*). Bilateral renal parapelvic cysts causing distortion of the infundibuli and the calices and enlargement of the kidney have occasionally been mistaken for ADPKD. With the use of computed tomography, the distinction of these two conditions is easy; in the cystic disease of the renal sinus or multiple parapelvic cysts, the cysts are confined to the renal sinus, although in some cases they can herniate out of the hilar space into the interstitium of the renal parenchyma (Vela Navarrete and Garcia Robledo, 1983).

Treatment

The therapeutic approach to parapelvic cysts should be conservative, since this is a benign condition.

Pelvicaliceal diverticula

These are cystic cavities that contain urine and are lined by transitional epithelium (Abeshouse and Abeshouse, 1963; Williams, Blandy and Tresidder, 1968; Devine *et al.*, 1969; Timmons *et al.*, 1975). They may be contained in the renal parenchyma and originate from the fornix of a minor calyx by a narrow isthmus (caliceal

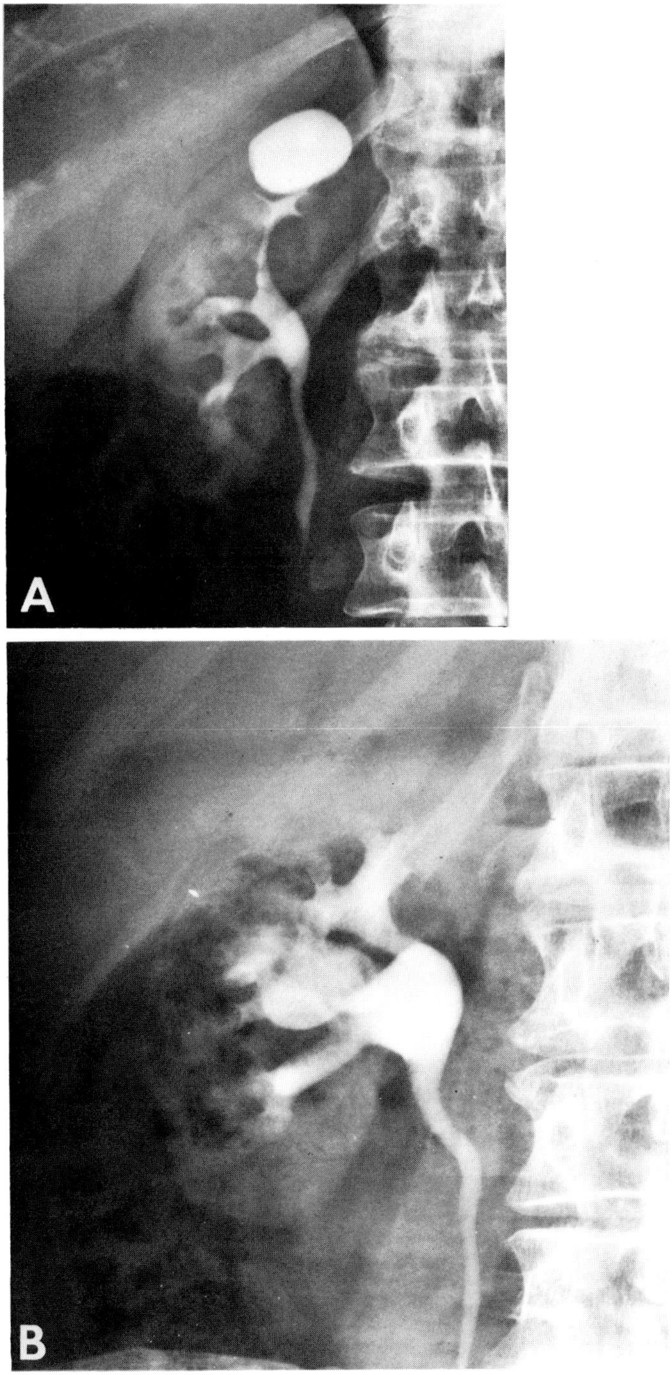

Figure 17.20 (A) Large caliceal diverticulum in the upper pole of the right kidney; (B) late filling of a pelvic diverticulum during excretory urography; (C) the pe!vic diverticulum cannot be seen in an early film

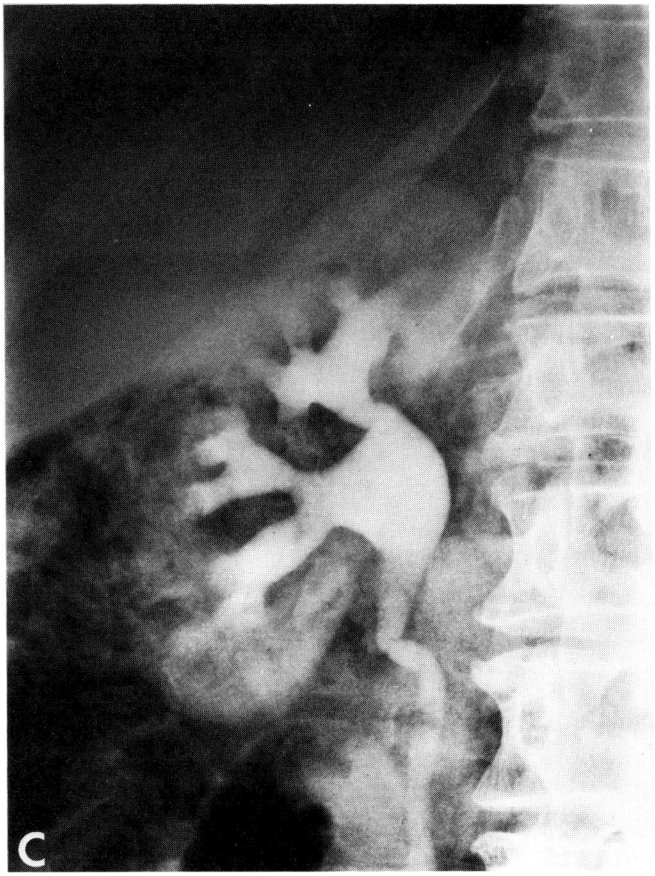

Figure 17.20 *continued*

diverticulum) or be extrarenal and in direct communication with the renal pelvis (pelvic diverticulum) (*Figure 17.20*). It is uncertain whether these diverticula are of congenital or acquired origin. They are usually better demonstrated by retrograde pyelography than by excretory urography. They are usually asymptomatic unless complicated by nephrolithiasis or infection. The frequency of stone formation in the caliceal diverticulum has been reported to be between 10 and 50 per cent. Surgical intervention is indicated rarely when conservative management of these complications fails.

Neoplastic cysts

These have been covered in previous sections.

Inflammatory cysts

Medullary cavities resulting from analgesic-related papillary necrosis or from mycobacterial or other bacterial infections sometimes need to be considered in the differential diagnosis of medullary sponge kidney and caliceal diverticula. Detailed discussion of these disorders is not in the scope of this chapter.

A rare cystic renal disorder that has been known for centuries is the renal infection by *Echinococcus granulosus* (hydatid cysts). Renal hydatid cysts are rare even in countries where hydatid cysts are common (Kretschmer, 1923; Raffii and Dutz, 1967). The frequency of renal involvement in large series of *Echinococcus* infections has ranged between 1 and 3 per cent. The clinical manifestations are flank pain and pressure sensation and occasionally the cysts may rupture into the peritoneal cavity or into the renal pelvis. Calcified inactive hydatid cysts have a characteristic radiological appearance. Percutaneous aspiration should not be performed when a hydatid cyst is suspected. In these cases, a Cassoni skin test and the complement fixation test for *Echinococcus* should be done and the surgeon alerted to the possible nature of the cyst. The treatment of an active hydatid cyst is surgical, with special care to prevent spillage of the cyst content and, whenever possible, minimize the loss of renal mass.

References

ABESHOUSE, B.S. and ABESHOUSE, G.A. (1963). Calyceal diverticulum: a report of sixteen cases and review of the literature. *Urologia Internationalis,* **15,** 329–357

ABREO, K. and STEELE, T.H. (1982). Simultaneous medullary sponge and adult polycystic kidney disease. *Archives of Internal Medicine,* **142,** 163–165

ADVISORY COMMITTEE TO THE RENAL TRANSPLANT REGISTRY (1977). The 13th report of the human renal transplant registry. *Transplantation Proceedings,* **9,** 9–26

AKHTAR, M. and QADEER, A. (1980). Multilocular cyst of kidney with embryonic tissue. *Urology,* **16,** 90–94

ALTEMUS, R., SALAZAR, H. and ROTHERAM, E.B. Jr. (1968). Infected solitary cyst of the kidney. *Vascular Diseases,* **5,** 125–129

ANDERSON, R.J., MILLER, P.D. and LINAS, S.L. (1979). Role of the renin–angiotensin system in hypertension of polycystic kidney disease. *Mineral and Electrolyte Metabolism,* **2,** 137–141

BABKA, J.C., COHEN, M.S. and SODE, J. (1974). Solitary intrarenal cyst causing hypertension. *New England Journal of Medicine,* **291,** 343–344

BAERT, L. (1978). Hereditary polycystic kidney disease (adult form): a microdissection study of two cases at an early stage of the disease. *Kidney International,* **13,** 519–525

BAERT, L. and STEG, A. (1977). Is the diverticulum of the distal and collecting tubules a preliminary stage of the simple cyst in the adult? *Journal of Urology,* **118,** 707–710

BALDAUF, M.C. and SCHULZ, D.M. (1975). Multilocular cyst of the kidney. Report of three cases with review of the literature. *American Journal of Clinical Pathology,* **65,** 93–102

BANNER, M.P., POLLACK, H.M., CHATTEN, J. and WITZLEBEN, C. (1981). Multilocular renal cysts: radiologic–pathologic correlation. *American Journal of Roentgenology,* **136,** 239–247

BARBARIC, Z.L., SPATARO, R.F. and SEGAL, A.J. (1977). Urinary tract obstruction in polycystic renal disease. *Radiology,* **125,** 627–629

BARRIE, H.J. (1953). Paracalyceal cysts of the renal sinus. *American Journal of Pathology,* **29,** 985–991

BECKER, J.A. and ROBINSON, T. (1970). Congenital multicystic disease in the adult. *Journal of the Canadian Association of Radiologists,* **21,** 165–168

BELL, E.T. (1950). *Renal Diseases,* 2nd edn. Philadelphia; Lea and Febiger

BERNSTEIN, J. (1976). A classification of renal cysts. In *Cystic Diseases of the Kidney,* edited by K.D. Gardner, Jr., pp. 7–30. New York; Wiley

BIGELOW, N.H. (1953). The association of polycystic kidneys with intracranial aneurysms and other related disorders. *American Journal of Medical Sciences,* **225,** 485–494

BJERLE, P., LINDQVIST, B. and MICHAELSON, G. (1971). Pressure measurements in renal cysts. *Scandinavian Journal of Clinical and Laboratory Investigation,* **27,** 135–138

BOLLACK, C., JURASCHECK, F., OBERLING, F., RIEFFEL, R. and SUHLER, A. (1967). Les kystes essentiels du rein. Etude histologique. *Journal d'Urologie et de Néphrologie,* **73,** 425–432

BOURGEOIS, N., KINNAERT, P., VEREERSTRAETEN, P., SCHOUTENS, A. and TOUSSAINT, C. (1983). Infection of hepatic cysts following kidney transplantation in polycystic disease. *World Journal of Surgery,* **7,** 629–631

BRAASCH, W.F. (1916). Clinical data of polycystic kidney. *Surgery, Gynecology and Obstetrics,* **23,** 697–702

BRAASCH, W.F. and HENDRICK, J.A. (1944). Renal cysts, simple and otherwise. *Journal of Urology*, **51**, 1–10

BRAASCH, W.F. and SCHACHT, F.W. (1933). Pathological and clinical data concerning polycystic kidney. *Surgery, Gynecology and Obstetrics*, **57**, 467–475

BRICKER, N.S. and PATTON, J.F. (1955). Cystic disease of the kidneys. A study of dynamics and chemical composition of cyst fluid. *American Journal of Medicine*, **18**, 205–219

BROWN, C.D. (1978). Massive spontaneous renal cyst hemorrhage. *Journal of American Medical Association*, **239**, 1418–1419

BROWN, R.A.P. (1951). Polycystic disease of the kidneys and intracranial aneurysms: the etiology and interrelationship of these conditions: review of recent literature and report of seven cases in which both conditions coexisted. *Glasgow Medical Journal*, **32**, 333–348

BUNTING, C.H. (1906). Congenital cystic kidney and liver with family tendency. *Journal of Experimental Medicine*, **8**, 157–167

CACCHI, R. and RICCI, V. (1948). Sopra una rara è forse ancora non descritta affezioine cistica delle piramidi renali ('rene e spugna'). *Atti della Societa Italiana di Urologia*, **5**, 59–63

CAIRNS, H.W.B. (1925). Heredity in polycystic disease of the kidney. *Quarterly Journal of Medicine*, **18**, 359–392

CALABRESE, G., VAGELLI, G., CRISTOFANO, C. and BARSOTTI, G. (1982). Behaviour of arterial pressure in different stages of polycystic kidney disease. *Nephron*, **32**, 207–208

CAMEY, M. and LE DUC, A. (1972). Un cas d'insuffisance rénale aiguë par syndrome bilatéral de jonction sur reins polykystiques. *Journal d'Urologie et de Néphrologie*, **78**, 720–726

CARONE, F.A., ROWLAND, R.G., PERLMAN, S.G. and GANOTE, C.E. (1974). The pathogenesis of drug-induced renal cystic disease. *Kidney International*, **5**, 411–421

CASE RECORDS OF THE MASSACHUSETTS GENERAL HOSPITAL, Case 16–1982, edited by R.E. Scully, E.J. Mark and B.U. McNeely (1982). *New England Journal of Medicine*, **306**, 975–984

CHANARD, J., SZYMANOWICZ, A., BRUNOIS, J.P., TOUPANCE, O., BIREMBAUT, P. and BOREL, P.J. (1980). Urinary 3-hydroxyproline in renal disease. *Renal Physiology*, **3**, 163–168

CHAPMAN, J.R. and HILSON, A.J.W. (1980). Polycystic kidneys and abdominal aortic aneurysms. *Lancet*, **1**, 646

CHURCHILL, D.N., BEAR, J.C., MORGAN, J., PAYNE, R.H., McMANAMON, P.J. and GAULT, M.H. (1984). Prognosis of adult onset polycystic kidney disease re-evaluated. *Kidney International*, **26**, 190–193

CHURCHILL, D., KIMOFF, R., PINSKY, M. and GAULT, M.H. (1975). Solitary intrarenal cyst: correctable cause of hypertension. *Urology*, **6**, 485–488

CLARKE, B.G., HURWITZ, I.S. and DUBINSKY, E. (1956). Solitary serous cysts of the kidney: biochemical, cytologic and histologic studies. *Journal of Urology*, **75**, 772–775

CLAYMAN, R.V., SURYA, V., MILLER, R.P., REINKE, D.B. and FRALEY, E.E. (1984). Pursuit of the renal mass: is ultrasound enough? *American Journal of Medicine*, **77**, 218–223

COMFORT, M.W., GRAY, H.K., DAHLIN, D.C. and WHITESELL, F.B. (1952). Polycystic disease of the liver: a study of 24 cases. *Gastroenterology*, **20**, 60–78

CRUMMY, A.B. and MADSEN, P.O. (1966). Parapelvic renal cyst: the peripheral fat sign. *Journal of Urology*, **96**, 436–438

CUPPAGE, F.E., HUSEMAN, R.A., CHAPMAN, A. and GRANTHAM, J.J. (1980). Ultrastructure and function of cysts from human adult polycystic kidneys. *Kidney International*, **17**, 372–381

DALGAARD, O.Z. (1957). Bilateral polycystic disease of the kidneys: a follow-up of two hundred and eighty-four patients and their families. *Acta Medica Scandinavica (Suppl.)*, **328**, 1–255

D'ANGELO, A., MIONI, G., OSSI, E., LUPO, A., VALVO, E. and MASCHIO, G. (1975). Alterations in renal tubular sodium and water transport in polycystic kidney disease. *Clinical Nephrology*, **3**, 99–105

DANIEL, W.W. Jr., HARTMAN, G.W., WITTEN, D.M., FARROW, G.M. and KELALIS, P.P. (1972). Calcified renal masses: a review of ten years experience at the Mayo Clinic. *Radiology*, **103**, 503–508

DARMADY, E.M., OFFER, J. and WOODHOUSE, M.A. (1973). The parameters of the ageing kidney. *Journal of Pathology*, **109**, 195–207

DECK, M.D.F. (1965). Medullary sponge kidney with renal tubular acidosis: a report of 3 cases. *Journal of Urology*, **94**, 330–335

DELANEY, V.B., ADLER, S., BRUNS, F.J., LICINIA, M., SEGAL, D.P. and FRALEY, D.S. (1985). Autosomal dominant polycystic kidney disease: presentation, complications, and prognosis. *American Journal of Kidney Diseases*, **5**, 104–111

DELIVELIOTIS, A. and KAVADIS, C. (1969). Parapelvic cysts of the kidney: report of seven cases. *British Medical Journal*, **41**, 386–393

DELIVELIOTIS, A., ZORZOS, S. and VARKARAKIS, M. (1967). Suppuration of solitary cyst of the kidney. *British Journal of Urology*, **39**, 472–478

DEVINE, C.J. Jr., GUZMAN, J.A., DEVINE, P.C. and POUTASSE, E.F. (1969). Calyceal diverticulum. *Journal of Urology*, **101**, 8–11

DIMATTEO, J., PICARD, R., VACHERON, A. and BENSAID, J. (1965). Polykystose rénale associée a un syndrome de Marfan fruste avec dilatation de l'aorte initiale et insuffisance aortique. *Bulletins et Mémoires de la Société Médicale des Hôpitaux de Paris,* **116,** 1665–1673

DLABAL, P.W., JORDAN, R.M. and DORFMAN, S.G. (1979). Medullary sponge kidney and renal-leak hypercalciuria. A link to the development of parathyroid adenoma? *Journal of the American Medical Association,* **241,** 1490–1491

DUNCAN, K.A. CUPPAGE, F.E. and GRANTHAM, J.J. (1985). Urinary lipid bodies in polycystic kidney disease. *American Journal of Kidney Diseases,* **5,** 49–53

DUNNILL, M.S., MILLARD, P.R. and OLIVER, D. (1977). Acquired cystic disease of the kidneys: a hazard of long-term intermittent maintenance haemodialysis. *Journal of Clinical Pathology,* **30,** 868–877

EGGERS, P.W., CONNERTON, R. and McMULLAN, M. (1984). The Medicare experience with end-stage renal disease: trends incidence, prevalence, and survival. *Health Care Financing Review,* **5,** 69–88

EKSTRÖM, T., ENGFELDT, B., LAGERGREN, C. and LINDVALL, N. (1959). *Medullary Sponge Kidney.* Stockholm; Almqvist and Wiksell

ELLIOTT, H.L., MACDOUGALL, A.E. and BUCHANAN, W.M. (1977). Acquired cystic disease of kidney. *Lancet,* **2,** 1359

EPSTEIN, L. WACKSMAN, J., DAUGHTRY, J. and STRAFFON, R.A. (1978). Multilocular cysts of kidney: a diagnostic dilemma. *Urology,* **11,** 573–576

EVAN, A.P., GARDNER, K.D. Jr. and BERNSTEIN, J. (1979). Polypoid and papillary epithelial hyperplasia: a potential cause of ductal obstruction in adult polycystic disease. *Kidney International,* **16,** 743–750

EVANS, A.T. and COUGHLIN, J.P. (1970). Urinary obstruction due to renal cysts. *Journal of Urology,* **103,** 277–280

FAYEMI, A.O. and ALI, M. (1980). Acquired renal cysts and tumors superimposed on chronic primary kidney diseases: an autopsy study of 24 patients. *Pathology Research and Practice,* **168,** 73–83

FEINER, H.D., KATZ, L.A. and GALLO, G.R. (1981). Acquired cystic disease of kidney in chronic dialysis patients. *Urology,* **27,** 260–264

FERGUSSON, J.D. (1949). Observations on familial polycystic disease of the kidney. *Proceedings of the Royal Society of Medicine,* **42,** 806–814

FRANZ, K.A. and REUBI, F.C. (1983). Rate of functional deterioration in polycystic kidney disease. *Kidney International,* **23,** 526–529

FUNCK-BRENTANO, J.L., VANTELON, J. and LOPEZ-ALVAREZ, R. (1964). Les accidents évolutifs de la maladie polykystique des reins: 154 observations personnelles. *La Presse Medicale,* **72,** 1583–1588

GABOW, P.A., IKLÉ, D.W. and HOLMES, J.H. (1984). Polycystic kidney disease: prospective analysis of nonazotemic patients and family members. *Annals of Internal Medicine,* **101,** 238–247

GARDNER, K.D. Jr. (1984). Acquired renal cystic disease and renal adenocarcinoma in patients on long-term hemodialysis. *New England Journal of Medicine,* **310,** 390

GARDNER, K.D. Jr. and EVAN, A.P. (1979). The nephronophthis-cystic renal medulla complex. In *Nephrology,* edited by J. Hamburger, J. Crosnier and J.-P. Grünfeld, pp. 893–908. New York; Wiley

GARDNER, K.D. and EVAN, A.P. (1984). Host-microbe interaction in nordihydroguaiaretic acid induced renal cystic disease. *Kidney International,* **25,** 244

GESUNDHEIT, N., KENT, D.L., FAWCETT, H.D., EFFRON., M.K. and MAFFLY, R.H. (1982). Infected liver cyst in a patient with polycystic kidney disease. *Western Journal of Medicine,* **136,** 246–249

GRANTHAM, J.J. (1983). Polycystic kidney disease: a predominance of giant nephrons. *American Journal of Physiology,* **244,** F3–F10

GRANTHAM, J.J. and SLUSHER, S.L. (1984). Management of renal cystic disorders. In *Therapy of Renal Diseases and Related Disorders,* edited by W.N. Suki and S.G. Massry, pp. 383–404. Boston; Nijhoff

GREEN, J., SZYLMAN, P., SZNAJDER, I.I., WINAVER, J. and BETTER, O.S. (1984). Renal tubular handling of potassium in patients with medullary sponge kidney: a model of renal papillectomy in humans. *Archives of Internal Medicine,* **144,** 2201–2204

GREENE, L.F., FEINZAG, W. and DAHLIN, D.C. (1971). Multicystic dysplasia of the kidney: with special reference to the contralateral kidney. *Journal of Urology,* **105,** 482–487

HALE, J.E. and MORGAN, M.N. (1969). Simple renal cysts. *Postgraduate Medical Journal,* **45,** 767–772

HELLWEG, G. (1954). Über Hiluscysten der Nieren. *Virchows Archiv,* **325,** S.98–108

HEPPLER, A.B. (1930). Solitary cysts of kidney: report of seven cases and observations on pathogenesis of these cysts. *Surgery, Gynecology and Obstetrics,* **50,** 668–670

HIGASHIHARA, E., NUTAHARA, K., TAGO, K., UENO, A. and NIJIMA, T. (1984). Medullary sponge kidney and renal acidification defect. *Kidney International,* **25,** 453–459

HIGGINS, C.C. (1952). Bilateral polycystic kidney disease: review of 94 cases. *AMA Archives of Surgery,* **65,** 318–329

HINMAN, F., Jr. (1978). Obstructive renal cysts. *Journal of Urology,* **119,** 681–683

HOARD, T.D. and O'BRIEN, D.P., III (1976). Simple renal cyst and high renin hypertension cured by cyst decompression. *Journal of Urology,* **115,** 326–327

HOOVER, R. and FRAUMENI, J.F., Jr. (1973). Risk of cancer in renal-transplant recipients. *Lancet*, **2**, 55–57

HUGHSON, M.D., HENNIGAR, G.R. and McMANUS, J.F.A. (1980). Atypical cysts, acquired renal cystic disease, and renal cell tumors in end stage dialysis kidneys. *Laboratory Investigation*, **42**, 475–480

HURWITZ, R.S., BENJAMIN, J.A. and COOPER, J.F. (1978). Excessive proliferation of peripelvic fat of the kidney. *Urology*, **11**, 448

HUSEMAN, R., GRADY, A., WELLING, D. and GRANTHAM, J. (1980). Macropuncture study of polycystic disease in adult human kidneys. *Kidney International*, **18**, 375–385

IGLESIAS, C.G., TORRES, V.E., OFFORD, K.P., HOLLEY, K.E., BEARD, C.M. and KURLAND, L.T. (1983). Epidemiology of adult polycystic kidney disease, Olmsted County, Minnesota: 1935–1980. *American Journal of Kidney Diseases*, **2**, 630–639

ISHIKAWA, I., SAITO, Y., ONOUCHI, Z., KITADA, H., SUZUKI, S., KURIHARA, S. *et al.* (1980). Development of acquired cystic disease and adenocarcinoma of the kidney in glomerulonephritic chronic hemodialysis patients. *Clinical Nephrology*, **14**, 1–6

ISHIKAWA, I., YURI, T., KITADA, H. and SHINODA, A. (1983). Regression of acquired cystic disease of the kidney after successful renal transplantation. *American Journal of Nephrology*, **3**, 310–314

JAYASINGHE, K.S.A., MOHIDEEN, R., SHERIFF, M.H.R., MENDIS, B.L.J., EKANAYAKE, R. and DHARMADASA, K. (1984). Medullary sponge kidney presenting with hypokalaemic paralysis. *Postgraduate Medical Journal*, **60**, 303–304

JOHNSON, J.D. and RADWIN, H.M. (1976). High renin hypertension associated with renal cortical cyst. *Urology*, **7**, 508–511

KALA, R., FYHRQUIST, F., HALTTUNEN, P. and RAUSTE, J. (1976). Solitary renal cyst, hypertension and renin. *Journal of Urology*, **116**, 710–711

KARANICOLAS, S., OREOPOULOS, D.G., DOMBROS, N., PIERRATOS, A., MATHEWS, R.E. and VAS, S. (1979). Intestinal obstruction and bowel perforation in patients undergoing chronic peritoneal dialysis (Abstract). *16th European Dialysis and Transplantation Association Meeting* (Amsterdam)

KERESZTURY, S. and MEGYERI, L. (1962). Histology of renal pyramids with special regard to changes due to ageing. *Acta Morphologica Academiae Scientiarum Hungaricae*, **11**, 205–215

KISSANE, J.M. (1983). Congenital malformations. In *Pathology of the Kidney*, 3rd edn, edited by R.H. Heptinstall, pp. 83–140. Boston; Little, Brown

KONISHI, F., MUKAWA, A. and KITADA, H. (1980). Acquired cystic disease of the kidney and renal cell carcinoma on long term hemodialysis. *Acta Pathologica Japonica*, **30**, 847–858

KRAMER, P., BROYER, M., BRUNNER, F.P., BRYNGER, H., DONCKERWOLCKE, R.A., JACOBS, C. *et al.* (1982). Combined report on regular dialysis and transplantation in Europe. *Proceedings of the European Dialysis and Transplantation Association*, **19**, 4–59

KREMPIEN, B. and RITZ, E. (1980). Acquired cystic transformation of the kidneys of haemodialyzed patients. *Virchows Archiv A. Pathological Anatomy and Histology*, **386**, 189–200

KRETSCHMER, H.L. (1923). Echinococcus disease of the kidney. *Surgery, Gynecology and Obstetrics*, **36**, 196–207

KUIPER, J.J. (1976). Medullary sponge kidney. In *Cystic Diseases of the Kidney*, edited by K.D. Gardner, Jr., pp. 151–171. New York; Wiley

KYAW, M.M. and NEWMAN, H. (1971). Adult multicystic renal disease. *British Journal of Radiology*, **44**, 881–882

LAMBERT, P.P. (1947). Polycystic disease of the kidney: a review. *Archives of Pathology*, **44**, 34–58

LANG, E.K. and GERSHANIK, J.B. (1978). Multicystic dysplastic kidney: diagnostic considerations and management. *Southern Medical Journal*, **71**, 888–891

LAUCKS, S.P., Jr. and McLACHLAN, M.S.F. (1981). Aging and simple cysts of the kidney. *British Journal of Radiology*, **54**, 12–14

LEIER, C.V., BAKER, P.B., KILMAN, J.W. and WOOLEY, C.F. (1984). Cardiovascular abnormalities associated with adult polycystic kidney disease. *Annals of Internal Medicine*, **100**, 683–688

LEJARS, F. (1888). *Du gros rein polykystique de l'adulte*, pp. 5–55. Paris; Steinheill

LENARDUZZI, G. (1939). Reperto pielografico poco commune (dilatazione delle vie urinarie intrarenali). *Radiologia Medica*, **26**, 346–347

LEVEY, A.S., PAUKER, S.G. and KASSIRER, J.P. (1983). Occult intracranial aneurysms in polycystic kidney disease: when is cerebral arteriography indicated? *New England Journal of Medicine*, **308**, 986–994

LEVINE, E. and GRANTHAM, J. (1981). The role of computed tomography in the evaluation of adult polycystic kidney disease. *American Journal of Kidney Diseases*, **1**, 99–105

LEVINE, E., GRANTHAM, J.J., SLUSHER, S.L., GREATHOUSE, J.L. and KROHN, B.P. (1984). CT of acquired cystic kidney disease and renal tumors in long-term dialysis patients. *American Journal of Roentgenology*, **142**, 125–131

LIMJOCO, U.R. and STRAUCH, A.E. (1966). Infected solitary cyst of the kidney: report of a case and review of the literature. *Journal of Urology*, **96**, 625–630

LLOYD, L.K., WITTEN, D.M., BUESCHEN, A.J. and DANIEL, W.W. (1978). Enhanced detection of asymptomatic renal masses with routine tomography during excretory urography. *Urology*, **11**, 523–528

McMANUS, J.F.A. and HUGHSON, M.D. (1979). New therapies and new pathologies: end-stage-dialysis kidneys. *Archives of Pathology and Laboratory Medicine,* **103,** 53–57

MARTINEZ-MALDONADO, M. (1985). Functional aspects of adult polycystic kidneys: electrolyte and uric acid excretion with a comment on stone formation. In *Proceedings of International Workshop on Polycystic Kidney Disease: Problems in Diagnosis and Management.* Kansas City; Polycystic Kidney Research Foundation (in press)

MANG, H.Y.L., MARKOVIĆ, P.R., CHOW, S. and MARUYAMA, A. (1978). Solitary intrarenal cyst causing hypertension. *New York State Journal of Medicine,* **78,** 654–656

MASCHIO, G., TESSITORE, N., D'ANGELO, A, FABRIS, A., CORGNATI, A., OLDRIZZI, L. *et al.* (1982). Medullary sponge kidney and hyperparathyroidism—a puzzling association. *American Journal of Nephrology,* **2,** 77–84

MAYALL, G.F. (1970). The incidence of medullary sponge kidney. *Clinical Radiology,* **21,** 171–174

MELAND, E.L. and BRAASCH, W.F. (1933). Multilocular cysts of the kidney. *Journal of Urology,* **29,** 505–519

MICKISCH, O., BOMMER, J., BACHMANN, S., WALDHERR, R., MANN, J.F.E. and RITZ, E. (1984). Multicystic transformation of kidneys in chronic renal failure. *Nephron,* **38,** 93–99

MILUTINOVIC, J. and AGODOA, L.Y. (1983). Potential causes and pathogenesis in autosomal dominant polycystic kidney disease. *Nephron,* **33,** 139–144

MILUTINOVIC, J., FIALKOW, P.J., RUDD, T.G. *et al.* (1980). Liver cysts in patients with autosomal dominant polycystic kidney disease. *American Journal of Medicine,* **68,** 741–744

MILUTINOVICH, J., FOLLETTE, W.C. and SCRIBNER, B.H. (1977). Spontaneous retroperitoneal bleeding in patients on chronic hemodialysis. *Annals of Internal Medicine,* **86,** 189–192

MILUTINOVIC, J., PHILLIPS, L.A., BRYANT, J.I., AGODOA, L.Y. *et al.* (1980). Autosomal dominant polycystic kidney disease. Early diagnosis and data for genetic counselling. *The Lancet,* **1,** 1203

MINDELL, H.J. (1975). Percutaneous renal cyst puncture: unusual results in 2 cases. *Journal of Urology,* **114,** 332–336

MITCHESON, H.D., WILLIAMS, G. and CASTRO, J.E. (1977). Clinical aspects of polycystic disease of the kidneys. *British Medical Journal,* **1,** 1196–1199

MONTOLIU, J., TORRAS, A. and REVERT, L. (1980). Polycystic kidneys and abdominal aortic aneurysms. *Lancet,* **1,** 1133–1134

MOORTHY, A.V. and BEIRNE, G.J. (1978). Acquired cystic disease of kidney. *Lancet,* **1,** 663

MUTHER, R.S. and BENNETT, W.M. (1981). Cyst fluid antibiotic concentrations in polycystic kidney disease: differences in proximal and distal cyst permeability. *Kidney International,* **20,** 519–522

NASH, D.A. Jr. (1977). Hypertension in polycystic kidney disease without renal failure. *Archives of Internal Medicine,* **137,** 1571–1575

NEMOY, N.J. and FORSBERG, L. (1968). Polycystic renal disease presenting as medullary sponge kidney. *Journal of Urology,* **100,** 407–411

NEWMAN, H.R. (1950). Congenital polycystic kidney disease. *American Journal of Surgery,* **80,** 410–418

NG, R.C.K. and SUKI, W.N. (1980). Renal cell carcinoma occurring in a polycystic kidney of a transplant recipient. *Journal of Urology,* **124,** 710–712

O'NEILL, M., BRESLAU, N.A. and PAK, C.Y.C. (1981). Metabolic evaluation of nephrolithiasis in patients with medullary sponge kidney. *Journal of the American Medical Association,* **245,** 1233–1236

OPPENHEIMER, G.D. (1934). Polycystic disease of the kidney. *Annals of Surgery,* **100,** 1136–1158

OSATHANONDH, V. and POTTER, E.L. (1964). Pathogenesis of polycystic kidneys: type 3 due to multiple abnormalities of development. *Archives of Pathology,* **77,** 485–501

PALUBINSKAS, A.J. (1963). Renal pyramidal structure opacification in excretory urography and its relation to medullary sponge kidney. *Radiology,* **81,** 963–970

PARAMO, P.G. and SEGURA, A. (1972). Hilioquistosis renal. *Revista Clinica Española,* **126,** 387–396

PARKS, J.H., COE, F.L. and STRAUSS, A.L. (1982). Calcium nephrolithiasis and medullary sponge kidney in women. *New England Journal of Medicine,* **306,** 1088–1091

PATEL, N.P., PITTS, W.R. Jr. and WARD, J.N. (1978). Solitary infected renal cyst: report of 2 cases and review of literature. *Urology,* **11,** 164–167

QUINBY, W.C. and BRIGHT, E.F. (1977). Solitary renal cysts; their symptoms when situated at the upper pole of the right kidney. *Journal of Urology,* **33,** 201–214

RAFFII, P. and DUTZ, W. (1967). Hydatid cysts of the kidney. *Journal of Urology,* **97,** 815–817

RALL, J.E. and ODEL, H.M. (1949). Congenital polycystic disease of the kidney: review of the literature and data in 267 cases. *American Journal of the Medical Sciences,* **218,** 399–407

RASKIN, M.M., POOLE, D.O., ROEN, S.A. and VIAMONTE, M., Jr. (1975). Percutaneous management of renal cysts: results of a four-year study. *Radiology,* **115,** 551–553

RAYER, P.F.Q. (1837–41). *Traité des maladies des reins. Etudiées en elles-mêmes et dans leur rapports avec les maladies des uretères, de la vessie, de la prostate, de l'urete, etc.* Paris; Ballière

REED, J.R., RUTSKY, E.A. and WITTEN, D.M. (1984). Medullary sponge kidney presenting as polycystic renal disease. *Southern Medical Journal,* **77,** 909–912

REEDERS, S.P., BREUNING, M.H., CORNEY, G., JEREMIAH, S.J., MEERA KAHN, P., DAVIES, K.E., HOPKINSON, D.A., PEARSON, P.L. and WEATHERALL, D.J. (1986). Two genetic markers closely linked to adult polycystic kidney disease on chromosome 16. *British Medical Journal,* **292,** 851–853

REID, R.E. (1966). Pyelocalyceal obstruction due to a renal cyst. *Journal of the National Medical Association,* **58,** 342–344

ROCKSON, S.G., STONE, R.A. and GUNNELLS, J.C. Jr. (1974). Solitary renal cyst with segmental ischemia and hypertension. *Journal of Urology,* **112,** 550–552

ROSE, H.J. and PRUITT, A.W. (1976). Hypertension, hyperreninemia and a solitary renal cyst in an adolescent. *American Journal of Medicine,* **61,** 579–582

ROTH, J.K. Jr. and ROBERTS, J.A. (1980). Benign renal cysts and renal function. *Journal of Urology,* **123,** 625–628

SADLOWSKI, R.W., SMEY, P., WILLIAMS, J. and TAXY, J. (1979). Adenocarcinoma in multilocular renal cyst. *Urology,* **14,** 512–514

SAGALOWSKY, A. and SOLOTKIN, D. (1980). Infected renal mass successfully treated by ultrasound-guided needle aspiration. *Southern Medical Journal,* **73,** 957

SCHACHT, F.W. (1931). Hypertension in cases of congenital polycystic kidney. *Archives of Internal Medicine,* **47,** 500–509

SCHEFF, R.T., ZUCHERMAN, G., HARTER, H., DELMEZ, J. and KOEHLER, R. (1980). Diverticular disease in patients with chronic renal failure due to polycystic kidney disease. *Annals of Internal Medicine,* **92,** 202–204

SCHWAB, S., HINTHORN, D., DIEDERICK, D., CUPPAGE, F. and GRANTHAM, J. (1983). pH-dependent accumulations of clindamycin in a polycystic kidney. *American Journal of Kidney Diseases,* **3,** 63–66

SELGAS, R., TEMES, J.L., SOBRINO, J.A., VIGUER, J.M., OTERO, A. and SANCHEZ, S.L. (1981). Enfermedad poliquistica renal del adulto asociada con una forma incompleta de sindrome de Marfan. *Medicina Clinica (Barcelona),* **76,** 311–313

SHAPIRO, I.J. (1929). Congenital polycystic kidneys. *Journal of Urology,* **21,** 308–339

SIMON, H.B. and THOMPSON, G.J. (1955). Congenital renal polycystic disease: a clinical and therapeutic study of 366 cases. *Journal of American Medical Association,* **159,** 657–662

SMITH, D.C., RICH, D.H. and BARNES, R.W. (1977). Hematuria and massive calycovenous reflux secondary to benign renal cyst. *Urology,* **9,** 698–700

SPENCE, H.M. (1955). Congenital unilateral multicystic kidney: an entity to be distinguished from polycystic kidney disease and other cystic disorders. *Journal of Urology,* **74,** 693–706

SPENCE, H.M. and SINGLETON, R. (1972). Cysts and cystic disorders of the kidney: types, diagnosis, treatment. *Urologic Survey,* **22,** 131–158

STABLES, D.P. and JACKSON, R.S. (1974). Management of an infected simple renal cyst by percutaneous aspiration. *British Journal of Radiology,* **47,** 290–292

STEELE, B.T., LIRENMAN, D.S. and BEATTIE, C.W. (1980). Nephronophthisis. *American Journal of Medicine,* **68,** 531

STEG, A. (1975). Etio-pathogénie et classification des affections kystiques du rein de l'adulte. In *Les Affections Kystiques du Rein de l'adulte. Journal d'Urologie et de Nephrologie,* **81** (9 bis), 11–40

STEG, A. (1976a). Renal cysts. I. Current pathogenic approach. *European Urology,* **2,** 161–163

STEG, A. (1976b). Renal cysts. II. Chemical and dynamic study of cyst fluid. *European Urology,* **2,** 164–167

STEG, A. (1976c). Renal cysts in adults. III. Clinical aspects and diagnostical approach, based on the analysis of 2,342 cases. *European Urology,* **2,** 209–212

STEG, A. (1976d). Renal cysts in adults. IV. Therapeutic problems. *European Urology,* **2,** 213–215

SUTER, W. (1949). Das kongenitale Aneurysma der basalen Gehirnarterien und Cystennieren. *Schweizerische Medizinische Wochenschrift,* **79,** 471–476

SWENSON, R.S., KEMPSON, R.L. and FRIEDLAND, G.W. (1974). Cystic disease of the renal medulla in the elderly. *Journal of American Medical Association,* **228,** 1401–1404

TADROS, P. (1979). Unilateral renal shutdown: uncommon complication of polycystic disease. *Canadian Medical Association Journal,* **121,** 597–598

TAXY, J.B. and MARSHALL, F.F. (1983). Multilocular renal cysts in adults. Possible relationship to renal adenocarcinoma. *Archives of Pathology and Laboratory Medicine,* **107,** 633–637

TIMMONS, J.W., Jr., MALEK, R.S., HATTERY, R.R. and DEWEERD, J.H. (1975). Caliceal diverticulum. *Journal of Urology,* **114,** 6–9

TORRES, V.E., HOLLEY, K.E. and OFFORD, K.P. (1985). Epidemiology of adult polycystic kidney disease. In *Proceedings of Internal Workshop on Polycystic Kidney Disease: Problems in Diagnosis and Management.* Kansas City; Polycystic Kidney Research Foundation (in press)

TSAI, S.Y. and SHIMIZU, A.G. (1975). Spontaneous perirenal hemorrhage in patients on hemodialysis. *Urology,* **5,** 523–525

TUTTLE, R.J., MINIELLY, J.A. and FAY, W.P. (1971). Spontaneous renal hemorrhage in chronic glomerular nephritis and dialysis. *Radiology,* **98,** 137–138

VANICHAYAKORNKUL, S., CIOFFI, R.F., HARPER, E., O'CONNELL, J.M.B. and SHALHOUB, R.J. (1974). Spontaneous retroperitoneal hematoma: a complication of hemodialysis. *Journal of the American Medical Association,* **230,** 1164–1165

VELA NAVARRETE, R. and GARCIA ROBLEDO, A. (1982). Identification nosológica de la enfermedad poliquística del seno renal: datos clínicos, analíticos y estructurales. *Revista Clínica Española,* **166,** 15–22

VELA NAVARRETE, R. and GARCIA ROBLEDO, A. (1983). Polycystic disease of the renal sinus: structural characteristics. *Journal of Urology,* **129,** 700–703

VELA NAVARRETE, R., GARCIA DE LA PEÑA, E., VILLALOBOS, C.A. and DELATTE, L.C. (1973). Quistes no nefrogenicos del seno renal: expresividad radiográfica y consideraciones diagnósticas. *Revista Clinica Española,* **132,** 29–39

VESTBY, G.W. (1967). Percutaneous needle puncture of renal cysts: new methods in therapeutic management. *Investigative Radiology,* **2,** 449–462

WAKABAYASHI, T., FUJITA, S., OHBORA, Y. *et al.* (1983). Polycystic kidney disease and intracranial aneurysms: early angiographic diagnosis and early operation for the unruptured aneurysm. *Journal of Neurosurgery,* **58,** 488–491

WALKER, D., FENNELL, R., GARIN, E. and RICHARD, G. (1978). Spectrum of multicystic renal dysplasia. *Urology,* **11,** 133–146

WALTERS, W. and BRAASCH, W.F. (1934). Surgical aspects of polycystic kidney. *Surgery, Gynecology and Obstetrics,* **58,** 647–650

WARD, J.N., DRAPER, J.W. and LAVENGOOD, R.W., Jr. (1967). A clinical review of polycystic kidney disease in 53 patients. *Journal of Urology,* **98,** 48–53

WERDER, A.A., AMOS, M.A., NIELSEN, A.H. and WOLFE, G.H. (1984). Comparative effects of germfree and ambient environments on the development of cystic kidney disease in CFW sd mice. *Journal of Laboratory and Clinical Medicine,* **103,** 399–407

WIEBERS, D.O., WHISNANT, J.P. and O'FALLON, W.M. (1981). The natural history of unruptured intracranial aneurysms. *New England Journal of Medicine,* **304,** 696–698

WILLIAMS, G., BLANDY, J.P. and TRESIDDER, G.C. (1968). Communicating cysts and diverticula of the renal pelvis. *British Journal of Urology,* **41,** 163–170

WILLIAMSON, B., Jr., HARTMAN, G.W., CHARBONEAU, J.W., JOHNSON, C.M., BROWN, M.L. *et al.* (1985). Diagnostic imaging of renal masses: an update. *Archives of Clinical Imaging* (in press)

WRIGLEY, K.A., SHERMAN, R.L., ENNIS, F.A. and BECKER, E.L. (1973). Progressive hereditary nephropathy: a variant of medullary cystic disease? *Archives of Internal Medicine,* **131,** 240–244

YENDT, E.R. (1982). Medullary sponge kidney and nephrolithiasis. *New England Journal of Medicine,* **306,** 1106–1107

Chapter 18

Renal malignancies in the elderly

Juan Montero Gomez, Manuel Urrutia Avisrror and Juan Corrales Hernandez

Introduction

In general, the incidence of tumours rises with age, at least until 80 years, when thereafter there may be a true fall-off in the incidence of total cancers. Given the aging of the Western population as a whole, a high proportion of patients with malignant tumours will be over the age of 60 at diagnosis.

Some 2 per cent of all cancer deaths in the USA arise from carcinoma of the kidney, the great majority in older individuals. Thus, renal tumours are an important topic among renal diseases of the elderly. Renal carcinomata may be very slow growing, and the presentation is commonly non-specific or through some paraneoplastic syndrome. For this reason, underdiagnosis or late diagnosis of renal tumours in the elderly is a frequent finding.

Most of the malignancies of the kidney in the elderly are represented by the epithelial tumours derived from the tubular tissue and those tumours arising from the mucous membrane lining the pelvic and calyces. Less common are the mesenchymal tumours, accounting for only 2–3 per cent of all malignant renal tumours. In this group leiomyosarcoma is by far the most frequently observed, but with no more than 100 cases reported in the medical literature. Other mesenchymal tumours include rhabdomyosarcoma, liposarcoma, osteogenic carcinoma, fibroxanthosarcoma and primary malignant lymphoma.

Unlike some other authors, on the basis of their distinct anatomical and histological origin as well as the clear differentiation in their aetiological and pathogenetic features, we consider in this review adenocarcinoma of the kidney and cancer of the renal pelvis as separate entities. For both tumours, an updated description of their most outstanding clinical and diagnostic features as well as a detailed exposition of the different therapeutic options are developed. For renal adenocarcinoma, a special section is devoted to an analysis of the experience of our group in the newest and promising field of steroid hormone receptors, with special regard to their possible value as a parameter for assessing the benefits that could be expected from the hormonal treatment and as a prognostic statement for the disease.

Epidemiology

In the past, most major epidemiological surveys used to group the malignant tumours of the kidney together with malignant tumours from the renal pelvis, under the common denomination of 'upper urinary tract tumours'.

This trend has been modified in recent years, rendering more information available to clinicians as to the influence of age, sex, race and environmental and geographical factors for the prevalence of each histological type.

Age

The incidence of renal adenocarcinoma is closely related to age, and as with prostatic cancer could be regarded as a process associated with aging.

Figures taken from standarized cancer rates per 100 000 (population (1.5/ 100 000, all ages) show that prior to the third decade epithelial cancers of the kidney are rare, but after this age there is a steady increase in frequency with each passing decade.

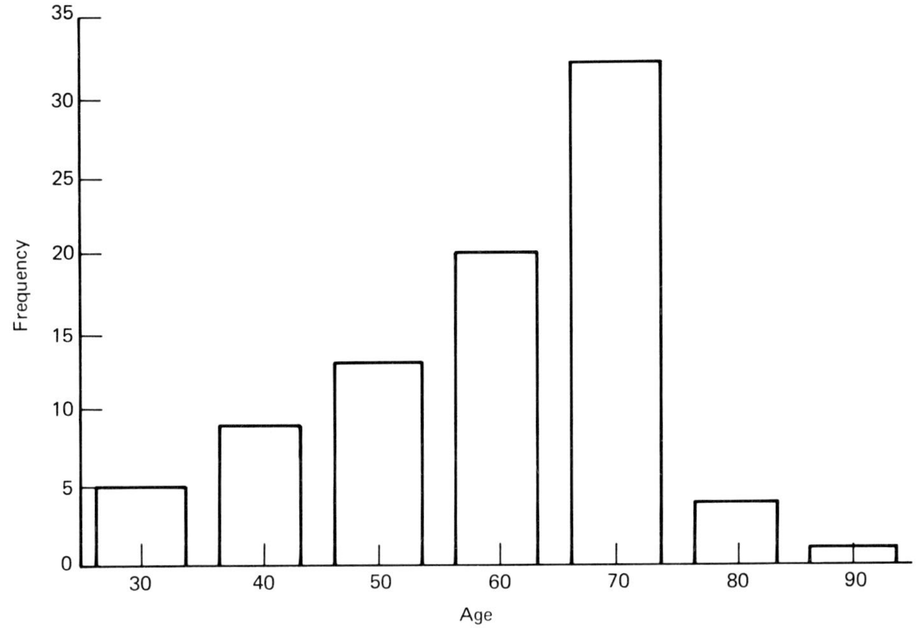

Figure 18.1 Age distribution of 84 cases of renal adenocarcinoma studied in the Urology Department of the Hospital Clinico Universitario of Salamanca

If data are taken from a non-standardized population, the percentage of distribution by age groups has a peak at the seventh decade, appearing as if the disease decreased after 70 years (*Figure 18.1*). This represents a biased estimation, due to a significant decrease of the population after that age and, probably, by less accurate diagnosis in the older patients.

Sex

The different reported series reveal that the incidence of renal adenocarcinoma is 2.5–3 times as great in males as in females, after compensating the cumulative frequency curves for more females in the population. The male:female ratio remains constant up to the fifth decade and after menopause tends to increase, reaching a ratio of 4:1

Race and geographical distribution

Unlike prostatic cancer, the racial factor does not seem to play a major role for adenocarcinoma of the kidney. Epidemiologic studies in countries like the USA, whose population is from different origins, have demonstrated only minor fluctuations in the incidence rate among the different ethnic groups.

The participation of an environmental factor may be indirectly deduced comparing the mortality rates from renal malignancies in different countries (Paganini-Hill, Ross and Henderson, 1983), which permits a clear distinction of three different groups: (1) countries showing high rates, such as Denmark, Scotland, Norway and New Zealand; (b) countries with low rates, such as Ireland, Italy, Japan and Spain; (c) countries with an intermediate incidence, such as the USA, England, France, Holland, Belgium, Wales and Australia.

It seems obvious, with the only exception of Japan and Italy, that the highest frequencies of malignant tumours of the kidney are found in the industrialized countries and appear to be associated with urbanization, food intake, habits and exposure to different industrial carcinogenic agents.

Heredity

Genetic factors are known to play a definite role in rats, mice and rhesus monkeys (Ratcliffe, 1940). In humans, the theories of a genetic determinant, especially in cases of bilateral tumours, are supported by several observations of renal adenocarcinomas in different members of the same family throughout consecutive generations (Brinton, 1960) and its high incidence in subjects with blood group A. They have also been reported in association with certain hereditary diseases, such as polycystic disease, von Hippel–Lindau disease and with colour blindness (Griffin, Hughes and Peeling, 1967).

Aetiology

In recent years, many agents have been postulated as possible aetiological factors in renal adenocarcinoma. At the present time, most of them have been convincingly demonstrated to play an important role for experimental carcinogenesis in different animal models but, unfortunately, the problem of the aetiology of renal cancer in humans remains still unsolved.

Physical agents

Whole-body irradiation with X-rays and fast neutrons induces renal adenocarcinoma in mice and rats (Guerin, Chouroulinikov and Riviere, 1969). In humans, the only radioactive product known to induce renal adenocarcinoma and squamous cell carcinomas of the pelvis is thorotrast, a weak alpha emitter utilized many decades ago as a radio-opaque substance for pyelographic studies (Alken *et al.*, 1960; Ruiz-Marcellan *et al.*, 1979).

Chemical agents

Since the induction of the first experimental adenocarcinoma in rats by systemic administration of beta-anthraquinoline (Sempronj and Morelli, 1939), it has been demonstrated that several exogenous chemical carcinogens have the capability to produce malignant renal tumours in various laboratory animals, which appear to be the counterpart of spontaneous human renal adenocarcinoma.

The long list of these substances include aromatic hydrocarbons, aliphatic compounds, aromatic amines and amides, metals, anti-cancer chemotherapeutic agents and natural compounds. Special attention is drawn to the N-nitroso compounds, e.g. dimethylnitrosamine, and some metals, like cadmium and lead. The former is known to be a potent oncogenic agent in rats and other animal species, and is widely employed in the rubber and textile industries.

Recent epidemiologic studies reveal that chronic exposure to cadmium, as may occur in the manufacture of almost all industrial products, is associated with a relatively high incidence of both renal and prostatic cancer (Pavone-Macaluso, 1983).

Lead poisoning has also been incriminated as a possible inducing agent and would explain the higher incidence of renal cancer in urban than in rural areas. This hypothesis is supported by the experimental induction of renal tumours in rats fed with lead acetate (Van Esch and Kroes, 1969). This fact has also been observed in wild rats living in suburban areas whose soil, because of contamination from the surrounding industries, has a high lead content. In humans, however, follow-up studies of workers exposed to lead vapour inhalation have failed to demonstrate a significant greater incidence of malignant renal tumours than in the general population.

Aflotoxins B_1 and B_2 produced by the fungus *Aspergillus flavus* are also to be considered in the aetiology of human renal tumours, since they contaminate a variety of foodstuffs and contain lactone moieties capable of producing renal adenocarcinoma and pelvic carcinoma in rats (Epstein, Bartus and Farber, 1969). Other natural compounds identified as potent renal carcinogens are cyscain, streptozotocin, daunomycin and ochratoxin A.

The role of endogenous carcinogens such as tryptophan metabolites, which are involved in the induction of urothelial tumours, is a hypothesis still to be investigated, since only one case of adenocarcinoma of the kidney, without further confirmation, has been reported in association with increased urinary excretion of this product (Kerr *et al.*, 1963).

Hormones

Prolonged administration of large doses of oestrogens is known to produce renal adenomas and adenocarcinomas in male and castrated female hamsters (Kirkman, 1959). Production of the tumour is inhibited by concurrent administration of testosterone, progesterone, deoxycorticosterone, bromoergocryptine, 20-methylcholanthrene and nafoxidine, and the induction period is shortened if the animals undergo unilateral nephrectomy before oestrogen treatment.

Tumours so induced are histologically similar to adenocarcinomata of the human kidney and provide a unique tumour model in the absence of naturally occurring renal adenocarcinomas. In hamsters, the resistance of the species to induction of renal tumours by physical and chemical agents makes their induction all the more striking.

Human renal adenocarcinoma is considered to be a hormone-dependent tumour on the basis of its higher frequency in males than females, and the recent finding of hormone receptors in normal kidney tissue and renal tumours. However, positive facts obtained with hormonal manipulation in both oestrogen-dependent and oestrogen-independent animal models have been challenged with rather poor results obtained using hormonal treatment in humans; therefore, its relationship with the hormonal environment remains a controversial issue.

Viruses

A herpes simplex virus has been identified as the aetiological agent of a well-differentiated adenocarcinoma in the North American leopard frog (Granoff, 1973). Renal tumours with a sarcomatous pattern can also be produced by the adenovirus-7, the polyoma virus and the SV 40 virus in some species of rodents. Although herpes simplex virus specific antigens have been identified in human renal tumours, this finding is far from representing the demonstration of the viral aetiology of kidney adenocarcinoma.

Habits

Smoking is the only risk factor which has been consistently linked to cancer of the kidney, in several epidemiologic studies. The risk is also greater for pipe and cigar smokers. The mechanism by which this habit might induce kidney cancer is unclear, but the possible participation of the numerous carcinogens present in the smoke, especially N-nitroso compounds, has been considered. The greater use of tobacco by men may account in part for the observed sex differentiation in the frequency of the disease, and it could be expected that with increased smoking by females the sex ratio should begin to fall.

Heavy usage of phenacetin-containing analgesgics is a well-documented risk factor for transitional cell carcinoma of the pelvis and it has been demonstrated that persons taking analgesics on a daily basis have a tenfold risk of developing adenocarinoma, compared to those who never use the drugs (Armstrong, Garrod and Doll, 1976).

Coffee consumption as an aetiological factor for adenocarcinoma deserves to be re-examined, taking into account that this habit is closely related to smoking and the use of artificial sweeteners.

Pathologic features

Histogenesis of renal adenocarcinoma was the subject of controversy for nearly 70 years, until Oberling, Riviere and Haguenau (1960), by a combination of immunofluorescent and ultrastructural studies, demonstrated its unequivocal origin from epithelial cells of the proximal convoluted tubule of the nephron.

The term 'renal adenocarcinoma' is considered to be sufficiently descriptive of the epithelial origin of the tumour, but in the medical literature, terms like 'Grawitz' tumour and 'hypernephroma', as it is often called, testify to the long-held misconception of its histogenetic origin.

Another controversial topic is the so-called 'renal adenoma', a term arbitrarily applied to well-differentiated epithelial tumours less than 3 cm in greatest diameter. This size-based definition arises from Bell's original publication (Bell, 1950) which showed that renal cortical epithelial tumours less than 3 cm in diameter rarely metastasize. This misconception disregards the fact that in his series two tumours less than 2 cm in diameter had metastasized, and a large percentage of tumours greater than 10 cm had not. Additionally, as Bennington and Kradjian (1967) claim, there are no proven, gross, histologic, histochemical, immunologic or ultrastructural features which will reliably distinguish a renal adenocarcinoma from what is supposed to be its benign counterpart. For this reason, the most recent definition of renal adenoma applies to well-differentiated, encapsulated tumours, devoid of haemorrhage and necrosis and unlikely to metastasize.

Renal adenocarcinoma occurs with equal frequency in either kidney and bilateral tumours are found in 0.5–1.5 per cent of patients. There is no predilection for the distribution in any portion of the kidney, although the middle portion is somewhat more commonly affected.

The size of the tumour is, in general terms, directly related to the presence and duration of symptoms and histological grade. Irrespective of size, the gross appearance is of an irregular, greyish, often haemorrhagic, bosselated mass, that in large tumours protrudes from the renal cortex.

The cut surface has a lobulated appearance, varying according to the vascularization and histological type. The surface is glistening and yellow in the clear cell type (*Figure 18.2*) and grey in the sarcomatoid one. In large tumours, the blood supply is outgrown by the mass, and degenerative changes appear as necrotic areas of gelatinous, cystic or fibrous aspect. Some tumours may be totally or predominantly cystic as a result of extensive central necrosis.

At the periphery, the renal parenchyma is compressed, forming a pseudocapsule of condensed connective tissue. Invasion of the main renal vein and infiltration of

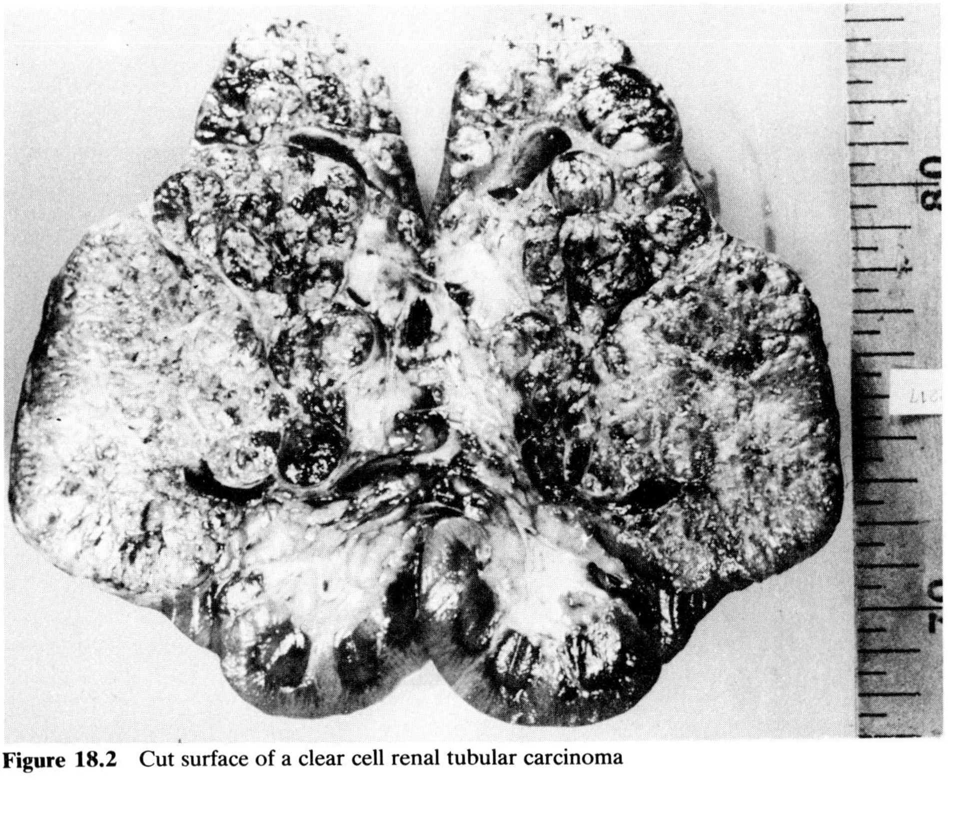

Figure 18.2 Cut surface of a clear cell renal tubular carcinoma

the calyces and pelvis is a common feature in advanced tumours. Casts of tumour thrombi may extend into the lumen of the inferior vena cava, sometimes reaching up the level of the right atrium.

The overall histological patterns found in renal adenocarcinoma are variable and they may change from area to area in the same growth. The tumour may be composed of three different cell types, which are fairly uniform in appearance. The most frequent are relatively large cells with a clear cytoplasm due to a high content of lipids and glycogen. The cells have a polygonal, cubical or columnar form; the nuclei are characteristically small, round-shaped and have a dense and evenly distributed chromatin. Another type are cells whose cytoplasm is brightly eosinophilic and granular, due to the large content of organelles, principally mitochondria. In some cases, the least in frequency, the bulk of the tumour is formed by fusiform cells arranged in an irregular fashion and intermixed with a collagenous stroma and may be erroneously interpreted as rhabdomyosarcoma or fibrosarcoma (*Figure 18.3*).

The fibrous stroma of the tumour is richly vascular and contains foam cells and scattered foci of calcification. Characteristically, in areas of necrosis cholesterol clefts surrounded by foreign body giant cells are found.

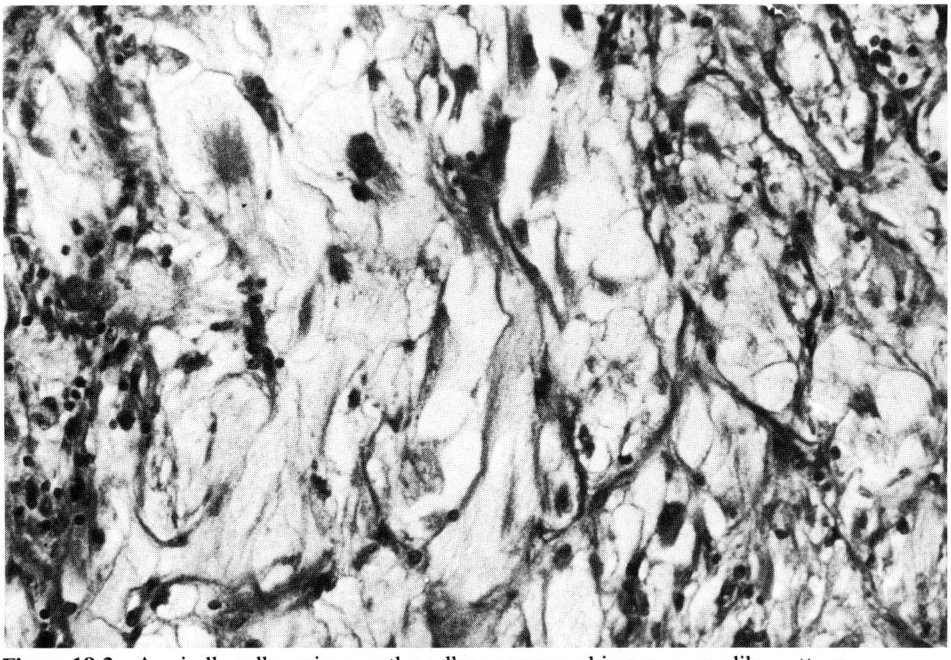

Figure 18.3 A spindle cell carcinoma; the cells are arranged in a sarcoma-like pattern

Renal adenocarcinoma spreads via three main routes: lymphogenous, haematogenous and lymphohaematogenous. Advanced tumours also spread by direct extension through the renal capsule to adjacent structures. Lymphogenous spread implies primarily the proximal regional lymph nodes and less frequently other retroperitoneal, abdominal, mediastinal, supraclavicular, cervical, axillary and inguinal lymph nodes. Haematogenous spread is more important in renal adenocarcinoma than for most other cancers and accounts for the many unusual sites of metastases observed; systemic involvement is preceded by a primary extension of the tumour into the renal vein with further dissemination to the lungs and axial skeleton by way of Batson's plexus; the pelvic structures are involved by retrograde flow via the left spermatic or ovarian vein. After bypassing the pulmonary circulation, the tumour cells may gain access to multiple organs and tissues by the arterial circulation. Besides the lungs and regional lymph nodes, the organs involved by decreasing frequency are liver, bones, adrenal glands, contralateral kidney, brain, heart, spleen, intestinal tract and skin. Metastases to breast and other organs, like tonsils, vagina, orbit, tongue, larynx and thyroid have also been reported and in some cases may simulate primary carcinoma of these organs. In lymphohaematogenous spread, the tumour cells reach the lung via the thoracic duct, bypassing the liver.

The frequency of direct extension of the tumour and distant metastases appears to be directly related to the size of the primary tumour. It has been reported that at time of nephrectomy 40 per cent of the patients have capsular invasion, 36 per cent renal vein invasion and approximately 40 per ent distant metastases, unsuspected prior to surgery (Riches, Griffiths and Thackray, 1951).

The microscopic features of the tumour, i.e. clear, granular or spindle cell carcinoma, and the degree of differentiation helps very few in assessing prognostic statements, although different groups of workers have attempted to correlate it with nuclear grade, size and growth pattern (Petkovic, 1959; Rauschmeier *et al.*, 1983).

Table 18.1 Renal adenocarcinoma: pathological findings (n = 84)

Affected side:		
right	40	47.6%
left	44	52.4%
Location:		
upper	25	29.8%
middle	31	36.9%
lower	28	33.3%
Cell type:		
clear	75	89.3%
granular	6	7.1%
spindle	3	3.6%
Histological type:		
solid	32	38.1%
tubular	26	31.1%
papillary	15	17.8%
mixed	11	13.1%
Cell differentiation:		
well diff.	53	63.1%
moderate–poorly diff.	31	36.9%

In our series, there is a predominance of clear cell type tumours, with a 63.1 per cent of well-differentiated cells and 36.9 per cent ranging from intermediate to poorly differentiated. For statistical purposes, the last two are grouped together as a single histological type. The most outstanding gross and microscopic findings are presented in *Table 18.1*

Symptoms and clinical findings

In many medical textbooks, adenocarcinoma of the kidney is usually referred to as the 'internist's tumour' or the 'great imitator in medicine', based on the known fact that most of the early presenting symptoms are non-urological. The often-mentioned classical triad of haematuria, flank pain and palpable mass is only found in about 11-16 per cent of the patients and is always indicative of advanced disease, half of these patients already having distant metastases at the time of the diagnosis. Nevertheless, all of the above-mentioned symptoms are observed as isolated features in more than 50 per cent of the patients and an association of two is reported in about one-third, thus giving a global incidence which is comparatively higher than in any other non-urological symptoms (*Table 18.2*).

Table 18.2 Renal adenocarcinoma: clinical findings (n = 84)

Haematuria	52	62.0%
Pain	48	57.0%
Palpable mass	22	26.0%
Fever	12	14.0%
Hypertension	8	9.5%
Increased ESR	32	38.0%
Anaemia	38	45.0%
Thrombocytosis	10	12.0%
Hypercalcaemia	2	2.3%
Hepatic dysfunction	3	3.6%

Haematuria in our series was the initial symptom in 62 per cent of the patients. This symptom is produced by extension of the tumour into the lumen of the excretory or intrarenal circulation. Characteristically, haematuria in renal tumour is painless, total and intermittent in nature; usually it is gross, although instances of microhaematuria can also be observed. These semeiotic features may help to differentiate it on a clinical basis from haematuria whose origin is the bladder or another organ of the lower urinary tract. Sometimes, worm-like clots corresponding to casts of the ureteric wall can be identified in freshly voided urine, and represent a valuable sign which suggests its origin in some point of the upper urinary tract. As a general rule in clinical practice, *any haematuria with these features should be considered a renal tumour until otherwise demonstrated.*

Pain is a late and inconstant symptom, especially in older patients. The reported incidence as an isolated symptom ranges from 20 per cent to more than 45 per cent of patients. Dull and continuous pain is the most frequent modality and is due to distension of the renal capsule or compression and traction of perinephric structures. In gross significant haematuria, passing clots may lead to acute ureteric obstruction and give symptoms simulating a typical renal colic. In this instance, a differential feature is given by the fact that in acute ureteric obstruction by urinary calculous disease haematuria is preceded by pain, whereas in renal cancer pain, if present, it always follows haematuria.

A *palpable mass* is also a late symptom and usually indicates an advanced stage of the disease. The estimates of the frequency of this symptom in patients with renal adenocarcinoma varies from less than 6 per cent to over 50 per cent, but clinicians must bear in mind that the incidental discovery of a flank mass is a *very* rare event and only possible in lean patients with large tumours arising at the lower pole of the kidney.

Acute *varicocele* due to spermatic or caval vein obstruction by a tumour thrombus is another companion symptom of renal carcinoma, and it should always lead to the search for a renal tumour in the absence of other major symptoms.

Although local or distant metastases are present in about one-third of the patients at the time of the diagnosis, no more than 5 per cent have presenting symptoms directly related to metastases. Solitary soft tissue metastases may involve most organs of the body, giving several non-specific symptoms: paraplegia, pathological fractures, vaginal bleeding, melana, priapism, etc. For similar reasons, physical findings other than a flank mass do not suggest the diagnosis of a renal tumour in the context of an otherwise asymptomatic patient. Physical findings include, among others, hepatomegaly, oedema of the lower extremities, thyroid and skin nodules, enlarged left supraclavicular lymph nodes, and pulsating bony masses.

As previously mentioned, adenocarcinoma of the kidney may have its clinical debut with a relatively large variety of early non-specific signs and symptoms, that may be found alone or in combination and sometimes associated with a large spectrum of abnormal laboratory findings.

Non-specific systemic manifestations of renal cancer are known to be dependent on some kind of humoral or endocrine activity, since they may disappear with nephrectomy and may reappear with the development of metastases. If they are detected in an otherwise asymptomatic patient, they can also act as valuable clinical markers.

These paraneoplastic syndromes have been classified in three main groups on the basis of either the principal abnormality or the aetiology. Because of their clinical interest, they are treated to some extent in the next paragraphs.

Non-specific syndromes

Metabolic syndromes

Asthenia, anorexia and weight loss. This triad is a common feature in all malignant tumours that seems to be related to either a systemic toxic effect, as result of the liberation of an unknown factor by the tumour cells, or a side effect secondary to the immunologic reaction of the host. Severe pain, intestinal obstruction and a specific malabsorption mechanism may also be involved in the presentation of these symptoms.

Fever. Pyrexia in association with renal tumour has been observed in 14 per cent of our patients, although some series have reported a higher incidence (Marshall and Walsh, 1977). We believe that it must always be considered as a bad prosnostic sign.

The occurrence of fever seems to depend upon an endogenous pyrogen secreted by the tumour cells, or leucocytes within the tumour (Rawlins, Luff and Cranston, 1970). Characteristically, fever disappears after nephrectomy; its persistence or recurrence after radical operation is almost always indicative of residual tumour or the development of metastases.

Haematological syndromes

Anaemia. The incidence of anaemia in our series was 45 per cent. Anaemia is usually of the normochromic, normocytic type and its aetiology remains still unclear. The possibility of a micro-angiopathic haemolytic anaemia can be discarded if one takes into account the normal to high levels of serum haptoglobin found in these patients; even more, an extrarenal triad consisting of fever, anaemia and hyperhaptoglobinaemia has been described in association with renal adenocarcinoma (Bowman and Martinez, 1968). Ferrokinetic patterns found in patients with non-metastatic renal carcinoma are quite similar to those observed in chronic disease and share some features of ineffective erythropoiesis.

Increased erythrocyte sedimentation rate. A raised ESR is a common and non-specific finding in renal adenocarcinoma, as in other types of malignancies and in chronic inflammatory diseases. The supposed correlation of ESR levels with the tumour cell type has not been confirmed so far in our observations.

Other haematological syndromes described in association with renal adenocarcinoma include thrombocytosis, thrombocytopenia, leukaemoid reactions and disorders of coagulation.

Biochemical syndromes

Reversible hepatic dysfunction. Stauffer (1961) first reported a syndrome characterized by non-metastatic hepatic dysfunction in patients with renal adenocarcinoma. The clinical and biochemical manifestations of this syndrome include: (a) non-tender non-nodular hepatomegaly; (b) normal levels of serum bilirubin; (c) increased alkaline phosphatase; (d) increased bromosulphthalein retention; (e) hypoprothrombinaemia; (f) increased alpha-2 globulin levels. Histologic examination of the liver reveals non-specific mild reactive hepatitis, characterized by Kupffer cell hyperplasia with or without fatty change. Although an increased lysosomal activity in liver tissue has been postulated to explain these changes, its pathogenesis remains uncertain.

At the beginning, this syndrome was considered to be specific of renal adenocarcinoma, but so far it has also been reported in association with gastrointestinal tract malignancies and xanthogranulomatous pyelonephritis. We have observed a similar syndrome in two patients with prostatic cancer and bone metastases. The chemical and morphologic abnormalities return to normal after nephrectomy in the absence of metastases.

Specific syndromes related to endocrine or humoral activity

Hypertension. The role of renin hypersecretion in systemic hypertension observed in some patients with renal tumour remains controversial since its frequency is about that expected for the age group and is not greater than in patients without renal disease or with benign lesions. Nevertheless, there are clinical instances of hypertension associated with elevated serum renin levels that are relieved by nephrectomy. Renin elevation unrelated to blood pressure has also been reported in one-third of patients with high grade and high stage tumours; this feature seems to be associated with a poor prognosis (Sufrin *et al.*, 1977). Polycythaemia, arteriovenous shunts and hypercalcaemia are other factors suggested to contribute to hypertension.

Polycythaemia. Renal adenocarcinoma is but one among the various clinical conditions that may be associated with erythrocytosis, leukocytosis and thrombocytosis, either alone or in combination, due to an increased secretion of erythropoietin or an erythropoietin-like substance. The estimated incidence of polycythaemia in renal adneocarcinoma ranges from 1.8 to 6 per cent of all cases, a rather low figure taking into account that up to 63 per cent of patients may have raised levels of this enzyme (Sufrin *et al.*, 1977).

Different mechanisms have been postulated to explain the elevated levels of erythropoietin in renal carcinoma: local ischaemia, mechanical stimulation by the tumour growth of juxtaglomerular apparatus, ectopic production by the tumour cells of erythropoietin or an erythropoietin-like substance, and substrate activation by a substance produced by the tumour cells. Recurrence with the development of metastases after nephrectomy excludes ischaemia and mechanical stimulation as factors promoting the increased levels of erythropoietin in renal adenocarcinoma.

Hypercalcaemia. Production by the tumour of a substance indistinguishable antigenically from parathormone might explain elevated serum levels found in some patients, in the absence of osteolytic bony metastases. Evidence that prostaglandins of the A and E series might also play an important role have been reported by Brereton *et al.* (1974). Hypercalcaemia may present as an isolated laboratory finding or be associated with a severe, rapidly progressive, occasionally fatal clinical syndrome with symptoms of polyuria, polydypsia, dysphagia, constipation, muscular weakness, mental depression and hypokalaemic alkalosis. Serum levels return to normal after nephrectomy and reappear with the development of metastases.

Other endocrine syndromes observed in renal carcinoma are associated with ectopic production of different hypophyseal hormones and include Cushing's syndrome, galactorrhoea, male feminization and female masculinization. Their evidence has been based only on the regression of the symptoms after nephrectomy.

Miscellaneous syndromes

A broad range of clinical entities have been linked with renal adenocarcinoma. Only a few of them have been specifically correlated to the development of the tumour, whereas others seem to be coincidental associations. The first group include amyloidosis, neuromyopathy, salt-losing nephritis and gastrointestinal disorders. They have been extensively reviewed elsewhere and hence a further description of their clinical features is omitted in this chapter.

Biological markers

Besides the biochemical changes associated with the specific paraneoplastic syndromes mentioned above, other substances may also show increased values in serum concentrations in renal adenocarcinoma. They include carcino-embryonic antigen, acute phase reactant proteins, urinary polyamines and prostaglandins. None of these substances has proven diagnostic reliability, but they might play a role in detecting relapses and monitoring the reponse to treatment. In our experience, increased serum activity of alkaline phosphatase in the absence of a concomitant hepatic disease is the best non-specific biological marker for the detection of early bone metastases, since at least 40–45 per cent of bone structural involvement is needed to become evident on radiological examination. Its reliability is increased to almost absolute levels if combined with radionuclide scanning with ^{99m}Tc diphosphonate (Urrutia *et al.,* 1977).

Diagnosis of renal adenocarcinoma

The most important factor in the diagnosis of renal tumours in the elderly is a high level of suspicion, especially in those with haematuria and renal masses.

The introduction of new non-invasive techniques, represented by radionuclide scanning, ultrasonography and computed tomography (CT), has increased the preoperative diagnostic accuracy of malignant renal tumours almost to absolute levels, and has promoted the development of different algorithms which are claimed by their respective authors as the best tools for the differential diagnosis of renal masses.

Herein we describe the sequential procedure utilized in our own department, which has a diagnostic accuracy that approaches 100 per cent, and has been designed to maximize the diagnostic reliability while minimizing the costs and discomfort to the patient. A diagnostic flow chart of renal masses is given in *Figure 18.4.*

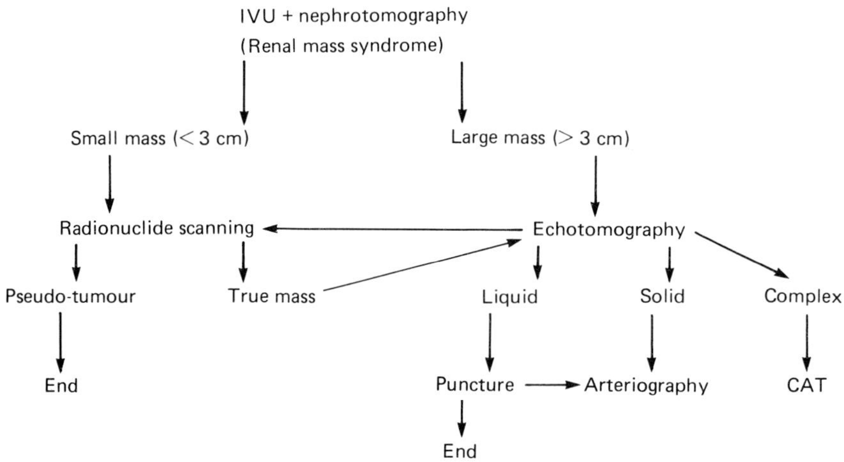

Figure 18.4 Diagnostic flow chart of renal masses

Plain films of the abdomen and combined infusion *excretory urography* with nephrotomography give by themselves several signs which are characteristic enough for detecting a mass developed in the kidney and to assess whether it is solid or liquid. To minimize the possibility of missing a mass that involves the anterior or posterior surface of the kidney, radiographs should always be obtained in oblique as well as the standard anteroposterior projections.

All renal masses produce distortion of the renal contour and/or the collecting system (*Figure 18.5*). At nephrotomography, simple renal cysts appear as a lucent mass sharply demarcated from the adjacent renal parenchyma and surrounded by a thin wall, if at least 25 per cent of the mass extends beyond the renal cortex. At the site where the cyst bulges through the kidney surface, the parenchyma has a typical triangular 'beak-like' shape (*Figure 18.6*); this sign is still considered in many textbooks as pathognomonic of a benign renal cyst, but we have observed it in poorly vascularized and slow-growing tumours. Small and central cysts are not clearly visualized at nephrotomography and require other, more sensitive methods for their diagnosis.

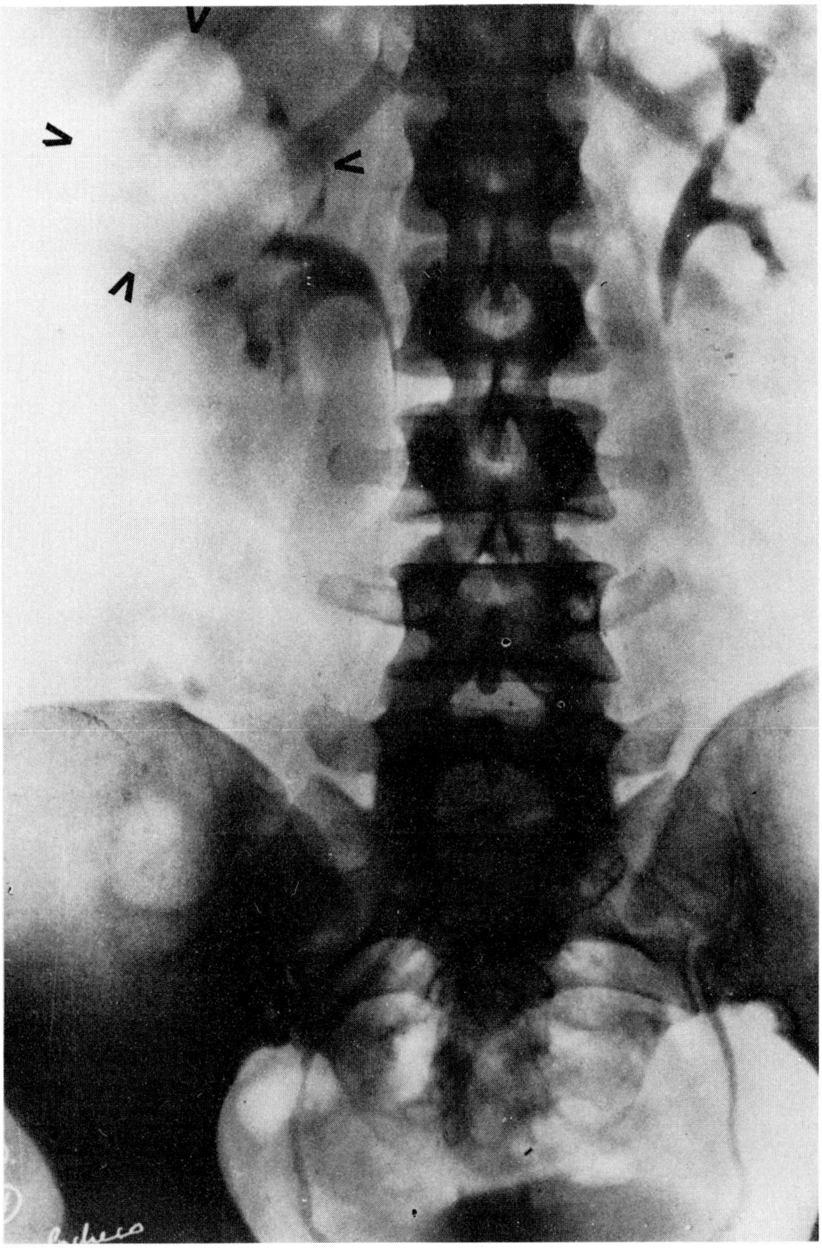

Figure 18.5 An intravenous urogram showing a mass at the upper pole of the kidney (arrows) with calyceal distortion

A solid mass must be suspected if calcifications with a mottled pattern are observed in the plain films and urography shows an irregularly shaped mass whose density increases in successive films. Necrotic tumours or abscesses have a translucent centre with a thick wall, and usually lack the 'beak sign'. Calyceal

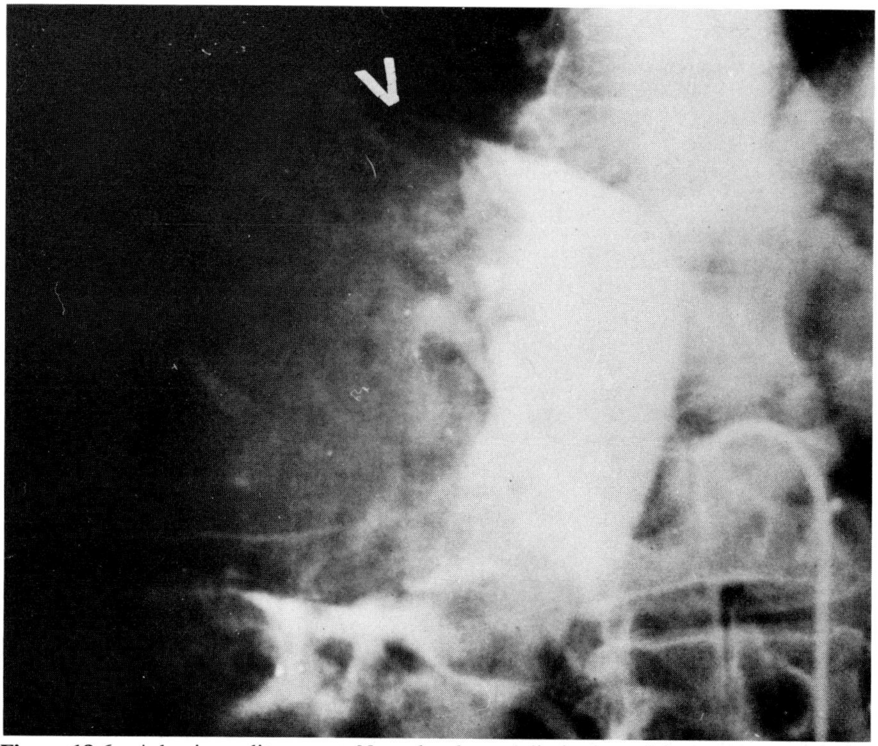

Figure 18.6 A benign solitary cyst. Note the sharp delimitation of the mass and the 'beak sign'

amputation is another radiological feature characteristic of malignant renal tumours, and is never observed in simple renal cysts.

Once a mass is identified, the steps to follow depend upon its size and radiological appearance. In small masses we perform first a *radionuclide scanning* with ^{99m}Tc DTPA, which helps to differentiate true renal masses from different clinical entities known as renal pseudo-tumours, that are due to congenital structural anomalies or hypertrophied renal tissue. Congenital pseudo-tumours include atypical persistent fetal lobation, septa of Bertin and protrusion of the upper lip of the renal hilum associated with accessory renal arteries. Acquired pseudo-tumours are observed in kidneys with chronic pyelonephritis and extensive scarring as nodules of hypertrophied tissue that bulges from the surrounding contracted parenchyma. Radionuclides are concentrated by renal pseudo-tumours since they are composed of normal functioning renal tissue, and do not need further exploration. True masses are identified by the absence of isotopic activity (*Figure 18.7*), but we must consider the possibility of false negatives since the minimal resolution level is within the range of 2–2.5 cm in diameter.

As congenital pseudo-tumours are unlikely to give prominent radiological signs, masses greater than 3 cm in diameter are explored with *grey scale nephrosonography* as a second step after excretory urography. This method is highly sensitive to differentiate solid tissue from fluid. A liquid mass, as occurs in simple renal cysts (*Figure 18.8*), can be identified in B-mode scan by three main features: (a) they are sonolucent, even at high gain settings; (b) the far wall has a sharply defined appearance as a smooth curved line; (c) the density of echoes from

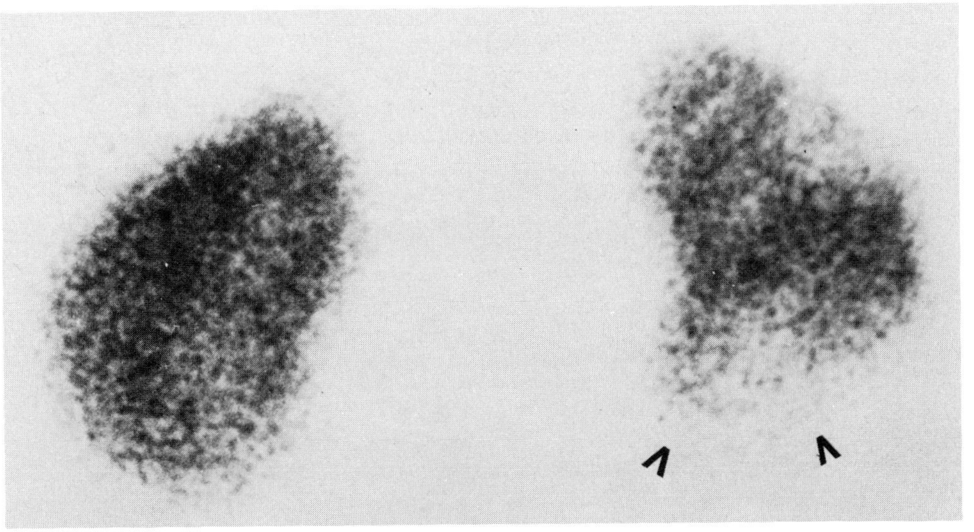

Figure 18.7 ^{99m}Tc DTPA radionuclide scan of a true mass at the lower pole of the left kidney (arrows). There is also a 'cold spot' near the upper pole

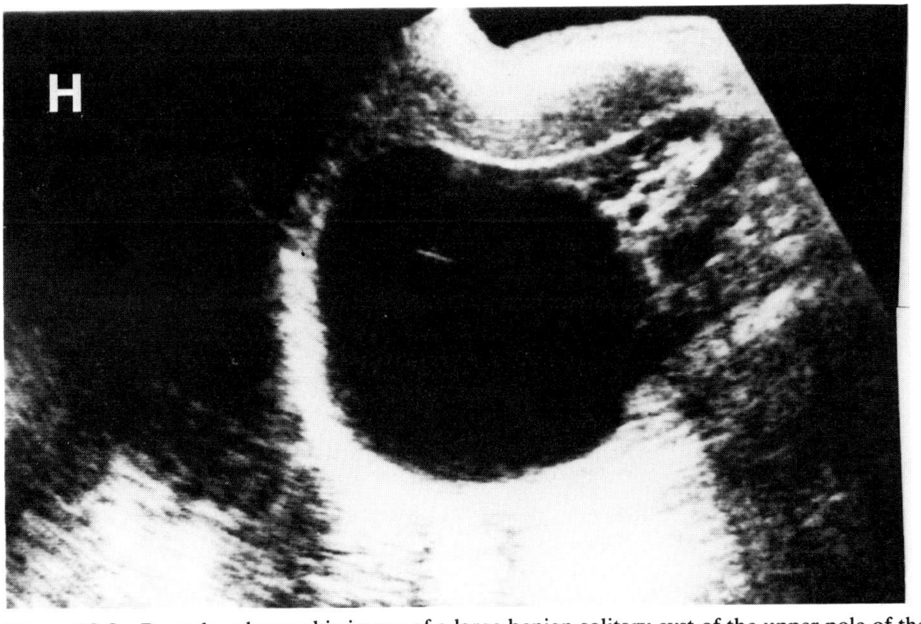

Figure 18.8 B-mode echographic image of a large benign solitary cyst of the upper pole of the kidney; H indicates the head end of the patient

the back wall have a characteristic acoustic enhancement, whose intensity is directly related to the cyst diameter. Since the diagnostic reliability of a cystic pattern with sonography is approximately 95 per cent, to avoid the 5 per cent possibility of a non-cyst mass being overlooked, we are of the opinion that cyst puncture with ultrasound guidance should always be performed for diagnostic confirmation. The combination of cyst aspiration, chemical and cytological studies of the aspirate and double contrast cystography has an accuracy that approaches 100 per cent and, hence, the exploration can be stopped.

Solid masses are identified by two main sonographic signs: (a) attenuation of ultrasonic beam; (b) presence of scattered echoes within the mass (*Figure 18.9*).

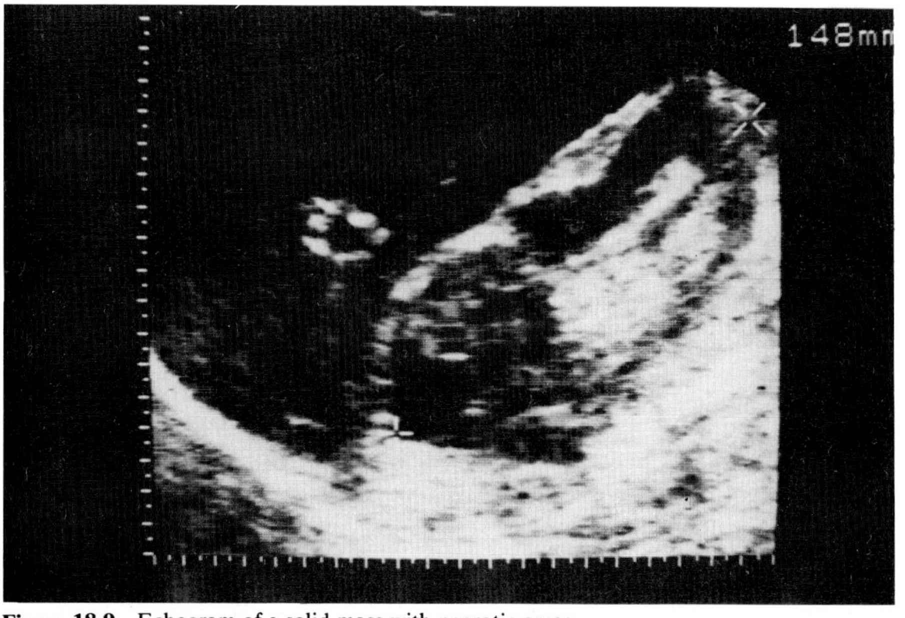

Figure 18.9 Echogram of a solid mass with necrotic areas

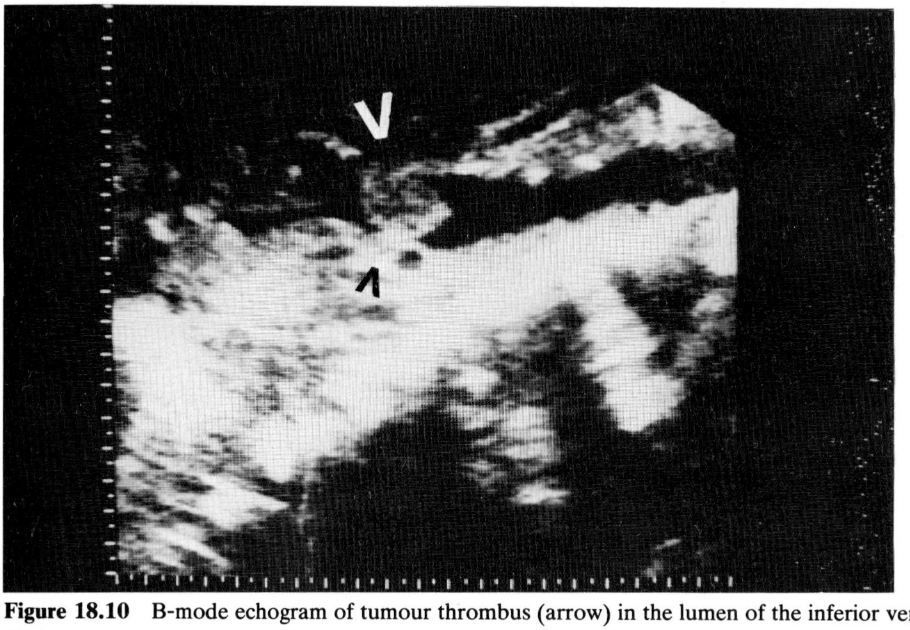

Figure 18.10 B-mode echogram of tumour thrombus (arrow) in the lumen of the inferior vena cava

Ultrasound attenuation by the mass is an almost constant feature of renal carcinoma and is better demonstrated by A-mode scan at variable gain settings as a decreased amplitude of the back wall echoes, compared with the anterior wall; in B-mode scan they lack the posterior enhancement observed in cystic lesions. The number and intensity of internal echoes are related to the mass vascularity and the tissue pattern of the mass. Ultrasound exploration can also detect renal vein extension of the tumour, inferior vena cava involvement (*Figure 18.10*) and the presence of hilar and retroperitoneal enlarged lymph nodes. Pitfalls associated with ultrasonography in the diagnoses of solid masses include cystic tumour, haemorrhagic cyst, abscesses and papillary cystoadenocarcinoma.

All solid or indeterminate masses at ultrasonography should undergo an *angiographic exploration.* Arteriographic findings in hypervascular tumours are highly characteristic and are represented by an increase in the diameter of the renal artery, large vessels with irregular course and varying calibre, microaneurysms, arteriovenous shunts, diffuse tumour blush, pooling and puddling of contrast material and early filling of the renal vein (*Figure 18.11*). Invasion of perinephric tissues is indicated by a parasitic blood supply that may arise from the lumbar, phrenic, inferior suprarenal and gonadal arteries. Renal adenoma and

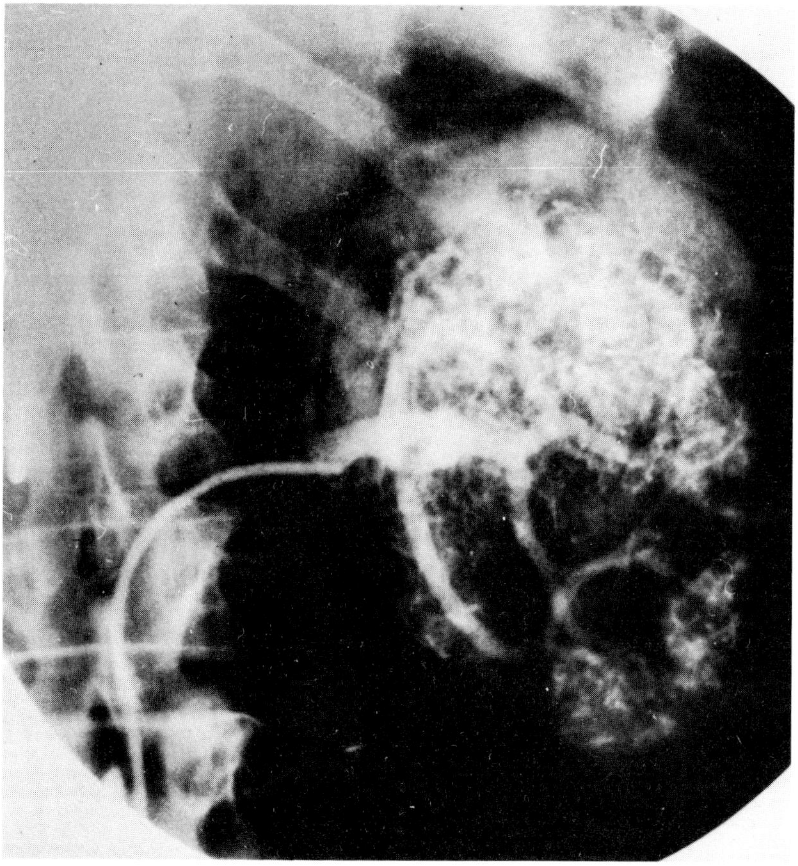

Figure 18.11 Selective renal arterial angiography showing a hypervascular renal adenocarcinoma

angiomyolipoma ('hamartoma') are also hypervascular benign neoplasms, and must be distinguished from true adenocarcinoma.

Large tumours usually outgrow their blood supply and become necrotic, giving an angiographic appearance that may simulate a cystic tumour. Hypovascular renal neoplasms also include some mesenchymal benign and malignant tumours, metastatic neoplasms, lymphoma, spindle cell carcinoma and tumours of the renal pelvis infiltrating the adjacent parenchyma. Inflammatory abscesses and chronic haematoma may also give pseudo-tumour patterns, similar to those observed in malignant disease.

Computed tomography (CT) is another alternative method for the diagnosis of renal masses, with an accuracy of 100 per cent in angiomyolipoma because of the low attenuation values registered (−20 to −80 Hn) due to their high fat content. Its diagnostic confidence level in cystic masses is the same as ultrasonography combined with cystic puncture, and is as reliable as this last method in the assessment of solid tumours. Since CT is still an expensive procedure for the systematic screening of renal masses, we are of the opinion that it should only be used in the diagnosis of renal carcinoma when the other methods so far mentioned render equivocal or complex images, or when angiography is formally contraindicated. It seems also to be useful in the follow-up of the patient after nephrectomy to detect early recurrence of tumour.

Staging

Two staging systems are in use for adenocarcinoma of the kidney in an attempt to study its incidence and clinical behaviour and to enable randomized trials of different therapeutic modalities according to the extent of the disease. The main system was popularized by Robson in 1969 and is based mainly on the pathological findings (*Table 18.3*); for this reason, its accuracy is strongly influenced by the extent of the operative procedure.

Table 18.3 Staging of renal adenocarcinoma (After Robson *et al.*, 1969)

Stage 1 :	Tumour confined within the capsule of the kidney
Stage 2 :	Invasion of the perinephric fat but tumour still confined within Gerota's fascia
Stage 3 :	Involvement of regional nodes and/or renal vein and cava
Stage 4 :	Involvement of adjacent organs and distant metastases

An alternative classification has been introduced by the International Union Against Cancer (UICC) using the TNM categories applied to other tumours (T = tumour; N = node; M = metastases). This system relies on preoperative information obtained from the different investigative techniques available to detect the extent of the tumour. Inaccuracy of radiological studies and lymphography to assess the size of the tumour and lymph node involvement together with the lack of specific tumour markers have limited the diffusion of this system.

Treatment of renal adenocarcinoma

Surgery

Surgical removal of the tumorous kidney with perinephric fat, adrenal gland and regional lymph nodes is the first step to be undertaken for a rational approach to the treatment of renal adenocarcinoma. This radical approach has proved to increase the 10-year survival rates significantly when compared to simple nephrectomy, with a relatively low operative mortality (Robson, Churchill and Anderson, 1969).

If the objective of surgery is limited to the *removal of the kidney*, without lymph node dissection, an anterior retroperitoneal approach gives enough exposure and good control over the vascular pedicle and is suitable for the management of most of the tumours, even for those located at the upper pole of the kidney. We prefer this route to the extended flank approach, which is still advocated by some authors, but adequate only for relatively small cancers.

When retroperitoneal *lymphadenectomy* is programmed, the thoraco-abdominal nephrectomy, as first described by Mortensen (1948), is the approach of choice and it does not represent a major insult to the patient. With the patient placed in the flank position, an incision is made between the tenth or eleventh intercostal space; the pleura is opened and the diaphragm is divided laterally to avoid injury to the phrenic nerve. After the peritoneal cavity is opened, the abdomen is explored for the presence or absence of metastases and the retroperitoneal space is entered after reflection of the colon towards the middle line. The most important step at time of operation is the dissection of the renal pedicle and its occlusion without manipulation of the kidney. The renal artery should be ligated first, followed by the renal vein after its careful palpation to determine the presence of a tumour thrombus. If the vein is ligated first, there is a risk of excessive bleeding; moreover, this manoeuvre does not seem to prevent the spread of metastases and is only acceptable if preoperative embolization has been performed. The lymph nodes should be dissected before removing the kidney with Gerota's fascia and adrenal gland.

The true benefit of lymphadenectomy in renal adenocarcinoma has been questioned. An argument against lymphadenectomy is the possibility of impairing the immunological defences of the host against the tumour by abolishing the regional lymph barrier. The extent of the lymphatic dissection is also controversial due to the unpredictable patterns of nodal involvement. Extensive lymphadenectomy as advocated by Robson, Churchill and Anderson (1969) implies major morbidity for the patient and does not seem to improve the survival compared with a more limited dissection, which must extend from the diaphragm down the level of aortic bifurcation and includes the ipsilateral lumbar nodes, the retroaortic, the retrocaval and the interaorticocaval nodes. Our experience with lymphadenectomy is still too limited to draw any conclusion, but considering the high percentages of regional node involvement at time of surgery, we believe that its practice might always have a beneficial effect in the outcome of the disease, without adding any significant morbidity.

The indication for *surgery in the presence of distant metastases* is a matter judged differently by various authors. Sometimes it is performed with the hope of a spontaneous regression of the metastases, a fact that has only been carefully documented in a limited number of patients as to become too solid an argument. Since positive effects on the cellular immunity of the host have been reported after palliative nephrectomy, we are of the opinion that in these cases nephrectomy and lymphadenectomy should be performed with the purpose of reductive surgery only, which by itself gives better possibilities of further chemotherapeutic or immunotherapeutic treatment.

Surgical resection of solitary metastases is not in dispute and must always be attempted by an experienced surgeon, if the anatomical site permits a radical excision without excessive risk of massive bleeding because of their usually increased vascularity.

Sometimes we have to face the management of patients with *bilateral tumours* or single tumours arising in a solitary kidney. In the first instance, there is a justified reluctance to perform bilateral nephrectomy followed by transplantation because of the possible adverse effects of immunosuppressive therapy. The alternative option is the radical removal of one kidney, whereas the other side undergoes an organ-saving operation or an extracorporeal bench surgery with the same basic principles as used in autotransplantation of the kidney.

The natural history and therapeutic options for tumour occurring in a solitary kidney has been extensively reviewed by Wickham (1975) and Novick *et al.* (1977). In general terms, all the patients are potential candidates for curative surgery, but the results obtained are strongly influenced by the stage of the disease and the original cause of the contralateral nephrectomy. The prognosis is poor for patients whose opposite kidney was removed because of renal tumour or those with asynchronous tumours that developed recurrences within 5 years of the original nephrectomy. The use of *in vivo* or extracorporeal bench surgery has no influence on the survival rates.

Embolization

Transcatheter embolization of the kidney has gained acceptance as a palliative procedure in inoperable renal cancer with massive haematuria, or as a previous step in the surgical treatment of largely vascularized tumours to prevent bleeding at time of operation (Alferez and Diaz-Alferez, 1980). Different embolic materials have been utilized, including fragments of autologous muscle, microspheres, gelatin foam, metallic coils and cyano-acrylates.

Complications observed with embolization are, among others, lumbar pain, fever, acute renal failure and ectopic embolization. These side effects, which can sometimes be severe, have decreased the initial enthusiasm for this method and limited its use to certain patients with advanced tumours or when the aim is to enable a more easy removal of the tumorous kidney. If practised before surgery, temporary balloon occlusion of the renal artery until the pedicle is ligated is preferred to permanent embolization.

Chemotherapy

Experience accumulated in the treatment of advanced or recurrent renal carcinoma has revealed that only a small benefit can be expected from the use of the current chemotherapeutic antiblastic agents in the control of the symptoms and progression of the disease.

Objective response rates reported in several reviews range from 4 per cent up to 28 per cent (Garnick, 1983). No single agent seems to be effective but vinblastine and CCNU alone are associated with higher rates of response than the other drugs.

Drug combinations are more effective than single agents in the treatment of most malignancies, but this fact has not been convincingly demonstrated in renal cancer. Merrin *et al.* (1975) reported 10 per cent of objective response and 50 per cent of subjective improvement with the association of vinblastine and CCNU. With this same schedule, Davis and Mamalo (1978) reported a 24 per cent objective response rate in a group of 29 patients with metastatic disease. Bleomycin, methotrexate and cis-platinum have been assayed in various combinations, but the limited number of patients does not permit us to draw any conclusions as to the therapeutic value. Any combination studied so far seems not be superior to vinblastine or CCNU when used as single agents.

These poor results have promoted the evaluation of new chemotherapeutic agents in renal carcinoma. Recently, the EORTC Urological Group (Child *et al.*, 1983) formulated a protocol to study the effect of methyl-GAG in a group of 45 patients with metastatic disease not amenable to surgery, and to assess the morbidity of the treatment. Methyl-GAG is a drug synthesized in 1958 and used in the treatment of the leukaemias. Its anti-proliferative effect depends upon the combined mechanism of selective binding to mitochondria and inhibition of polyamine synthesis. The drug was administered in a weekly schedule at a dose of 500 mg/m^2 intravenously to reduce its toxicity. Of the total of 30 fully evaluated patients only 3 achieved partial remission, whose duration in no case exceeded 8 weeks; 11 showed no significant change and in the remaining 16 the disease followed a progressive course. The side effects varied from mild to severe and by far surpassed the transitory and limited benefit obtained with the treatment. The commonest were anorexia, vomiting, neuropathy, myopathy and myalgia.

Another drug tested in metastatic renal cancer is 4′-epi-Adriamycin, a stereoisomer of Adriamycin and devoid of severe side effects, with the single exception of cardiomyopathy if higher cumulative doses are used, as with Adriamycin itself. Preliminary reports seemed to show some activity (Fossa *et al.*, 1983), but they have not been confirmed in other clinical trials.

Attempts at intra-arterial chemotherapy with 5-fluorouracil, methotrexate and actinomycin D have also been performed (Leiter, Edelmas and Brandler, 1966; Wiley *et al.*, 1975), with no conclusive results due to the limited number of patients evaluated.

Radiotherapy

The lack of consistent clinical trials, together with the assumed low radiosensitivity of the renal tubular elements, are the factors that have restricted to a minimum the utilization of radiotherapy in the treatment of kidney adenocarcinoma. More recently, nevertheless, prospective and randomized studies designed with definite criteria have demonstrated that significant benefits can be expected of its use as an adjuvant therapeutic modality.

Some authors (Riches, 1966) are of the opinion that radiotherapy should be administered in all the tumours which at time of operation are found to extend beyond the kidney, and also if after radical surgery are presumed to have residual microscopic disease, in order to prevent local recurrences.

Preoperative irradiation achieves mass reduction of more than 50 per cent and is useful to significantly reduce the number of primarily inoperable tumours.

Another application of radiotherapy is the treatment of selected solitary metastases found postoperatively and in the control of haemorrhages or severe pain produced by tumour growth.

Immunotherapy

Adenocarcinoma of the kidney is considered to be ideal for attempts at immunotherapy since its clinical behaviour strongly suggests an important role of host immunity in the growth of the primary tumour and development of metastases (Thatcher *et al.*, 1977).

Active immunotherapy with intradermal BCG injections and other non-specific immunostimulants has been the object of many clinical trials as adjuvant therapy after surgical removal of the bulk of the tumour. The results reported are irregular, and the overall rates of tumour stabilization or temporary regression are rather poor (Minton, Pennline and Nowrocki, 1976).

The first attempts at passive immunotherapy were in the form of serotherapy, but they did not expand into specific protocols for clinical trials. More extensive use has received the technique of adoptive immunotherapy with transfer factor and immune RNA extracted from lymphoid tissue. Lack of randomized studies with a significant number of patients, however, does not permit any assessment to be made as to its real value in the treatment of renal cancer.

For some authors, a significant increase of the survival and objective regression of pulmonary metastases is obtained with the use of a soluble fraction of autologous tumour injected intradermally with PPD tuberculin or *Candida* antigen as adjuvants (Tykka *et al.,* 1978). This technique of specific immunotherapy, which has been applied with many other antigen adjuvants, seems to be promising, but its use is limited by the necessity of obtaining autologous tumour cells.

Results obtained with immunotherapy are not so good as would be expected from its theoretical basis; in some cases, however, they are much better than current chemotherapy and, therefore, its use should be considered in the treatment of patients with metastatic disease, as a complement to radical nephrectomy.

Steroid receptors and hormonal management of renal adenocarcinoma

As previously mentioned, experimental and clinical evidence suggests that steroid hormones might play a definite role in the induction of human renal carcinoma. In the search for a practical application of these findings, quantification of steroid receptors in various endocrine-dependent neoplasias has been performed. More recently, different studies have been undertaken to investigate the existence and the possible clinical application of the quantification of steroid receptors in both normal and tumorous human kidney. Objectives were orientated to assess the endocrine substrate of renal carcinoma, its character as a hormone-dependent tumour and the possible therapeutic usefulness of the steroid hormone receptor assay.

Bojar *et al.* (1975) and Concolino *et al.* (1976) first demonstrated the existence of oestrogen and progesterone receptors in normal renal tissue; soon they were also detected in human renal tumour tissue (Concolino *et al.,* 1978; Giuliani *et al.,* 1978). More recently, the presence of androgen receptors in normal and tumorous human kidney tissue (Pertschuk *et al.,* 1980; Bojar *et al.,* 1980; Ghanadian *et al.,* 1982; Corrales *et al.,* 1984) has been demonstrated. Although steroid receptors are only found in about 60 per cent of all adenocarcinomas, these findings seem to be indicative enough of certain hormone dependence of human renal tumours.

Taking into account that this large number of patients with advanced disease on adjuvant endocrine therapy does not respond objectively to treatment, and that many of the patients lack steroid receptors in the tumour cells, it is tempting to detect and quantify these receptors; the goal is to avoid empirical hormone therapy and to reserve this treatment only for those cases where definite criteria of possible hormone sensitivity exists.

Preliminary studies by Concolino *et al.* (1978) suggested a greater sensitivity to treatment with progestogens in those patients with positive progesterone receptors in tumour cytosol. Likewise, preliminary observations by Giuliani *et al.* (1978) appear to indicate a greater efficacy of treatment with anti-oestrogens in patients with oestrogen receptors, albeit the limited number of the series avoids the drawing of any valid conclusion. These preliminary results promoted different therapeutic approaches based on the use of either progesterone or anti-oestrogens, whose choice is based upon the prior quantification of oestrogen and progesterone receptors (Concolino, 1978, 1979). Further studies have not confirmed the validity or usefulness of this protocol, considering that positive responses have been observed in patients with negative progestogen receptors and lack of response to treatment with anti-oestrogens in patients with positive oestrogen receptors (Concolino *et al.*, 1981).

The lack of concordance between the presence of progesterone receptors and the clinical response to the adjuvant treatment with medroxyprogesterone has not yet been convincingly explained. One possible factor would be the absence of biochemical and cellular homogeneity among the different parts of the tumour. It has also been suggested that positive response to medroxyprogesterone treatment is closely linked to its androgenic activity (Concolino *et al.*, 1976) and depends upon the presence of androgen receptors in the tumorous tissue (Concolino *et al.*, 1981). For these authors, the quantification of androgen receptors would therefore be the best approach for the hormonal therapeutic selection of patients with kidney adenocarcinoma.

On the basis of this hypothesis, we have concluded a preliminary study to evaluate the possible effectiveness of adjuvant medroxyprogesterone therapy (1 g/day over 7 days, followed by 1 g/week over 1 year, as a minimum) in a group of 15 randomly selected patients affected by renal adenocarcinoma in different clinical stages (*Table 18.4*). The presence or absence of androgen receptors in tumour cytosol was analysed using the method of dextran-charcoal and methyltrienolone as a radioactive ligand (Corrales *et al.*, 1983). Results obtained were compared against another group with androgen receptor quantification, but without progestogen treatment.

Androgen receptors were detected in 60 per cent of all patients, a level similar to that previously reported by Concolino *et al.* (1981). Of 7 patients with local or distant metastases treated with medroxyprogesterone, 3 followed a downhill course and died within a few months after radical nephrectomy due to their neoplasia. A fact to emphasize is that 3 of the patients had low to undetectable receptor levels. The clinical outcome of the remaining patients who had receptors levels well above 3 fmol/mg of cytosol protein were good to excellent. One showed complete disappearance of metastases, normalization of laboratory tests and a spectacular clinical recovery, having the highest level of androgen receptors registered in the series.

Although this series is small, the observed trends seem to point towards an absence of response to medroxyprogesterone in the majority of patients with low to undetectable levels of androgen receptors, and some degree of remission — partial or complete — in those patients with positive receptor values. The observation of an objective response to progestogens in a patient whose tumour was lacking in receptors and in an advanced stage of the disease suggests that medroxyprogesterone treatment may occasionally be valuable in the absence of androgen receptors.

Table 18.4 Clinical follow-up of patients with renal cell carcinoma and quantification of androgen receptors in their cytosol

Patient	*Sex*	*Age* (yr)	B_{max} fmol/g	B_{max} fmol/mg	K_d nmol/l	*Treatment**	*Stage of disease*†	*Evolution*‡	*Survival* (months)
1. C.H.H.	F	58	147	6.9	2.4	MPA	II	TFI	32+
2. A.F.A.	F	49	34	1.6	8.7	MPA	IV	Progression	15 exitus
3. L.G.M.	M	49	N.D.	N.D.	N.D.	MPA	IV	Progression	2 exitus
4. M.E.P.	F	47	136	9.1	4.8	MPA	IV	Complete remission	13+
5. S.C.A.	M	76	N.D.	N.D.	N.D.	MPA	IV	Objective response	10+
6. E.I.P.	F	63	45	2.1	2.1	MPA	IV	Partial remission	6+
7. M.C.E.	F	48	175	5.6	0.5	MPA	I	TFI	16+
8. M.M.T.	F	53	N.D.	N.D.	N.D.	MPA	IV	Progression	2 exitus
9. P.G.E.	F	51	N.D.	N.D.	N.D.	MPA	II	TFI	22+
10. L.B.S.	M	56	75	5.1	6.8	MPA	III	Stabilization	12+
11. A.G.C.	F	60	N.D.	N.D.	N.D.	No	III	Complete remission	18+
12. D.L.P.	M	57	49	2.7	1.2	No	No	TFI	40+
13. V.G.A.	F	35	N.D.	N.D.	N.D.	No	I	TFI	19+
14. M.J.G.	M	60	30	2.3	1.2	No	II	TFI	19+
15. J.P.M.	M	70	64	3.6	3.4	No	I	TFI	16 exitus due to intercurrent disease

*Medroxyprogesterone acetate.
†Before nephrectomy (according to Robson, Churchill and Anderson, 1969).
‡ According to Hahn *et al.* (1977).

B_{max}, receptor content in cytosol; TFI, time free interval; N.D., non-detectable; K_d, dissociation constant.

Carcinoma of the renal pelvis

Owing to space restrictions, this section is exclusively devoted to analysis of the most important epidemiologic, aetiologic, diagnostic and therapeutic features of malignant tumours arising from the transitional epithelium of the renal pelvis and calyces. They account for more than 80 per cent of all tumours in this category and are represented by papillary transitional cell carcinoma, squamous cell carcinoma, undifferentiated carcinoma and adenocarcinoma.

General epidemiology

Malignant tumours of the renal pelvis and calyces share with renal adenocarcinoma the same epidemiologic determinants so far as the age distribution is concerned (*Figure 18.12*) and there is also a male sex predominance. The parenchyma to pelvis incidence ratio is about 5:1.

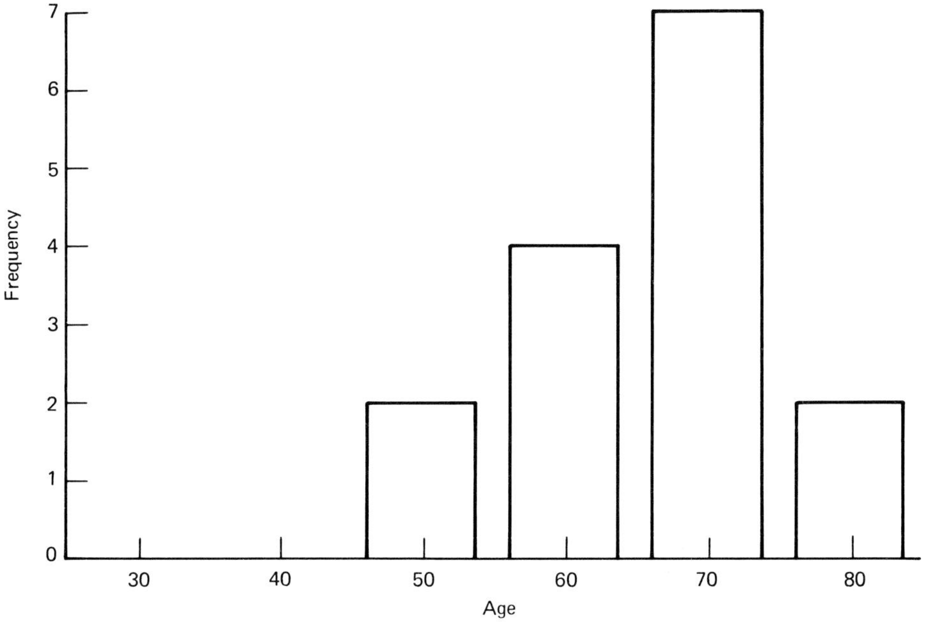

Figure 18.12 Age distribution in 15 cases of renal pelvic cancer in the Urology Department of the Hospital Clinico Universitario of Salamanca

Because carcinoma of the pelvis is included with kidney adenocarcinoma as 'tumours of the kidney' in most of the major epidemiologic studies, no extensive data are available as to racial and geographic influences on its occurrence. The only known fact is its unusually high incidence in localized areas of Bulgaria, Yugoslavia and Roumania, where it is observed in association with an endemic chronic renal disease, referred to as Balkan nephropathy (Muir and Nectoux, 1980). Patients with this chronic disease have an 88-fold higher risk of urinary tract cancer compared to persons living in the non-endemic area, and the incidence of pelvic cancer observed is about the same as that of bladder cancer.

Aetiology

Due to their common histologic origin, the same aetiologic factors involved in bladder and ureteric transitional tumours are applied to transitional tumours of renal pelvis.

Among chemical agents, the most common carcinogens are a group of aromatic substances that share a common ortho-aminophenol radical, utilized in the aniline dye, rubber, plastic and gas industries (Poole-Wilson, 1969). They include beta-naphthylamine, benzidine, 4-aminodiphenyl and 2-acetylaminofluorane. Chronic exposure to these substances is known to add a 30-fold risk compared to an unexposed population for the development of transitional tumours, especially bladder tumours (Lower, 1982).

These compounds are absorbed by cutaneous, pulmonary and digestive routes and metabolized through N-hydroxylation, producing different carcinogenic by-products. They are detoxified in the liver by conjugation with sulphuric and glucuronic acid, giving rise to non-carcinogenic metabolites that are excreted in the urine. Once in the urine they may be split back to their unconjugated, active state by beta-glucuronidase and sulphatase activity, which has been demonstrated to be increased in the urine of patients with bladder and pelvic tumours (Boyland, 1963). The enzymatic activity of beta-glucuronidase is reduced by 1->4-glucosaccharolactone (Boyland *et al.*, 1964). The question that arises is whether intermediate metabolites of tryptophan excreted by urine having an ortho-aminophenol radical, such as 3-hydroxyanthranilic acid and 3-hydroxykynurenin, are involved by similar mechanism in the induction of these tumours (Kerr and Barkin, 1970). The extent of the epithelial surface and the time of exposure to these substances might account for the observed differences in the incidence rates between tumours of the bladder, renal pelvis and ureter, whose ratio is approximately 50 : 3 : 1 (Bennington and Beckwith, 1975).

Heavy use of phenacetin-containing analgesics has been linked to cancer of the renal pelvis in many epidemiologic surveys (Bengtsson *et al.*, 1968). Evidence also supports smoking, coffee drinking and use of artificial sweeteners as predisposing factors in the development of carcinoma of the renal pelvis (Weir and Dunn, 1970; Cole, 1971).

The aetiology of renal pelvic cancer occurring in patients affected with Balkan nephropathy has been discussed by many authors, but a convincing explanation for both diseases has not been postulated so far. Due to the fact that distribution of this endemic nephropathy follows that of streams and rivers, a high content of silicate, nickel and chromium in drinking water has been incriminated as possible inducing agents. Such a hypothesis is supported by experimental induction of both nephropathy and tumours in rats by the administration of water containing quartz, nickel and chromium during a period of 2–12 months (Muir and Nectoux, 1980). Ochratoxin-A, a toxin of fungal origin and a contaminant of different foodstuffs, has also been suggested as a possible aetiological agent in Balkan nephropathy and associated pelvic tumours (Kanisawa and Suzuki, 1978).

The only physical agent known to induce malignant epithelial tumours of the renal pelvis is a radioactive thorium compound (thorotrast) utilized many decades ago in retrograde pyelographic studies (Hubman and Hoer, 1964; Ott, Weyeneth and Tuchschmid, 1977).

Chronic inflammation promoted by calculi or *Schistosoma haematobium* has been observed in association with carcinoma of the urinary tract. Glandular, cystic and squamous metaplasia occur in areas of inflammation as a reactive response of the urothelium, but the interrelationship of these pathologic alterations is not yet clearly established.

Pathology

Malignant epithelial tumours of the renal pelvis share the same pathologic features with the transitional tumours arising from the ureteric and bladder wall.

Papillary carcinoma accounts for about 85 per cent of all tumours in this category. They present a variable growth pattern which seems to be closely related to the degree of anaplasia of the tumour cells.

Although squamous metaplasia can be observed in over 20 per cent of papillary transitional carcinomas, true squamous tumours occur in only 8 per cent and in most cases they tend to be solid with an infiltrative and ulcerative growth pattern, similar to that observed in undifferentiated carcinoma.

Adenocarcinoma of the renal pelvis is an extremely rare tumour, with only a few cases reported in the world literature (Quattlebaum and Shirley, 1968). Grossly, they have the appearance of colonic adenocarcinoma and usually are reported in association with staghorn calculi and chronic pyelonephritis.

Clinical findings

Gross *macroscopic haematuria* is the most common presenting symptom, and unlike kidney adenocarcinoma seems usually to be an early clinical finding, due to the continuity of the tumour with the excretory system. Haematuria may be persistent or intermittent in nature with long remission periods; in some instances, terminal haematuria because of concomitant bladder tumour may confuse the clinical suspicion of upper urinary tract tumour.

Pain is the second major symptom. It may be acute and paroxysmal due to ureteric obstruction by passing clots; or dull and continuous in cases of local extension of the tumour or the development of chronic progressive hydronephrosis (see Chapter 19).

A *palpable flank mass* is observed in about 10 per cent of all cases and is evidence of far advanced tumours or a hydronephrotic kidney secondary to ureteric obstruction.

Recurrent urinary infection is another common finding, but is more common in ureteric than pelvic tumours.

Paraneoplastic syndromes as observed in renal carcinoma have not been convincingly documented in association with pelvic tumours, although isolated instances of secondary amyloidosis, hypercalcaemia and high levels of human chorionic gonadotrophins have been reported. Asthenia, anorexia and weight loss are late symptoms, and are indicative of either disseminated disease or the presence of an infected hydronephrosis.

Some patients may have increased serum levels of carcino-embryonic antigen and LDH. Increased urinary excretion of tryptophan metabolites and lysosomal enzymes have also been reported, but all these findings do not have a high enough specificity to be considered as of diagnostic value.

Diagnosis

Infusion excretory urography, either alone or combined with nephrotomography, is the initial diagnostic procedure. Pelvic tumours appear as radiolucent filling defects with irregular contours, sometimes showing a clear implantation stalk in the wall of the pelvis. The most common radiologic pelvic filling defects that may be confused with a tumour include clots, non-opaque renal stones, fungus balls and cholesteatoma. Hydronephrosis and non-visualization of the affected kidney is observed with relative frequency in advanced tumours.

Retrograde pyelography may contribute to the clarification of filling defects in poorly functioning kidneys or demonstrate a ureteric tumour overlooked on the IVP (*Figure 18.13*).

The value of ultrasonography is limited to the differential diagnosis of pelvic tumours from radiolucent uric acid stones or to the evaluation of a 'silent' kidney.

Selective angiography is also of little benefit in the diagnosis of pelvic tumours, but may help to assess the preoperative extent of the disease. The most common arteriographic findings include encasement of intrarenal arteries, hypertrophy of renal pelvic artery and tumour blush.

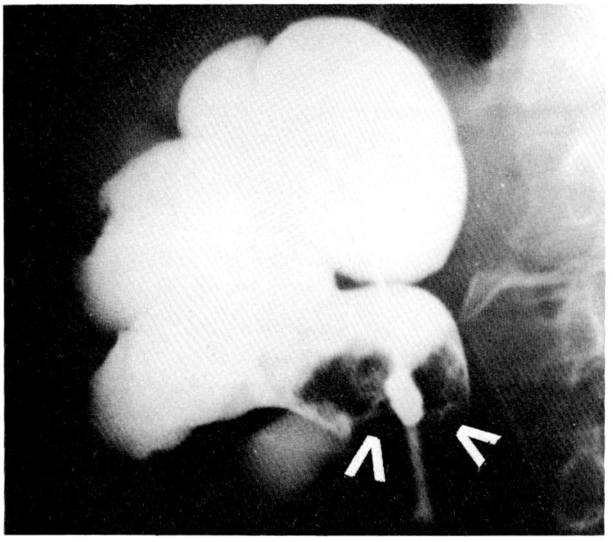

Figure 18.13 Retrograde pyelogram showing a filling defect of the renal pelvis and hydronephrosis, both arising from an infiltrating transitional cell tumour

Urinary cytology has a high rate of false negative results in cases of pelvic transitional carcinoma (Hawtrey, 1971). Retrograde brushing of the pelvis and calyces, as first described by Gill, Lu and Thomasen (1973), significantly increases preoperative diagnostic accuracy.

Treatment

The treatment of choice is radical nephroureterectomy that must always include regional lymph nodes and a cuff of bladder to prevent recurrences at the ureteral stump (Cummings *et al.*, 1975). Conservative therapy may be considered in patients with low grade, low stage tumours and is mandatory in solitary kidney, bilateral tumours and endemic Balkan nephropathy.

The role of adjuvant radiotherapy and chemotherapy remains controversial in the absence of extensive clinical trials. Some authors advocate the systematic use of postoperative radiotherapy to prevent local recurrences or as a palliative procedure in inoperable tumours.

References

ALFEREZ, C. and DIAZ ALFEREZ, F. (1980). Embolizacion en Urologia. In *Ponencia al XLV Congreso Nacional de Urologia* (Oviedo, 1980), edited by Asociacion Española de Urologia, pp. 154–161. Madrid; ENE Ediciones

ALKEN, C.E., ROUCAYROL, J.C., OBERHAUSEN, E., TAUPITZ, A. and UEBERBERG, H. (1960). On the problem of carcinogenesis following Thorotrast pyelography. *Urologia Internationalis,* **10,** 137–156

ARMSTRONG, B., GARROD, A. and DOLL, R. (1976). A retrospective study of renal cancer with special reference to coffee and animal protein consumption. *British Journal of Cancer,* **33,** 127–136

BELL, E.T. (1950). *Renal Diseases,* 2nd edn. Philadelphia; Lea and Febiger

BENGTSSON, U., ANGERVALL, L., EKMAN, H. and LEHMANN, L. (1968). Transitional cell tumors of the renal pelvis in analgesic abusers. *Scandinavian Journal of Urology and Nephrology,* **2,** 145–150

BENNINGTON, J.L. and BECKWITH, J.B. (1975). *Tumors of the Kidney, Renal Pelvis, and Ureter,* pp. 243–336. Washington D.C.; Armed Forces Institute of Pathology

BENNINGTON, J.L. and KRADJIAN, R.M. (1967). *Renal Carcinoma.* Philadelphia; Saunders

BOJAR, H., BALZER, K., DREYFURST, R. and STAIB, W. (1975). Identification and partial characterization of specific estrogen-binding components in human kidney. *Journal of Clinical Chemistry and Clinical Biochemistry,* **14,** 515–520

BOJAR, H., MAAR, K. and STAIB, W. (1980). The endocrine background of human renal cell carcinoma. V. Binding of the highly potent androgen methyltrienolone (R 1881) by tumor cytosol. *Urologia Internationalis,* **35,** 154–160

BOWMAN, H.S. and MARTINEZ, E.J. (1968). Fever, anemia and hyperhaptoglobinemia an extrarenal triad of hypernephroma. *Annals of Internal Medicine,* **68,** 613–620

BOYLAND, E. (1963). *The Biochemistry of Bladder Cancer.* Springfield, Illinois; Thomas

BOYLAND, E., WALLACE, M., AVIS, P.R.D. and KINDER, C.H. (1964). Attempted prophylaxis of bladder cancer with 1→4 glucosaccharolactone. *British Journal of Urology,* **36,** 563–569

BRERETON, H.D., HALUSHKA, P.V., ALEXANDER, R.W., MASON, D.M., KEISER, H.R. and DE VITA, U.T. (1974). Indomethacin responsive hypercalcemia in a patient with renal cell adenocarcinoma. *New England Journal of Medicine,* **291,** 83–85

BRINTON, L.F. (1960). Hypernephroma familial occurrence in one family. *Journal of the American Medical Association,* **173,** 888–890

CHILD, J.A, STOTER, G., FOSSA, S.D., BONO, A.V., DE PAUW, M. and THE EORTC UROLOGICAL GROUP (1983). Chemotherapy of advanced renal cell carcinoma: results of treatment with methyl-glyoxal-*bis*-guanylhydrazone (methyl-GAG): an EORTC study. In *Cancer of the Prostate and Kidney,* edited by M. Pavone-Macaluso and J. Smith, pp. 693–697. New York; Plenum Press

COLE, P. (1971). Coffee drinking and cancer of the lower urinary tract. *Lancet,* **1,** 1335–1337

CONCOLINO, G., DI SILVERIO, F., MAROCCHI, A. and BRACCI, U. (1979). Renal cancer steroid receptors: biochemical basis for endocrine therapy. *European Urology,* **5,** 90–93

CONCOLINO, G., MAROCCHI, A., CONCOLINO, F., SCIARRA, F., DI SILVERIO, F. and CONTI, C. (1976). Human kidney steroid receptors. *Journal of Steroid Biochemistry,* **7,** 831–835

CONCOLINO, G., MAROCCHI, A., CONTI, C., TENAGLIA, R., DI SILVERIO, F. and BRACCI, U. (1978). Human renal carcinoma as a hormone-dependent tumor. *Cancer Research,* **38,** 4340–4344

CONCOLINO, G., MAROCCHI, A., TOSCANO, V. and DI SILVERIO, F. (1981). Nuclear androgen receptor as marker of responsiveness to medroxyprogesterone acetate in human renal cell carcinoma. *Journal of Steroid Biochemistry,* **15,** 397–402

CORRALES, J.J., MIRALLES, J.M., HOISAETER, P.A., MARTIN, T., GARCIA, L.C. and MONTERO, J. (1983). Relations between circulating levels of testosterone, 17-beta estradiol, androstenedione, dehydroepiandrosterone sulfate and androgenic receptor content of cytosol in benign prostatic hyperplasia. *Urologia Internationalis,* **38,** 109–115

CORRALES, J.J., PASTOR, I., GARCIA, L.C., BUITRAGO, J.M., MERCADO, F. and MIRALES, J.M. (1984). Receptores androgenicos en el rinon humano. Efectos de los niveles circulantes de androgenos. *Endrocrinologia,* **71,** 106

CUMMINGS, K.B., CORREA, R.J., GIBBONS, R.P., STOLL, H.M., WHEELIS, R.F. and MASON, J.T. (1975). Renal pelvic tumors. *Journal of Urology,* **113,** 158–162

DAVIS, T.E. and MAMALO, F.B. (1978). Combination chemotherapy of advanced renal cancer with CCNU and Vinblastine. In *Proceedings of the American Society of Clinical Oncology,* edited by American Association for Cancer Research Inc., vol. 19, p. 316. Baltimore; Waverly Press

EPSTEIN, S.M., BARTUS, B. and FARBER, E. (1969). Renal epithelial neoplasm induced in male wistar rats by oral Aflotoxin B-1. *Cancer Research,* **29,** 1045–1050

FOSSA, S.D., WIK, B., BAE, E. and ANDLIEN, H.H. (1983). 4′Epi-Adriamicin in metastatic renal cancer. In *Cancer of the Prostate and Kidney,* edited by M. Pavone-Macaluso and J. Smith, pp. 699–703. New York; Plenum Press

GARNICK, M.B. (1983). Renal cell carcinoma — diagnostic workup and natural history. In *Urologic Cancer,* edited by M.B. Garnick and J.P. Richie, pp. 41–50. New York; Plenum Press

GHANADIAN, R., AUF, G., WILLIAMS, G. and COLEMAN, A.P.M. (1982). Steroid receptors in kidney tumours. *Progress in Clinical and Biological Research,* **100,** 245–254

GILL, W.B., LU, C.T. and THOMASEN, S. (1973). Retrograde brushing: a new technique for obtaining histologic and cytologic material from ureteral, renal pelvic and renal calyceal lesions. *Journal of Urology,* **109,** 573–578

GIULIANI, L., PESCATORE, D., GIBERTI, C. and MARTARONA, G. (1978). Usefulness and limitation of estrogen receptor protein (ERP) assay in human renal cell carcinomas. *European Urology,* **4,** 342–347

GRANOFF, A. (1973). Herpes virus and the Lucke tumor. *Cancer Research,* **33,** 1431–1433

GRIFFIN, J.P., HUGHES, G.V. and PEELING, W.B. (1967). A survey of the familial incidence of adenocarcinoma of the kidney. *British Journal of Urology,* **39,** 63–66

GUERIN, M., CHOUROULINIKOV, I. and RIVIERE, M.R. (1969). Experimental kidney tumors. In *The Kidney: Morphology, Biochemistry, Physiology,* vol. II, edited by C. Rouiller and A.F. Muller, pp. 199–268. New York; Academic Press

HAHN, D.M., SCHIMPFF, S.C., RUCKDESCHEL, J.C. and WIERNICK, P.H. (1977). Single-agent therapy for renal cell carcinoma: CCNU, vinblastine, thio-tepa or bleomycin. *Cancer Treatment Reports,* **61,** 1585–1587

HAWTREY, C.E. (1971). Fifty-two cases of primary ureteral carcinomas: a clinical pathology study. Journal of Urology, **105,** 188–193

HUBMANN, R.H. and HOER, P.W. (1964). Nierenbecker Carcinoma nach retrograder Pyelographie mit Thorotrast. *Urologe,* **3,** 27–32

KANISAWA, M. and SUZUKI, S. (1978). Induction of renal and hepatic tumors in mice by ochratoxin-A, a mycotoxin. *Gann,* **69,** 599–600

KERR, W.K. and BARKIN, M. (1970). Aetiology and biochemistry of cancer of the bladder. In *Modern Trends in Urology—3,* edited by E. Riches, pp. 163–179. New York; Appleton-Century-Crofts

KERR, W.K., BARKIN, M., TODD, J.A.D. and MENCZYK, Z. (1963). A hypernephroma associated with elevated levels of bladder carcinogens in the urine: case report. *British Journal of Urology,* **35,** 263–266

KIRKMAN, H. (1959). Estrogen induced tumors of the kidney. *National Cancer Institute Monographs,* **1,** 1–91

LEITER, E., EDELMAS, S. and BRANDLER, H. (1966). Continuous preoperative intra-arterial perfusion of renal tumors with chemotherapeutic agents. *Journal of Urology,* **95,** 169–175

LOWER, G.M. (1982). Concepts in causality. Chemically induced human urinary bladder cancer. *Cancer,* **49,** 1056–1066

MARSHALL, F.F. and WALSH, P.C. (1977). Extrarenal manifestation of renal cell carcinoma. *Journal of Urology,* **117,** 439–440

MERRIN, C., MITTLEMAN, A., FANOUS, A., WAJSMAN, Z. and MURPHY, G.P. (1975). Chemotherapy of advanced renal cell carcinoma with Vinblastine and CCNU. *Journal of Urology,* **113,** 21–23

MINTON, J.P., PENNLINE, K. and NOWROCKI, J.F. (1976). Immunotherapy of human kidney cancer. In *Proceedings of the American Society of Clinical Oncology,* edited by American Association for Cancer Research Inc., vol. 17, p. 301. Baltimore; Waverly Press

MORTENSEN, H. (1948). Transthoracic nephrectomy. *Journal of Urology,* **60,** 855–858

MUIR, C.S. and NECTOUX, J. (1980). Geographical distribution and aetiology of kidney cancer. In *Renal Adenocarcinoma,* edited by G. Sufrin and S.A. Beckley, pp. 133–155. Geneva; UICC Technical Report Series

NOVICK, A.C., STEWARD, B.H., STRAFFON, R.A. and BANOWSKY, L.H. (1977). Partial nephrectomy in the treatment of renal adenocarcinoma. *Journal of Urology,* **118,** 932–936

OBERLING, C., RIVIERE, M. and HAGUENAU, F. (1960). Ultrastructure of the clear cells in renal carcinoma and its importance for the demonstration of their renal origin. *Nature,* **186,** 402–403

OTT, R., WEYENETH, R. and TUCHSCHMID, D. (1977). Les cancers de la voie excrètice superieure aprés pyélographie au thorotrast. *Journal d'Urologie et Néphrologie,* **12,** 225–230

PAGANINI-HILL, A., ROSS, R.K. and HENDERSON, B.E. (1983). Epidemiology of kidney cancer. In *Urological Cancer,* edited by D.G. Skinner, pp. 393–407. New York; Grune and Stratton

PAVONE-MACALUSO, M. (1983). Aetiology of kidney tumors. In *Cancer of the Prostate and Kidney,* edited by M. Pavone-Macaluso and J.H. Smith, pp. 475–488. New York; Plenum Press

PERTSCHUK, L.P., CARVOUNIS, E.E., TOBIN, E.H. and GAETJENS, E. (1980). Renal glomerular steroid hormone binding. Detection by fluorescent microscopy. *Journal of Steroid Biochemistry,* **113,** 1115–1120

PETKOVIC, S.D. (1959). An anatomical classification of renal tumors in the adult as a basis for prognosis. *Journal of Urology,* **81,** 618–623

POOLE-WILSON, D.S. (1969). Occupational tumours of the renal pelvis and ureter arising in the dye-making industry. *Proceedings of the Royal Society of Medicine,* **62,** 93–94

QUATTLEBAUM, R.B. and SHIRLEY, S.W. (1968). Adenocarcinoma of the renal pelvis. *Journal of Urology,* **99,** 384–386

RATCLIFFE, H.L. (1940). Familial occurrence of renal carcinoma in Rhesus monkeys (*Macaca mulatta*). *American Journal of Pathology,* **16,** 619–624

RAUSCHMEIER, H., HOFSTADTER, F. and JAKSE, G. (1983). Prognostic relevance of cytologic grading in metastatic renal cell carcinoma. In *Cancer of the Prostate and Kidney,* edited by M. Pavone-Macaluso and J. Smith, pp. 587–593. New York; Plenum Press

RAWLINS, M.D., LUFF, R.H. and CRANSTON, W.I. (1970). Pyrexia in renal carcinoma. *Lancet,* **1,** 1371–1373

RICHES, E. (1966). The place of radiotherapy in the management of parenchymal carcinoma of the kidney. *Journal of Urology,* **95,** 313–317

RICHES, E.W., GRIFFITHS, I.H. and THACKRAY, A.C. (1951). New growths of the kidney and ureter. *British Journal of Urology,* **23,** 297–356

ROBSON, C.J., CHURCHILL, B.M. and ANDERSON, W. (1969). The results of radical nephrectomy for renal cell carcinoma. *Journal of Urology,* **101,** 297–301

RUIZ-MARCELLAN, F.J., QUINTANILLA, B., RUIZ-MARCELLAN, M.C., COSME, M.A. and BERSHTAM, J. (1979). Efectos tardios de la pielografia ascendente con Thorotrast. *Actas Urologicas,* **5,** 283–286

SEMPRONJ, A. and MORELLI, E. (1939). Carcinoma of the kidney in rats treated with beta-anthraquinoline. *American Journal of Cancer,* **35,** 534–537

STAUFFER, M.H. (1961). Nephrogenic hepatosplenomegaly (Abstract). *Gastroenterology,* **40,** 694

SUFRIN, G., MIRANDA, E.A., MOORE, R.H., CHU, T.M. and MURPHY, G.P. (1977). Hormones in renal cancer. *Journal of Urology,* **117,** 433–438

THATCHER, N., BARNARD, R., GASINNAS, N. and GROWTHER, P. (1977). Changes in cellular immunity following nephrectomy for localized and metastatic hypernephroma. *European Journal of Cancer,* **13,** 951–956

TYKKA, H., ORAVISTO, K.J., LEHTONEN, T., SHARNA, S. and TALLBER, T. (1968). Active specific immunotherapy of advanced renal cell carcinoma. *European Urology,* **4,** 250–258

URRUTIA, M., MONTERO, J., GANDE, J. and LLOPIS, M. (1977). Fosfatasas y scan oseo en el carcinoma de prostata. *Actas Urologicas Españolas,* **4,** 207–212

VAN ESCH, G.J. and KROES, R. (1969). The induction of renal tumors by feeding basic lead acetate to mice and hamsters. *British Journal of Cancer,* **23,** 765–771

WEIR, J.M. and DUNN, J.E. (1970). Smoking and mortality. A prospective study. *Cancer,* **25,** 105–112

WICKHAM, J.E.A. (1975). Conservative renal surgery for adenocarcinoma. The place of bench surgery. *British Journal of Urology,* **47,** 25–36

WILEY, A.L., WIRTANEN, G.W., ANSFIELD, F.J. and RAMIREZ, G. (1975). Combined intra-arrterial Actinomycin D and radiation therapy for surgically unresectable hypernephroma. *Journal of Urology,* **114,** 198–201

Chapter 19

Obstructive uropathy in the elderly

Saulo Klahr

Introduction

The changes in renal function that occur with normal aging have an important impact on the routine clinical management of urinary tract obstruction in the geriatric patient. There are greater risks of volume overload, from continuous salt intake, of hyperkalaemia and acid-base disturbances in older patients during the period of obstruction. The salt-losing tendency and abnormalities of water conservation that occur after relief of obstruction may be more severe in the geriatric patient. The increased susceptibility of the kidney to injury in elderly patients requires the cautious use of contrast material in the diagnosis of obstruction in these individuals. There is a greater propensity to develop congestive heart failure or pulmonary oedema during the period of obstruction or dehydration following relief of obstruction in geriatric patients. Since causes of lower urinary tract obstruction are more common and instrumentation more frequent in the elderly, infections of the urinary tract are seen quite often in geriatric patients with obstruction.

All of the above factors, and others not mentioned here but discussed in other chapters of this book, should be kept in mind when managing geriatric patients with urinary tract obstruction. Due to space limitations, certain areas of pathophysiology and diagnostic approach to obstruction have not been addressed in this chapter. The reader is referred to a recent review and chapter on obstructive uropathy for additional details (Klahr, 1983; Klahr, Buerkert and Morrison, 1986). However, none of these reviews deals specifically with the problems of urinary tract obstruction in the elderly.

Incidence

Urinary tract obstruction is a relatively common disorder. The incidence and causes of obstructive uropathy differ according to the age and sex of the patient. Bell (1946) found 1226 cases of hydronephrosis in an analysis of 32 360 autopsies, an overall frequency of 3.8 per cent. For the whole group, the frequency of urinary tract obstruction in males (3.9 per cent) and females (3.8 per cent) was similar, and before the age of 20 years no striking differences were found between the sexes. However, between 20 and 60 years of age, hydronephrosis was considerably more frequent in females, principally due to pregnancy and pelvic cancer. Over the age of 60 years the great majority of cases were found in males and this preponderance was related to the frequency of prostatic hypertrophy. The incidence of clinically apparent renal disease or symptoms of obstruction prior to death was not reported in the series of Bell, and hydronephrosis may have been an incidental finding at post mortem in many of these patients. A common, usually non-fatal, cause of hydronephrosis in the male is acute ureteral obstruction due to stones, and such cases would not be apparent in autopsy surveys. It has been estimated that nephrolithiasis is the cause of hospitalization in 1 of every 1000 Americans per year (Boyce and Strawcutter, 1956).

Classification

Obstruction of the urinary tract may be classified according to the following:

(1) *Duration. Acute obstruction* is said to occur when it is of short duration and abrupt in onset, as may occur with the passage of a stone, blood clot or sloughed papillae; *chronic obstruction* is used to describe those lesions present for months or years as, for example, in long-standing urolithiasis and hydronephrosis due to benign hyperplasia.

(2) *Location.* Obstruction may be located at the level of the renal tubules, as, for example, in uric acid nephropathy, or deposition of abnormal proteins (multiple myeloma). Obstruction of the *upper urinary tract* is most frequently unilateral. It may be located at the level of the renal infundibulum and pelvis, at the ureteropelvic junction, ureter or ureterovesical junction. Obstruction of the *lower urinary tract* is that occurring at the level of the bladder or posterior urethra or at the urethra. Obstruction at this level is by definition bilateral in nature and therefore affects the upper urinary tract of both kidneys.

(3) *Degree.* The obstruction is said to be *complete, high grade* or *total* when the lumen of the affected segment of the urinary tract is completely occluded. *Incomplete, partial* or *low grade obstruction* are those lesions that produce only partial occlusion of the lumen of the urinary tract.

This classification has important connotations both in terms of clinical presentation and therapeutic approach.

Causes of urinary tract obstruction in the elderly

The causes of urinary tract obstruction in the elderly are listed in *Table 19.1* and discussed in the text below.

Intrinsic causes of urinary tract obstruction

Intraluminal causes

Intraluminal obstruction can be intrarenal or extrarenal. A common cause of *intrarenal obstruction* is the deposition of uric acid crystals in the tubular lumen (uric acid nephropathy). This condition is seen most commonly in haematological malignancies, particularly during treatment with alkylating agents, and bears a direct relationship to the levels of uric acid in plasma (Conger, 1981). Renal failure is the second cause of death in patients with multiple myeloma (DeFronzo *et al.*,

Table 19.1 Causes of urinary tract obstruction in the elderly

- I Intrinsic causes
  - A. Intraluminal
    - 1. Intrarenal:
      uric acid
      multiple myeloma
    - 2. Extrarenal:
      calculi
      blood clots
  - B. Intramural
    - 1. Functional
      - (a) Neurogenic bladder:
        diseases of the brain, spinal cord or of peripheral innervation
      - (b) Bladder neck dysfunction
    - 2. Anatomical
      - (a) Tumours (polyps, carcinoma)
      - (b) Infections
      - (c) Strictures (post-radiation)
- II. Extrinsic causes
  - A. Reproductive system
    - 1. Males: prostatic enlargement either benign prostatic hyperplasia or adenocarcinoma
    - 2. Females: uterus, prolapse, fibro-adenoma, carcinoma of the cervix
  - B. Gastrointestinal tract
    Malignancies
  - C. Vascular system
    Aneurysmal dilatation
  - D. Retroperitoneal space
    - 1. Fibrosis
    - 2. Surgical complications
    - 3. Tumours: primary or metastatic
    - 4. Haemorrhage (haematomas)

1975). Deposition of Bence-Jones protein in the lumen of the renal tubule may play a significant role in this disease since histological studies of end-stage kidneys of patients with multiple myeloma show a lamellar deposition in the tubule of a protein which is immunologically similar to Bence-Jones protein. In support of this concept is the observation that the incidence of renal failure is higher in patients with multiple myeloma and Bence-Jones proteinuria. Further, the severity of the renal disease correlates well with the quantity of Bence-Jones protein excreted. Against this concept, however, is the observation that most patients with early renal failure have striking alterations in renal tubule cell morphology, but no histological evidence of protein deposition. Thus, renal insufficiency in these patients may be related to the toxic rather than the obstructive effects of Bence-Jones protein. Further, extrinsic obstruction of the ureter may occur in multiple myeloma as a consequence of large retroperitoneal myelomatous masses (Talreja *et al.*, 1980).

Renal calculi and blood clots are probably the most common *extrarenal cause* of intraluminal obstruction. Renal calculi composed of magnesium ammonium sulphate (struvite) occur in patients with persistently alkaline urine and frequent urinary tract infections (Williams, 1974), a clinical setting often observed in the elderly (Dontas *et al.*, 1966; Adler *et al.*, 1968; Sourander and Kasanen, 1972). The prevalence of this type of renal stone in the elderly is unknown, but 15 per cent of all renal calculi are struvite stones (Williams, 1974). Whether an abnormality in urinary acidification or infection with urea-splitting organisms is the primary event leading to stone formation is unclear. Indeed, the frequency of urinary tract infections is significantly greater in all types of kidney stone disease, and struvite stones may occur in individuals on chronic alkali therapy alone (Williams, 1974; Smith, 1979). Regardless of the exact mechanism of stone formation, infection with urea-splitting organisms, most commonly *Proteus* and less frequently *Klebsiella, Pseudomonas* and *Providentia* (Williams, 1974; Smith, 1979), leads to alkalinization of the urine and increased concentration of ammonia (Smith, 1979). This environment favours the precipitation of triple phosphate crystals (Williams, 1974).

Intramural causes

These causes of urinary tract obstruction can be (1) *functional* or (2) *anatomical.* The functional causes are related to dynamic abnormalities in the urinary tract. In the elderly, the two major functional abnormalities observed are neurogenic bladder and bladder neck dysfunction.

NEUROGENIC BLADDER

Abnormalities of urine storage in the bladder are characterized by incontinence and not infrequently by sustained increases in intravesical pressure which can adversely affect ureteral and renal function (McGuire, 1983). Alterations in the elastic properties of the bladder wall may result in a non-compliance state wherein the bladder resists filling at a higher pressure than normal. Pathological processes which damage the musculature of the bladder and its elastic fibres alter the normal bladder accommodation response. Prolonged catheterization, drainage via suprapubic tubes, chronic infection, interstitial cystitis and radiation therapy can result in permanent transmural injury and fibrosis. Increased vesical pressures (greater than 40–50 cm of water) are usually associated with ureteral dilatation and the development of vesico-ureteral reflux. There is, in addition, evidence that inflammation and ultimately fibrosis of the trigone which follows long-term chronic catheterization leads to vesico-ureteral reflux even at moderate bladder pressures (McGuire, 1983). These complications may occur, particularly in elderly patients, in whom chronic catheterization is frequently used for the management of incontinence.

In addition to changes in the anatomic characteristics of the bladder wall, neural abnormalities may also alter the storage ability of the bladder (Bradley, 1979). Interruption of the pelvic nerve, as may occur, for example, during radical pelvic surgery for carcinoma of the cervix, rectum or prostate, results with time in a subtle abnormality of storage function which appears to be due to injury of the preganglionic parasympathetic motor axon. The bladder becomes 'hypertonic' and resists filling with a pressure greater than normal. The pressure/volume relationship is controlled by the strength of the urethral continence mechanism which determines the intravesical pressure at which urethral urinary leakage occurs. As soon as intravesical pressure equals urethral pressure, urine loss from the urethra occurs. Therefore, the peak intravesical pressure is approximately equal to peak intra-urethral pressure. After pelvic neural transection, there is no neural mechanism to affect sphincteric relaxation with an increase in intravesical pressure. Ureteral pressure remains fixed and intravesical pressure, as a result of increasing volume, rises until urethral leakage occurs. Therefore, the magnitude of urethral pressure has a direct bearing on ureteral function since ureteral dilatation and vesico-ureteral reflux will develop at sustained intravesical pressures which are greater than 40 cm of water. While these pressures are unusual in females, pressures of 60–85 cm of water within the urethral sphincter are not unusual in males. To differentiate lesions which induce alterations in the elastic properties of the bladder wall from injuries affecting the innervation, a cystometrogram is required and usually the concurrent administration of cholinergic and/or anticholinergic agents. These drugs will induce a neuromuscular response in cases of neural injury, but will not influence the pressure/volume curve in fibrotic end-stage bladders.

Injuries or lesions at the level of the sacral plexus resemble those seen after pelvic neural injury and extensive sacral cord or root lesion may also injure alpha motor neurons to the external sphincter which will decrease urethral pressure. Dilatation of the bladder and increased pressures can also occur in patients who have isolated sensory denervation of the bladder. This occurs particularly commonly in patients with diabetes (Andersen and Bradley, 1976) and can also result from a posterior spinal cord compression syndrome. The bladder deprived only of its sensory innervation stores urine to great volumes with very little change in pressure. The principal problem here is the asymptomatic character of the neural injury which often prevents early diagnosis until the lesion is far advanced. The cystometrogram shows a flat pressure response to overfilling and there is lack of appreciation of bladder events by the patient.

Invasion of the lumbar and sacral dorsal roots by the virus of herpes zoster may result in urinary retention. The course of this disease is self-limited and resolves spontaneously in 1–2 months. Finally, in elderly individuals a definite relationship exists between the incidence of *cerebrovascular disease* and advanced *Parkinson's disease* and urinary bladder dysfunction. During the initial phase of a cerebrovascular accident, urinary retention is quite common (Marks and Bahr, 1977). In patients with Parkinson's disease hesitancy, difficulty in initiating voiding and retention of urine may occur. Obstructive symptoms may occasionally result from therapy with anti-parkinsonian agents (Bradley, 1979).

BLADDER NECK DYSFUNCTION

This abnormality has a peak incidence in the fourth to sixth decades of life (Gillenwater, 1978) and is an infrequent cause of obstructive nephropathy. Contracture of the vesical neck with difficulty in urination may be a complication of any form of prostatectomy, but more commonly of transurethral resection.

Anatomical causes

Anatomical lesions of the urinary tract resulting in obstruction are less common in the elderly. Strictures of the ureter have been described as a consequence of retroperitoneal surgery, although this is rare and as a complication of radiation therapy in patients with cervical carcinoma (0.3–1.6 per cent of treated patients) (Graham and Abad, 1967; Cushing *et al.*, 1968; Shingleton *et al.*, 1969). Rarely, strictures have been reported in association with analgesic nephropathy (McGregor *et al.*, 1973) and as a consequence of treatment of granulomatous diseases involving the ureter. Urethral strictures secondary to chronic instrumentation or surgery are infrequent causes of obstructive uropathy.

Extrinsic causes of urinary tract obstruction

Reproductive system — males

PROSTATIC ENLARGEMENT

Enlargement of the prostate to the extent that it produces obstruction of the urethra is an almost universal finding in aging men (Moore, 1943; Moore, 1944; Grayhack *et al.*, 1975; Walsh, 1979). Because of considerable progress in prostatic surgery, benign prostatic hyperplasia is not a leading cause of death, but it remains a major cause of morbidity in the elderly (Grayhack *et al.*, 1975). The prostate weighs approximately 1 g at birth, increases to about 4 g prior to puberty, and then grows to about 20 g by age 20. On average, there is no further change for approximately 20–30 years. A second growth spurt then commences and results in a mean weight of approximately 60 g by age 70 (Swyer, 1944). The frequency of symptomatic prostatic hyperplasia in American men above the age of 50 varies from 50 to 75 per cent in most series (Rotkin, 1975). In a small fraction of men the gland atrophies with age, presumably because of atherosclerosis of the arteries that supply the gland (Swyer, 1944).

In white men it is unusual for symptoms of urethral obstruction to be noted before 55 years of age; however, the disorder appears to be more common and to become manifest approximately 10 years earlier in black men. Japanese men have a lower incidence than do European and American men. There is no close relationship between the degree of enlargement and the development of symptoms, and severe obstruction to the urethra can occur as a result of regional changes within the gland in the absence of generalized growth (Chapman, Lapi and Fethiere, 1964). The discrepancy between the size of the gland and symptoms is due to the fact that benign prostatic hyperplasia begins in the peri-urethral area of the gland. The exact age at which the process commences is uncertain but is probably after 40 years. As the tissue in the peri-urethral area enlarges, it compresses the urethra and may cause obstructive symptoms prior to enlargement beyond the limits of the prostatic capsule. This may account for the fact that obstruction may occur before an increase in prostatic weight can be documented (Deming and Wolf, 1939; Semple, 1963).

Clinical manifestations. The symptoms of prostatic hypertrophy usually include disturbances in micturition (urgency, frequency, decreased urinary stream) and the finding of an enlarged prostate on rectal examination. Rarely, the enlargement of the prostate may be accompanied by symptoms which are so mild that the patients are unaware of them or choose to ignore them. Mild disturbances in micturition usually are discovered only after careful and direct questioning (Ewert and Summons, 1951). With progressive obstruction, the residual urine increases and eventually results in overflow incontinence. An enlarged prostate causing obstruction may result in hypertrophy of the detrusor with eventual detrusor decompensation, trabeculae formation and bladder diverticuli. This hypertrophy of the detrusor may also cause obstruction of the intramural ureter and dilatation of the upper urinary tract with progressive renal damage (Blandy, 1976). Reflux of urine into the ureters (found in up to 14 per cent of such patients) also contributes to the development of renal damage (Kogan and Freed, 1974).

One of the manifestations sometimes associated with prostatic obstruction is polyuria. This polyuria may mislead the physician with respect to the diagnosis of prostatic obstruction. Since polyuria with retention of urine in an atonic bladder may also occur in diabetes mellitus, the diagnosis of diabetes must be excluded (Motzkin,

1968). The generally accepted, but erroneous belief, that obstruction is associated with a decrease in urinary volume can seriously delay a correct diagnosis in these patients. With more advanced renal impairment as a consequence of prostatic obstruction, symptoms related to advanced renal failure may occur: generalized weakness, anorexia, nausea, constipation or diarrhoea, and weight loss. The abnormal rise in the levels of serum creatinine and blood urea nitrogen usually appears late in the development of renal failure, a fact which may also contribute to late diagnosis. Correct diagnosis is facilitated by a combination of these findings (Dick, 1952):

(1) A change in micturition habits and daily urine volumes (increase or decrease) indicative of an obstructive lesion in the lower urinary tract.
(2) The presence of an enlarged prostate on rectal examination, although the presence of a normal-sized prostate does not rule out the diagnosis.
(3) The presence of residual urine.
(4) Evidence of renal impairment, as demonstrated by a decrease in creatinine clearance or an increase in the serum creatinine level.
(5) Bilateral dilatation of the urinary collecting system with diverticula of the bladder, as shown by intravenous pyelography.

Mukamel *et al.* (1979), in reviewing the case histories of 345 patients who underwent prostatectomy, found that 1.7 per cent (6 patients) had progressive renal insufficiency secondary to prostatic hypertrophy. All these men were over the age of 60 and the disturbances in micturition were so mild that the patients were unaware of or chose to ignore them. The presenting symptoms were non-specific and included weakness, anorexia, nausea, constipation, and weight loss. Investigation revealed impaired renal function of varying degrees. Prostatectomy was associated with a dramatic improvement in all 6 patients. It should be remembered, therefore, that uraemia can develop with minimal urinary symptoms in patients who are elderly and have prostatic hypertrophy. Elderly men often suppress or deny their symptoms because of the fear of operation.

Pathogenesis. Any hypothesis that explains the pathogenesis of benign prostatic hypertropohy has to account for the following observations. First, the growth of the prostate, normal and abnormal, seems to be mediated by testicular hormones and it is generally believed that prostatic hyperplasia does not develop following castration. Secondly, it is widely believed that benign prostatic hypertrophy is a manifestation of aging. This belief awaits rigorous proof; although the symptoms of prostatic hyperplasia become manifest late, a pathologic process that gives rise to the symptoms may, in fact, have its onset many years earlier. Thirdly, there is a remarkable species specificity in that benign prostatic hyperplasia occurs only in men and dogs (Wilson, 1980). Thus, prostatic physiology in these two species may be different from that in other species. What these differences are remains to be established.

From studies of plasma hormone levels as a function of age, measurements of the concentration of androgen and of androgen–receptor proteins within the prostate and studies of the effects of administering various hormones on prostatic growth in the castrated dog, it is possible to provide a working hypothesis as to the pathogenesis of benign prostatic hyperplasia (Wilson, 1980; Horton, 1982). Dehydrotestosterone accumulation within the gland serves as the hormonal mediator for the hyperplasia in both species; the accumulation probably occurs in part because of decreased catabolism of the molecule and in part because of enhanced intracellular binding of the molecule. The process is accelerated by oestrogen which enhances the level of the androgen receptor in the gland; increase in the androgen receptor allows for androgen-mediated growth, even in the face of declining androgen production, and decreased circulating levels of androgens in advanced age.

Treatment. Provided the underlying model of the endocrine pathology is valid, then potentially exciting therapeutic implications can be drawn for the human disease. Transurethral resection of the prostate is generally safe, effective and associated with minimal side effects, and any alternative therapy for routine use would have to be clearly superior to surgical therapy. However, there is a group of poor risk patients in whom medical therapy would be desirable. To the present, non-extirpative therapy has been directed towards either surgical or medical castration, the latter with the use of drugs that block the synthesis or the action of androgens. In either case, hypogonadism and impotence are common side effects. Therapy directed either at inhibiting 5α-reductase activity (and consequently dehydrotestosterone formation) or blocking the synthesis or action of 17β-oestradiol might inhibit further prostatic growth and/or induce regression of the prostate without causing impotence or other manifestations of hypogonadism. To be effective, such therapy need not cause disappearance of the hyperplastic process but only enough regression to mitigate the symptoms of obstruction.

CANCER OF THE PROSTATE

In 1982, approximately 65 000 new cases of prostatic cancer were diagnosed in the USA. During this same period of time, approximately 24 000 patients died secondary to prostatic cancer (Cassady, 1982). The prompt diagnosis and optimal management of prostatic cancer is thus a major challenge to urologists, medical oncologists and radiation therapists. Carcinoma of the prostate is an important cause of urinary tract obstruction (Grayhack and Wendel, 1979). The probability of developing cancer of the prostate increases with age. Gaynor (1938) studied 1050 autopsies and found a correlation between the incidence of prostatic carcinoma and the age of the patient. Goldberg *et al.* (1956), utilizing data gathered in New York State (excluding the City of New York), calculated a 0.16 per cent probability of developing prostatic carcinoma at the age of 60, a 0.84 per cent chance at age 70, a 1.43 per cent chance at age 75, and a 2.55 per cent chance at age 85. The mortality rate of carcinoma of the prostate varies from 22.3 per 100 000 in non-white males in the USA to 1.1 per 100 000 males in Japan (Nesbit and Baum, 1950).

The spread of carcinoma of the prostate is by direct extension, lymphatic invasion or venous dissemination. When first discovered, most carcinomas of the prostate have already invaded locally with direct extension into the base of the bladder, into the perivesical fascia or laterally into the elevator ani muscles. Carcinoma of the prostate is often asymptomatic until it reaches an advanced state. Kimbrough (1956) states that when clinical symptoms are present only about 5 per cent of patients with prostatic carcinoma are amenable to surgical cure. The frequency of prostatic carcinoma in the absence of symptoms is demonstrated by discovery of 65 instances of localized carcinoma and 12 of metastatic carcinoma on random perineal prostatic biopsies of 686 virtually asymptomatic men, 78 per cent of whom were 50–60 years of age (Hudson, 1957). These observations emphasize the asymptomatic nature of early carcinoma of the prostate. When the disease does become symptomatic, complaints associated with bladder neck obstruction are most frequent, followed by pain in the back, bladder or perineum. Symptoms include dysuria, slow stream and urinary frequency. In one large series, complete urinary retention was the initial complaint in 24 per cent (Grayhack and Wendel, 1979).

The rectal examination is the principal resource in the diagnosis of carcinoma of the prostate. The seemingly increased rate of recognition of early carcinoma of the prostate (56 per cent) when prostatic examination is a mandatory routine (Kimbrough, 1956) would tend to support the value of the rectal examination as a screening device. Those carcinomas not suspected on rectal examination are probably overlooked because they are lacking in stroma or are soft or because they develop in an area which is not reached by posterior palpation. With more advanced disease, suspicion of carcinoma because of induration and irregularity of the prostate on examination becomes more accurate. Histologic study is the only presently available method to establish a definitive diagnosis of carcinoma of the prostate. Prostate fluid smears, transureteral punch, and open transrectal and punch and open perineal biopsies have been employed to obtain tissue to establish the diagnosis of carcinoma of the prostate. As a general rule, the more extensive the lesion, the easier it is to establish the diagnosis (Kaufman and Schultz, 1962). The determination of serum acid phosphatase levels has proved to be a valuable adjunct in assessing the cancer stage and the results of therapy in patients with carcinoma of the prostate. The failure of a rapid significant fall of an elevated serum acid phosphatase with therapy has usually heralded an unsatisfactory response. When the acid phosphatase returns to abnormal levels after a fall to or near normal, it is usually an indication of recurrent tumour activity or so-called relapse.

Treatment. Therapeutic attempts to modify the natural history of carcinoma of the prostate have utilized surgical excision, endocrine manipulation, radiation therapy, chemotherapeutic agents and combinations of these. The results obtained vary with the stage at which these therapeutic modalities are employed.

In summary, the combination of benign prostatic hypertrophy and adenocarcinoma of the prostate account for the greater occurrence of obstructive uropathy over the age of 60 in males than in females.

Reproductive system — females

In elderly females, uterine prolapse and pelvic masses, benign or malignant, account for most of the cases of hydronephrosis. The incidence of hydronephrosis associated with uterine prolapse is in the vicinity of 5 per cent (Persky, Kursh and Feldman, 1970). The mechanism is not clearly understood, but may be due to compression of the ureters outside the bladder (Rudin, Megalli and Lattimer, 1974). When the bladder, uretus and ureters are herniated through the weakness in the elevator ani muscles, the ureters may be compressed between the uterus and the bladder against elevators. Urinary infection, sepsis or pyonephrosis and renal insufficiency have all been reported with uterine prolapse. Benign pelvic masses, such as fibroids of the uterus and cysts of the ovary, may cause deviation and intrinsic compression of the ureter (Persky, Kursh and Feldman, 1970). This incidence of obstruction increases as the size of the mass enlarges, especially if it projects above the pelvic brim. Inadvertant ligation of the ureter may occur during abdominal or retroperitoneal surgery and more than 50 per cent of cases develop during gynaecologic procedures. The incidence of accidental ureteral damage in routine hysterectomy is less than 0.5

per cent, but alarmingly when it occurs is bilateral in approximately 16 per cent of cases (Donovan and Gibson, 1973). Less commonly, ureteral ligation may occur during general surgical procedures, particularly during colon–rectal surgery.

Another common cause of extrinsic urinary obstruction in females are pelvic malignancies, particularly adenocarcinoma of the cervix (Beach, 1952). In early studies, both clinical and post mortem, it has been shown that untreated patients with carcinoma of the cervix commonly die of uraemia (60–90 per cent). Of patients with adenocarcinoma of the cervix presenting to clinics, one-third have major urologic damage. Usually, the spread of cervical carcinoma first results in distortion of the base of the bladder, with later involvement of the lower portion of the ureters. Ureteral obstruction is the most common urinary tract complication of cervical carcinoma. Obstruction almost always occurs in the distal ureter; in one series the obstruction was found to be at or near the ureterovesical junction in 96 per cent of cases in which the site of obstruction could be localized (Van Nagell, Sprague and Roddeck, 1975). Ureteral obstruction is found at diagnosis in approximately 15 per cent of patients with cervical carcinoma. The incidence of ureteral obstruction is correlated with increasing stage of disease. Of 86 patients in one series who had ureteral obstruction, the incidence ranged from 2.2 per cent in patients with stage I disease to 38 per cent in those with stage IV disease. In addition, while bilateral ureteral obstruction did not occur in the early stages, it was found in 7.6 per cent of patients with stage IV disease.

Gastrointestinal tract

Malignancies of the gastrointestinal tract, particularly colon and rectum, may result in extrinsic compression of the ureter due to invasion or metastasis to the retroperitoneum. Occasionally, bladder dysfunction may occur as a complication of surgical procedures for cancer of the rectosigmoid (see above).

The vascular system

Abdominal aortic aneurysms are the most common vascular cause of obstructive uropathy in the elderly (Labardini and Ratliff, 1967; Abercrombie and Hendry, 1971; Abbott *et al.*, 1973; Peck *et al.*, 1973). As many as 10 per cent of patients with aneurysms may develop urological complications. The compromise of the ureter is usually unilateral, although bilateral ureteral obstruction secondary to aortic aneurysm has been reported (Wagenkecht and Madsen, 1970). Traction displacement of the ureter may be a sign of aortic aneurysm (Peck *et al.*, 1973). Aneurysms of both external and common iliac arteries are rare causes of ureteral obstruction (Mehl, 1969).

Diseases of the retroperitoneum

Diseases which involve the retroperitoneal space can give rise to obstructive uropathy. Tumour invasion from cervix, prostate, bladder, colon, ovary and uterus account for 70 per cent of the extrinsic causes of obstruction in the retroperitoneum (Abrams *et al.*, 1950; Persky *et al.*, 1970; Adams, 1974; Khan and Utz, 1975). Less commonly, retroperitoneal fibrosis may result in ureteral obstruction (Utz and Henry, 1966; Hewitt *et al.*, 1969). A growing number of cases of unknown aetiology, so-called *idiopathic retroperitoneal fibrosis,* have been described in recent years (Jones and Alexander, 1966). These cases occur with equal frequency in both sexes and have been described over a wide age range, but predominate in the fifth and sixth decades of life, with the oldest cases having been reported at age 85. The fibrosis appears to involve the middle third of the ureter pulling it toward the mid-line. Such fibrosis can also involve the aorta, vena cava and psoas muscles and may extend from the renal pedicle to below the psoas major. The aetiology is unclear. Long-term administration of methysergide (Sansert) may favour the development of this disease (Graham, 1964; Kunkel, 1971) which occurs in 1 per cent of patients taking the drug.

Retroperitoneal fibrosis may also be the consequence of other disease processes, inflammatory processes of the lower extremities with ascending lymphangitis, and multiple surgical procedures in the abdomen. Biliary tract disease, chronic urinary tract infection and tuberculosis have been all associated with retroperitoneal fibrosis on rare occasions.

Pathophysiology of urinary tract obstruction

Due to space limitations, the pathophysiology of urinary tract obstruction will not be discussed in detail in this chapter. The reader is referred to recent reviews on this subject for additional information (Klahr, 1983; Klahr, Buerkert and Morrison, 1986).

Normal urine production and flow depend on (1) hydrostatic pressure which progressively decreases from the kidney to the bladder, and (2) ureteral peristalsis. Obstruction to urine flow anywhere in the system causes an increase in pressure and volume of urine proximal to the obstruction. Significant obstruction impairs renal function, and if the obstruction is severe enough the kidney may be destroyed. Renal injury is probably due to elevated ureteral pressure and decreased renal blood flow causing ischaemia, cellular atrophy and necrosis. Ureteral peristalsis allows for the generation of high intraluminal pressures necessary for the propulsion of a bolus of urine, with contraction of the circular muscular fibres of the ureter preventing this pressure from being transmitted to the kidney (Struthers, 1982). With obstruction this phenomenon, called coaptation, is lost and high intraluminal pressures can be transmitted upwards to the kidney (Whitaker, 1982). An increase in ureteral pressure is reflected in increases in intratubular pressure. The rise in intratubular pressure in turn decreases the net hydrostatic filtration pressure. By 24 h of obstruction, intratubular pressures have returned to normal in animals with unilateral ureteral obstruction, but remain elevated in animals with bilateral ureteral obstruction, although values are less than the peak levels obtained at 6–8 h after obstruction (Klahr, 1983).

RENAL BLOOD FLOW

Although there is an increase in renal blood flow in the first few hours after the onset of obstruction, this is followed by a progressive decrease in renal blood flow such that after 8 weeks of obstruction in the dog renal blood flow in the obstructed kidney is only 20 per cent of control values. The initial rise in renal blood flow is mediated by increased prostaglandin synthesis, particularly PGE_2 (Blacksear and Wathen, 1978). The subsequent decrease in blood flow is probably due to the effects of vasoconstrictor substances such as thromboxane A_2 and angiotensin II (Yarger, Schocken and Harris, 1980).

GLOMERULAR FILTRATION RATE

In the first few hours after the onset of obstruction, there is a fall in net hydrostatic pressure which is due almost exclusively to a marked increase in intratubular pressure. This is the main mechanism responsible for the initial decrease in GFR. After 24 h of obstruction, a decrease in renal blood flow and a fall in hydrostatic glomerular capillary pressure are the main mechanisms responsible for the decrement in GFR. Partial obstruction of the urinary tract may lead to similar alterations in renal blood flow and GFR, but in addition tubular defects may be prominent. These include: a concentrating defect and decreased excretion of hydrogen ions and potassium.

CONCENTRATING DEFECT

The concentrating defect is due in part to the inability to generate a high osmolality gradient in the renal medulla and is probably related to decreased sodium reabsorption in the thick ascending limb of Henle. There is also a diminished hydro-osmotic response of the collecting duct to vasopressin (Hanley and Davidson, 1982).

ACIDIFYING DEFECT AND ALTERED POTASSIUM EXCRETION

The acidifying defect and the decrease in potassium excretion may be due to decreased hydrogen ion and potassium secretion in distal segments of the nephron, presumably related to decreased responsiveness of these segments to aldosterone (Campbell, Bello-Reuss and Klahr, 1984). In elderly individuals, low levels of aldosterone in plasma due to decreased renin secretion as a consequence of interstitial renal disease may contribute further to the decrease in hydrogen ion and potassium secretion seen in obstructive uropathy (Batlle, Arruda and Kurtzman, 1981).

Clinical manifestations

The symptoms and signs of urinary tract obstruction are often non-specific, and the clinical manifestations may be dominated by the degree of renal functional impairment, by the presence of urinary tract infection, and sometimes by extrarenal signs and symptoms of the underlying pathological process, for example, local and

Table 19.2 Clinical manifestations and laboratory findings in urinary tract obstruction

1. Alteration in urine output:
   changes in volume (anuria, oliguria, polyuria)
   difficulties in micturition (hesitancy, decreased force or calibre of urinary stream, urgency, etc.
2. Pain
3. Recurrent infections or infections of the urinary tract refractory to appropriate therapy
4. Impaired renal function or deterioration of renal function without apparent cause
5. Systemic hypertension
6. Polycythaemia
7. Gross haematuria
8. Hyperchloraemic hyperkalaemic acidosis

distant metastases from tumours producing obstruction of the urinary tract. Some clinical features of urinary tract obstruction, when present, however, are sufficiently distinctive to suggest the proper diagnosis (*Table 19.2*). The clinical manifestations of urinary tract obstruction will be conditioned by the duration, location and degree of obstruction.

Alterations in urine output

If obstruction is bilateral and complete or unilateral in a patient with a solitary kidney, total anuria results. However, with partial obstruction urine output may be normal. Polyuria may occur in this setting and, when marked, it may be a prominent presenting symptom (Roussak and Oleesky, 1954; Knowlan *et al.*, 1960; Mees, 1960). A finding characteristic of intermittent obstruction is the sequential occurrence of oligo-anuria and polyuria. When anuria occurs, obstruction should be suspected. The clinical setting of its occurrence is important and obstruction should be considered with precedent pelvic surgery where inadvertent ligation of the ureters can occur, pelvic malignancy where extension of the tumour with invasion of the ureters may result in obstruction, long-standing bladder neck obstruction, recent ureteric transplant, recent ileal bladder construction, recent retrograde pyelography, and in the presence of an indwelling bladder catheter which has not been irrigated.

Obstruction of the lower urinary tract may cause difficulties in micturition such as a decrease in the force and/or calibre of the urinary stream, intermittency, post-void dribbling, hesitancy and nocturia. Urgency, frequency and urinary incontinence (overflow incontinence) can result from inability to empty the bladder completely.

Pain

Pain is often a presenting complaint in patients with obstructive uropathy. The pain is secondary to stretching of the collecting system or renal capsule and it is not caused by increased peristalsis. The pain subsides when the distension is eliminated and its severity correlates with the rate of distension rather than the degree of dilatation. Thus, acute obstruction, as seen with renal calculi, is often associated with excruciating pain whereas marked, long-standing hydronephrosis may be asymptomatic. Acute ureteral obstruction may cause a steady crescendo pain radiating downward towards the groin and into the testicles or labia (Risholm, 1954). The onset of pain is often insidious. The pain usually is steady, continuous and crescendo in character, with minor fluctuations in intensity. Thus, the name 'renal colic' is a misnomer. The acute attack may be as brief as 30 min or as long as 24 h. Chronic ureteral obstruction may be associated with no pain or with intermittent mild non-radiating back or flank discomfort. Costovertebral angle pain after ingestion of large volumes of fluids or after diuretic therapy is suggestive of intermittent hydronephrosis secondary to ureteropelvic junction narrowing (Covington and Reeser, 1950). Pain radiating into the flank with micturition is said to be pathognomonic of ureterovesical reflux. Acute ureteral obstruction may cause a paralytic ileus and hence gastrointestinal manifestations. It should also be noted that obstruction at any level of the urinary tract can be painless and asymptomatic.

Recurrent or refractory urinary tract infection

Infection is a frequent complication in patients with lower urinary tract obstruction. Hasner (1962) found an infection rate of 8.6 per cent in 221 men with benign prostatic hypertrophy and post-void residual volume of greater than 50 ml who had not been instrumented. Obstruction of the upper urinary tract is not necessarily associated with infection, although experimental evidence indicates that the obstructed kidney is more easily infected than an unobstructed kidney (Guze and Beeson, 1956, 1958). Repeated infections without apparent cause should raise the suspicion of obstruction. Moreover, as long as the obstruction persists, eradication of the infection may prove exceedingly difficult. Therefore, obstructive uropathy must be considered in patients with a history of repeated urinary tract infections or with a persistent infection that is refractory to antibiotic therapy.

Deterioration of renal function without apparent cause

A number of patients who present with manifestations of chronic uraemia may have unrecognized long-standing urinary tract obstruction. Obstructive uropathy may occur in patients with underlying kidney disease of another aetiology and manifest itself by a change in the rate of progression of renal insufficiency. In some patients, however, obstruction is the only cause of end-stage renal failure. Occasionally, in patients with retroperitoneal fibrosis, where the onset of obstruction is slow and progressive, far-advanced renal failure may be an initial presenting complaint. Urinary tract obstruction should be considered in patients with uraemia with no previous history of renal disease and relatively benign urine sediment and in patients with known renal disease who develop an abrupt decrease in renal function that is otherwise unexplained. The added complication of urinary tract obstruction can result in serious and sometimes life-threatening exacerbation of renal failure if the glomerular filtration rate is already markedly reduced. Two special circumstances serve to predispose the elderly patient to obstruction: (1) the use of parasympatholytic drugs prescribed for the control of nausea and vomiting or for depression can lead to bladder atony, and (2) failure to respond appropriately to bladder distension. Partial bladder neck obstruction due to an enlarged prostate will enhance the predisposition to urinary tract obstruction in elderly patients.

Hypertension

Acute or chronic hydronephrosis, either unilateral or bilateral, may be accompanied by a significant elevation in blood pressure (Belman *et al.*, 1968; Schwartz, 1969; Garrett *et al.*, 1970; Palmer *et al.*, 1970; Nemoy *et al.*, 1973; Vaughan *et al.*, 1974; Weidmann *et al.*, 1977). The hypertension could be coincidental or could be due to the hydronephrosis causing either impaired sodium excretion or abnormal renin release.

In cases of bilateral hydronephrosis, the demonstration of increased exchangeable sodium and the usual prompt decrease of blood pressure after adequate drainage and diuresis would suggest that the hypertension is due primarily to expansion of the extracellular fluid volume as a consequence of abnormal retention of salt and water during the period of obstruction. These patients appear to have a volume-dependent form of hypertension, since renin levels in renal and peripheral venous blood are normal.

The hypertension seen in patients with unilateral ureteral obstruction may be renin related, since elevated renal vein renin concentrations from unilateral hydronephrotic kidneys have been reported (Belman *et al.*, 1968; Nemoy *et al.*, 1973; Squitieri *et al.*, 1974). After corrective surgery, the hypertension abated and the renin values returned to normal. Animal studies have demonstrated increased renin release following acute ureteral obstruction (Vander, 1967; Eide *et al.*, 1977; Oliw, 1978). In contrast, chronic studies in animals with prolonged unilateral ureteral occlusion have shown that plasma renin is normal. Although it has been suggested that, in unilateral obstruction, renin release is responsible for the hypertension, other studies in patients with chronic hydronephrosis revealed normal or low values for peripheral renin, suggesting that established hydronephrosis is not a cause of increased renin secretion. In addition, in these studies, differential measurements did not reveal increased renin levels in the renal vein of the hydronephrotic kidney or contralateral suppression of renin secretion. Since corrective surgery may improve the hypertension, some other abnormalities not related to renin may occur in obstruction. Whether these abnormalities relate to subtle changes in volume or the lack of release of vasodepressor substances by the kidney has not been established.

Polycythaemia

The association of polycythaemia and hydronephrosis has been reported and, in a few instances, the inreased red blood cell count decreased after relief of the obstruction (Jaworski and Wolan, 1963). The relation of hydronephrosis to increased erythropoietin levels in men is not clear. However, unilateral hydronephrosis in experimental animals has been shown to result in elevated plasma levels of erythropoietin which preceded an increase in haemoglobin levels (Mitus *et al.*, 1968).

Other clinical manifestations and laboratory findings

Gross haematuria may be associated with urinary tract obstruction. Obstruction may impair the ability of the kidney to acidify and result in a *hyperchloraemic hyperkalaemic acidosis* (Batlle *et al.*, 1981; Pelleya *et al.*, 1983). In patients with incomplete partial obstruction, a marked polyuria may occur leading to the development of hypertonic (*hypernatraemic*) dehydration and the clinical manifestations of such an electrolyte derangement (Landsberg, 1970).

Diagnostic approach

Clearly, the approach to a patient with urinary tract obstruction will depend on the clinical setting and presenting symptoms, the spectrum of which extends from those patients presenting with the acute onset of pain to those patients with acute renal failure and anuria (Klahr, 1984). Thus, the diagnostic approach and the urgency with which the diagnosis must be made will be highly variable. When urinary tract obstruction is suspected, certain preliminary information is essential. The past history of similar symptoms, urinary tract infection and the kinds of drugs ingested are important. Eliciting previous symptoms of lower urinary tract obstruction is clearly important. In hospitalized patients, an attempt should be made to characterize the pattern of urinary output, whether it has changed abruptly, gradually declined, or fluctuates. Such information may be obtained from input and output records.

Physical examination with particular reference to the abdomen and prostatic size is of obvious importance. In elderly patients, urinary outlet obstruction should be suspected when a suprapubic mass is found.

Urinalysis and blood studies

Analysis of the urinary sediment provides important information. The presence of haematuria alone may suggest that the obstructing lesion is a calculus, sloughed papilla or tumour. When haematuria is found in conjunction with bacteriuria, one might suspect that if urinary tract obstruction exists it is of a more chronic nature. Bacteriuria alone may suggest stasis, especially in males. When the bacteriuria is associated with numerous white blood cell casts, pyelonephritis should be suspected. At this point, the differential diagnosis would include chronic obstruction, perhaps as a consequence of calculi, and if the patient is septic, the diagnosis of papillary necrosis must be ruled out. The urinary sediment should be examined carefully for the presence of crystals. Uric acid crystals may be the first indication that an episode of acute renal failure is due to intrarenal obstruction. Laboratory studies should include measurements of renal function (serum creatinine and urea nitrogen levels) in addition to the usual haematological determinations.

Diagnostic procedures

Once the above information is obtained, the course of the diagnostic evaluation will be determined by the symptom complex and results obtained during the preliminary evaluation of the patient. Two important factors are pain and whether or not there is evidence of diminished renal function. In patients presenting with pain but no evidence of a decrease in GFR, the diagnostic emphasis should be focused on the presence or absence of a renal calculus. In these patients, the next step is a radiological evaluation of the abdomen without the injection of contrast media. In most cases, plain films of the abdomen will allow evaluation of the size and contour of the kidneys. Frequently, a calculus can be seen at some juncture along the urinary tract. If a calculus is found, or if the clinical evidence strongly suggests the passage of a stone, the next step is to perform an intravenous pyelogram. Such a study will be important for two reasons: (1) it will allow the clinician to establish the degree of obstruction caused by the stone, and (2) it will ascertain if the pain is a result of a radiolucent stone. Once a diagnosis of an obstructing calculus has been made, radiological techniques are essential in the follow-up care of such patients. Whether or not the stone is to be removed surgically will be determined in large part by the chronicity of the obstruction. An aid in this decision should be sought from a urologist. Subsequent studies should involve characterization of the aetiology of the calculus and an attempt should be made to control those factors which gave rise to the stone. In elderly patients, however, radiographic evaluation using contrast material should be performed with caution. Using renographic techniques, obstruction can be inferred if the excretory decay curves are different, right versus left. Ultrasound may also be used in centres where expertise with this technique is available.

When renal function is impaired and there is no clear aetiology or when renal insufficiency exists for a known reason but abruptly declines, the diagnosis of urinary obstruction should be considered. The diagnostic approach to these patients will depend in large part on the facilities and expertise available to the physician. In most centres, the standard approach is to evaluate renal size and function with the use of plain film X-rays of the abdomen, followed by intravenous pyelography (*Figure 19.1A*). If obstruction exists, it may be discerned at two points in the study. The nephrogram phase of the study is the first point. This may be delayed, but in most cases occurs within the first hour after the injection of the contrast media. At this time, the calyces will be outlined as a negative shadow. Tomographic patterns of the fat near the renal pelvis will also be helpful. If it is present, under normal circumstances it appears as well-defined finger-like projections radiating from the renal hilum. When obstruction is present, this fat is displaced by the hydronephrotic calyces. The second point in time when obstruction may be ascertained is in the delayed films. At this interval, the radio-opaque dye enters the renal pelvis. It is important to remember that using the combination of the plain films, high dose either drip or bolus intravenous injections of radio-opaque dye and tomography, renal size and calyceal dilatation can be adequately assessed independent of the level of renal function.

In choosing this approach to a patient with renal insufficiency, the clinician must be aware of the possible risks involved (Shedahi and Toniolo, 1980). There is an accumulating body of information which suggests that acute renal failure, usually reversible, can follow *intravenous pyelography* (Harkonen and Kjellstrand, 1981). The risk of this complication is greatest in patients with diabetes mellitus, with or without renal insufficiency, in chronic renal insufficiency of any type, and in patients with hypertension, cardiovascular disease or haematological disorders such as polycythaemia vera. Dehydration probably constitutes the single most important factor influencing further renal impairment after intravenous pyelography (Harkonen and Kjellstrand, 1981). There is a strong relationship between renal failure and multiple studies using any of the four contrast media procedures (intravenous and oral cholecystography, angiography and computed tomography). Finally, there is an increased risk in patients in the older age group, with or without azotaemia (Greenberger *et al.*, 1980). Because of this risk, less invasive procedures to diagnose ureteral obstruction have been developed.

Of these procedures, *ultrasonography* is the least invasive. In the proper hands, the diagnosis of a dilated calyceal system can be made using ultrasonography in nearly 100 per cent of cases. Exceptions would include patients with end-stage kidneys or patients with high urine output states. It is important to remember that with this technique one demonstrates ureteral (*Figure 19.1B*) and calyceal dilatation. Thus, the diagnosis of obstruction is implied and further studies are indicated to determine if the dilatation is a consequence of obstruction at some point along the urinary tract or whether the dilatation is a consequence of reflux, urinary tract infection or primary mega-ureter and megacalycosis. Hence, a positive finding from ultrasound would lead one to intravenous pyelography.

Computed tomography scanning (CT scan) can be a valuable adjunct to ultrasonography in the evaluation of the azotaemic patient. It provides additional information in that it better defines space-occupying lesions in the retroperitoneum. Computed tomography may be utilized in the preliminary evaluation of patients with suspected urinary tract obstruction.

With this armamentarium of diagnostic tools, it is seldom necessary, as a diagnostic technique, to perform retrograde pyelography which is associated with a significant morbidity, although such an approach may be important to characterize a

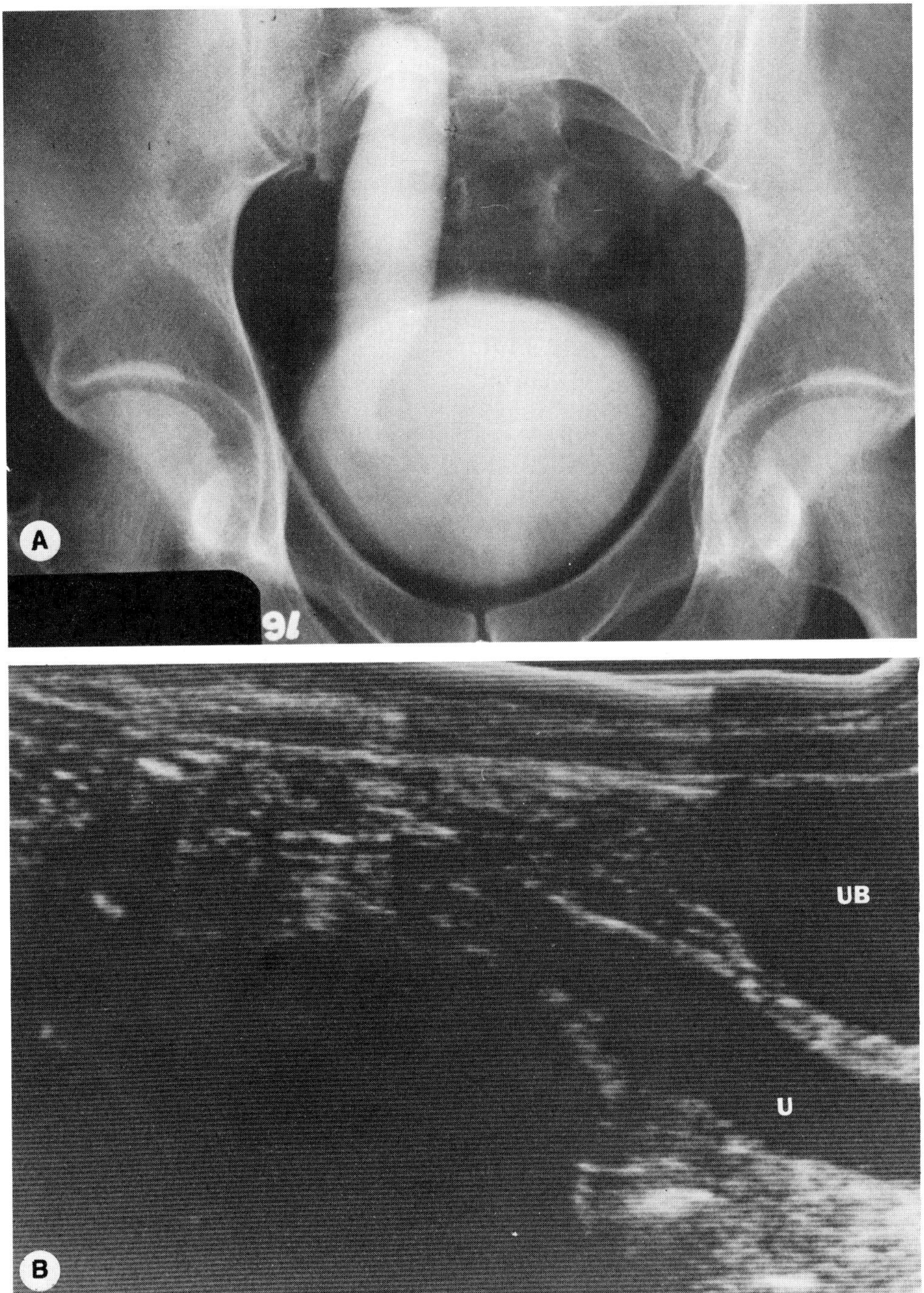

Figure 19.1 (A) Intravenous pyelogram; (B) pelvic ultrasonogram showing a dilated ureter to the level of the bladder. Ultrasonography may occasionally elucidate the level of ureteral obstruction (U, ureter; UB, urinary bladder) (From Kaye and Pollack, 1982, reproduced with permission)

lesion, relieve obstruction or determine whether the observed dilatation is a consequence of obstruction.

While non-invasive techniques are helpful in making the diagnosis of ureteral dilatation or hydronephrosis, it is frequently difficult to differentiate non-obstructing from obstructing causes of hydronephrosis. Radiological evaluation may be helpful; a non-visualized kidney is an extreme example of complete obstruction. Failure of the dye to pass through a point of narrowing produces additional information. Retrograde evaluation may be necessary to determine whether a standard-sized ureteral catheter can be easily passed through a point of narrowing and whether the passage through this site is associated with a 'gush' of urine. Frequently, the diagnosis of obstruction may only be made in retrospect; that is, once the stenotic lesion is removed, renal function improves.

Treatment and management

After establishing the diagnosis of urinary tract obstruction, a decision should be made whether to undertake surgical or instrumental procedures. Complete bilateral obstruction presenting as acute renal failure requires intervention as soon as possible. In these patients, the site of obstruction will frequently determine the approach. If the obstructive lesion is distal to the bladder, passage of a urethral catheter may suffice, although this may require the aid of a urological surgeon. In some cases, suprapubic cystostomy may be necessary. On the other hand, if there is an upper tract lesion (e.g. malignant infiltration of the trigone by cervical or prostatic adenocarcinoma), then nephrostomy tubes should be placed at the time of ultrasonography. It is worth emphasizing that tubes should be placed in *both* renal calyces since the potential for recovery of function by either kidney cannot be predicted at the time of the procedure. Such an approach may avoid the need for dialysis and allows the physician time to determine the specific site and character of the obstructing lesion. Further, the nephrostomy tube may be useful for the local infusion of pharmacologic agents with which to treat infection, malignancy or calculi (Pfister and Newhouse, 1979). In patients with obstruction complicated by urinary infection and generalized sepsis, appropriate antibiotics and other supportive therapy is indicated.

In patients with low grade acute obstruction or partial chronic obstruction, surgical intervention could be delayed for a few weeks or even months, especially when infection is present. In such patients, elective repair of obstruction is indicated when: (1) there are multiple repeated episodes of urinary tract infection; (2) there is persistent pain; (3) urinary retention; and (4) recurrent or progressive renal damage documented by sequential renal function studies. It should be remembered that the presence of post-void residual urine, ureterovesical reflux or dilatation of the collecting system is not in itself an indication for surgical intervention.

Management of lower urinary tract obstruction

Bladder neck and urethral obstruction should be surgically repaired in ambulatory patients who have recurrent infections, especially when associated with reflux, evidence of renal parenchymal damage, total urinary retention, repeated bleeding or severe symptoms. Difficulties with voiding secondary to benign prostatic hypertrophy do not always follow a progressive course. Therefore, the patient with minimal symptoms, no infection and a normal upper urinary tract may be followed safely until he and his physician agree that surgery is desirable. The incidence of bladder neck and urethral obstruction in females is low and has been overestimated in the past; therefore, urethral dilatation, internal urethrotomies, meatotomies and bladder neck plasties are seldom indicated. Urethral stricture secondary to infection or trauma are frequently treated by simple dilatation, subsequent to which follow-up care is essential to rule out recurrence. Suprapubic cystostomy, for bladder drainage, may be indicated in patients who are unable to void after sustaining injury to the urethra or who have an impassable urethral stricture.

When obstructive uropathy is due to a neurogenic bladder, urodynamic studies are essential to determine a treatment regimen. In all cases, the main therapeutic goals are to establish the bladder as a site of urine storage without causing renal parenchymal injury, continence, and to provide a mechanism for bladder emptying which is acceptable to the patient (Wein *et al.*, 1976). In general, these patients fall into two general groups: those with bladder atony secondary to lower motor neuron injury, and those with unstable bladder function due to upper motor neuron disease. In both cases ureteral reflux and renal parenchymal injury may occur. This may be potentiated by sphincter–detrusor dyssynergia. Patients with neurogenic bladder function due to diabetes mellitus are classic examples of lower motor neuron disease (Andersen and Bradley, 1976). Voiding at regular intervals, followed by external compression (Crede manoeuvre) and increased abdominal pressure (Valsalva manoeuvre), may result in satisfactory bladder emptying in such patients. Occasionally, these individuals will respond to cholinergic medications. Bethanechol chloride (urecholine) 50 mg orally is most frequently used, although a subcutaneous dose of 1–10 mg is more effective. In such patients, overdistension of the bladder impairs emptying since detrussor contraction is essential to sphincter relaxation. Thus, bladder outlet obstruction may be a major problem, the best treatment for which is the institution of clean intermittent catheterization at regular intervals (Lapides *et al.*, 1972, 1974; Pearman, 1976). This technique has met with considerable success in almost all age groups, but requires patient acceptance and careful training. Alpha adrenergic drugs, such as phenoxybenzamine, relax sphinter tone but have only limited success because of their side effects and because the patient may be rendered incontinent. External sphincterostomy by transurethral resection is equally as successful as clean intermitten catheterization, but also has the disadvantage of urine incontinence (Morrow and Bogaard, 1977). In males, this problem can be obviated by the use of a penile clamp. In females, incontinence is a major problem. In both sexes, implantation of artificial sphincters have been partially successful and are a promising alternative.

In patients with neurogenic bladders due to upper motor lesions, the major goal is to improve the storage function of the bladder. Pharmacologic manoeuvres include the use of anticholinergic agents like propantheline bromide (Pro-Banthine), 15 mg every 4–6 h, which block uninhibited contractions. Adjunctive therapy such as intermittent catheterization or the Crede manoeuvre are frequently necessary to ensure complete bladder emptying.

In all these patients, chronic indwelling catheters are to be avoided if at all possible (Perkash, 1975, 1976). Surgical diversions are seldom indicated (less than 1 per cent of patients with neuropathic bladder function undergo this procedure). The major indications for such a procedure are (1) deterioration of renal function despite conservative measures, (2) intractable incontinence in the female, (3) small contracted bladder, and (4) multiple bladder fistulae. Intermittent bacteriuria is seldom an indication, since it is common to all therapeutic approaches to the neurogenic bladder. The ileal conduit is the operation of choice for permanent diversion. Although many individuals do well after this procedure, operative mortality, postoperative intestinal obstruction and stomal obstruction are complications that make the operation far from ideal. Further, recent studies indicate a progressive decline in renal function in as many as 80 per cent of these patients.

The indications for chronic urethral catheterization include: (1) facilitation of bladder drainage, (2) monitoring the urinary output, (3) enhancement of X-ray procedures, and (4) facilitation of lower abdominal or pelvic surgery. Indiscriminate use of chronic urethral catheterization has been properly criticized because of the risk of suppurative infection of the urogenital tract and renal parenchymal injury which could lead to chronic renal failure. Chronic catheter drainage should be replaced by intermittent catheterization as soon as feasibly possible (Donnelly, Hackler and Bunts, 1972). This latter technique should be performed under sterile conditions while in the hospital and under clean conditions after discharge. The use of intermittent catheterizations significantly reduces the incidence of pyelonephritis and suppurative lesions in the genital tract (e.g. prostatic and testicular abscesses). Further, it virtually eliminates chronic bacteriuria. Adequate patient selection and proper technique for self-catheterization and catheter drainage are essential.

Good care is necessary to prevent urinary tract infections in patients requiring an indwelling urethral catheter. Using specific indications for catheter drainage, proper patient selection, aseptic technique, closed urinary drainage, the judicious use of systemic antimicrobials and proper catheter care of the indwelling urethral catheter is a satisfactory means of short-term diversion and in certain instances long-term urinary diversion. The principles of closed drainage should be rigorously adhered to. The author prefers not to break the drainage system for catheter irrigation or for the use of antibiotic irrigating solutions to reduce infection, as has been advocated by some. In patients requiring long-term catheter drainage, use of intermittent irrigation with an acid citrate solution is useful in reducing encrustation and frequent catheter changes.

Renal function after release of obstruction in man

Clinical course

Several studies of renal function in man after release of chronic hydronephrosis or correction of partial unilateral ureteral obstruction indicate that the post-obstructed kidney has reduced renal blood flow, glomerular filtration rate, concentrating ability, hydrogen ion excretion and phosphate excretion. Sodium reabsorption is mildly impaired, while urinary dilution is not affected (Platts and Williams, 1963; Better *et al.*, 1973; Gillenwater *et al.*, 1975; McDougal and Persky, 1975).

Glomerular filtration and renal blood flow

In man, the relationship between the duration of obstruction and the degree of recovery of renal function after release is not known. In most instances, where renal function has been studied before and after correction of chronic, partial ureteral obstruction, there is a tendency for renal blood flow to increase and glomerular filtration rate either to remain the same or increase slightly. Clearly, such studies do not provide information on the relationship between the duration of obstruction and the recovery of function. Recovery of significant renal function after complete ureteral obstruction is largely anecdotal and consists of a few reported cases. However, in all cases there was some return in function, usually as judged by the appearance of radiographic contrast in the renal pelvis. Whether the degree of recovery of renal function after release of obstruction in the elderly is comparable to that seen in younger individuals is not known.

However, return of function depends upon many factors other than duration of obstruction, such as absence of infection, presence of an intrarenal or extrarenal pelvis in the obstructed kidney or the degree of pyelolymphatic and pyelovenous flow. Presumably, incomplete ureteral obstruction will destroy renal function slowly, but it certainly can destroy all renal function. This loss of renal function due to partial obstruction is seen clinically with 'silent' prostatism or ureteropelvic junction obstruction. Currently, there is little objective evidence which allow the clinician to predict the severity of damage or potential for recovery in an obstructed kidney. It should be noted that many kidneys that radiographically appear to have a thin cortex, suggesting almost complete loss of function, will recover some degree of glomerular filtration.

Renal tubular function

The functional alterations in the renal tubule following release of obstruction will be partially dependent upon whether the occlusion is bilateral or unilateral. However, certain functional changes are seen with either form of obstruction.

Impairment of urinary concentration

A concentrating defect is the most consistent and probably the first derangement of physiologic function that occurs with urinary tract obstruction (Olbrick *et al.*, 1957; Berlyne, 1961; Berlyne and Macken, 1962). Berlyne (1961) described some improvement in concentrating ability with time after correction of the obstruction. The concentrating defect is presumably due to a decrease in solute content of the medulla, resulting from decreased sodium transport in the thick ascending limb of Henle and/or increased vasa recta blood flow which will wash out the medullary gradient. In addition, the hydro-osmotic response of the cortical collecting duct to the action of vasopressin is decreased so that both failure to maintain medullary hypertonicity and failure of equilibration of fluid in the collecting duct with interstitial fluid could contribute to the concentrating defect observed.

Alterations in the process of renal acidification

In man, acid excretion is impaired before and following release of bilateral or unilateral ureteral obstruction. Berlyne (1961) described a defect in the acidifying capacity in 6 of 7 patients with chronic hydronephrosis. These patients failed to appropriately acidify their urine following an ammonium chloride load, and ammonium and titratable acid excretion were low. In 1 patient, the defect in acidification was partially corrected following surgical intervention. Batlle *et al.* (1981) have characterized the acidifying defect in 13 patients with chronic obstructive uropathy. All patients manifested a hyperkalaemic metabolic acidosis. Three defects were found. In all patients, ammonium ion and titratable acid excretion was reduced and failed to respond to an acid load. In 4 patients, there was a selective deficiency of aldosterone. These patients appropriately acidified their urine in response to an ammonium chloride load. The remaining patients had evidence of a classic distal renal tubular acidosis or a combined defect.

Following release of obstruction, the defect in acidification may persist. Two mechanisms may be responsible for the impaired capacity of the post-obstructed kidney to acidify the urine. First, there is a marked increase in the excretion of bicarbonate (Falls and Stacy, 1973), presumably related to decreased reabsorption of bicarbonate in the proximal tubule. Secondly, there is considerable evidence to suggest that the intrinsic capacity of the kidney to acidify at more distal sites is impaired. This defect is most apparent after release of unilateral ureteral obstruction when there is no diuretic phase (Better *et al.*, 1973).

Effects of obstructive uropathy on renal potassium handling

In man (Bricker *et al.*, 1957; Massry *et al.*, 1967; Better *et al.*, 1972), there is an increase in potassium excretion after relief of bilateral ureteral obstruction. In addition, potassium excretion may be impaired by ureteral obstruction. In the report of Batlle *et al.* (1981), all 13 patients were hyperkalaemic. In fact, frequently the diagnosis of obstructive uropathy was suspected in patients who presented with a hyperkalaemic metabolic acidosis. In these patients, fractional potassium excretion was lower than would be predicted for their level of GFR. As stated previously, a distal defect in potassium was suspected in these patients. Subsequent studies indicated that two-thirds of these patients had intrinsic defects in distal acidification. In the remaining one-third, an isolated deficiency in aldosterone was found.

Effects of ureteral obstruction on cation reabsorption by the kidney

The effect of ureteral obstruction on *calcium* excretion by the kidney has not been well studied. Falls and Stacy (1973) measured the rate of calcium excretion during a post-obstructive diuresis which occurred in a patient who had been completely obstructed for 3 weeks. Within 12 h after ureteral release, calcium excretion was 3 times greater than predicted values. In this case, calcium excretion roughly paralleled sodium excretion and decreased four-fold during the period of observation. Similar results were reported by Better *et al.* (1972). When ureteral obstruction is unilateral, calcium excretion from the post-released kidney is reduced out of proportion to the decrease in filtered load (Better *et al.*, 1973).

Magnesium excretion is inappropriately increased after release of both bilateral and unilateral ureteral obstruction. As with calcium, urinary losses of magnesium may be striking following release of bilateral obstruction (Falls and Stacy, 1972; Better *et al.*, 1972). The increase in excretion of magnesium seems to parallel the increase in sodium excretion seen during the post-obstructive diuretic phase (Falls and Stacey, 1972; Better *et al.*, 1972) and may cause profound magnesium deficiency (Davis *et al.*, 1975). In the patient studied by Better *et al.* (1973) after release of unilateral ureteral obstruction, fractional and absolute magnesium excretion were significantly greater from the post-released kidney than from a normally functioning kidney.

Phosphate handling after relief of ureteral obstruction

In man, phosphate excretion after release of ureteral obstruction depends on two factors: (1) whether the obstruction is bilateral or unilateral, and (2) the duration of the obstruction. After release of bilateral ureteral obstruction, both fractional and absolute excretion of phosphate are increased and parallel the excretion of sodium and water (Falls and Stacy, 1972; Better *et al.*, 1972). Absolute phosphate excretion declines coincident with that of sodium and water excretion. Subsequent changes in fractional phosphate excretion depend in part on the level to which renal function is restored. If glomerular filtration rate does not return to normal, then renal phosphate excretion will be increased as needed to maintain phosphate balance.

A consistent observation in man is that phosphate excretion from the post-released kidney is markedly reduced following release of unilateral obstruction (Better *et al.*, 1973, 1975). The decrease in phosphate excretion is out of proportion to the reduction in the filtered load. Thus, when compared to the normally functioning kidney, fractional excretion of phosphate is markedly reduced. Further, the phosphate excretion from the normally functioning kidney is actually increased. The pathogenesis of this defect has been extensively studied in experimental animals (Purkerson *et al.*, 1974).

Post-obstructive diuresis

Obstruction of the urinary tract, even after it has been relieved, can alter the ability of the kidneys to modulate water and solute excretion in response to the homeostatic needs of the body. Indeed, under certain circumstances, a dramatic loss of salt and water in the urine can occur after release of obstruction. The mechanisms underlying this syndrome, usually referred to as post-obstructive diuresis, are not completely clear (Vaughan and Gillenwater, 1973).

Many factors may be causing this phenomenon. One is the volume status of the patient prior to the relief of obstruction. Individuals who have been treated with large amounts of intravenous fluid prior to the release of obstruction are often volume expanded. Thus, part of the increased polyuria after relief of obstruction may be a physiologic response to an expanded volume of the extracellular space. Another factor is the accumulation during obstruction of osmotic agents such as urea. Finally, the inappropriate natriuresis and diuresis that occurs after release of obstruction may result from either an intrinsic defect in renal tubule function or a humoral agent that accumulates during the period of anuria and directly affects sodium and water reabsorption by the renal tubule.

The management of this entity should include careful and adequate fluid replacement with frequent determinations of body weight and plasma and urine electrolytes. These latter measurements provide a rational basis for the amount and composition of fluid to be administered as replacement. Urinary losses of fluid and electrolytes should be replaced only to the extent necessary to prevent hypovolaemia, hypotension, hypokalaemia, hypomagnesaemia, and hypo- or hypernatraemia.

References

ABERCROMBIE, G.F. and HENDRY, W.F. (1971). Ureteral obstruction due to peri-aneurysmal fibrosis. *British Journal of Urology,* **43,** 170–173

ABBOTT, D.L., SKINNER, D.G., YALOWITZ, P.A. and MULDER, D. (1973). Retroperitoneal fibrosis associated with abdominal aortic aneurysms: an approach to management. *Journal of Urology,* **109,** 987–989

ABRAMS, H.L., SPIRO, R. and GOLDSTEIN, N. (1950). Metastases in carcinoma. *Cancer,* **3,** 74–85

ADAMS, J.T. (1974). Retroperitoneal tumors. In *Principles of Surgery,* edited by S. Schwartz, pp. 1339–1341. New York; McGraw-Hill

ADLER, S., LINDEMAN, R.D., YIENGST, M.J. *et al.* (1968). Effect of acute acid loading on urinary acid excretion by the aging human kidney. *Journal of Laboratory and Clinical Medicine,* **72,** 278–289

ANDERSEN, J.T. and BRADLEY, W.E. (1976). Abnormalities of bladder innervation in diabetes mellitus. *Urology,* **7,** 442–448

BATLLE, D.C., ARRUDA, J.A.L. and KURZMAN, N.A. (1981). Hyperkalemic distal renal tubular acidosis associated with obstructive uropathy. *New England Journal of Medicine,* **304,** 373–380

BEACH, E.W. (1952). Urologic complications of cancer of the uterine cervix. *Journal of Urology,* **68,** 178–189

BELL, E.T. (1946). *Renal Diseases,* pp. 113–139. Philadelphia; Lea and Febiger

BELMAN, A.B., KROPP, K.A. and SIMON, N.M. (1968). Renal-pressor hypertension secondary to unilateral hydronephrosis. *New England Journal of Medicine,* **278,** 1133–1136

BERLYNE, G.M. (1961). Distal tubular function in chronic hydronephrosis. *Quarterly Journal of Medicine,* **30,** 339–355

BERLYNE, G.M. and MACKEN, A. (1962). On the mechanism of renal inability to produce a concentrated urine in chronic hydronephrosis. *Clinical Science,* **22,** 315–324

BETTER, O.S., ARIEFF, A.I., MASSRY, S.G., KLEEMAN, C.R. and MAXWELL, M.H. (1973). Studies on renal function after relief of complete unilateral ureteral obstruction of three months' duration in man. *American Journal of Medicine,* **54,** 234–240

BETTER, O.S., TUMA, S., KEDAR, S. and CHAIMOWITZ, C. (1975). Enhanced tubular reabsorption of phosphate. *Archives of Internal Medicine,* **135,** 245–248

BETTER, O.S., TUMA, S., RICHTER-LEVIN, D., SZYLMAN, P., GERESH, Y., ELBAZ, S. and CHAIMOVITZ, C. (1972). Intrarenal resetting of glomerulotubular balance in a patient with postobstructive uropathy. *Nephron,* **9,** 131–145

BLACKSHEAR, J.L. and WATHEN, R.L. (1978). Effects of indomethacin or renal blood flow and renin secretory responses to ureteral occlusion in the dog. *Mineral and Electrolyte Metabolism,* **1,** 271–278

BLANDY, J. (1976). Benign enlargement of the prostate gland. In *Urology,* vol. 2, edited by J. Blandy, pp. 878–879. Oxford; Blackwell

BOYCE, W.H. and STRAWCUTTER, H.E. (1956). Incidence of urinary calculi in general hospitals, 1948 to 1952. *Journal of the American Medical Association,* **161,** 1437–1446

BRADLEY, W.E. (1979). Neurologic disorders affecting the urinary bladder. In *Clinical Neuro-Urology,* edited by R.J. Krane and M.B. Siroky, pp. 245–255. Boston; Little, Brown

BRICKER, N.S., SHWAYRI, E.I., REARDAN, J.B., KELLOG, D., MERRILL, J.P. and HOLMES, J.H. (1957). An abnormality in renal function resulting from urinary tract obstruction. *American Journal of Medicine,* **23,** 554–564

CAMPBELL, H.T., BELLO-REUSS, E. and KLAHR, S. (1984). Effects of unilateral obstruction on hydraulic water permeability and transepithelial potential in isolated perfused cortical collecting tubule. *Kidney International,* **25,** 228 (abstract)

CASSADY, J.R. (1982). External beam irradiation for carcinoma of prostate. In *Urologic Cancer — A Multidisciplinary Perspective,* edited by M.B. Garnick and J.P. Richie, pp. 23–30. New York; Plenum

CHAPMAN, I., LAPI, N. and FETHIERE, W. (1964). Prostatic enlargement and lower urinary tract obstruction. *Geriatrics,* **19,** 231–239

CONGER, J.D. (1981). Acute uric acid nephropathy. *Seminars in Nephrology,* **1,** 69–74

COVINGTON, T. Jr. and REESER, W. (1950). Hydronephrosis associated with overhydration. *Journal of Urology,* **63,** 438–440

CUSHING, R.M., TOVELL, H.M.M. and LIEGNER, I.M. (1968). Major urologic complications following radion and x-ray therapy for carcinoma of the cervix. *American Journal of Obstetrics and Gynecology,* **101,** 750–755

DAVIS, B.B., PREUSS, H.G. and MURDAUGH, H.V. Jr. (1975). Hypomagnesemia following the diuresis of post-renal obstruction and renal transplant. *Nephron,* **14,** 275–280

DEFRONZO, R.A., HUMPHREY, R.L., WRIGHT, J.R. and COOKE, C.R. (1975). Acute renal failure in multiple myeloma. *Medicine,* **54,** 209–223

DEMING, C.L. and WOLF, J.S. (1939). The anatomical origin of benign prostatic enlargement. *Journal of Urology,* **42,** 566–580

DICK, V.S. (1952). Unrecognized prostatism. *Journal of the American Medical Association*, **148**, 925–928

DONNELLY, J., HACKLER, R.H. and BUNTS, R.C. (1972). Present urologic status of the World War II paraplegic: 25-year follow-up. Comparison with status of the 20-year Korean War paraplegic and 5-year Vietnam paraplegic. *Journal of Urology*, **108**, 558–562

DONOVAN, A.J. and GIBSON, R.A. (1973). Identification of ureteral ligation during gynecologic operation. *American Journal of Obstetrics and Gynecology*, **116**, 793–794

DONTAS, A.S., PAPANAYIOTOU, P., MARKETOS, S., PAPANICOLAOU, N. and ECONOMOU, P. (1966). Bacteriuria in old age. *Lancet*, **1**, 305–306

EIDE, I., LOYNING, E., LANGARD, O. and KIIL, F. (1977). Mechanism of renin release during acute ureteral constriction in dogs. *Circulation Research*, **40**, 293–299

EWERT, E.E. and SUMMONS, H.J. (1951). 'Silent' prostatism. *Surgical Clinics of North America*, **31**, 659–670

FALLS, W.F., Jr. and STACY, W.K. (1973). Postobstructive diuresis. Studies in a dialyzed patient with a solitary kidney. *American Journal of Medicine*, **54**, 404–412

GARRETT, J., POLSE, S.L. and MORROW, J.W. (1970). Ureteral obstruction and hypertension. *American Journal of Medicine*, **49**, 271–273

GAYNOR, E.P. (1938). Zur Frage des Prostatakrebses. *Virchows Archives (Pathology and Anatomy)*, **310**, 602–652

GILLENWATER, J.Y. (1978). Pathophysiology of obstructive uropathy. In *Prevention of Kidney and Urinary Tract Diseases*, DHEW (NIH 78–855), vol. 5, edited by C.H. Coggins and N.B. Cummings, pp. 169–187. Washington D.C.; US Department of Health, Education and Welfare

GILLENWATER, J.Y., WESTERVELT, F.B., Jr., VAUGHAN, E.D., Jr. and HOWARDS, S.S. (1975). Renal function after release of chronic unilateral hydronephrosis in man. *Kidney International*, **7**, 179–186

GOLDBERG, I.D., LEVIN, M.L., GERHARDT, P.R., HANDY, V.H. and CASHMAN, R.E. (1956). The probability of developing cancer. *Journal of the National Cancer Institute*, **17**, 155–173

GRAHAM, J.R. (1964). Methysergide for prevention of headache; experience in five hundred patients over three years. *New England Journal of Medicine*, **270**, 67–72

GRAHAM, J.B. and ABAD, R.S. (1967). Ureteral obstruction due to radiation. *American Journal of Obstetrics and Gynecology*, **99**, 409–412

GRAYHACK, J.T. and WENDEL, E.F. (1979). Carcinoma of the prostate. In *Urology*, vol. 2, edited by A.R. Kendall and L. Karafin, pp. 1–32. New York; Harper and Row

GRAYHACK, J.T., WILSON, J.D. and SHERBENSKE, M.J. (1975). *Benign Prostatic Hyperplasia*, DHEW (NIH) 76-1113. Washington D.C.; US Department of Health, Education and Welfare

GREENBERGER, P., PATTERSON, R., KELLY, J., STEVENSON, D.D., SIMON, R. and LIEBERMAN, P. (1980). Administration of radiographic contrast media in high-risk patients. *Investigative Radiology*, **16**(6 Suppl.), S40–S43

GUZE, L.B. and BEESON, P.B. (1956). Experimental pyelonephitis. I. Effect of ureteral ligation on the course of bacterial infection in the kidney of the rat. *Journal of Experimental Medicine*, **104**, 803–815

GUZE, L.B. and BEESON, P.B. (1958). Experimental pyelonephritis. II. Effect of partial ureteral obstruction on the course of bacterial infection in the kidney of the rat and the rabbit. *Yale Journal of Biology and Medicine*, **30**, 315–319

HANLEY, M.J. and DAVIDSON, K. (1982). Isolated nephron segments from rabbit models of obstructive nephropathy. *Journal of Clinical Investigation*, **69**, 165–174

HARKONEN, S. and KJELLSTRAND, C. (1981). Contrast nephropathy. *American Journal of Nephrology*, **1**, 69–77

HASNER, E. (1962). Prostatic urinary infection. *Acta Chirurgica Scandinavica Supplementum*, **285**, 1–40

HEWITT, C.B., NITZ, G.L., KISER, W.S., STRAFFON, R.A. and STEWART, B.H. (1969). Surgical treatment of retroperitoneal fibrosis. *Annals of Surgery*, **169**, 610–615

HORTON, R. (1982). Benign prostatic hyperplasia: a disorder of androgen metabolism in the male. *American Journal of Nephrology*, **2**, 157–163

HUDSTON, P.B. (1957). Prostatic cancer. XIV. Its incidence, extent and behaviour in 686 men studied by prostatic biopsy. *Journal of the American Geriatrics Society*, **5**, 338–350

JAWORSKI, Z.F. and WOLAN, C.T. (1963). Hydronephrosis and polycythemia. *American Journal of Medicine*, **34**, 523–534

JONES, E.A. and ALEXANDER, M.K. (1966). Idiopathic retroperitoneal fibrosis associated with arteritis. *Annals of Rheumatological Diseases*, **25**, 356–360

KAUFMAN, J.J. and SCHULTZ, J.I. (1962). Needle biopsy of the prostate: a re-evaluation. *Journal of Urology*, **87**, 164–168

KAYE, A.D. and POLLACK, H.M. (1982). Diagnostic imaging approach to the patient with obstructive uropathy. *Seminars in Nephrology*, **2**, 55–73

KHAN, A.U. and UTZ, D.C. (1975). Clinical management of cancer of prostate associated with bilateral ureteral obstruction. *Journal of Urology,* **113,** 816–819

KIMBROUGH, J.C. (1956). Carcinoma of the prostate: five-year followup of patients treated by radical surgery. *Journal of Urology,* **76,** 287–291

KLAHR, S. (1983). Pathophysiology of obstructive nephropathy. *Kidney International,* **23,** 414–416

KLAHR, S. (1984). Approach to the patient with renal and electrolyte disorders. In *Differential Diagnosis of Renal and Electrolyte Disorders,* 2nd edn, edited by S. Klahr, pp. 1-3. Norwalk; Appleton-Century-Crofts

KLAHR, S., BUERKERT, J. and MORRISON, A. (1986). Urinary tract obstruction. In *The Kidney,* 3rd edn, pp. 1443–1490, edited by B.M. Brenner and F.C. Rector, Jr. Philadelphia; Saunders

KNOWLAN, D., CORRADO, M., SCHREINER, G.D. and BAKER, R. (1960). Periureteral fibrosis, with a diabetes insipidus-like syndrome occurring with progressive partial obstruction of a ureter unilaterally. *American Journal of Medicine,* **28,** 22–31

KOGAN, S.J. and FREED, S.Z. (1974). Post-operative course of vesicoureteral reflux associated with benign obstructive prostatic disease. *Journal of Urology,* **112,** 322–325

KUNKEL, R.S. (1971). Fibrotic syndromes with chronic use of methysergide. *Headache,* **11,** 1–5

LABARDINI, M.M. and RATLIFF, R. (1967). Abdominal aortic aneurysm and the ureter. *Radiology,* **68,** 590

LANDSBERG, L. (1970). Hypernatremia complicating partial urinary tract obstruction. *New England Journal of Medicine,* **283,** 746–748

LAPIDES, J., DIOKNO, A.C., LOWE, B.S. and KALISH, M.D. (1974). Follow-up on unsterile, intermittent self-catheterization. *Journal of Urology,* **111,** 184–187

LAPIDES, J., DIOKNO, A.C., SILBER, S.J. and LOWE, B.S. (1972). Clean intermittent self-catheterization in the treatment of urinary tract disease. *Journal of Urology,* **107,** 458–461

McDOUGAL, W.S. and PERSKY, L. (1975). Renal function abnormalities in post-unilateral ureteral obstruction in man. A comparison of these defects to post-obstructive diuresis. *Journal of Urology,* **113,** 601–604

MacGREGOR, G.A., JONES, N.F., BARRACLOUGH, M.A., WING, A.J. and CRANSTON, W.I. (1973). Ureteric stricture with analgesic nephropathy. *British Medical Journal,* **5,** 271–272

McGUIRE, E.J. (1983). Physiology of the lower urinary tract. *American Journal of Kidney Diseases,* **2,** 402-408

MARKS, R.L. and BAHR, G.A. (1977). How to manage neurogenic bladder after stroke. *Geriatrics,* **32,** 50–54

MASSRY, S.G., SCHAINUCK, L.I., GOLDSMITH, C. and SCHREINER, G.E. (1967). Studies on the mechanism of diuresis after relief of urinary tract obstruction. *Annals of Internal Medicine,* **66,** 149–158

MEES, E.J.D. (1960). Reversible water losing state, caused by incomplete ureteric obstruction. *Acta Medica Scandinavica,* **168,** 193–196

MEHL, R.L. (1969). Retro-iliac ureter. *Journal of Urology,* **102,** 27–29

MITUS, W.J., TOYAMA, K. and BRAUER, M.J. (1968). Erythrocytosis, juxtaglomerular apparatus (JGA) and erythropoietin in the course of experimental unilateral hydronephosis in rabbits. *Annals of the New York Academy of Science,* **149,** 107–113

MOORE, R.A. (1943). Benign hypertrophy of the prostate. A morphological study. *Journal of Urology,* **50,** 680–710

MOORE, R.A. (1944). Benign hypertrophy and carcinoma of the prostate. *Surgery,* **16,** 152–167

MORROW, J.W. and BOGAARD, T.P. (1977). Bladder rehabilitation in patients with old spinal cord injuries with bladder neck incision and external sphincterotomy. *Journal of Urology,* **117,** 164–167

MOTZKIN, D. (1968). The significance of deficient bladder sensation. *Journal of Urology,* **100,** 445–450

MUKAMEL, E., NISSENKORN, I., BONER, G. and SERVADIO, C. (1979). Occult progressive renal damage in the elderly male due to benign prostatic hypertrophy. *Journal of the American Geriatrics Society,* **24,** 403–406

NEMOY, N.J., FICHMAN, M.P. and SELLERS, A. (1973). Unilateral ureteral obstruction. A cause of reversible high renin content hypertension. *Journal of the American Medical Association,* **225,** 512–513

NESBIT, R. and BAUM, W.C. (1950). Endocrine control of prostatic carcinoma. *Journal of the American Medical Association,* **143,** 1317–1320

OLBRICH, O., WOODFORD, W.E., IRVINE, R.E. and WEBSTER, D. (1957). Renal function in prostatism. *Lancet,* **1,** 1322–1324

OLIW, E. (1978). Acute unilateral ureteral occlusion increases plasma renin activity and contralateral urinary prostaglandin excretion in rabbits. *European Journal of Pharmacology,* **53,** 95–102

PALMER, J.M., ZWEIMAN, F.G. and ASSAYKEEN, T.A. (1970). Renal hypertension due to hydronephrosis with normal plasma renin activity. *New England Journal of Medicine,* **283,** 1032–1033

PEARMAN, J.W. (1976). Urological follow-up of 99 spinal cord injured patients initially managed by intermittent catheterization. *British Journal of Urology,* **48,** 297–310

PECK, D.R., BHATT, G.M. and LOWMAN, R.M. (1973). Traction displacement of the ureter: a sign of aortic aneurysm. *Journal of Urology*, **109**, 983–986

PELLEYA, R., OSTER, J.R. and PEREZ, G.O. (1983). Hyporeninemic, hypoaldosteronism, sodium wasting and mineralocorticoid-resistant hyperkalemia in two patients with obstructive uropathy. *American Journal of Nephrology*, **3**, 223–227

PERKASH, I. (1975). Intermittent catheterization and bladder rehabilitation in spinal cord injury patients. *Journal of Urology*, **114**, 230–233

PERKASH, I. (1976). An attempt to understand and to treat voiding dysfunctions during rehabilitation of the bladder in spinal cord injury patients. *Journal of Urology*, **115**, 36–40

PERSKY, L., KURSH, E.D. and FELDMAN, S. (1970). Extrinsic obstruction of the ureter. In *Urology*, 3rd edn, edited by M.F. Campbell and J.H. Harrison. Philadelphia; Saunders

PFISTER, R.C. and NEWHOUSE, J.H. (1979). Interventional percutaneous pyeloureteral techniques. II. Percutaneous nephrostomy and other procedures. *Radiology Clinics of North America*, **17**, 351–363

PLATTS, M.M. and WILLIAMS, J.L. (1963). Renal function in patients with unilateral hydronephrosis. *British Medical Journal*, **2**, 1243–1247

PURKERSON, M.L., ROLF, D.B., CHASE, L.R., SLATOPOLSKY, E. and KLAHR, S. (1974). Tubular reabsorption of phosphate after release of complete ureteral obstruction in the rat. *Kidney International*, **5**, 326–336

RISHOLM, L. (1954). Studies on renal colic and its treatment of posterior splanchnic block. *Acta Chirurgica Scandinavica Supplementum*, **184**, 1–64

ROTKIN, I.D. (1975). Epidemiology of benign prostatic hypertrophy: review and speculations. In *Benign Prostatic Hyperplasia*, DHEW (NIH 76–1113), edited by J.T. Grayhack, J.D. Wilson and M.J. Sherbenske, pp. 105–117. Washington, D.C.; US Department of Health, Education and Welfare

ROUSSAK, N.J. and OLEESKY, S. (1954). Water-losing nephritis: syndrome simulating diabetes insipidus. *Quarterly Journal of Medicine*, **23**, 147–164

RUDIN, L.J., MEGALLI, M.R. and LATTIMER, J.K. (1974). Obstructive uropathy associated with uterine prolapse. *Urology*, **4**, 73–79

SCHWARTZ, D.T. (1969). Unilateral upper urinary obstruction and arterial hypertension. *New York Journal of Medicine*, **69**, 668–671

SEMPLE, J.E. (1963). Surgical capsule of benign enlargement of prostate: its development and action. *British Medical Journal*, **1**, 1640–1643

SHEDAHI, W.H. and TONIOLO, G. (1980). Adverse reactions to contrast media. *Radiology*, **137**, 299–302

SHINGLETON, H.M., FOWLER, W.C. Jr., PEPPER, F.D. Jr. and PALUMBO, I. (1969). Ureteral strictures following therapy for carcinoma of the cervix. *Cancer*, **24**, 77–83

SMITH, L. (1979). Urolithiasis. In *Strauss and Welt's Diseases of the Kidney*, 3rd edn, edited by L.E. Earley and C.W. Gottschalk, pp. 921–923. Boston; Little, Brown

SOURANDER, L.B. and KASANEN, A. (1972). A 5-year follow-up of bacteriuria in the aged. *Gerontology Clinic*, **14**, 274–281

SQUITIERI, A.P., CECCARELLI, R.E. and WURSTER, J.C. (1974). Hypertension with elevated renal vein renins secondary to ureteropelvic junction obstruction. *Journal of Urology*, **111**, 284–287

STRUTHERS, N.W. (1982). The physiology of the ureter. In *Scientific Foundations of Urology*, 2nd edn, edited by G.D. Chisholm and D.I. Williams, pp. 385–389. Chicago; Year Book

SWYER, G.I.M. (1944). Postnatal growth changes in human prostate. *Journal of Anatomy (London)*, **78**, 130–145

TALREJA, D., SLATER, L.M., DARA, P., BRANSON, H. and ARMENTROUT, S.A. (1980). Multiple myeloma complicated by myelomatous obstructive uropathy. *Cancer*, **46**, 1893–1895

UTZ, D.C. and HENRY, J.D. (1966). Retroperitoneal fibrosis. *Medical Clinics of North America*, **50**, 1091–1099

VAN NAGELL, J.R. JR., SPRAGUE, A.D. and RODDECK, J.W. (1975). The effect of intravenous pyelography and cystoscopy on the staging of cervical cancer. *Gynecology and Oncology*, **3**, 87–91

VANDER, A.J. (1967). Control of renin release. *Physiological Review*, **47**, 359–382

VAUGHAN, E.D. Jr., BUCHLER, F.R. and LARAGH, J.H. (1974). Normal renin secretion in hypertensive patients with primarily unilateral chronic hydronephrosis. *Journal of Urology*, **112**, 153–156

VAUGHAN, E.D. Jr. and GILLENWATER, J.Y. (1973). Diagnosis, characterization and management of post-obstructive diuresis. *Journal of Urology*, **109**, 286–292

WAGENKNECHT, L.V. and MADSEN, P.O. (1970). Bilateral ureteral obstruction secondary to aortic aneurysm. *Journal of Urology*, **103**, 732–736

WALSH, P.C. (1979). Benign prostatic hyperplasia. In *Campbell's Urology*, 4th edn, vol. 2, edited by J.H. Harrison *et al.*, pp. 949–966. Philadelphia; Saunders

WEIDMANN, P., BERETTA-PICCOLI, C., HIRSCH, D., REUBI, F.C. and MASSRY, S.G. (1977). Curable hypertension with unilateral hydronephrosis. Studies of the role of circulating renin. *Annals of Internal Medicine*, **87**, 437–440

WEIN, A.J., RAEZER, D.M. and BENSON, G.S. (1976). Management of neurogenic bladder dysfunction in the adult. *Urology,* **8,** 432–443

WHITAKER, R.W. (1982). Pathophysiology of ureteric obstruction. In *Scientific Foundations of Urology,* 2nd edn, edited by G.D. Chisholm and D.I. Williams, pp. 390–394. Chicago; Year Book

WILLIAMS, H.E. (1974). Nephrolithiasis. *New England Journal of Medicine,* **290,** 33–38

WILSON, J.D. (1980). The pathogenesis of benign prostatic hyperplasia. *American Journal of Medicine,* **68,** 745–756

YARGER, W.E., SCHOCKEN, D.D. and HARRIS, R.H. (1980). Obstructive nephropathy in the rat; possible roles for the renin–angiotensin system, prostaglandins, and thromboxanes in postobstructive renal function. *Journal of Clinical Investigation,* **65,** 400–412

Chapter 20

Acute renal failure in old people

Juan F. Macias Nuñez and Jose A. Sanchez Tomero

Introduction

Acute renal failure (ARF) is defined as the abrupt interruption of renal function to the extent that the kidney is unable to maintain the control of the internal milieu. The aging kidney is more susceptible to develop ARF due to the morphological and functional renal changes occuring with age (Frey, 1973; Griffiths *et al.*, 1976; Graux and Metstdagh, 1977; Schramm, Jenett and Gerhardt, 1981; Hering and Carlson, 1982; Kafetz, 1983). The high incidence of systemic illnesses such as hypertension, diabetes mellitus, arteriosclerosis (Chrysont, Frohlich and Papper, 1976; Rosenfeld, 1983; Samiy, 1983; Frocht and Fillit, 1984) is also responsible for ARF, as is the polypharmacological treatment often administered to the elderly. The pathogenesis of ARF is frequently multifactorial and thus renal failure is much more common in an older hospitalized population. This chapter will give a general presentation of ARF, paying special attention to its peculiarities in the elderly.

Aetiology

There are three fundamental mechanisms involved in the production of ARF: diminution of renal blood flow (pre-renal ARF), acute lesions of the renal parenchymal (renal or intrinsic ARF) and obstruction of the urinary flow (obstructive ARF) (*Table 20.1*).

Pre-renal ARF (acute reversible renal hypoperfusion)

Any situation leading to hypovolaemia and hypotension, accompanied by a drop in renal blood flow (RBF), can result in ARF. The elderly are more prone to develop this form of ARF due to hypodipsia (Miller *et al.*, 1982) and the impairment of the aging kidney in conserving sodium (Epstein and Hollenberg, 1976; Macias Nuñez *et al.*, 1978; Macias Nuñez *et al.*, 1980) (see Chapter 3), which induces water and sodium depletion easily. Because of the ease of volume depletion, diuretic intake, mild diarrhoea, vomiting, profuse sweating or simply the diminution of fluid intake can produce oliguria in the elderly, which when maintained for relatively short periods results first in an acute reversible uraemia, then in established ARF (Kumar, Hill and McGeown, 1973; Epstein and Hollenberg, 1976; Macias Nuñez *et al.*, 1978, 1980, 1981; Montoliu *et al.*, 1981; Prinseau *et al.*, 1983). Dehydration and

Table 20.1 The aetiology of ARF

PRE-RENAL ARF

A. Hypovolaemia

1. Fluid loss: sweating, burns
   Gastrointestinal: diarrhoea, vomiting, fistulae
   Renal: diuretic, intake, salt wasting
2. Redistribution of the extracellular volume
   Distributive shock (septic shock), hypoalbuminaemia, nephrotic syndrome, liver diseases, malnutrition
3. Haemorrhage
4. Fluid restriction

B. Cardiac failure

1. Acute: arrhythmias, trauma, acute valvular diseases, malignant hypertension, acute myocardial failure, cardiac tamponade
2. Chronic: myocardiopathies (ischaemic, hypertension), valvulopathies

RENAL OR INTRINSIC ARF

A. Acute glomerulonephritis

Post-infectious
Mesangiocapillary
Rapidly progressive
(idiopathic, Goodpasture's syndrome, SLE, etc.)

B. Vasculitis

Polyarteritis nodosa
Hypersensibility angiitis
(classic, serum sickness, mixed cryoglobulinaemia, Schönlein–Henoch, Wegener, scleroderma, haemolytic–uraemic syndrome

C. Acute interstitial nephritis

1. Drugs: methicillin, ampicillin, allopurinol, diphenylhydantoin, cimetidine, thiazides
2. Infections: acute pyelonephritis
3. Infiltrative: lymphoma, leukaemia, sarcoidosis
4. Idiopathic

D. Intratubular deposition

Urates
Myoglobin
Myeloma
Sulphonamides

E. Severe hypercalcaemia

F. Hepatorenal syndrome

G. Vascular obstruction

1. Arterial: athero-embolic disease, aneurysms
2. Venous: thrombosis of vena cava, diffuse small thrombosis in amyloidosis

H. Cellular tubular damage

1. Post-ischaemic: all conditions listed in the pre-renal section maintained in time
2. Haem pigments
   (a) Intravascular haemolysis: transfusion reactions, haemolysis due to toxins or immunological damage, malaria
   (b) Rhabdomyolysis and myoglobinuria: trauma, muscle diseases, prolonged coma, seizures, heat stroke, excessive exercise
3. Nephrotoxin related: antibiotic (aminoglycosides, cephalosporins, tetracyclines), metals (Hg, Ag, Pt, Bi), organic solvents, sulphonamides, iodinated contrast media, etc.)

OBSTRUCTIVE ARF

A. Ureteral and pelvic

1. Intrinsic obstruction: blood clots, stones, sloughed papillae, fungus balls
2. Extrinsic obstruction: malignancy, retroperitoneal fibrosis, iatrogenic (inadvertent) ligation

B. Bladder

Stones, blood clots, prostatic hypertrophy as in malignancy, bladder carcinoma, neuropathic

C. Urethra

Strictures, phimosis

hydroelectrolytic imbalance account for 50 per cent of the incidence of reversible or irreversible ARF in the elderly (Kumar, Hill and McGeown, 1973) and 44 per cent in an early revision of our own cases (Macias Nuñez *et al.*, 1981). The current incidence of dehydration as a cause of ARF is 23 per cent (*Table 20.2*). Another

Table 20.2 Aetiology of acute renal failure

Aetiologic factor	*Young* (*n* =67) (%)	*Elderly* (*n* =298) (%)
Nephrotoxic	6.8	10.8
Dehydration desalination	15.1	23.4
Septic shock	20.5	25.8
Surgical	8.2	5.1
Cardiogenic shock	11.0	5.8
Multifactorial	15.1	11.9
Obstructive	5.5	10.5
Hepatorenal syndrome	4.1	1.0
Glomerular	5.5	0.7
Others	8.2	5.8

important aetiologic factor of ARF in our unit is septic shock (*Table 20.2*), probably related to the diminution of the immunity against bacterial agents observed in the elderly (Wardle, 1982).

Renal or intrinsic ARF (established ARF, acute tubular necrosis)

The aetiologic agents responsible for acute incompetence of the kidney acting primarily upon the renal tissue as the target organ seem to provoke renal damage by a direct lesion of the tubular cells, by acute injury to the interstitium, by intratubular deposition of some insoluble substances or by acute attack on the glomerular tuft. All the situations included in the 'pre-renal' section, maintained for a long enough period, will lead to failure of the renal parenchyma. Nephrotoxic drug-induced renal failure is also a very common aetiologic cause of ARF in the aged population (Crooks, O'Malley and Stevenson, 1976; Ritschel, 1976; Douhoux and Sraer, 1982; Greenblatt, Sellers and Shader, 1982). Due to the increasing number of aged patients treated with non-steroidal anti-inflammatory drugs, the incidence of ARF due to them is becoming more frequent (Clive and Stoff, 1984). Another cause of ARF is interstitial nephritis (Burton *et al.*, 1974; Hyman, Ballow and Knieser, 1978; Van Ypersele de Strihou, 1979).

Myoglobinuria or haemoglobinuria following arterial embolectomies in the limbs and mismatched blood transfusions are also frequently seen in the eldery. Athero-embolic illness can produce ARF in the elderly by releasing atheromatous material during surgery of the aorta, or during radiological studies (Thurlbeck and Castleman, 1957; Harrington, Sommer and Kassirer, 1968; Kassirer, 1969). All the above clinical pictures correlate histopathologically with acute tubular necrosis on renal biopsy or autopsy, particularly among hospitalized patients (Anderson *et al.*, 1977).

Ten to 20 per cent of intrinsic ARF is due to glomerular injury (see Chapters 15 and 16). There are many illnesses that can damage the renal parenchyma, reducing acutely the glomerular filtration rate (GFR) (*Table 20.1*). Some of the more common causes of intrinsic ARF in the elderly are rapidly progressive idiopathic glomerulonephritis, mesangiocapillary glomerulonephritis and the proliferative variety of systemic lupus erythematosus. Vasculitis, extensively discussed in Chapter 16, scleroderma and haemolytic uraemic syndrome are also responsible for intrinsic ARF in the elderly.

Obstructive ARF

The incidence of obstructive ARF is from 17 to 38 per cent of the total incidence of ARF in the elderly (Kumar, Hill and McGeown, 1973; Almaraz *et al.*, 1976), in comparison to 1.15 per cent when global series are considered (Miller *et al.*, 1978). When obstructive ARF coexists with urinary tract infection, the risk of sepsis greatens and worsens the patient's prognosis (Basso, 1974; Carty, Brocklehurst and Carty, 1981).

The cause of ARF in a single patient, as we have seen, can be multifactorial; dehydration, hydroelectrolytic imbalance, major surgery, hypotension, various infections, pharmacological treatments (particularly aminoglycosides), diuretics, contrast media and urological problems are the most frequent precipitating factors of ARF in the elderly (Kumar, Hill and McGeown, 1973).

Pathophysiology

From the observations drawn from ischaemic and nephrotoxic experimental models of ARF, the following mechanisms have been proposed as responsible for the establishment and maintenance of ARF: reduction of RBF by persistent vasoconstriction, tubular obstruction, tubular back-leak and diminution of the glomerular ultrafiltration coefficient (K_f). The influence of these factors varies depending on the experimental model, but some of the factors can act simultaneously (Andreucci, 1984).

Renal blood flow is diminished in all experimental models of ARF, preferentially in the superficial cortex (Solez *et al.*, 1976), although other groups have found a homogeneous reduction through the superficial and deep cortex (Hsu *et al.*, 1976). Recently, it has been pointed out that the function of the superficial nephrons remains intact after an ischaemic injury. The functional alteration of the deep nephrons is responsible for the deterioration of the entire renal function and the inability to concentrate urine (Masson, Welsch and Takabatoke, 1983). Although ischaemia is an induction mechanism for ARF, RBF returns to normal levels within 24–48 h (Eisenbach, Klitzlinger and Steinhausen, 1974), whereas GFR remains low. Therefore, ischaemia is not the main cause for *maintenance* of ARF (Oken, 1976). There is no general agreement regarding the role of haemodynamics. It has been said that the decrease of RBF is provoked by afferent and efferent arteriolar vasoconstriction (Daugharty *et al.*, 1974). Other authors have found afferent vasoconstriction and efferent vasodilatation (Reubi, 1974; Balint and Szocs, 1976). Finally, it has been proposed that the incapacity to filtrate is reached when preglomerular resistance decreases 74 per cent or more, provoking diminution of GFR (Oken, 1983).

Some authors have attributed the decrease of GFR to intrarenal renin activity (Thurau, Vogt and Dahlheim, 1976; Flamembaum *et al.*, 1976). It has been proved that volume expansion, which lowers the intrarenal renin content, improves the outcome of some models of experimental ARF (Bondia *et al.*, 1979). In contrast, in some other experimental models such as intrarenal infusion of norepinephrine or occlusion of the renal artery, it is known that volume expansion does not prevent ARF. Blockade of angiotensin II with saralasin does not block the appearance of ARF following occlusion of the renal artery (Arendshorst *et al.*, 1976), but it protects against ARF due to gentamicin (Shor *et al.*, 1981) or that induced by uranyl nitrate (Blantz, 1982). Acute renal failure has been related to the intrarenal renin–angiotensin system through the tubuloglomerular feedback mechanism (Thurau and Boylan, 1976; Mason, 1976). This theory postulates an inverse relationship between RBF and the intrarenal renin–angiotensin system, along with the reabsorption of sodium by the macula densa. The lesion of the proximal tubule and loop of Henle diminishes the capacity of these segments to reabsorb sodium, allowing the arrival of higher amounts of sodium to the macula densa. This stimulates the release of intrarenal renin and arteriolar vasoconstriction mediated by intrarenal angiotensin II. This tubuloglomerular feedback reduces the RBF and GFR of the damaged nephron. This mechanism is pictured as acting to defend the maintenance of the extracellular volume, although this theory remains under question by many groups.

Prostaglandins can act directly upon vascular resistance or modulate the response to other vasoconstrictor agents (angiotensin II, catecholamines and bradykinin). Also, the activation of the renin–angiotensin system stimulates, locally, the release of prostaglandins. Because of this, the interaction among both renin–angiotensin system and prostaglandins may be of importance in the development of ARF (Gerber, Olson and Nies, 1981; Henrich, 1981). Indomethacin inhibits prostaglandin synthesis and reduces the renal autoregulation capacity by 60 per cent (Schnermann, Briggs and Weber, 1984). Intrarenally infused PGE_1 in situations of ARF increases RBF, but provokes efferent vasodilatation. Because of this, GFR does not increase (Reubi and Vorbuger, 1976). The above finding makes it seem unlikely that ARF is due to a deficit in prostaglandin secretion, although in some cases it has been observed that following indomethacin administration, ARF worsens (Torres *et al.*, 1975; Clive and Stoff, 1984).

It is also possible that pre-glomerular vasoconstriction is due to abnormal intrinsic vascular contractility or to a hypersensibility of the pre-glomerular vessels to normal vasoconstrictor stimuli. Another possibility is a deficit of vasodilator substances such as prostaglandins or kinins, or an insensitivity of the pre-glomerular vasculature to these substances, thus accounting for an abnormal vascular pre-glomerular tone (Oken, 1976). A well-known cause of established ARF is *tubular obstruction* (Tanner and Steinhausen, 1976; Neugarten, Aynedjian and Bank, 1983), produced by cellular detritus coming from the tubular epithelial cells that fall inside the tubular lumen (Donohoe *et al.*, 1978). Tamm–Horsfall mucoprotein, myoglobin, phosphate or urates may precipitate into the tubular lumen and are all further causes of ARF related to intratubular obstruction. It is not always possible to record an increase in the intratubular hydrostatic pressure because the obtruction produces a glomerular vasoconstriction, creating a consequent fall in the GFR. These factors combined with tubular leakage produce a diminution of the intratubular hydrostatic pressure (Arendshorts, Finn and Gottschalk, 1974).

The damaged tubular epithelium may also be abnormally permeable, favouring *tubular back-leak*, which can be responsible for the leakage of 50% of the GFR (Myers *et al.*, 1980), although other groups argue that this leakage is only a technical artefact (Oken, 1975).

The existence of a *fall in the glomerular ultrafiltration coefficient, K_f* (Torres *et al.*, 1975; Baylis, Rennke and Brenner, 1977), changes in the foot processes (Stein *et al.*, 1975) and a diminution of the number and total surface of the fenestrae of the capillary endothelium (Avasthi, Evan and Hay, 1980) have been suggested from the experimental field to be other possible explanations for the diminution of GFR. The pathophysiological significances of these alterations are still under discussion.

Two interesting hypotheses have been proposed recently. One concerns the deleterious role of *oxygen-free radicals* in ischaemic ARF (Paller, Hoidal and Ferris, 1984). These authors found that when ischaemic kidneys were pretreated with superoxide dismutase or allopurinol (both substances inhibit the formation of oxygen-free radicals), the renal damage which followed kidney revascularization was much less severe than in the group not treated in this manner. It is well known that the amount of oxygen-free radicals increases with age, and ARF can appear more easily or in a shorter period of time after the same ischaemic renal insult in the elderly. The other possibility is that the medullary thick ascending limb of Henle's loop has a precarious oxygen supply, and this segment is particularly vulnerable to ischaemic injury during renal hypoperfusion (Brezis *et al.*, 1984). As has been discussed in Chapter 3, the ascending limb of Henle's loop is damaged, functionally at least, in the elderly, making the aged population more susceptible to ischaemic injury than younger persons.

The aging kidney has a reduced blood supply, a tendency to develop volume depletion, a liability to intercurrent illnesses, and is subject to polypharmacy. All these circumstances make the aging kidney more prone to suffer from ARF (Kumar, Hill and McGeown, 1973; Epstein and Hollenberg, 1976; Macias Nuñez *et al.*, 1978, 1980, 1981).

Clinical spectrum of acute tubular necrosis (ATN)

Oliguric phase

The most common initial phase is with oliguria. The oliguric phase has a variable duration, but diuresis usually recovers in 1–2 weeks, although in the elderly this period is sometimes prolonged (Hall *et al.*, 1970). Biochemically, uraemia and a raised serum creatinine (more than 1.5 mg/dl in the elderly) are found. Hyperkalaemia (more pronounced following trauma or sepsis) (Adrogue and Madias, 1981), metabolic acidosis with elevated anion gap due to an increase of phosphates, sulphates and organic anions (Relman, 1972), hyperphosphataemia, hypoalbuminaemia, hypermagnesaemia and hypocalcaemia (Massry *et al.*, 1974) are also usually present in ARF. If patients have been treated with an excessive amount of fluids, dilutional hyponatraemia is common, particularly when they are treated with solutions, such as glucose or laevulose without electrolytes. Among elderly patients, hyponatraemia is more frequent due to their inability to reabsorb sodium.

A normochromic, normocytic anaemia of multifactorial aetiology (diminution of the synthesis of erythropoietin, haemolysis, haemodilution), leukocytosis with an increase in granulocytes and alterations of platelet function are found in ARF (Anagnostou, Fried and Kurtzman, 1981; Eknoyan and Brown, 1981). Cardiac arrhythmias, congestive cardiac failure and oedema occur when patients are volume overloaded. Severe anaemia or hypertension make cardiac failure refractory to conventional treatment (Ianhez, Lowen and Sabbaga, 1975). Neurological manifestations such as lethargy and agitation are present, and even coma can accompany these neurological complications (Guisado, Arieff and Massry, 1975; Raskin and Fishman, 1976). Gastrointestinal complications such as haematemesis, mainly due to stress ulcers, have been recognized as common in our own series. Gastrointestinal complications are diminished if dialytic treatment is performed early in the treatment of ARF (Kleinknecht *et al.*, 1972) and prophylaxis with ranitidine or cimetidine should be given to all patients. Superimposed infectious diseases, due to the depression of cell-mediated immune response, create one of the most serious complications in ARF, although phagocytic activity and antibody production remain relatively normal (Boulton-Jones *et al.*, 1973). If diuresis has not appeared with 3 weeks, a renal biopsy should be performed.

Polyuric phase

Following the oliguric period diuresis increases, although creatinine and urea may continue to rise for several days. Hypopotassaemia, hypomagnesaemia and hyponatraemia continue to complicate ARF as before. Twenty-five per cent of all the deaths caused by ARF happen during the polyuric phase, even if dialysis has been performed early and frequently (McMurray *et al.*, 1978).

Recovery phase

Renal function slowly recovers for variable periods, ranging between a few weeks and as long as 12 months. Various renal functions have the same rate of recuperation, and there is a certain degree of established renal deterioration which may occur as permanent damage in the elderly (Hall *et al.*, 1970; Merino, Buselmeier and Kjellstrand, 1975). Sodium handling and concentration capacity are the last functions to recover, particularly in the elderly. When there is no previous history of renal disease, recuperation of renal function is more complete. In general, recovery of renal function in the elderly is less complete in older patients than in the young, but one must remember the lower levels of renal function in the elderly when interpreting the data (see Chapter 2).

Non-oliguric acute tubular necrosis

In a variable number of patients (10–40 per cent), depending somewhat on the study population, a diuresis greater than 500 ml/day in the initial phase of ARF may be observed (Bhat *et al.*, 1976; Anderson *et al.*, 1977), but with identical urine composition and fixed urinary output. Tubular injury is less severe, and the clinical course more benign, requiring less dialysis (Anderson *et al.*, 1977; Sanchez Tomero *et al.*, 1984). This picture of non-oliguric ARF is more frequent after open heart surgery, aminoglycoside treatment and extensive burns.

Differential diagnosis

History

A careful search for high temperature, thirst, loss of appetite, high fluids loss (vomiting, profuse sweating, diarrhoea, gastrointestinal aspiration, etc.), low water intake, recent surgery, prostatism, gynaecological or urological neoplasia and drug intake is necessary, as these are the commonest causes of renal failure in the aged population.

If none of these conditions is found responsible for ARF the remaining illnesses listed in *Table 20.1* must be investigated.

Physical examination

The dehydrated patient of a young age exhibits skin-fold signs, dryness of the tongue and axillae, and diminution of eye turgor, when dehydration is pronounced. Malnourished and elderly patients have diminished elasticity of the skin, therefore making skin-fold signs difficult to evaluate. This sign can best be read from the skin on the anterior part of the forearm, and in the area of the breastbone. Axillary dryness is helpful in diagnosing dehydration in the elderly. Tachycardia and postural hypotension are present in more severe states of dehydration. Hypovolaemia stimulates sympathetic nerves which results in coolness of the limbs. If the condition progresses, paleness due to peripheral vascoconstriction and cyanosis can occur. Vesical enlargement, prostatic enlargement by rectal examination and gynaecological malignancies in women must always be considered and sought.

Laboratory findings

A urinary output of less than 100 ml/24 h often suggests an obstructive pathology. In ischaemic and intrinsic ARF, diuresis is usually slightly higher than in obstructive uropathy — between 100 and 400 ml/day — although this amount of urine can be passed despite obstructions. The creatinine clearance is an accurate clinical index of renal function: when plasma creatinine increases by 1.5–2 mg/day, this indicates the existence of a ARF. An increase larger than this is an expression of a hyperproduction of creatinine, such as is seen in situations of rhabdomyolysis (Grossman, Hamilton and Marse, 1974). A quotient U_{Cr}/P_{Cr} superior to 40 indicates the presence of renal hypoperfusion, but when this quotient is less than 20,

Table 20.3 Indices of acute renal failure in the elderly

Parameter	*'Pre-renal' renal hypoperfusion*	*'Intrinsic' established 'ATN'*
Urine osmolality (mosmol/kg)	>500	<350
Urinary Na^+ output (mmol/l)	< 70	> 70
FE_{Na^+} (%)*	< 1	> 3
U_{urea}/P_{urea}	> 8	< 3
U_{Cr}/P_{Cr}	> 40	< 20
P_{BUN}/P_{Cr}	> 15/1	10–15/1

*See text for calculation.

this may suggest the presence of intrinsic ARF, although there are many exceptions; therefore, the creatinine index must be carefully evaluated (Espinel, 1976; Miller *et al.*, 1978) (*Table 20.3*). The clearance of urea is not a good index of renal function because of the extrarenal origin of the production of urea (protein intake, gastrointestinal bleeding, hypercatabolic states such as trauma, sepsis) (Walser, 1980). But the relation between urinary urea/blood urea is a reliable index in differentiating intrinsic from ischaemic ARF. Normal values for this index are always higher than 8. When this relationship is <3, this may mean that an intrinsic or obstructive ARF is present (Miller *et al.*, 1978). During oliguric ARF, the blood urea (or BUN) increases 10–25 mg/day or possibly more in hypercatabolic states. The relation P_{BUN}/P_{Cr} is 10–15/1 because P_{BUN} and P_{Cr} may increase in intrinsic ARF.

The relationship between urinary and plasma osmolarity is an accurate index for differential diagnosis. A urinary osmolarity higher than 500 mosmol/kg suggests acute reversible renal hypoperfusion, but when plasma osmolarity is 350 mosmol/kg or less, intrinsic ARF may be present. Intermediate levels remain undefined (Miller *et al.*, 1978). When the relationship between urinary osmolarity and plasma osmolarity ranges between 1.29 and 1.35 or more, this indicates acute reversible renal hypoperfusion, but when the relationship between urinary and plasma osmolarity is that of 1.04 or less, this failure is usually due to a lesion of the renal parenchyma in a young population. Nevertheless, these figures are not conclusive in the elderly, due to the inability to conserve sodium and concentrate urine that exists even in healthy aged people. These are precisely some of the reasons why old people are able to go into ARF more easily than younger adults (Abel *et al.*, 1976; Rowe, Shock and De Fronzo, 1976; Schrier, 1979; Beck and Yu, 1982; Macias Nuñez, 1983).

The urinary pH is lower in the ischaemic than in the intrinsic ARF. In obstructive ARF, pH may be alkaline as an expression of renal tubular acid impairment (Battle, Arruda and Kurtzman, 1981). In reversible ischaemic ARF, acute urinary obstruction and in the initial phase of the acute glomerulonephritis the tubular reabsorption of sodium increases; therefore, the urinary sodium content is lowered. In established intrinsic ARF and in the late phase of urinary obstruction, urinary sodium elimination is high. The fractional excretion of sodium (FE_{Na^+}) correlates the excretion of sodium with the degree of renal function, assessed as creatinine clearance. The following formulae will illustrate the steps involved in calculating the amount of filtered sodium and the fractional excretion of sodium:

$$\text{Amount of filtered sodium} = C_{Cr} \,.\, P_{Na^+} = (U_{Cr} \,.\, V/P_{Cr}) \,.\, P_{Na^+}$$

where C_{Cr} is the creatinine clearance; P_{Na^+} the plasma sodium concentration; V the urinary volume (ml/min); P_{Cr} the creatinine plasma concentration; and U_{Cr} the urinary creatinine concentration.

$$\text{Total sodium excretion} = V \,.\, U_{Na^+}$$

$$\text{Fraction excretion of sodium} = (U_{Na^+} \,.\, P_{Cr})/(P_{Na^+} \,.\, U_{Cr})$$

$$\%\ \text{Fractional excretion of sodium} = [(U_{Na^+} \,.\, P_{Cr})/(P_{Na^+} \,.\, U_{Cr})] \,.\, 100$$

where U_{Na^+} is the urinary sodium concentration.

In acute reversible renal hypoperfusion, FE_{Na^+} is usually less than 1 per cent. An oliguric patient with $U_{Na^+} > 20$ mmol/l and $FE_{Na^+} > 3$ per cent suggests intrinsic ARF or established obstructive ARF. Although this is the rule, some exceptions can be found. FE_{Na^+} can be low in azotaemic situations triggered by a non-volume-dependent process such as hepatic or cardiac failure, acute glomerulonephritis, polyuric renal failure associated with burns, acute obstruction, and occasionally non-oliguric ARF. Conversely, in patients on diuretics a high FE_{Na^+} can be seen in oliguria due to volume depletion (Steiner, 1984). The intermediate values of FE_{Na^+} have no significance in the differential diagnosis (Espinel, 1976; Miller *et al.*, 1978; Espinel and Gregory, 1980; Oken, 1981). Again, these values are not completely valid for determining ARF in the elderly because they normally have an increased FE_{Na^+} (Epstein and Hollenberg, 1976), due to the incompetence of the diluting segment (Macias Nuñez *et al.*, 1978) and low aldosterone levels.

The most common parameters in differential diagnosis, for the aged population, are given in *Table 20.3*. In the elderly, ARF shows a $U_{Na^+} < 70$ mmol/l when due to hypoperfusion, and higher than this when intrinsic. Acute renal failure produced by contrast media, acute glomerulonephritis and the hepatorenal syndrome, during the early stage of acute tubular necrosis, in the first 24–48 h of obstructive ARF and even in patients with ARF and sepsis when there is a concomitant volume depletion, may all have low U_{Na} (Hoffman and Suki, 1976; Miller *et al.*, 1978; Van Ypersele de Strihou, 1979; Espinel and Gregory, 1980; Fang *et al.*, 1980; Vaz, 1983). The urinary sediment may be normal in renal hypoperfusion, but in established acute tubular necrosis, epithelial cells either alone, or pigmented casts of these cells, are frequently found. In the obstructive ARF, haematuria, triple phosphate, calcium oxalate or uric acid crystals can be found (Wahlin, 1977). In acute interstitial nephropathy, leukocytes, red cells and white cell casts may be seen in urinary sediment. In allergic interstitial nephropathy, eosinophils may be seen (Galpin *et al.*, 1978). Red cells of glomerular origin, when they lose their haemoglobin, acquire a distorted shape. Red cells from the rest of the urinary tract maintain their normal form (Birch and Fairley, 1979).

Positive blood reactions with orthotoluidine-impregnated dipsticks indicate the presence of haem pigments in the urine. This becomes positive in the presence of myoglobin, haemoglobin and lysed red cells. If this reaction is positive and there are no red cells in the microscopic examination of the urinary sediment, the presence of other illnesses producing pigmenturia must be considered in relation to ARF.

Proteinuria is usually minor (1–4 g/l) except when ARF is caused by proliferating glomerulonephritis and occasionally in cases of a congestive cardiac failure (Carrie *et al.*, 1980). A myeloma with light chains in the urine can be suspected when ARF caused by proteinuria is present, by using the thermal test of precipitation of Bence-Jones protein, along with a negative dipstick test.

Radiology

Plain abdominal radiography can provide valuable information regarding the localization, shape, size of the kidneys and the presence of urinary tract stones.

Intravenous urography (IVU) has been widely used in the past as a diagnostic tool. As GFR and RBF are diminished in ATN, concentrations 2–3 times higher are needed of the contrast media to visualize the kidney. The risk of cardiac failure as a result of the osmotic load and volume expansion is always present (Fry and Catell, 1971). The appearance of a negative pyelogram and late filling of the pyelocaliceal system (10–12 h later than the contrast is injected) are consistently found in obstructive uropathy, as well as dilatation of the pelvis and/or ureter, depending on the location of the obstruction. A few different patterns can help with the diagnosis of intrinsic ARF. One of them is the prompt appearance of a faint nephrogram that becomes progressively more prominent. Another is the complete absence of any nephrogram (Catell *et al.*, 1973). Although intravenous urography is a widely used technique, its side effects must be considered. Retrograde urography has now been almost completely replaced by newer techniques in the diagnosis of obstructive uropathy.

Anterograde percutaneous pyelo-ureteral urography in conjunction with ultrasonographic procedures are successfully used in simultaneously diagnosing and locating the obstruction, which allows the use of a drainage catheter, thus avoiding the surgical nephrostomy (Burnett, Correa and Bush, 1976). The renal arteriogram is of very little value in the aetiologic diagnosis of ARF, except in cases of cortical necrosis, where a patchy cortical nephrogram is discovered, or when a renal artery embolism, aneurysm of the aorta or renal trauma are suspected to be responsible for ARF.

Ultrasonography is now the preferable technique to use in the differential diagnosis of ARF, not the least because of its lack of morbidity. This procedure can accurately measure the size and shape of the kidney, dilatation of the excretory systems as well as any accompanying structural pathology. Ultrasonography is highly sensitive, about 98 per cent; the accuracy in diagnosing obstructive uropathy is 74 per cent (Sanders, 1975; Ellenbogen *et al.*, 1978). Studies made with a gamma camera and radioactive isotopes such as ^{125}I radiohippuran or with pertechnate ^{99m}Tc, are not specific in the differential diagnosis of ARF, but can be useful in cases of unilateral processes, because this technique may be performed in selective studies on the injured kidney without risk to the patient.

Renal biopsy

Renal biopsy can be a precise indicator in diagnosing ARF. In general, the aetiologic diagnosis can be made with conservative procedures. The indications to perform a renal biopsy are when (a) the oliguric phase extends for more than 3–4 weeks (Sraer *et al.*, 1975; Wilson *et al.*, 1976; Solez, Morel-Maroger and Sraer, 1979; Kourilsky *et al.*, 1982); (b) other indications are when ARF is accompanied by extrarenal manifestations that are expressions of systemic illnesses such as vasculitis, systemic lupus erythematosus, rapidly progressive glomerulonephritis or acute interstitial nephropathy, or (c) in complete anuria not the result of obstruction.

Influence of age on the survival of ARF

There is a considerable disagreement regarding the influence of age on ARF. Mortality in young patients is 50–60 per cent. Some authors have found that there is a direct relationship between age and the prognosis of ARF, mortality of the elderly from ARF being much greater, at about 70–80 per cent (Hall *et al.*, 1970; Stott *et al.*, 1972; Abel *et al.*, 1976; Almaraz *et al.*, 1976; McMurray *et al.*, 1978; Schrier, 1979; Orofino *et al.*, 1984) (*Table 20.4*). Other authors have found that the prognosis is independent of age, attributing the mortality rate of 60–70 per cent to the aetiology of ARF (Kumar, Hill and McGeown, 1973; Montoliu *et al.*, 1981; Rasmussen and

Table 20.4 Survival of different series of acute renal failure in the elderly

Series	*Survival* (%)	
Stott *et al.* (1972)	20	(*n* = 26)
Kumar, Hill and McGeown (1973)	43	(*n* = 122)
Almaraz *et al.* (1976)	31	(*n* = 45)
McMurray *et al.* (1978)	40	(*n* = 135)
Rasmussen and Ibels (1982)	46	(*n* = 81)
Brivet *et al.* (1983)	34	(*n* = 64)
Orofino *et al.* (1984)	35	(*n* = 107)
Macias *et al.* (1985)	31	(*n* = 295)

Ibels, 1982; Sanchez Tomero *et al.*, 1984). In our own experience, the mortality is higher in the elderly, conditioned by the higher incidence of associated illnesses prior to the beginning of ARF (coronary ischaemia, uropathies, previous lung diseases, etc.) in patients with septic shock. All the above-mentioned complications of ARF are more severe in oliguric ARF (Rasmussen and Ibels, 1982).

The disagreement among the different authors of the role played by age itself as a risk factor may be due to various circumstances. In the first place, some authors give results of ARF from people aged 70 years and over (Orofino, 1984). Others refer to aging patients as 60 and older (Stott, 1972).

Also, the criteria used by various authors to divide the illnesses leading to ARF into groups has been very heterogeneous. A few groups present results of ARF in the elderly, dividing aetiological causes into medical, surgical, obstructive and 'multifactorial'. Even so, it remains rather difficult to evaluate and compare series. It is easily understandable that under the heading of 'medical', a broad spectrum of illnesses (from dehydration to shock) is included. Only selected patients are admitted to some intensive care units, and there are units where patients aged 70 or more are in practice not accepted even when they suffer from severe illnesses. All these circumstances make it very difficult to evaluate the effect of age as a risk factor in terms of survival. The same is true for post-surgical ARF. Acute renal failure following urological surgery carries a better prognosis than that following cardiovascular surgery. But the worst prognosis is when ARF appears after abdominal surgery, particularly when bowel is involved. If bowel surgery is complicated by sepsis and artificial ventilation is needed, mortality reaches a value of 90 per cent or more (Brown, 1973). Other authors say nothing about the aetiology of ARF in the elderly, giving a global percentage of mortality only.

Table 20.5 Prognosis of acute renal failure in the elderly compared with the young

Associated illness	*Survival* *Young* (%)	*Elderly* (%)
Nephrotoxic	40.0	25.0
Dehydration	90.9	43.5
Septic shock	40.0	15.8
Surgical	83.3	66.7
Cardiogenic shock	12.5	0.0
Multifactorial	9.1	11.4
Obstructive	75.0	67.7
Hepatorenal syndrome	0.0	0.0
Glomerular	75.0	100.0
Others	66.7	17.6
Survival (mean)	47.9	30.5

Table 20.5 shows the prognosis, in terms of survival, of 298 elderly patients aged 65–96 years, treated at the nephrology unit of the University Hospital of Salamanca for ARF, during 1974–85. All of them fulfil the diagnostic criteria of established ATN (see above), and none was rejected on the basis of age, aetiologic cause or clinical situation. The global survival of the elderly group was 30.5 per cent versus 47.9 per cent in the younger patients. Therefore, age does seem to influence the outcome of ARF in our own data. This global survival does not take into account the influence of the different therapeutical strategies introduced during the period of study. For instance, the use of dopamine was begun in 1976, and standard intensive

intravenous feeding in 1979 to all critically ill patients. From 1974 to 1979 we provided a nutritional support of low protein intake either by mouth or via nasogastric tube. When the digestive tract was unsuitable for nutrition (gastrointestinal surgery, stress ulcers, etc.), albumin, hypertonic glucose and occasionally amino acid solutions (in a non-standard regimen) were used with nutritional purposes. During these years, the interdialytic period was prolonged as much as the metabolic status allowed it; on average, two haemodialyses or 48 h of peritoneal dialysis per week were given. Total parenteral nutrition, high calorie, high protein and/or oral intake, when possible, increased the survival from 28.7 to 40.3 per cent in old patients (*Table 20.6*). This nutritional regimen has been especially helpful on septic shock outcome, having increased the survival from 9.6 to 30 per cent in our cases of elderly patients.

Table 20.6 Influence of total parenteral nutrition on ATN survival

Regimen	*Young* (%)	*Elderly* (%)	*Total* (%)
Without TPN	41.4	28.8	31.2
With TPN	66.7	40.4	46.3

TPN, total parenteral nutrition.

Septic shock accounts for 25.7 per cent of ARF in the elderly (*Table 20.2*). This high incidence of septic shock may be due, first, to the deterioration of the immune system which accompanies the aging process; and secondly, that we do not refuse for dialytic treatment any elderly patients with septic shock as defined by prostration, hypotension (systolic blood pressure lower than 80 mmHg), pallor, cold moist skin, collapsed superficial veins, mental confusion, oliguria with criteria of established ATN, and a positive bacteriological culture either from blood or from a major primary source of infection (Ledingham and McArdle, 1978; Sanchez Tomero *et al.*, 1984). As this ominous entity accounts for the majority of ARF in our unit, we have put special effort into trying to improve its prognosis.

In other situations, therapeutical manoeuvres are of little, or at least doubtful, help regarding survival of ARF in the elderly. When ARF is superimposed on cardiogenic shock or hepatorenal syndrome, survival in our series is zero.

This brings into discussion another factor apart from age: 'multiple organ failure'. Although there is no trial specifically focused on the mortality of aged patients with ARF, both from post-surgical and medical causes, it is well known that when one patient has two organs malfunctioning (kidney and another organ) mortality dramatically increases, reaching 89–100 per cent in our own series: multifactorial (89 per cent) and liver or heart failure (100 per cent) (*Table 20.5*). In surgical series, the effect of multiple organ system failure in worsening prognosis after emergency operations of all types ranged from 23 per cent (one organ) to 100 per cent (3–5 organ) failure (Fry, 1980; Pine, 1983). In view of this it seems reasonable not to begin dialysis treatment to elderly patients (65 years or more) who develop an established ATN in the course of cardiogenic shock. Before taking this decision, the patient should be carefully evaluated in order to differentiate cardiogenic shock from the treatable condition of congestive heart failure with oliguria and/or ATN. Nevertheless, remarkable individual cases of recovery have been recorded, and decision is never easy.

When ATN is superimposed on a hepatorenal syndrome, dialysis is of no benefit in improving survival. Again, this picture must be differentiated from the appearance of an oliguric glomerulonephritis in the course of a liver cirrhosis, which should be treated by all available means; and the conditions of liver cirrhosis and oliguria, which respond to pharmacological treatment (plasma or albumin together with dopamine in beta-dose and frusemide). In any situation, a medical pharmacological support should be provided.

Another organ failure which may accompany kidney failure is lung dysfunction. The need for ventilation and ATN following surgery carries a poor prognosis, 91 per cent mortality (Brown, 1973), but currently has diminished to 71 per cent (Neild and Cameron, unpublished observation). We think that if a third organ fails in the presence of ATN and lung failure, dialysis is virtually useless in altering the fatal outcome.

Before finishing this section of risk factors in ARF, it is necessary to emphasize that in general ATN in the elderly is a treatable condition. This means that patients should be intensively treated regardless of age in the presence of reversible conditions. When multiple organ failure appears, or multifactorial causes are responsible for ATN, prognosis worsens considerably; but in this situation, it is these factors and not age that are the major determinants of outcome. Aged people, in the case of multiple causes for renal failure, have a survival of 11.4 per cent and young people of 9 per cent in our own series (*Table 20.5*).

Prophylaxis of ARF

The most important aspect of acute renal failure in the elderly is prevention: ARF in the elderly, once established, is always a serious condition, carrying a poor prognosis (*Table 20.5*). Therefore, it is always preferable to try and *prevent* ARF. Taking into account that the elderly are prone to develop extracellular volume depletion, due to their inability to conserve sodium and water, in order to avoid the establishment of ARF the appropriate amount of fluid and electrolyte replacement must be provided when lacking, because of the mental or physical incapacity in the elderly to provide for themselves. When oral intake is forbidden for some hours prior to surgery, particularly in aggressive operations, in order to prevent ARF it is helpful to infuse 2 litres of isotonic saline solution during this 12 h period. The avoidance of abrupt hypotension during anaesthesia, even for a very short time, may prevent some of the ARF seen following surgery, in cases without surgical complications during the operation period.

After surgery, it is necessary to maintain a correct balance of electrolytes. The prescription of solutions containing no electrolytes (laevulose, glucose), as the only fluid therapy, may be dangerous if blood electrolytes are not monitored. If after a few hours at the end of the surgical treatment the patient remains oliguric, a central venous pressure (CVP) catheter must be used to establish CVP at 8–10 cm of water. If low, further fluids are needed; if above, and diuresis does not appear, a dose of 40 mg of frusemide or more is advisable (Epstein, Schneider and Befeler, 1975; Olivero *et al.*, 1975; Kleinknecht *et al.*, 1976; Hayes *et al.*, 1977; Patak *et al.*, 1979). Frusemide should be administered in the elderly *only if the patient is already correctly hydrated.* Using this simple protocol in tight conjunction with surgical and urological teams, the incidence of ATN following surgery, mainly abdominal vascular and urological, has been reduced (*Table 20.2*), improving the survival at the same time. We think that the reason for these encouraging results may be due to the fact that surgical patients are followed from the very beginning of ATN or even prior to its establishment (*Table 20.5*).

The use of nephrotoxic antibiotics is another cause of ARF in the elderly due to frequent overdose in relation to GFR. Although this point is extensively discussed in Chapter 9, we have found useful both the administration of 2 litres of liquids orally and no more than 80 mg of gentamicin every 12 h in the prevention of ARF, unless 'trough' blood levels suggest the need for more. Tobramycin or netilmicin may be preferable because of their lower nephrotoxicity, or ototoxicity in the case of netilmicin.

Contrast media can produce ARF, particularly in patients with previous deterioration in renal function (diabetes, myeloma, dehydration, peripheral arteriopathy and in the elderly) (Van Zee *et al.*, 1978). When this examination is needed, it is advisable to check the plasma creatinine before, and in the days immediately following radiological exploration. Old persons should *not* be dehydrated and/or purged before performance of an intravenous urogram; tomography renders this unnecessary.

Very recently, it has been shown that calcium channel blockers may avoid the reduction of RBF following intrarenal injection of contrast media in the renal artery of dogs (Bakris and Burnett, 1985). These authors pointed out that the diminution of RBF which followed the intrarenal infusion of contrast media may be mediated by adenosine. It has been proved that the vasoconstriction following intrarenal injection of adenosine in dogs is not modified by plasma renin content, intrarenal angiotensin II or captopril, but renal vasoconstriction is abolished in calcium channel blocker-pretreated dogs (Macias Nuñez *et al.*, 1985). Although these observations seem promising, it is still premature to use calcium channel blockers as a routine in order to avoid the deleterious renal haemodynamic changes provoked by the use of contrast media.

Treatment

Volume replacement

In order properly to treat ARF, the underlying cause must first be identified (nephrotoxic antibiotics, dehydration, obstruction, shock, etc.). A CVP catheter must be used for the replacement of fluid and electrolytes. If, after the replacement of fluid and electrolytes, the situation persists, 40 mg of frusemide should be administered. If diuresis does not appear within 1 h, 250 mg of frusemide must be given intravenously. In the elderly, diuresis can be restored as late as 12 h after the administration of the diuretic. Therefore, if the metabolic and clinical picture (acidosis, hyperpotassaemia, congestive cardiac failure) can be controlled during this period of time, it is advisable to delay dialytic treatment for 12 h. If the metabolic alteration worsens, regardless of diuretic response, a dialysis must be begun.

Dialysis/ultrafiltration/nutrition

It is preferable to use *peritoneal dialysis* whenever possible (Tzamaloukas *et al.*, 1973; Bartecchi, 1975), because heparinization is not necessary and nor is myocardial depression from the acetate of the dyalisate seen; these states are best avoided (Vincent *et al.*, 1982). Also, the volume of intravenous feeding is reduced because approximately 1200 kcal/24 h are provided by glucose content of the usual peritoneal dialysis fluid. Both problems are of special importance when dealing with elderly patients. Peritoneal dialysis is particularly useful when elderly patients are on vasoactive drugs, such as dopamine, for the treatment of septic shock. If peritoneal dialysis cannot be used (many cases of abdominal surgery, fistulae, etc.), *haemofiltration* is the second choice because it produces, in our experience at least, less hypotensive and haemodynamic disorders than conventional haemodialysis.

Another therapeutic approach which has proved useful in the treatment of ARF, especially in those patients in whom intensive intravenous feeding is needed, is the alternative dialysis–ultrafiltration scheduled treatment.

The new technique of *continuous arteriovenous haemofiltration* (CAVH) with a high permeability membrane is used in patients in whom the haemodynamic situation is very compromised. Perhaps because it is used mostly in these high risk patients, the results in terms of survival are not very encouraging at present. A major inconvenience of this variety of treatment is the necessity for continuous heparinization for relatively long periods (10–20 days) depending on the duration of recovery of the ARF, which can prove to be dangerous in the elderly.

With the exception of cases of non-oliguric ARF, patients who receive dialysis early do not seem to show an increased chance of survival than those who receive later treatment (Stott *et al.*, 1972; Sanchez Tomero *et al.*, 1984). Nevertheless, early dialysis can diminish the symptomatology of uraemia and contribute to the overall comfort of the patient. Early dialytic treatment allows proper nutrition, which is essential in the treatment of ARF of any aetiology. When intravenous feeding is needed, ultrafiltration dialysis can help to provide the volume necessary for calories, high protein parenteral nutrition, and avoid volume overload (Figueroa, 1969).

Regarding *nutritional support* in very ill oligo-anuric patients, who for one reason or another cannot be fed through the digestive tract, we have given 0.25 mg of nitrogen (essential and non-essential amino acids) per kg of body weight (an average of 15 g of casein hydrolysate per 60 kg of body weight) and 200 kcal of energy per gram of nitrogen (3000 kcal/24 h for a 60 kg person). This caloric supply consists of fats (soya oil emulsions) and carbohydrates. Fats must *not* be given in a quantity of more than 3 g/kg of the body weight of the patient, and the remaining calories should be given in the form of hypertonic glucose (20–30 per cent). Vitamins and trace elements are provided twice a week.

This is the basic scheme to begin with. In the following days, when urine output returns and dialysis ceases, it is necessary to monitor the nitrogen balance and increase the quantity of these elements until a positive balance of nitrogen is reached. The estimation of the amount of nitrogen needed to bring patients into a nitrogen-positive balance is calculated according to a modified Lee formula (Lee and Hartley, 1975):

$$\text{Nitrogen balance} = \text{Nitrogen intake (g/24 h)} - \text{Nitrogen elimination (NE) (g/24 h)}$$

$$\text{NE} = \text{Urinary urea (g/24 h)} \times (3.5 \pm \Delta \text{ blood urea}) \times \text{Body weight (kg)} \times 1.8$$

$$\text{Total protein catabolism} = \text{NE} \times 6.25$$

To this quantity it is necessary to add 10 per cent of NE as a rough estimate of the amount of nitrogen eliminated by sweating and faeces. Separate lines for intravenous feeding are not used, and we have not observed severe infections due to sepsis produced by the infection of the catheter.

Although the use of a single central venous line for both measurement and feeding is condemned by most writers on critical care medicine, we believe that this practice is not heterodox, in agreement with some others, who found fewer complications using one instead of two lines (Gray, 1982). We put our lines in under sterile conditions by percutaneous needling of an antecubital vein. The dressing is removed and changed once a week. The mean duration of our intravenous feeding period is 17 days (*Figure 20.1*). We believe that the short period that the catheters are in position, the use of a laminar flow hood, the use of a single line inserted under sterile conditions, the care of the venipuncture zone and the frequent use of cloxacillin account for the low incidence of sepsis due to the central line.

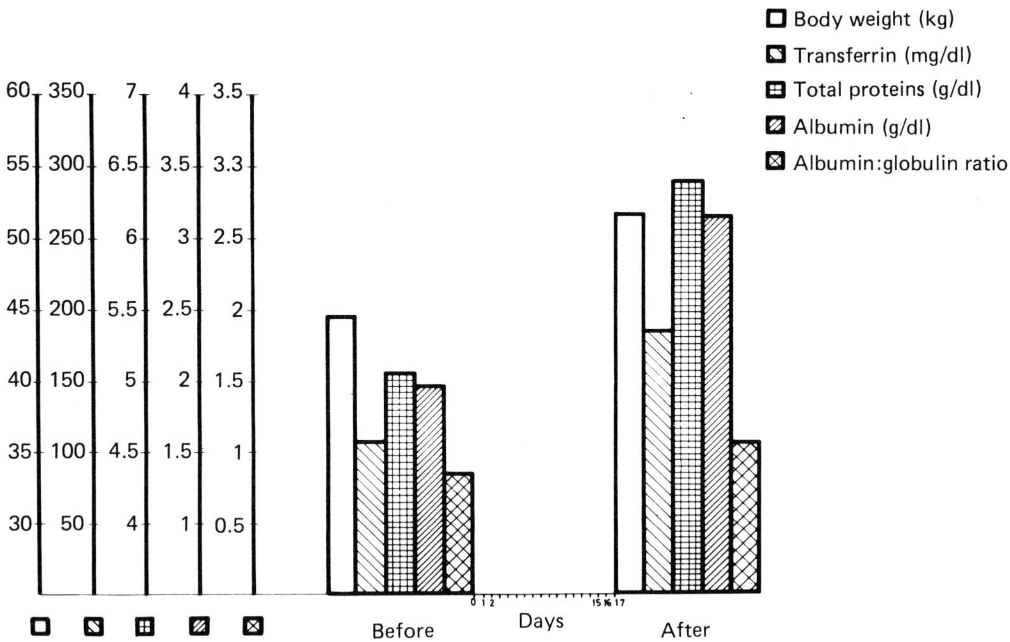

Figure 20.1 The effect of intravenous feeding on body weight and plasma proteins

Clinical, enzymatic or electrocardiographic manifestations of pulmonary embolism have not been observed in our series as a result of the use of fat in the intravenous feeding regimen. The total volume of the intravenous feeding is sometimes as high as 4 litres/24 h; because of this we dialyse and ultrafiltrate one day, and ultrafiltrate alone the next day, in order to make room for intravenous nutrition. Since we dialyse one day and ultrafiltrate the next day, lipids are infused in the last 2 h of dialysis or ultrafiltration. In this way, a reduced amount of fluid is given over the rest of the day. Insulin is not used routinely in this treatment, except in the diabetic patient.

Weight, proteins, albumin, albumin : globulin ratio, and transferrin as a biochemical index of nutrition were monitored (*Figure 20.1*). Blood glucose, uric acid, cholesterol, triglycerides and osmolarity were also determined. Interestingly enough, the blood levels of these substances do not increase during intravenous feeding. Using this technique, hyponatraemia, hypo-osmolarity, hypokalaemia and hypophosphataemia have recently been found (Macias Nuñez *et al.*, 1980; Sanchez Tomero *et al.*, 1984). These elements must be monitored daily in order to replace them according to need.

This type of nutrition may improve the survival of very ill elderly patients due to the impairment of intestinal absorption exhibited by people suffering from severe diseases. With these techniques our survival reaches from 41.4 to 66.7 per cent in young and from 28.7 to 40.4 per cent in the aged group (*Table 20.6*). Although this percentage is not very high, it should be taken into account that the incidence of well-established septic shock in our unit is 26 per cent. From this particular group of aged patients suffering from septic shock, the survival was 30 per cent in patients in whom intravenous feeding was used, but only 9.6 per cent in patients treated without parenteral nutrition. This is in agreement with the observation made by others (Knochel, 1985). Parenteral nutrition favours the recovery of ARF because it favours the synthesis of proteins, the peripheral utilization of glucose, the immune response and the synthesis of phospholipids from the tubular membrane (Dudrick, Steiger and Long, 1970; Abel *et al.*, 1973; Baek *et al.*, 1975; Toback, 1977; Toback, Teegarden and Havener, 1979; Feinstein *et al.*, 1981; Macias Nuñez *et al.*, 1981; Wesson, 1983). In patients able to tolerate oral feeding we obviously prefer this route; in these cases, a high calorie, high protein diet is given.

The maintenance of the water and electrolyte balance, providing the amount of electrolytes necessary for the maintenance of normal blood values in conjunction with the correction of acidosis and hypocalcaemia, are both part of necessary daily care. Drugs must be administered following the adequate correction of renal function or dialysis treatment (Bennet *et al.*, 1980; Tiller and Mudge, 1980).

Infection presents the greatest threat to life and the most severe complication of the elderly patient with ARF. It is useful, if possible, to mobilize the patient (from the bed to an armchair) as soon as possible. Chest infections can be prevented with the use of respiratory physiotherapy every 8 h while in bed. Samples of blood, urine, sputum, axillae and exudates from surgical wounds, when present, must all be taken before administering antibiotics if the patient is septic or when fever appears during the course of the treatment. It is advisable to start a broad-spectrum antibiotic therapy before the germ responsible for the infection can be identified (Sanchez Tomero *et al.*, 1984). Respiratory infections and the indirect effect of septicaemia on the lungs ('shock lungs') are particularly adverse prognosis features (*Table 20.7*).

Table 20.7 Prognosis of respiratory insufficiency on the survival of elderly patients with acute renal failure

Associated illness	*Number of patients*		
	Exitus	*Survival*	*Total*
Nephrotoxic	2		2
Dehydration	4	2	6
Septic shock	8		8
Cardiogenic shock	2		2
Multifactorial	10		10
Obstructive	1		1
Others	2		2
Total	29	2	31
Percentage	93.5%	6.5%	100%

Only 6 per cent of our elderly patients with respiratory problems previous to the beginning of the ARF, which started during the course of it (not all of whom required ventilation), survived.

During the stay of the elderly in the acute care unit, tremendous behavioural changes are the rule. By the fourth day of their admittance, 89 per cent capable of responding presented a low capacity for associative thought (subtest of Ways), and 73 per cent dissociative phenomena with disturbance of the personality (test of Bender). In 80 per cent of the patients there was a noticeable increase in negativism, together with seclusion and a tendency to aggression. There were, however, no major changes in the electroencephalogram, and we did not find any relationship between this and the behavioural alterations. All this abnormal behaviour disappeared a few days after the patients were moved back to the general ward (Macias Nuñez *et al.*, 1980).

References

ABEL, R.M., BECK, C., ABBOT, W.M., RYAN, J.A., BARNETT, G.D. and FISHER, J.E. (1973). Improved survival from acute renal failure after treatment with intravenous essential L-amino acids and glucose. *New England Journal of Medicine,* **288,** 695–699

ABEL, R.M., BUCKLEY, M.J., AUSTEN, W.G., BARNETT, G.O., BACK, G.H. and FISHER, J.E. (1976). Etiology, incidence and prognosis of renal failure following cardiac operations. Results of a prospective analysis of 500 consecutive patients. *Journal of Thoracic and Cardiovascular Surgery,* **71,** 323–333

ADROGUE, H.J. and MADIAS, N.E. (1981). Changes in plasma potassium concentration during acute acid-base disturbances. *American Journal of Medicine,* **71,** 456–467

ALMARAZ, M.A., MARTINEZ, J., RIBERO, M., MIGUEL, J.L., RINON, M.C., MONTERO, A. *et al.* (1976). Fracaso renal agudo en el anciano. *Revista Clinica Española,* **140,** 365–370

ANAGOSTOU, A. and KURTZMAN, N.A. (1986). Hematological consequences of renal failure. In *The Kidney,* edited by B.M. Brenner and F.C. Rector, pp. 1631–1656. Philadelphia; Saunders

ANDERSON, R.J., LINAS, S.L., BERNS, A.S., HENRICH, W.L., MILLER, T.R., GABOW, P.A. *et al.* (1977). Nonoliguric acute renal failure. *New England Journal of Medicine,* **296,** 1134–1138

ANDREUCCI, V. (1984). Pathophysiology of acute renal failure. In *Acute Renal Failure: Pathophysiology, Prevention and Treatment,* edited by V. Andreucci, pp. 1–50. The Hague; Martinus Hyhoff

ARENDSHORST, W.J., FINN, W.F. and GOTTSCHALK, C.W. (1974). Nephron stop-flow pressure response to obstruction for 24 hours in the rat kidney. *Journal of Clinical Investigation,* **53,** 1497–1500

ARENDSHORST, W.J., FINN, W.F., GOTTSCHALK, C.W. and LUCAS, H.R. (1976). Micropuncture study of acute renal failure following temporary renal ischemia in the rat. *Kidney International,* **10,** S100–S105

AVASTHYI, P.S., EVAN, A.P. and HAY, D. (1980). Glomerular endothelial cells in uranyl nitrate-induced acute renal failure in rats. *Journal of Clinical Investigation,* **65,** 121–127

BAEK, S.H., MAKABALI, G.G., BRYAN–BROWN, C.W., KUSEK, J. and SHOEMAKER, W.C. (1975). The influence of parenteral nutrition on the cause of acute renal failure. *Surgery, Gynecology and Obstetrics,* **141,** 405–408

BAKRIS, G.L. and BURNETT, J.C. (1985). A role for calcium in radiocontrast-induced reductions in renal hemodynamics. *Kidney International,* **27,** 465–468

BALINT, P. and SZOCS, E. (1976). Intrarenal hemodynamics following temporary occlusion of the renal artery in the dog. *Kidney International,* **10,** S128–S136

BARTECCHI, C.E. (1975). When should peritoneal dialysis be considered in elderly patients. *Geriatrics,* **30,** 47–51

BASSO, A. (1974). Genitourinary tract problems of the aged male. *Journal of the American Geriatric Society,* **22,** 352–354

BATTLE, D.C., ARRUDA, J.A.L. and KURTZMAN, N.A. (1981). Hyperkalemic distal renal tubular acidosis associated with obstructive uropathy. *New England Journal of Medicine,* **304,** 373–380

BAYLIS, C., RENNKE, H.R. and BRENNER, B.M. (1977). Mechanisms of the defect in the glomerular ultrafiltration associated with gentamicin administration. *Kidney International,* **12,** 344–353

BECK, N. and YUM, B.P. (1982). Effect of ageing on urinary concentrating mechanism and vasopressin-dependent cAMP in rats. *American Journal of Physiology,* **12/2,** F121–F125

BENNETT, W.M., MUTHER, R.S., PARKER, R.A., FEIG, P., MORRISON, G., GOLPER, T.A. and SINGER, I. (1980). Drug therapy in renal failure: dosing guidelines for adults. *Annals of Interenal Medicine,* **93,** 286–325

BHAT, J.C., GLUCK, M.C., LOWENSTEIN, J. and BALDWIN, D.S. (1976). Renal failure after open heart surgery. *Annals of Interenal Medicine,* **84,** 677–682

BIRCH, D.F. and FAIRLEY, K.F. (1979). Haematuria: glomerular or non-glomerular? *Lancet,* **2,** 845–846

BLANTZ, R.C. (1982). Amelioration of uranyl nitrate acute renal failure by converting enzyme inhibitor and plasma volume expansion (Abstract). *Kidney International,* **21,** 215

BONDIA, A., TABERNERO, J.M., CORBACHO, L., SANCHEZ TOMERO, J.A., MACIAS, J.F., FLORES, T. *et al.* (1979). Contribucion experimental al conocimiento patogenetico de la insuficiencia aguda. *Morfologia Normal y Patologica,* **3,** 575–581

BOULTON-JONES, J.M., VICK, R., CAMERON, J.S. and BLACK, P.J. (1973). Immune responses in uremia. *Clinical Nephrology,* **1,** 351–360

BREZIS, M., ROSEN, S., SILVA, P. and EPSTEIN, F.H. (1984). Renal ischemia: new perspective. *Kidney International,* **26,** 3375–383

BRIVET, F., DELFRAISSY, J.F., BALAVOINE, J.F., BIANCHI, A. and DORMONT, J. (1983). Insuffisance rénale aigüe: l'age n'intervient pas dans le prognostic. *Nephrologie,* **4,** 14–17

BROWN, C.B., CAMERON, J.S., BEWICK, M. and STOTT, R.B. (1973). Established acute renal failure following surgical operations. In *Proceedings of a Conference on Acute Renal Failure,* edited by E. Friedman and H. Eliahou, pp. 187–201. Washington DC.; Department of Health, Education and Welfare

BURNETT, L.L., CORREA, R.J. and BUSH, W.H. (1976). A new method for percutaneous nephrostomy. *Radiology,* **120,** 557–561

BURTON, J.R., LICHTENSTEIN, N.S., COLVIN, R.B. and HYSLOP, N.E. (1974). Acute renal failure during cephalothin therapy. *Journal of the American Medical Association,* **229,** 679–682

CARRIE, B.J., HILBERMAN, M., SCHROEDER, J.S. and MYERS, B.D. (1980). Albuminuria and the permselective properties of the glomerulus in cardiac failure. *Kidney International,* **17,** 507–514

CARTY, M., BROCKLEHURST, J.C. and CARTY, J. (1981). Bacteruria and its correlates in old age. *Gerontology,* **27,** 72–75

CATTELL, W.R., McINTOSH, C.S., MOSELEY, I.F. and FRY, I.K. (1973). Excretion urography in acute renal failure. *British Medical Journal,* **2,** 575–578

CLIVE, D.M. and STOFF, J.S. (1984). Renal syndromes associated with nonsteroidal anti-inflammatory drugs. *The New England Journal of Medicine,* **310,** 563–572

CHRYSONT, S.G., FROHLICH, E.D. and PAPPER, S. (1976). Why hypertension is so prevalent in the elderly and how to treat it. *Geriatrics,* **31,** 101–108

CROOKS, J., O'MALLEY, K. and STEVENSON, I.H. (1976). Pharmokinetics in the elderly. *Clinical Pharmacokinetics,* **1,** 288–296

DAUGHARTY, T.M., UEKI, I.F., MERCER, P.F. and BRENNER, B.M. (1974). Dynamics of glomerular ultrafiltration in the rat. Response to ischemic injury. *Journal of Clinical Investigation,* **53,** 105–116

DONOHOE, J.F., VENKATACHALAM, M.A., BERNARD, D.B. and LEVINSKY, N.G. (1978). Tubular leakage and obstruction in acute ischemic renal failure. *Kidney International,* **13,** 208–222

DOUHOUX, P. and SRAER, J.D. (1982). The pathology of acute renal failure due to interstitial nephritis in man, with comments on the role of interstitial inflammation and sex in gentamicin nephrotoxicity. *Medicine (Baltimore),* **61,** 258–268

DUDRICK S.J., STEIGER, E. and LONG, J.M. (1970). Renal failure in surgical patients. Treatment with intravenous essential amino acids and hypertonic glucosa. *Surgery,* **68,** 180–186

EISENBACH, G.M., KLITZLINGER, B. and STEINHAUSEN, M. (1974). Renal blood flow after temporary ischemia of rat kidneys: renal venous outflow and clearance techniques. *Pflugers Archives,* **347,** 223–234

EKNOYAN, G. and BROWN, C.H. (1981). Biochemical abnormalities of platelets in renal failure. *American Journal of Nephrology,* **1,** 17–23

ELLENBOGEN, P.H., SCHEIBLE, F.W., TALNER, L.B. and LEOPOLD, G.R. (1978). Sensitivity of grey scale ultrasound in detecting urinary tract obstruction. *American Journal of Roengenology,* **130,** 731–733

EPSTEIN, M. and HOLLENBERG, N.K. (1976). Age as a determinant of sodium conservation in man. *Journal of Laboratory and Clinical Medicine,* **87,** 411–417

EPSTEIN, M., SCHNEIDER, N.S. and BEFELER, B. (1975). Effect of intrarenal furosemide on renal function and intrarenal hemodynamics in acute renal failure. *American Journal of Medicine,* **58,** 510–516

ESPINEL, C.H. (1976). The FE_{Na} test; use in the differential diagnosis of acute renal failure. *Journal of the American Medical Association,* **236,** 579–581

ESPINEL, C.H. and GREGORY, A.W. (1980). Differential diagnosis of acute renal failure. *Clinical Nephrology,* **13,** 73–77

FANG, L.S.T., SIROTA, R.A., EBERT, T.H. and LICHTENSTEIN, N.S. (1980). Low-fractional excretion of sodium with contrast media-induced acute renal failure. *Archives of Internal Medicine,* **140,** 531–533

FEINSTEIN, E.I., BLUMENKRANTZ, M.J., HEALY, M., KOFFLER, A., SILVERMAN, H., MASSRY, S.G. *et al.* (1981). Clinical and metabolic responses to parenteral nutrition in acute renal failure. *Medicine,* **60,** 124–137

FIGUEROA, J.E. (1969). Dialysis in older patients. *Postgraduate Medicine,* **45,** 205–210

FLAMEMBAUM, W., HAMBURGER, M.J., HUDLESTON, M.L., KAUFMAN, J., McNEIL, J.S., SCHWARTZ, J.H. *et al.* (1976). The initiation phase of experimental acute renal failure: an evaluation of uranyl-nitrate-induced acute renal failure in the rat. *Kidney International,* **10,** S115–S122

FREY, J. (1973). Changes of clearance values in the aged. *Fortschritte der Medizin,* **91,** 96–99

FROCHT, A. and FILLIT, H. (1984). Renal disease in the geriatric patient. *Journal of American Geriatrics Society,* **32,** 28–43

FRY, D.E., GARRISON, R.N., HEITSCH, R.C., CALHOUN, K. and POLK, H.C. (1980). Determinants of death in patients with intra-abdominal abscess. *Surgery,* **88,** 517–522

FRY, I.K. and CATTELL, W.R. (1971). Excretion urography in advanced renal failure. *British Journal of Radiology,* **44,** 198–202

GALPIN, J.E., SHINABERGER, J.H., STANLEY, T.M., BLUMENKRANTZ, M.J. *et al.* (1978). Acute interstitial nephritis due to methicillin. *American Journal of Medicine,* **65,** 756–765

GERBER, J.C., OLSON, R.D. and NIES, A.S. (1981). Interrelationship between prostaglandins and renin release. *Kidney International,* **19,** 816–821

GRAUX, P. and METSTDAGH, M. (1977). The kidney in the elderly. *Annals of Anesthesiology,* **18,** 439—445

GRAY, G.E., DEBONIS, D., ROBINSON, G.W. and MEGUID, M.M. (1982). Multiple use of TPN catheter is not heresy: retrospective review and initial report of prospective study. *Nutritional Support Services,* **2,** 18–21

GREENBLATT, D.J., SELLERS, E.M. and SHADER, R.I. (1982). Drug therapy: drug disposition in old age. *New England Journal of Medicine,* **306,** 1081–1088

GRIFFITHS, G.T., ROBINSON, K.B., CARTWRIGHT, G.O. McLACHLAN, M.S. (1976). Loss of renal tissue in the elderly. *British Journal of Radiology,* **49,** 111–117

GROSSMAN, R.A., HAMILTON, R.W. and MARSE, B.M. (1974). Nontraumatic rhabdomyolisis and acute renal failure. *The New England Journal of Medicine,* **291,** 807–811

GUISADO, R., ARIEFF, A.I. and MASSRY, S.G. (1975). Changes in the electroencephalogram in acute uremia. *Journal of Clinical Investigation,* **55,** 738–745

HALL, J.W. JOHNSON, W.J., MAHER, F.T. and HUNT, J.C. (1970). Immediate and long-term prognosis in acute renal failure. *Annals of Internal Medicine,* **73,** 515–521

HARRINGTON, J.T., SOMMERS, S.C. and KASSIRER, J.P. (1968). Atheromatous emboli with progressive renal failure. Renal arteriography as the probable inciting factor. *Annals of Internal Medicine,* **68,** 152–159

HAYES, D.M., CVITKOVIC, E., GOLBEY, R.B., SCHEINER, E., HELSON, L. and KRAKOFF, I.H. (1977). High dose cis-platinum diamine dichloride. Amelioration of renal toxicity by mannitol diuresis. *Cancer,* **39,** 1372–1381

HENRICH, W.L. (1981). Role of the prostaglandins in renin secretion. *Kidney International,* **19,** 822–830

HERING, P.J. and CARLSON, R.E. (1982). Serum creatinine and renal function in the elderly. *Journal of the American Medical Association,* **248**(1), 31

HOFFMAN, L.M. and SUKI, W.N. (1976). Obstructive uropathy mimicking volume depletion. *Journal of the American Medical Association,* **236,** 2096–2097

HSU, C.H., KURTZ, T.W., GOLDSTEIN, R.D. and WELLER, J.M. (1976). Intrarenal hemodynamics in acute myoglobinuric renal failure. *Nephron,* **17,** 65–72

HYMAN, L.R., BALLOW, M. and KNIESER, M.R. (1978). Diphenylhydantoin interstitial nephritis. Roles of cellular and humoral immunologic injury. *Journal of Pediatrics,* **92,** 915–920

IANHEZ, L.E., LOWEN, J. and SABBAGA, E. (1975). Uremic myocardiopathy. *Nephron,* **15,** 17–28

KAFETZ, K. (1983). Renal impairment in the elderly: a review. *Journal of the Royal Society of Medicine,* **76,** 398–401

KASSIRER, J.P. (1969). Atheroembolic renal disease. *The New England Journal of Medicine,* **280,** 812–819

KLEINKNECHT, D., GENEVAL, D., GONZALEZ-DUQUE, L.A. and FERMANIAN, J. (1976). Furosemide in acute oliguric renal failure: a controlled trial. *Nephron,* **17,** 51–58

KLEINKNECHT, D., JUNGERS, P., CHANARD, J., BARBANEL, G. and GANEVAL, D. (1972). Uremic and non-uremic complications in acute renal failure. Evaluation of the early and frequent dialysis on prognosis. *Kidney International,* **1,** 190–196

KNOCHEL, J.P. (1985). Complications of total parenteral nutrition. *Kidney International,* **27,** 489–496

KOURILSKKY, O., SOLEZ, K., MOREL-MAROGER, L., WHELTON, A., DOHOUX, P. and SRAER, J.D (1982). The pathology of acute renal failure due to interstitial nephritis in man, with comments on the role of interstitial inflammation and sex in gentamicin nephrotoxicity. *Medicine,* **61,** 258–268

KUMAR, R., HILL, C.M. and McGEOWN, M.G. (1973). Acute renal failure in the elderly. *Lancet,* **i,** 90–91

LEDINGHAM, I.McA. and McARDLE, C.S. (1978). Prospective study of the treatment of septic shock. *Lancet,* **i,** 1194–1197

LEE, H.A. and HARTLEY, T.F. (1975). A method of determining daily nitrogen requirements. *Postgraduatae Medicine Journal,* **51,** 441—445

MACIAS NUÑEZ, J.F. (1983). Aspectos morfologicos, funcionales y patologicos del riñon del viejo. *Nefrologia,* **3,** 1–7

MACIAS NUÑEZ, J.F., CARCIA IGLESIAS, C., ACOSTA, A., GARCIA, P., GASCON, M. and TABERNERO, J.M. (1980). Psicopatologia clinica de pacientes geriatricos en unidades de cuidados intensivos. In *Resumés des Rapports et Communications* (Grenoble, 1980), 76pp. Paris; International Association of Gerontology

MACIAS NUÑEZ, J.F., GARCIA IGLESIAS, C., BONDIA, A., RODRIGUEZ, J.L., CORBACHO, L., TABERNERO, J.M. and DE CASTRO, S. (1978). Renal handling of sodium in old people: a functional study. *Age and Ageing*, **7**, 178–181

MACIAS NUÑEZ, J.F., GARCIA IGLESIAS, C., SANTOS, J.C., SANZ, E. and LOPEZ NOVOA, J.M. (1985). Influence of plasma renin content, intrarenal angiotensis II, captopril and calcium channel blockers on the vasoconstriction and renin release promoted by adenosine in the kidney. *Journal of Laboratory and Clinical Medicine*, **106**, 562–567

MACIAS NUÑEZ, J.F., GARCIA IGLESIAS, C. and TABERNERO, J.M. (1981). Fracaso renal agudo en el anciano. *Revista Española de Geriatria y Gerontologia*, **16**, 195–200

MACIAS NUÑEZ, J.F., GARCIA IGLESIAS, C., TABERNERO, J.M., DIAZ MOLINA, H. and YUSTE CHAVES, M. (1980). Experiencia en el tratamiento de pacientes geriatricos con insuficiencia renal mediante una tecnica de nutricion parenteral de facil aplicacion y manejo. *Revista Española de Geriatria y Gerontologia*, **15**, 343–352

McMURRAY, S.D., LUFT, F.C., MAXWELL, D.R., HAMBURGER, R.J., FUTTY, D., SZWED, J.J. *et al.* (1978). Prevailing patterns and predictor variables with acute tubular necrosis. *Archives of Internal Medicine*, **138**, 950–955

MASON, J. (1976). Tubulo-glomerular feedback in the early stages of experimental acute renal failure. *Kidney International*, **10**, S106–S111

MASSON, J., WELSCH, J. and TAKABATOKE, T. (1983). Disparity between surface and deep nephron function early after renal ischemia. *Kidney International*, **24**, 27–36

MASSRY, S.G., ARIEFF, A.I., COBURN, J.W., PALMIERI, G. and KLEEMAN, C.R. (1974). Divalent ion metabolism in patients with acute renal failure. Studies on the mechanism of hypocalcemia. *Kidney International*, **51**, 437–445

MERINO, G.E., BUSELMEIER, T.J. and KJELLSTRAND, C.M. (1975). Postoperative chronic renal failure: a new syndrome. *Annals of Surgery*, **182**, 37—44

MILLER, P.D., KREBS, R.A., NEAL, B.J. and McINTYRE, D.O. (1982). Hypodipsia in geriatric patients. *American Journal of Medicine*, **73**, 354—356

MILLER, T.R., ANDERSON, R.J., LINAS, S.L., HENRICH, W.L., BERNS, A.S., GABOW, P.A. *et al.* (1978). Urinary diagnostic indices in acute renal failure. A prospective study. *Annals of Internal Medicine*, **89**, 47–50

MONTOLIU, J., DARNELL, A., TORRAS, A. and REVERT, L. (1981). Acute and rapidly progressive forms of glomerulonephritis in the elderly. *Journal of the American Geriatrics Society*, **29**, 108–116

MYERS, B.D., CARRIE, B.J., YEE, R.R., HILBERMAN, M. and MICHAELS, A.S. (1980). Pathophysiology of hemodynamically-mediated acute renal failure in man. *Kidney International*, **18**, 495–504

NEUGARTEN, J., AYNEDJIAN, H.S. and BANK, N. (1983). Role of tubular obstruction in acute renal failure due to gentamicin. *Kidney International*, **24**, 330–335

OKEN, D.E. (1975). On the passive back flow theory of acute renal failure. *American Journal of Medicine*, **58**, 77–82

OKEN, D.E. (1976). Local mechanisms in the pathogenesis of acute renal failure. *Kidney International*, **10**, S94–S99

OKEN, D.E. (1981). On the differential diagnosis of acute renal failure. *American Journal of Medicine*, **71**, 916–920

OKEN, D.E (1983). Theoretical analysis of pathogenetic mechanisms in experimental acute renal failure. *Kidney International*, **24**, 16–26

OLIVERO, J.J., LOZANO-MENDEZ, J., GHAFARY, E.M., EKNOYAN, G. and SUKI, W.M. (1975). Mitigation of amphotericin B toxicity by mannitol. *British Medical Journal*, **1**, 550–551

OROFINO, L., MARTIN DEL YERRO, J., DIAZ, J., LIANO, F., ORTE, L. and ORTUÑO, J. (1984) Fracaso renal agudo en el viejo. *Nefrologia*, **4**, 191–195

PALLER, M.S., HOIDAL, J.R. and FERRIS, T.F. (1984). Oxygen-free radicals in ischemic acute renal failure in the rat. *Journal of Clinical Investigation*, **74**, 1156–1164

PATAK, R.V., FADEN, S.Z., LIFSCHITZ, M.D. and STEIN, J.H. (1979). Study of factors which modify the development of norepinephrine-induced acute renal failure in the dog. *Kidney International*, **15**, 227–237

PINE, R.W., WERTZ, M.J., LENNARD, E.S., DELLINGER, EP., CARNICO, C.J. and MINSHEW, B.H. (1983). Determinants of organ malfunction or death of patients with intra-abdominal sepsis. A discriminate analysis. *Archives of Surgery*, **118**, 242–249

PRINSEAU, J., GRANIER, F., BAGLIN, A., FENDLER, J.P. and FRITEL, D. (1983). Glomerulopathies in the aged (excluding diabetes). *Semaine des Hôpitaux*, **59**, 2813–2817

RASKIN, N.H. and FISHMAN, R.A. (1976). Neurologic disorders in renal failure. *New England of Medicine*, **294**, 204–210

RASMUSSEN, H.H. and IBELS, L.L.S. (1982). Acute renal failure: multivariate analysis of causes of risk factors. *American Journal of Medicine*, **73**, 211–219

RELMAN, A.S. (1972). Metabolic consequences of acid-base disorders. *Kidney International*, **1**, 347–359

REUBI, F.C. (1974). The pathogenesis of anuria following shock. *Kidney International,* **5,** 106–110

REUBI, F.C. and VORBURGER, C. (1976). Renal hemodynamics in acute renal failure after shock in man. *Kidney International,* **10,** S137–S143

RITSCHEL, W.A. (1976). Pharmacokinetic approach to drug dosing in the aged. *Journal of American Geriatic Society,* **24,** 344–354

ROSENFELD, J. (1983). Hypertension in the elderly. *Kidney International,* **23,** 540–547

ROWE, J.M., SHOCK, N.W. and DE FRONZO, R.A. (1976). The infuence of age on the renal response to water deprivation in man. *Nephron,* **17,** 270–278

SAMIY, A.H. (1983). Renal disease in the elderly. *Medical Clinics of North America,* **67,** 463–480

SANCHEZ-TOMERO, J.A., MARTIN, J., MACIAS NUÑEZ, J.F., BONDIA, A., RODRIGUEZ, J.L., CORBACHO, L. *et al.* (1984). Shock septico y fracaso renal agudo: analisis de los factores que intervienen en su evolucion. *Nefrologia,* **4,** 197–203

SANDERS R.C. (1975). Renal ultrasound. *Radiologic Clinics of North America,* **13,** 417–434

SCHNERMANN, J., BRIGGS, J.P. and WEBER, P.C. (1984). Tubulo-glomerular feedback, prostaglandins and angiotensin in the autoregulation of glomerular filtration rate. *Kidney International,* **25,** 53–64

SCHRAMM, A., JENETT, M. and GERHARDT, K.H. (1981). Changes in kidney function and morphology in the aged. *Zeitschrift für Gerontologie,* **14,** 354–369

SCHRIER, R.W. (1979). Acute renal failure. *Kidney International,* **15,** 205–216

SHOR, N., ICHICAWA, I., RENNKE, H.G., TROY, L.J. and BRENNER, B.M. (1981). Pathophysiology of altered glomerular function in aminoglycoside-treated rats. *Kidney International,* **19,** 288–296

SOLEZ, K., ALTMAN, J., RIENHOFF, H.Y., FINER, P.M. and HEPTINSTALL, R.H. (1976). Early angiographic and renal blood flow changes after $HgCl_2$ or glycerol administration. *Kidney International,* **10,** S153–S159

SOLEZ, K., MOREL-MAROGER, L. and SRAER, J.D. (1979). The morphology of 'acute tubular necrosis' in man: analysis of 57 renal biopsies and a comparison with the glycerol model. *Medicine (Baltimore),* **58,** 362–376

SRAER, J.D., KANFER, A., MARSAC, J., MIGNON, F., MOREL-MAROGER, L. and RICHET, G. (1975). Renal biopsy in acute renal failure. *Kidney International,* **8,** 60–61

STEIN, J.H., GOTTSCHALK, J., OSGOOD, R.W. and FERRIS, T.F. (1975). Pathophysiology of a nephrotic model of acute renal failure. *Kidney International,* **8,** 27–41

STEINER, R.W. (1984). Interpreting the fractional excretion of sodium. *The American Journal of Medicine,* **77,** 699–702

STOTT, R.B., CAMERON, J.S., OGG, C.S. and BEWICK, M. (1972). Why the persistent mortality in acute renal failure? *Lancet,* **2,** 75–78

TANNER, G.A. and STEINHAUSEN, M. (1976). Tubular obstruction in ischemia-induced acute renal failure in the rat. *Kidney International,* **10,** S65–S67

THURAU, K. and BOYLAN, J.W. (1976). Acute renal success. The unexpected logic of oliguria in acute renal failure. *American Journal of Medicine,* **61,** 308–315

THURAU, K., VOGT, C. and DAHLHEIM, H. (1976). Renin activity in the juxtaglomerular apparatus of the rat kidney during postischemic acute renal failure. *Kidney International,* **10,** S177–S182

THURLBECK, W.M. and CASTLEMAN, B. (1957). Atheromatous emboli to the kidney after aortic surgery. *New England Journal of Medicine,* **257,** 442–447

TILLER, D.J. and MUDGE, G.H. (1980). Pharmacologic agents used in the management of the acute renal failure. *Kidney International,* **18,** 700–711

TOBACK, F.G. (1977). Amino-acid enhancement of renal regeneration after acute tubular necrosis. *Kidney International,* **12,** 193–198

TOBACK, F.G., TEEGARDEN, D.E. and HAVENER, L.J. (1979). Amino-acid-mediated stimulation of renal phospholipid biosynthesis after acute tubular necrosis. *Kidney International,* **15,** 542–547

TORRES, V.E., STRONG, C.G., ROMERO, J.C. and WILSON, D.M. (1975). Indomethacin enhancement of glycerol-induced acute renal failure in rabbits. *Kidney International,* **7,** 170–178

TZAMALOUKAS, A.H., GARELLA, S., CHAZAN, J.A. and PROVIDENCE, R.I. (1973). Peritoneal dialysis for acute renal failure after major abdominal surgery. *Archives of Surgery,* **106,** 639–643

VAN YPERSELE DE STRIHOU, C. (1979). Acute oliguric interstitial nephritis. *Kidney International,* **16,** 751–765

VAN ZEE, B.D., HOY, W.E., TALLEY, T.E. and JAENIKE, J.R. (1978). Renal injury associated with intravenous pyelography in non-diabetic and diabetic patients. *Annals of Internal Medicine,* **89,** 51–54

VAZ, A.J. (1983). Low fractional excretion of urine sodium in acute renal failure due to sepsis. *Archives of Internal Medicine,* **143,** 738–739

VINCENT, J.L., VANHERWEGHEM, J.L., DEGAUTE, J.P., BERRE, J., DUFAYE, P. and KAHN, R.J. (1982). Acetate-induced myocardial depression during hemodialysis for acute renal failure. *Kidney International,* **22,** 653–657

WAHLIN, A. (1977). The urinary sediment in hydronephrosis. *Acta Medica Scandinavica,* **201,** 449–452

WALSER, M. (1980). Determinant of ureagenesis, with particular reference to renal failure. *Kidney International,* **17,** 709–721

WARDLE, N. (1982). Acute renal failure in the 1980's: the importance of septic shock and endotoxaemia. *Nephron,* **30,** 193–200

WESDORP, R.I.C., FALCAO, H.A., BANKS, P.B., MARTINO, J. and FISHER, J.E. (1981). Gastrin and gastric acid secretion in renal failure. *American Journal of Surgery,* **141,** 334–338

WESSON, D.E., MITCH, W.E. and WILMORE, C.W. (1983). Nutritional considerations in the treatment of acute renal failure. In *Acute Renal Failure,* edited by B.M. Brenner and M.G. Lazarus, pp.618–642. Philadelphia; Saunders

WILSON, D.M., TURNER, D.R., CAMERON, J.S., OGGS, C.H., BROWN,C.B. and CHANTLER, C. (1976). Value of renal biopsy in acute intrinsic renal failure. *British Medical Journal,* **2,** 459–461

Chapter 21

Aetiology and diagnosis of chronic renal insufficiency in the aged: the role of renal biopsy

Jeffrey L. Glickman, Donald L. Kaiser and W. Kline Bolton

Introduction

Before the availability of haemodialysis, chronic renal insufficiency had to be managed by conservative means alone, usually in the form of dietary manipulation and fluid restriction. The process was invariably fatal with eventual progression to end-stage renal disease (ESRD). With the advent of haemodialysis, the diagnosis of ESRD was no longer a death sentence, and patients who qualified for this treatment could continue to live a productive life. Due to an initial paucity of dialysis equipment and trained personnel, only a limited number of patients could be offered long-term support. Committees consisting of physicians, psychiatrists, clergymen and lay people were given the task of choosing who would benefit from this new technology. Generally, young patients who were felt to be contributing members of the community were selected. Few elderly patients were supported due to the limited resources. In the past 15 years, however, there has been a steady increase in the availability of dialytic support. With advances in dialysis technology, increases in the number of trained support personnel, advent of home dialysis training programmes and, in the USA, full government financial support of the ESRD programme, few patients are denied access to maintenance dialysis (see Chapter 22).

Age alone is no longer a major criterion for selecting patients in most programmes (Walker *et al.*, 1976). Initial fears that the technical aspects of haemodialysis would result in a prohibitively high mortality in the elderly population have been refuted by numerous studies over the past decade (Ghantous *et al.*, 1971; Bailey *et al.*, 1972; Walker *et al.*, 1976; Chester *et al.*, 1979; Taube *et al.*, 1983; Mallinson *et al.*, 1984). Elderly patients whose cardiovascular instability precludes haemodialysis can be effectively supported with various modes of home or in-centre peritoneal dialysis (see Chapter 22). Some centres are even performing renal transplantation in the elderly age group with very good results (Kjellstrand *et al.*, 1976; Walker *et al.*, 1976) (see Chapter 23).

The fact that the elderly age group comprises an increasing percentage of the general population (see Preface and Chapter 11), coupled with the widespread availability of medical support and dialysis, has resulted in a rise in the number of elderly patients with chronic renal insufficiency. Indeed, in 1982, 35 per cent of the 56 046 patients in the USA on chronic maintenance dialysis were age 60 or older (Department of Health and Human Services, 1984). One might expect that the aetiology of chronic renal insufficiency in the older age groups would be somewhat different when compared to a younger age group (see Chapter 22). Whereas primary renal diseases would affect both age groups, secondary renal diseases (i.e.

systemic diseases such as diabetes mellitus and essential hypertension, which have the kidneys as a target organ) would become more apparent the longer the disease was present, and would be expected to predominate in older age groups. It is generally accepted that the incidence of secondary diseases of the kidney increases in the elderly (Samiy, 1983).

Cystic diseases of the kidney are discussed in Chapter 17, and obstructive uropathies in Chapter 19. The present chapter deals principally with the diagnosis of patients with diffuse parenchymal disease causing renal failure in elderly subjects, and should be read in conjunction with Chapters 13–16 of this book which give accounts of glomerular diseases, tubulo-interstitial diseases and vasculitis in old people.

In view of the increasing incidence of chronic renal insufficiency in the elderly, and in spite of the fact that the aetiology of the underlying renal disease can have an effect on therapy (such as influencing the decision to transplant or what form of dialysis might be better tolerated), it is surprising that there are few studies looking specifically at the diagnosis of renal disease in this age group. Most available series suffer from the fact that the diagnosis is usually made on clinical grounds alone, without biopsy confirmation (see *Figure 22.3*, page 511). Moorthy and Zimmerman (1980) presented perhaps the best biopsy series to date, yet looked only at primary renal disease, excluding secondary causes of renal insufficiency from their study. It is the purpose of this chapter to present our findings on the aetiology of chronic renal insufficiency in an elderly population. We had three main objectives for the study. First, to define by tissue diagnosis the spectrum of renal disease in elderly patients relative to younger patients in our geographic region; secondly, to assess the accuracy of the clinical diagnosis of the aetiology of renal disease when compared to the 'gold standard' of renal biopsy; and thirdly, to ascertain the aetiology of renal insufficiency in our population aged 60 or greater and compare the incidence of various renal diseases with a geographically matched younger population with chronic renal insufficiency. Our indications for performing renal biopsy in the elderly are discussed later in this chapter.

Methods

Since the autumn of 1973, open and percutaneous renal biopsies have been processed at the University of Virginia School of Medicine, USA, for immunofluorescence and for light and electron microscopy. Tissue for immunofluorescence studies until 1978 has been processed, as previously described, by placing the tissue on cork and immersing it quickly into thoroughly pre-chilled isopentane (pre-chilled in dry ice) (Bolton *et al.*, 1976). This is followed by sectioning at 4 μm on a cryostat and staining with antisera directed against human IgG, IgA, IgE, IgM, Clq, C3, fibrinogen, alpha-2-macroglobulin, Tamm–Horsfall protein and kappa and lambda light chains. More recently, many biopsies, especially referral biopsies, have been processed by immersing the tissue in formol sucrose/gum sucrose solution for transport and fixing, after which it is paraffin embedded, sectioned at 4 μm, enzymatically digested and stained as noted above (Bolton and Mesnard, 1982). The results of these two techniques are comparable, with the latter being perhaps slightly superior in detail. Tissue for light microscopy has been processed by placing in buffered formalin or Zenker's solution, paraffin embedding, sectioning serially at 3 μm, and staining with haematoxylin and eosin and periodic acid Schiff's reagent. Tissue for ultrastructural analysis has been fixed in 2 per cent glutaraldehyde–paraformaldehyde–cacodylate buffer, followed by embedding in Araldite, thin sectioning with a glass knife, and post-fixing with osmium and lead tetroxide (Bolton and Sturgill, 1980, 1981).

One of the present authors (W.K.B.) has formulated a clinical information data sheet (*Figure 21.1*) which is requested for each biopsy, whether a referral or from

University of Virginia Hospital Data Sheet Renal Biopsy Immunofluorescence PHONE #804/924-5125	Patient's Name: History #:	
Referring M.D.:	Local Hospital:	Date:

Age:	Sex: M F	Duration of Renal Disease:	Previous biopsy: Yes No	Race:

Brief Clinical History, Including Significant Laboratory Findings
BUN Serum creatinine Creatinine clearance

Blood Pressure: Systolic / Diastolic
Clinical Diagnosis:

Clinical Manifestations of Renal Disease (circle yes or no):

Edema	yes no	Allergies	yes no
Gross hematuria	yes no	Diabetes	yes no
Flank pain	yes no	Renal masses	yes no
Stones	yes no	Arthritis	yes no
Dysuria	yes no	Skin rash	yes no
Polyuria	yes no	Upper respiratory infection	yes no
Family history	yes no		

Drug Therapy (circle yes or no):

Antibiotics	yes no	Other immunosuppressives	yes no
Steroids	yes no	Antihypertensives	yes no
Imuran	yes no	Non-steroidal agents	yes no
Cytotoxics	yes no	Other	yes no
Anticoagulants	yes no		

URINALYSIS					
Sg:	Proteinuria (circle one) 1+ 2+ 3+ 4+			Total urinary protein/24 hrs:	
RBC:	WBC:	Casts:	DRFB'S		
ASOT:	VDRL:	LE PREP (circle one) Pos Neg Not done	ANIF (circle one) Pos Neg Not done	COMPLEMENT: CH50 BETA 1C	

Pertinent Laboratory Data:

Kidney size & method:	Erythrocyte sed. rate:
Clq-precipitin test:	Total serum protein:
Rheumatoid factor:	Serum albumin:
Cryoglobulins:	Cholesterol:
	Other:

Figure 21.1 Data sheet for each patient with a kidney biopsy. Demographic information as well as clinical presentation, pertinent history, physical findings and laboratory values are requested

within the University of Virginia Hospital. This data sheet contains information about clinical presentation and duration of disease, renal function, age, clinical diagnosis as assessed by the referring physician, clinical manifestations of the renal disease, type of therapy and laboratory findings including urinalysis. The data sheet is used for interpretation of the biopsies by the three histologic methods. After the interpretation of the biopsy has been rendered, the aggregate of the data sheet, the pathology diagnosis from light and electron microscopy and the immunofluorescence diagnosis are compiled and the data is coded for entry into a data retrieval and analysis system. The format used for this is illustrated in *Figure 21.2.* Information includes demographic data on the patient, the type of biopsy and the immunofluorescence findings relative to proteins deposited, their distribution and pattern. Items 8–10 provide space for 3 pathologic codes and diagnoses, items 11–13 provide space for 3 fluorescence codes and diagnoses, and items 17–19 provide space for 3 clinical codes and diagnoses. Each of the biopsy's pathology, immunofluorescence and clinical reports is scanned by author W.K.B. or a trained technician and the most pertinent diagnoses are entered. The most likely clinical diagnosis is entered first, followed in succession by lesser choices. Similarly, the most likely pathologic or immunofluorescence diagnosis is entered first, followed then by second and third choices. Obviously, correlations between these entered data are dependent upon information provided by the referring physician, interpretation of

Fluorescence Microscopy

1. ________ FM Number 2-4. ________ Last Name, ________ First, ________ M.I.

5. ________ Hospital number 16. ________ Type: 1=open, 2=needle

6. ________ Location code 17-19. ____, ____, ____/________ Clin Dx

7. ________ Path number 20. ________ Days post-op

8-10. ____, ____, ____/________ Path Dx

11-13. ____, ____, ____/________ IF Dx

14. ________ Date of biopsy 21. ________ Fixative OK? (Y or N)

15. ________ Date of birth 22. ________ Formol sucrose (Y or N)

	THP (1)	ALPHA-2-MACRO (2)	K (3)	L (4)	IgG (5)	IgM (6)	IgA (7)	IgE (8)	C-4 (9)	C-3 (10)	C1q (11)	FIB (12)
Glomeruli (1)												
GBM-linear (2)												
GBM-granular (3)												
PCL (4)												
Mesang. (5)												
Other (6)												
G-focal (7)												
G-seg. (8)												
G-amorph. (9)												
Tubules (10)												
Casts (11)												
TBM-linear (12)												
TBM-gran. (13)												
T-focal (14)												
T-seg. (15)												
T-amorph. (16)												
Interstitium (17)												
Conn. (18)												
Cells (19)												
Medulla (20)												
Vessels:PTC (21)												
Arteries (22)												
Bowman's cap. (23)												
Crescents (24)												
Bowman's space (25)												

Figure 21.2 Data entry sheet for renal biopsies. The entry sheet provides information on the clinical diagnosis, pathologic and immunofluorescence findings, and the specific proteins deposited in the kidney, as well as their distribution and pattern

the histologic material and analysis of this data for entry into the computer. Once the data are entered into the computer, they are then available for analysis.

Entry data for renal biopsies at the University of Virginia Hospital and referring area encompass the 10-year period from August 1973 to December 1983. In the analysis of data for the present chapter, all of those patients 60 years of age and older (hereafter designated as 'elderly') were analysed in comparison with patients less than 60 years of age (hereafter designated as 'younger'). In order to assess the correlation between the clinical and pathologic diagnoses, data were analysed by matching the first and thus primary pathologic diagnosis with the first or primary clinical diagnosis, followed sequentially by matching of the first pathology diagnosis with any of the three clinical diagnoses, and finally assessment of any match between the three pathology diagnoses and the three clinical diagnoses. In addition, the reverse of this procedure was followed such that the first clinical diagnosis was matched with the first pathology diagnosis, first clinical with any pathology and finally any clinical with any pathology diagnosis to see the match. At the present time we are using 77 different histologic diagnoses in our programme. Histologic diagnoses that have the same nomenclature as clinical diagnoses have the same code in both of these categories, i.e. atheromatous emboli. In addition to these codes, which may be applicable to either pathology, clinical or both, there are 61 categories of clinical diagnoses that are not synonymous with the pathology diagnosis and 15 morphologic diagnoses which provide additional information applicable to ultrastructural analysis such as 'epimembranous deposits' or 'subepithelial humps'.

Initial analysis using each individual code and grouping of all patients who fall into that code illustrated that there was a wide scatter of patient diagnoses. After assessment of this information based upon the relative frequency of the individual codes, it was decided to combine those categories which provided similar clinical and/or histologic diagnoses to assist in analysing data. Therefore, clinical and pathologic diagnoses have been combined in categories, as illustrated in *Table 21.1*. Using this schema, for instance, pathology diagnosis group 11 would include all patients who had the pathologic diagnosis of multiple myeloma, light chain disease or amyloidosis. The other combination of categories is based on the type of overall histologic and clinical syndrome, i.e. systemic lupus erythematosus, chronic renal disease, membranoproliferative glomerulonephritis and mesangiocapillary glomerulonephritis, focal glomerulonephritis and Berger's disease, etc. Diagnoses that may not be present in *Table 21.1* remained as a single entity diagnosis, e.g. atheromatous emboli. The combining of the groups followed the same format for both the clinical and pathologic diagnoses; for example, multiple myeloma, light chain disease and amyloidosis are combined in the clinical as well as pathology as a single group. The authors are well aware that lumping of the categories in this fashion will lose some of the discrimination of keeping individual categories. However, the large number of different diagnoses renders analysis unmanageable and makes comparison between the elderly and younger patients essentially impossible. Therefore, in analysis of pathologic and clinical data, these groupings as well as the individual categories are used.

Results

Source of patients

Since the autumn of 1973, renal biopsies have been performed on 244 elderly individuals and 875 younger persons as defined above. Excluded from these

Table 21.1 Grouping categories

A. Clinical

1. Nephrotic syndrome, proteinuria
2. Acute renal failure, acute tubular necrosis
3. Rapidly progressive glomerulonephritis, crescentic glomerulonephritis, Goodpasture's syndrome
4. Chronic renal failure, end-stage renal disease, chronic glomerulonephritis
5. Glomerulonephritis, acute glomerulonephritis, cryoglobulinaemia
6. Vasculitis, polyarteritis nodosa, Henoch-Schönlein purpura, Wegener's granulomatosis
7. Rheumatoid arthritis, scleroderma, gold therapy, Sjögren's syndrome
8. Multiple myeloma, amyloidosis, light chain disease

B. Pathology diagnosis

1. Nephrosclerosis, hypertensive nephrosclerosis
2. Focal glomerular sclerosis, glomerular sclerosis
3. Chronic glomerulonephritis, end-stage kidney
4. Lupus nephritis — focal, proliferative, membranous, membranoproliferative types
5. Glomerulonephritis, diffuse glomerulonephritis, necrotizing glomerulonephritis, post-infectious glomerulonephritis, cryoglobulinaemia
6. Vasculitis, polyarteritis nodosa, Wegener's granulomatosis, Henoch-Schönlein purpura
7. Lipoid nephrosis, minimal change or normal (with proteinuria)
8. Mesangiocapillary glomerulonephritis, membranoproliferative glomerulonephritis, dense deposit disease
9. Berger's disease, focal proliferative glomerulonephritis, mesangial hypercellularity
10. Interstitial nephritis, acute pyelonephritis
11. Multiple myeloma, amyloid, light chain disease
12. Thrombotic thrombocytopenia, haemolytic uraemic syndrome, intrarenal coagulation
13. Chronic pyelonephritis, chronic interstitial nephritis
14. Diabetes, diabetic nodular sclerosis, diabetic glomerular sclerosis

considerations are any biopsies obtained from transplanted kidneys or nephrectomy specimens from transplanted patients, and each patient is considered only once; that is, if repeat biopsies were taken from the same patient, only the first biopsy is considered. Only patients with tissue available for light microscopic analysis are included. *Figure 21.3* shows the distribution of biopsies in our population in 10-year increments. The elderly are illustrated in the last three columns in *Figure 21.3*. The number of patients <10 years of age who were biopsied approximately equals those age 70–80, with each being approximately half of the number for the decades in between these extremes. Nearly equal numbers of biopsies were performed in the decades 10–70. The youngest patient who has been biopsied has been a few months of age, and the oldest 90 years of age.

The distribution of biopsies by year is shown in *Figure 21.4*. The total number of diagnostic biopsies increased until 1976 and then remained relatively stable until 1983, when a slight decline in the number of biopsies was observed. From 1976 to 1982 approximately 125–150 biopsies were performed yearly. The distribution of biopsies relative to the year of procurement of tissue and the age of the patient is given in *Figures 21.4(b)* and *21.4(c)*. In *Figure 21.4(b)* the number of biopsies per year is plotted for younger patients. As was the case for the total number of biopsies, the number obtained in the younger age group increased until 1976 and plateaued at that point for several years. Beginning in 1979 there appeared to be a slow but definite diminution in the total number of biopsies being performed on younger patients. On the other hand (*Figure 21.4c*) the total number of biopsies performed

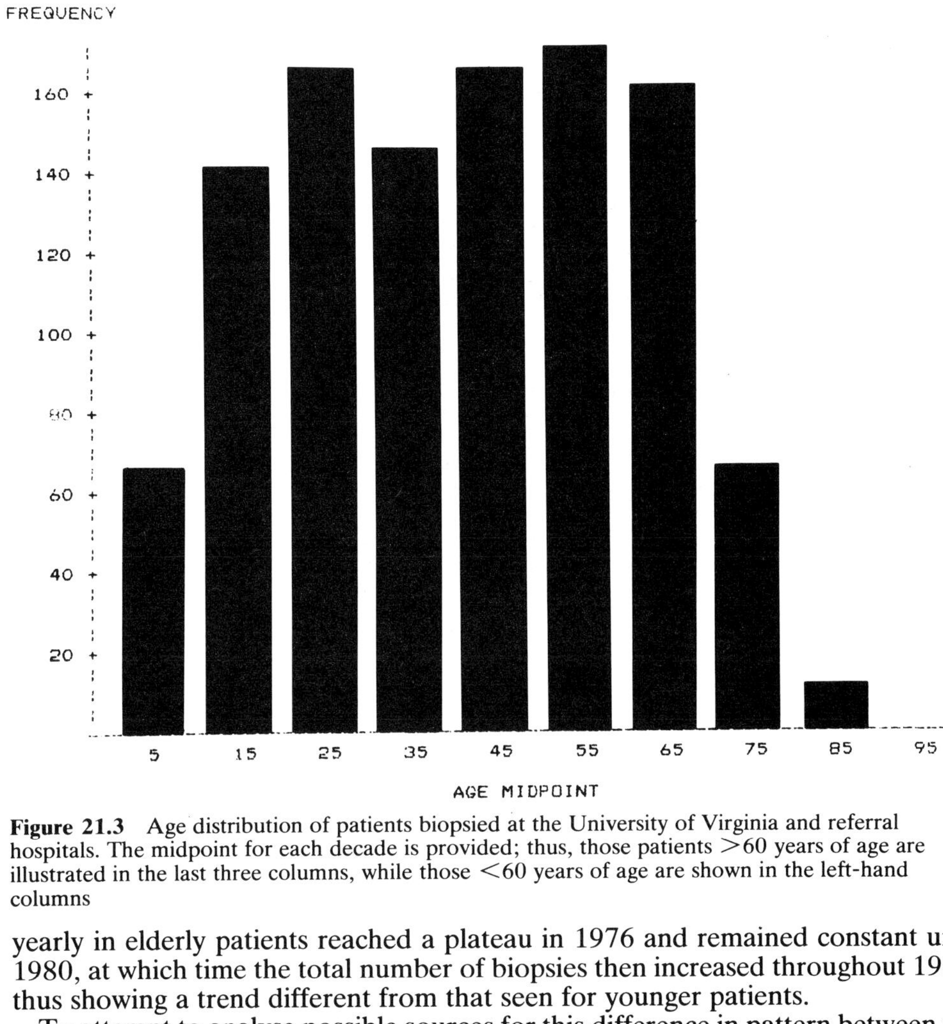

Figure 21.3 Age distribution of patients biopsied at the University of Virginia and referral hospitals. The midpoint for each decade is provided; thus, those patients >60 years of age are illustrated in the last three columns, while those <60 years of age are shown in the left-hand columns

yearly in elderly patients reached a plateau in 1976 and remained constant until 1980, at which time the total number of biopsies then increased throughout 1983, thus showing a trend different from that seen for younger patients.

To attempt to analyse possible sources for this difference in pattern between the younger and elderly groups, the number of biopsies performed by an open surgical procedure and percutaneous needle biopsy was examined in the two age groups (*Figures 21.5a* and *21.5b*). Other than the first two years on record, when open biopsies exceeded or were equal to percutaneous biopsies, the number of percutaneous needle biopsies in younger patients has been greater than open surgical biopsies at each time interval. Indeed, there is a decrease in proportion of open biopsies relative to percutaneous biopsies beginning in 1978 and continuing to the present time, when most tissue is obtained in this age group by a percutaneous approach. In the elderly group of patients (*Figure 21.5b*), tissue was obtained by the open surgical route with much greater relative frequency until 1981. However, in 1981 through to the present time the number of percutaneous needle biopsies greatly exceeded tissue obtained by the open surgical route in a distribution ratio not dissimilar to younger patients.

Thus, in the past several years the increased number of biopsies obtained in elderly

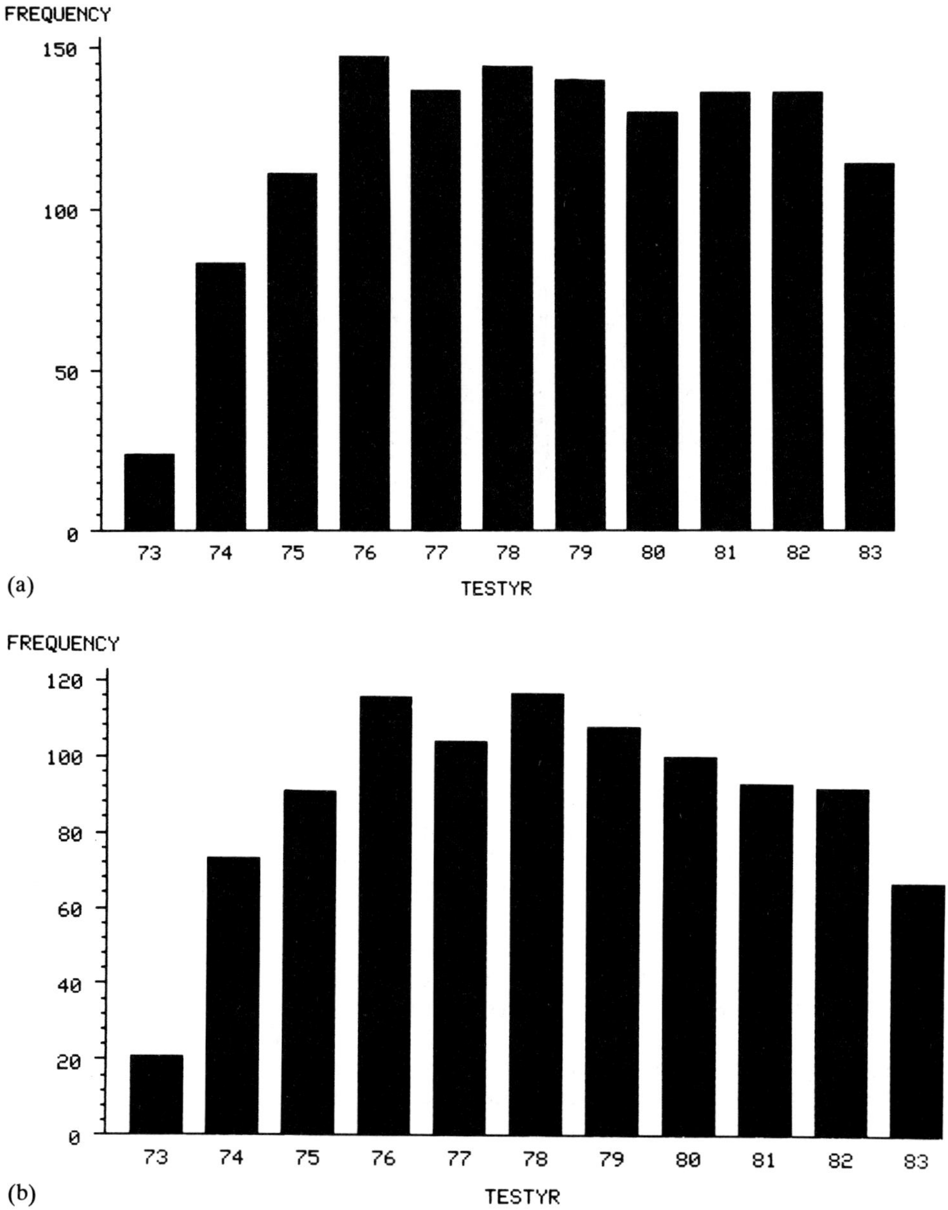

Figure 21.4 See caption opposite

patients has been attributable to increased use of percutaneous procurement of tissue. To examine whether this change in patterns of obtaining tissue might be related to the University of Virginia setting or from our referring physician, we investigated the pattern of referral biopsies and those obtained at the teaching institution (*Figure 21.6*). From 1974 onward the total number of biopsies obtained from our referring nephrologists has always exceeded those performed at the University of Virginia Hospital. This ratio was approximately 2:1 from 1976 to

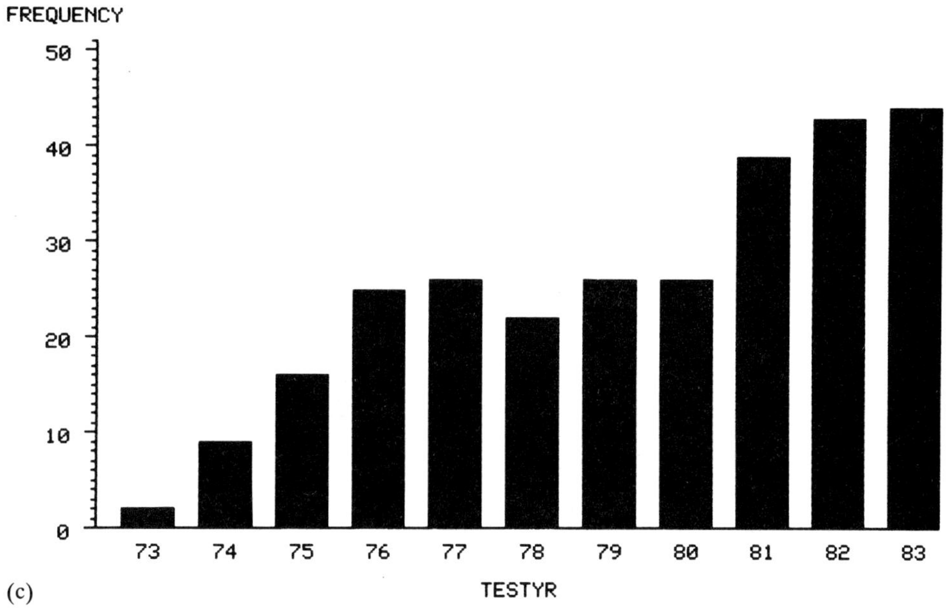

(c)

Figure 21.4 (a) Total number of biopsies performed by open surgical and percutaneous approach for the years 1973–83; (b) frequency of surgical and percutaneous biopsies obtained in patients <60 years of age for the time period of the study; (c) number of biopsies obtained in patients age 60 and over during the study period. An increasing number of elderly patients were biopsied in the last three years

1981. For 1981–83, a greater proportion of biopsies was performed in the University Hospital than in previous years. Information regarding the increased number of biopsies being performed in the elderly population was also examined by analysing the source of referral by year in elderly and younger patients. This information is provided in *Figures 21.6(b)* and *21.6(c)*. *Figure 21.6(a)* shows the increasing number of biopsies, with more biopsies referred from outside the University of Virginia than inside. However, for the last 3 years the differences for younger patients was slight, and thus approximately an equal number of patients were biopsied at the University's medical centre as outside. On the other hand (*Figure 21.6c*), there has been a rapid increase in the number of biopsies in the older population beginning in 1981, and this increase occurred both in the medical centre and referral biopsies.

Clinical diagnoses

We next examined the available data to ascertain the frequency of various clinical diagnoses in the two age groups of patients. These data are presented in *Table 21.2* which lists the most common clinical diagnoses in decreasing frequency (rank) for elderly patients. The table also provides the frequency of these diagnoses in the younger age population with their relative rank for that age group. There were 218 elderly patients who had both the pathologic and clinical diagnosis and there were 816 younger patients who fulfilled these two criteria. Nephrotic syndrome and/or proteinuria was the most frequent clinical diagnosis in both the elderly and younger

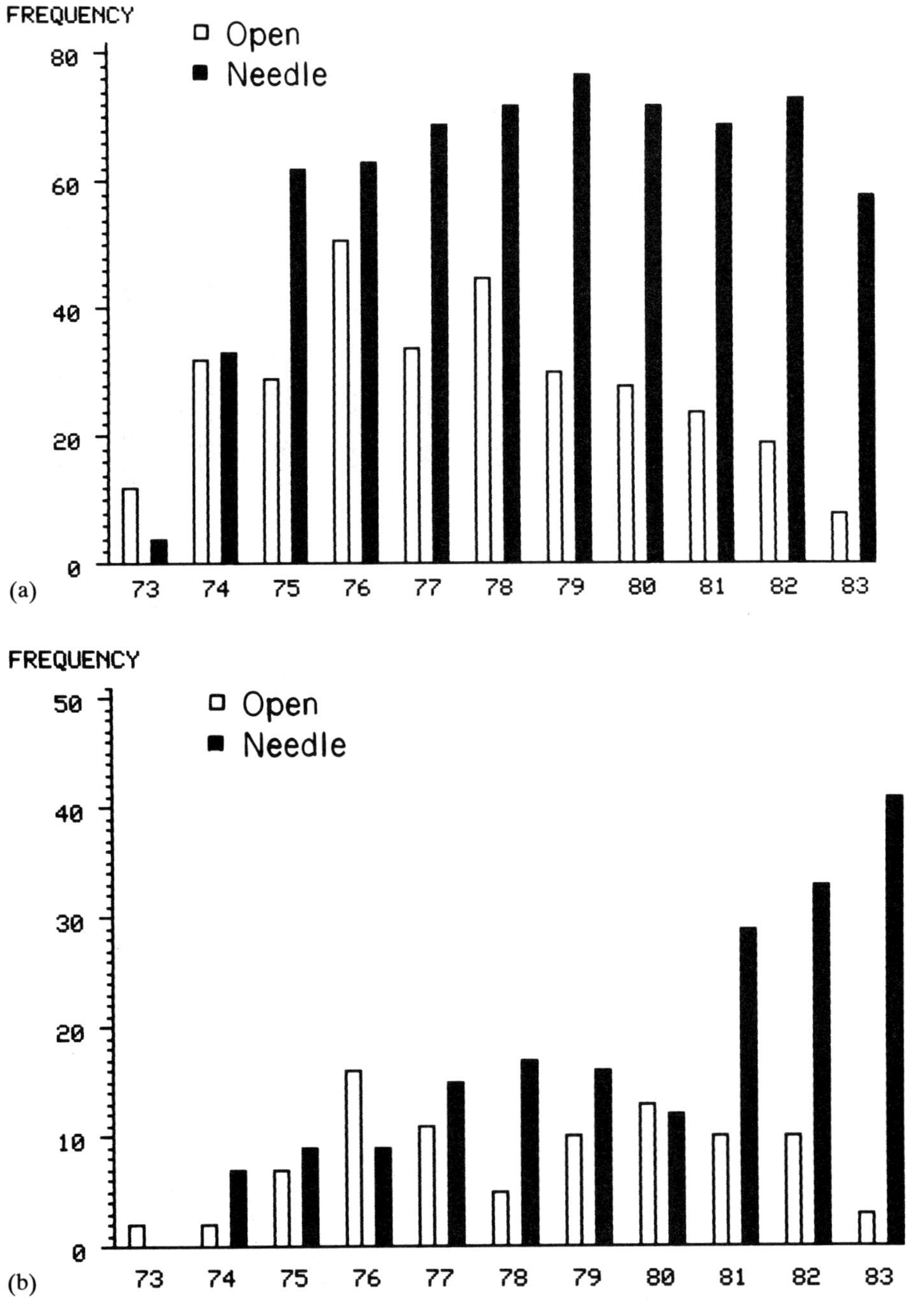

Figure 21.5 (a) Distribution of the type of renal biopsy obtained in patients <60 years of age. A decreasing number of surgical biopsies ('open') have been performed with a concomitant increase in the number of percutaneous ('needle') biopsies. (b) Type of renal biopsy performed on patients age 60 and over. The distribution ratio of open to needle biopsies had been approximately equal until the last three years, when a marked increase occurred in the number of needle biopsies obtained in this age group

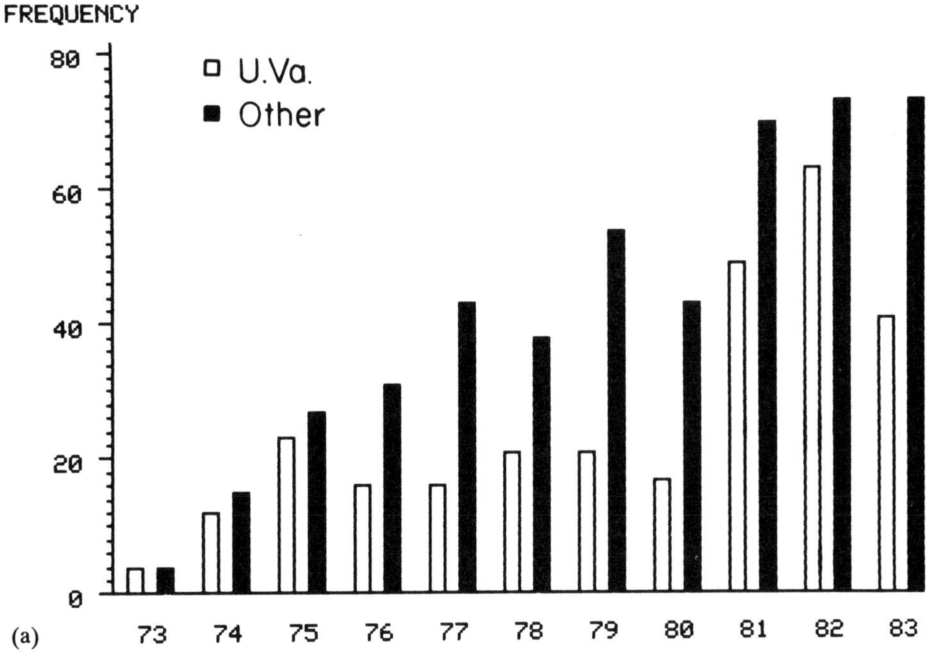

(a)

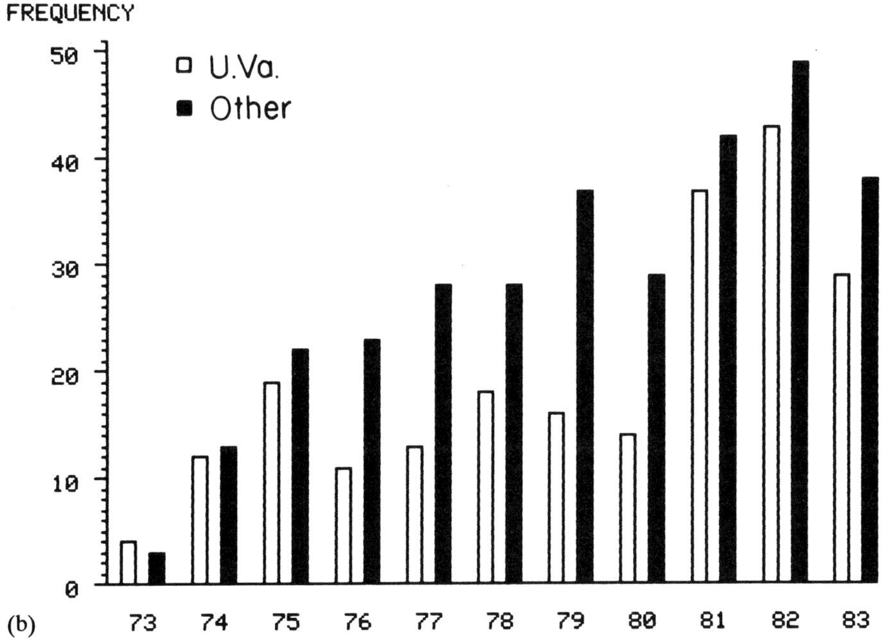

(b)

Figure 21.6 See caption on next page

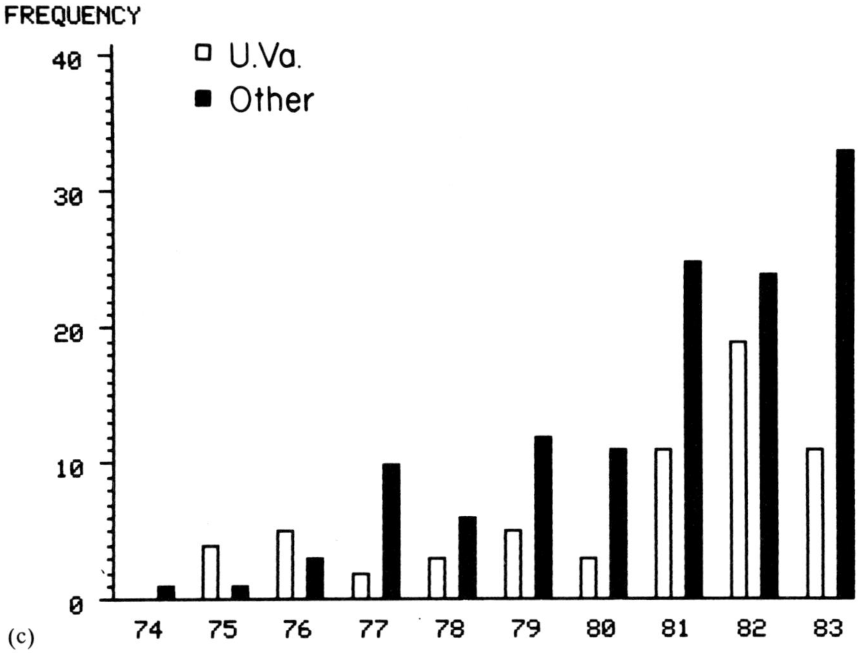

(c)

Figure 21.6 (a) Source of biopsies for all patients, illustrated by year, demonstrating a preponderance of both open and needle biopsies from referral nephrologists; (b) source of biopsies processed at the University of Virginia Hospital for patients under 60 years of age; (c) source of processed biopsies for patients age 60 and over — there has been a great increase in the number of biopsies performed in elderly patients in recent years, both in the University and referral settings, with a preponderance in the referral biopsies

population, accounting for approximately 30 per cent of cases. Acute renal failure was the second most common diagnosis and was approximately three times as frequent in the elderly as in the young patients. ESRD occurred with nearly equal frequency in the two age groups. Rapidly progressive glomerulonephritis was the fourth most common clinical diagnosis for the elderly compared with the ninth in the younger age group. Frequency of this diagnosis was about threefold greater in the elderly than in younger patients. Diabetes and acute glomerulonephritis occurred

Table 21.2 Clinical diagnoses in biopsied patients

Diagnosis	*≧60 yr old*	*≦ 60*	*Rank*
Number of patients	218	816	
1. Nephrotic syndrome, proteinuria	32.1%	31.4%	(1)
2. Acute renal failure	14.2	3.9	(7)
3. End-stage renal disease	13.3	11.4	(2)
4. Rapidly progressive glomerulonephritis	8.3	3.1	(9)
5. Acute glomerulonephritis	6.4	6.6	(5)
6. Diabetes mellitus	6.4	7.5	(3)
7. Vasculitis	3.7	2.6	(10)
8. Collagen vascular disease	2.8	1.7	(11)
9. Systemic lupus erythematosus	2.8	7.2	(4)
10. Hypertension	1.8	3.7	(8)
11. Haematuria	1.4	6.0	(6)

with approximately equal frequency in the two age groups, while vasculitis and non-lupus type collagen vascular diseases were slightly more common in elderly patients. Systemic lupus erythematosus and hypertension were twice as common in younger patients, and haematuria as an isolated finding was much more frequent in younger patients. A wide variety of other clinical diagnoses were present in the remaining patients, but those with a frequency of <1 per cent are not shown.

Pathologic diagnoses

Table 21.3 lists the pathologic diagnoses in biopsies in which tissue was adequate for interpretation. Once again, the diagnoses are listed in order of descending frequency for the elderly group of patients and the frequency and relative rank for the younger patients are provided in the last two columns. There were 244 patients in the older group and 875 in the younger group. Nephrosclerosis was the most frequent

Table 21.3 Pathologic diagnoses in biopsied patients

Diagnosis	*≧60 yr old*	*≦ 60*	*Rank*
Number of patients	244	875	
1. Nephrosclerosis	13.9%	10.7%	(1)
2. Membranous glomerulonephritis	11.9	7.5	(4)
3. Crescentic glomerulonephritis	11.1	4.1	(11)
4. Focal glomerular sclerosis	7.8	5.6	(9)
5. Amyloidosis	7.8	2.2	(14)
6. Diabetic nephropathy	7.8	8.1	(3)
7. Chronic glomerulonephritis	4.5	6.4	(7)
8. Acute glomerulonephritis	4.5	3.8	(12)
9. Focal glomerular obsolescence, tubular atrophy	4.5	5.5	(10)
10. Focal glomerulonephritis	4.1	6.7	(5)
11. Lipoid nephrosis	3.7	8.3	(2)
12. Interstitial nephritis	3.7	3.4	(13)
13. Membranoproliferative glomerulonephritis	2.9	6.3	(8)
14. Vasculitis	2.5	2.1	(15)
15. Systemic lupus erythematosus	2.0	6.6	(6)
16. Acute tubular necrosis	1.2	1.0	
Inadequate tissue	0.8	2.2	

diagnosis in the elderly as well as in the young, with approximately 14 per cent in the elderly and 11 per cent in young patients. Membranous nephropathy was the second most common diagnosis in the elderly, with 12 per cent compared to 7.5 per cent, and the fourth most common ranking for the younger patients. Crescentic glomerulonephritis was nearly three times as frequent in the elderly, with 11 per cent compared to 4 per cent in the young. Focal sclerosis was more frequently found in the elderly and amyloidosis was present in 8 per cent of older patients and only 2 per cent of those under the age of 60. Diabetic nephropathy was present in approximately the same percentage, and chronic glomerulonephritis, acute glomerulonephritis and focal glomerular obsolescence with tubular atrophy were all approximately of equal frequency. Focal nephritis was slightly more prevalent in younger patients and lipoid nephrosis was present in twice as great a frequency in the young patient as in the elderly. Membranoproliferative glomerulonephritis also was more common in the younger patient. Acute tubular necrosis was found in approximately 1 per cent of each of the two groups. Tissue inadequate for diagnosis was present in 0.8 per cent of elderly patients and in 2.2 per cent of younger patients. Lupus nephritis was three times as frequent in the younger population as in the older. Thus, in summary, in the older population membranous nephropathy, crescentic glomerulonephritis and amyloidosis were much more frequently present than in the younger age groups. On the other hand, younger patients were more likely to have lupus nephritis, membranoproliferative glomerulonephritis, lipoid nephrosis and focal glomerulonephritis.

Clinicopathologic correlations

Nephrotic syndrome and proteinuria

Seventy patients in the elderly group had nephrotic syndrome or proteinuria as the clinical diagnosis (*Table 21.2*). The corresponding pathologic diagnoses are listed in *Table 21.4*. Membranous nephropathy was the most common aetiology of abnormal proteinuria, with 30 per cent of the elderly population having this diagnosis. Amyloidosis accounted for 16 per cent of nephrotic patients with lipoid

Table 21.4 Nephrotic syndrome/proteinuria, patients aged ≧60

Diagnosis	*No. patients*	*Per cent*
Membranous nephropathy	21/70	30.0
Amyloidosis	11/70	15.7
Lipoid nephrosis	9/70	12.8
Focal glomerulosclerosis	7/70	10.0
Focal glomerular obsolescence and tubular atrophy	5/70	7.1
Diabetes	4/70	5.7
Membranoproliferative glomerulonephritis	4/70	5.7
Other	9/70	12.8

Total $n = 70$.

nephrosis in 13 per cent. Focal glomerulosclerosis was present in 10 per cent of this population and focal glomerular obsolescence with tubular atrophy was 7.1 per cent. The incidence of diabetes and membranoproliferative glomerulonephritis were each 5.7 per cent, while other aetiologies comprised the remaining 12.8 per cent. This obviously consists not only of primary glomerulopathies resulting in proteinuria, but secondary as well.

Acute renal failure

Acute renal failure (*Table 21.5*) was the second most common clinical diagnosis in the elderly group and consisted of 30 patients. A wide variety of histologic abnormalities were present including of noteworthy importance a 20 per cent incidence of crescentic glomerulonephritis. Membranous nephropathy and nephrosclerosis each accounted for 13 per cent of acute renal failure and focal glomerulosclerosis was present in 10 per cent of these patients. There was a wide variety of other aetiologies associated with acute renal failure, including atheromatous emboli, interstitial nephritis and coagulopathies. Interestingly, 18 of 30 or 60 per cent of patients with acute renal failure clinically had an associated glomerular lesion with proteinuria.

Table 21.5 Acute renal failure, patients aged ≥60

Diagnosis	*No. patients*	*Per cent*
Crescentic glomerulonephritis	6/30	20
Membranous nephropathy	4/30	13
Nephrosclerosis	4/30	13
Focal glomerulosclerosis	3/30	10
Other	13/30	43

Total $n = 30$.

End-stage renal disease

The third most common clinical diagnosis was ESRD and comprised 29 patients. Nephrosclerosis was present in 38 per cent of these patients with no other aetiologic findings on pathologic examination. Of importance relative to the clinical diagnosis of end-stage disease, 21 per cent of these patients did not have end-stage nephropathies but had potentially treatable lesions such as acute tubular necrosis, vasculitis, acute interstitial nephritis, focal glomerulonephritis and crescentic glomerulonephritis (see Chapters 15 and 16).

Rapidly progressive glomerulonephritis

The fourth most frequent clinical diagnosis in the elderly population was rapidly progressive glomerulonephritis. The accuracy of the clinician in diagnosing the histologic counterpart, i.e. crescentic nephritis, was greater than frequently seen with other syndromes and 10 of 17 or 59 per cent of these patients did indeed have crescentic glomerulonephritis. Other aetiologies associated with the clinical course of rapidly progressive glomerulonephritis were diabetes, glomerulonephritis, nephrosclerosis and chronic glomerulonephritis.

Diabetes mellitus

The fifth most frequent diagnosis was that of diabetes mellitus. Eleven of 14 (78.6 per cent) of these patients had diabetic glomerulosclerosis on biopsy. One additional patient had acute crescentic glomerulonephritis and 2 patients had sclerotic lesions without evidence of diabetes by light microscopic or ultrastructural analysis.

Acute glomerulonephritis

The next most frequent clinical diagnosis was acute glomerulonephritis. A variety of histologic diagnoses were present in this group of patients, including crescentic glomerulonephritis, interstitial nephritis, acute tubular necrosis, familial nephritis and, of course, acute glomerulonephritis. One patient had vasculitis associated with the clinical syndrome of glomerulonephritis. Vasculitis, the seventh most frequent clinical diagnosis, was the clinical diagnosis in 7 patients and was associated with crescentic glomerulonephritis in 3, focal nephritis in 1, and with overt vasculitis in only 2 patients (see Chapter 16). Additional individual analysis of the various categories will not be elaborated, except to note that the correlation between the clinical diagnosis and the pathologic diagnosis was imprecise at best.

Comparison of clinical with pathologic diagnoses

Although many of the pathologic diagnoses would be compatible with the clinical diagnosis, i.e. membranous nephropathy, diabetes, amyloidosis and lipoid nephrosis all being consistent with the clinical diagnosis of nephrotic syndrome, comparison of the exact clinical diagnosis to the exact pathologic diagnosis revealed marked disparities. If we allowed the clinician only one clinical diagnosis, only 12 of 244 patients had an exact match between clinical and pathologic diagnoses. However, since our referring physicians might not list all clinical diagnoses in their order of importance, we reanalysed the data allowing three clinical diagnoses; in other words, correct diagnosis with any of the three pathological diagnoses compared with any and all of the three clinical diagnoses. Use of this approach resulted in a dramatic change in the proportion of misdiagnoses. Only 23 of 244 patients had a total mismatch. Analysis of these cases indicated that they were indeed valid mismatches. Twelve of 242 or 5 per cent of clinical diagnoses matched with the first pathology diagnosis in elderly patients. Of younger patients, 84 or 10 per cent correlated with the exact pathologic diagnosis. When a match between any of the three pathology diagnoses and any of the three clinical diagnoses is considered a match in the elderly, 221 of 242 or 91.3 per cent of the biopsies correlated clinically with the histologic lesion. In the younger age groups, 839 of 875 or 95.9 per cent of the clinical and pathologic diagnoses correlated.

It is necessary to analyse the data relative to the maximum three specific clinical or pathologic diagnoses each inasmuch as some physicians might place the priority of their diagnosis in the correct order, others may not, and part of the secondary or tertiary diagnoses in either pathological or clinical categories might pertain to the actual 'true' diagnosis. For instance, a patient with diabetes, hypertension and nephrotic syndrome might well have diabetic glomerulosclerosis with nephrosclerosis and this would be a mismatch according to the computer if the pathology diagnoses were listed as diabetic sclerosis first with hypertension as the first clinical diagnosis. The true match would obviously be picked up using the combination of all three clinical and all three pathologic diagnoses. Therefore, in an attempt to characterize in a more valid fashion the association between the pathologic and clinical diagnoses, computer lists of pathologic and clinical mismatches were evaluated individually within each of the major pathologic diagnostic categories to ascertain if a mismatch was truly present or not.

For nephrosclerosis, a variety of different clinical aetiologies were present consistent with the pathologic diagnosis such as ESRD and hypertension, but other diagnoses made clinically were not present, such as multiple myeloma and crescentic glomerulonephritis. Using the broadest of inclusive acceptable clinical diagnoses, there was a 15 per cent mismatch for nephrosclerosis. In consideration of those patients with membranous nephropathy, most had nephrotic syndrome and proteinuria, but 25 per cent had a clinical diagnosis other than membranous nephropathy, such as lymphoma, glomerulonephritis, acute renal failure. In patients with crescentic glomerulonephritis, 22 per cent presented with a clinical diagnosis of acute renal failure of unknown aetiology and 11 per cent of others had the clinical diagnosis of end-stage disease, diabetes, etc. Focal glomerulosclerosis most frequently presented as nephrotic syndrome, but also presented as acute renal failure in 16 per cent of patients. Diabetes was correctly diagnosed as either nephrotic syndrome or diabetes in most patients, although 10 per cent had rapidly progressive glomerulonephritis or drug reactions. Amyloidosis was diagnosed as nephrotic syndome most frequently, but also presented as acute renal failure, ESRD and acute glomerulonephritis in 28 per cent of patients. Thus, using only the most frequent pathologic diagnoses and generous criteria for acceptance of a match between the pathologic and the clinical diagnosis, there was nevertheless a 15–33 per cent mismatch.

It seems appropriate to concentrate on pathologic diagnoses in the elderly which would normally progress to ESRD and dialysis if not diagnosed and appropriately treated. This is obvious in several areas. For instance, of 27 patients with the pathologic diagnosis of crescentic nephritis, 3 had the clinical diagnosis of end-stage disease or diabetes and might not have been biopsied. None of the 9 patients with interstitial nephritis carried that clinical diagnosis and might have progressed to end-stage disease otherwise.

Of 29 patients with ESRD, 6 or 21 per cent potentially treatable pathologic diagnoses were found including 2 with crescentic glomerulonephritis, 1 with vasculitis, 1 with interstitial nephritis, 1 with acute glomerulonephritis and 1 with acute tubular necrosis. Of 14 patients with the clinical diagnosis of diabetes, crescentic glomerulopathy was found in 1. Thus, if three clinical diagnoses were allowed, a high degree of accuracy in predicting histology was present. If less than three diagnoses were allowed, there was much less chance of accuracy. Reliance on clinical acumen to make a diagnosis would therefore have resulted in 'missing' a significant number of potentially treatable diseases correctly diagnosed by biopsy.

Analysis of patients progressing to ESRD resulting in dialysis or transplantation

In order to gain information about the outcome of elderly patients upon whom biopsy information was available, all of the records of the Transplantation and Dialysis Committee meetings were examined to obtain the names of patients presented who had progressed to ESRD. These data were then entered into the computer so that patients in our geographic region who had progressed to ESRD and who also had had renal biopsies could be accessed. After this subset of patients had been identified, the histopathologic diagnoses were ascertained using the combined pathology categories described in *Table 21.1*

Information regarding histologic diagnosis in patients accepted for dialysis and transplantation was available in 279 younger individuals and 87 elderly persons. The frequency of diagnoses are listed in descending order in *Table 21.6*. In the elderly population, nephrosclerosis accounted for 37 per cent of end-stage disease.

Table 21.6 Aetiology of end-stage renal disease in patients supported with dialysis/transplantation

Diagnosis	*≧60 yr old* (*n* = 87)	*≦60 and rank* (*n* = 279)	
1. Nephrosclerosis	36.8%	30.8%	(1)
2. Diabetes	25.3	11.8	(3)
3. Crescentic glomerulonephritis	12.6	6.8	(5)
4. Amyloidosis	6.9	1.1	(14)
5. Focal glomerular obsolescence with tubular atrophy	4.6	0.0	
6. Chronic glomerulonephritis	3.4	17.6	(2)
7. Membranous glomerulopathy	3.4	2.2	(9)
8. Other	7.0	29.7	

It likewise accounted for 31 per cent in younger patients and was also the most frequent cause of end-stage disease. Diabetes was the second most common diagnosis in the elderly group, with 25 per cent having this diagnosis, more than twice as frequent as younger patients. The age-related disparity between the histologic diagnosis associated with end-stage disease became much greater thereafter. Crescentic glomerulonephritis was the third most common cause of ESRD in the elderly patient, twice as frequent as in the younger. The fourth most common cause was amyloidosis, which was six times more frequent in the elderly population. Membranous glomerulopathy was present with approximately equal frequency in the two populations, while chronic glomerulonephritis was 5 times more frequent in the younger population than in the elderly. There were no patients in the younger population with the diagnosis of focal glomerular obsolescence and tubular atrophy alone in association with end-stage renal disease. Other diagnoses not found in the elderly which led to end-stage disease in younger patients included membranoproliferative glomerulonephritis, nephritis of lupus erythematosus, focal glomerular sclerosis and acute interstitial nephritis. These diagnoses together accounted for 18 per cent of cases of end-stage disease in the younger population, not present in the elderly.

Discussion

The present survey suggests that attitudes toward renal disease in the elderly are changing. An increasing number of elderly patients are undergoing biopsy, both in the University of Virginia and in our referral area, and procurement of tissue in both situations is more frequently by percutaneous approach than open surgical biopsy. Analysis of the patterns of referral and the types of biopsy suggest that there is an increasing overall awareness of the potential for treating renal disease in the elderly, both in the referral and the University sectors. This logically results in a decreased threshold for renal biopsy to evaluate the presence of renal disease in this age population. The present study has also demonstrated that the spectrum of clinical and pathologic diseases in the elderly is different from that in younger individuals, and as many as one-third of the pathologic lesions are incorrectly diagnosed clinically. Even more important was the observation that more than 20 per cent of patients designated as ESRD had a potentially treatable lesion when the biopsy was actually performed.

The increased awareness by the nephrologist of these facts clearly indicates an increasingly aggressive attitude toward diagnosing and treating renal disease in the elderly population. In those cases where ESRD was indeed present in the renal biopsy, the spectrum of disease in the young and elderly was quite different. As one might anticipate, this reflected the role of secondary renal disease possibly made by the passage of time and by renal disease that one might anticipate would occur from natural process of aging, i.e. changes in the humoral/cellular immune systems (Bolton, 1984b). Our study also provides information about the actual lesion that is present producing the ESRD, data not previously available. *Table 21.7* compares the aetiologies of ESRD in the elderly as found in our study, with the series available in the literature (Ghantous *et al.*, 1971; Bailey *et al.*, 1972; Kjellstrand *et al.*, 1976; Mallinson *et al.*, 1984; Department of Health and Human Services, 1984) (see also Chapter 22).

Several differences are apparent. First, since our study consisted only of biopsied patients, 'polycystic kidney disease' was not included as an aetiology, since the

Table 21.7 Reported aetiologies of ESRD in the elderly

	*Present series**	*Bailey* et al. *(1972)*	*Mallinson* et al. *(1984)*	*Chester* et al. *(1979)*	*Ghantous* et al. *(1971)*	*Kjellstrand* et al. *(1976)*	*Dept. of Health and Human Services (1984)*
No. of patients	87	100	93	45	60	69	19 748
Age of patients	≧60	>50	>50	>70	>50	>50	>60
Diagnosis							
Nephrosclerosis	37%	3%	3%	13%	10%	14%	22%
Diabetes	25	2	6	19	—	6	12
Chronic glomerulonephritis	16	59	17*	9	46	36	15
Amyloidosis	7	1	3	—	2	2	—
Chronic interstitial nephritis†	<1	8	12	29	12	19	—
Polycystic kidney disease	ND	21	—	7	25	19	6
Other‡	15	6	59	23	5	4	45

*Biopsy proven; ND, not done.
†Includes atrophic pyelonephritis, chronic pyelonephritis, analgesic nephropathy.
‡Includes myeloma, unknown, vasculitis, obstruction, Alport's, carcinoma, gouty nephropathy, tuberculosis, 'small kidneys'.

diagnosis of polycystic kidney disease is generally made on clinical and radiologic grounds, rarely by biopsy. This does not detract from our data, since well over 90 per cent of patients with polycystic kidney disease will have been diagnosed by the sixth decade of life (see Chapter 17); therefore, the incidence should not increase in a progressively more elderly population. Secondly, our study reveals that secondary renal diseases account for the majority of ESRD in the elderly population; 65 per cent of elderly patients in our study had ESRD consequent to diabetes or hypertension. All of the other studies demonstrated <50 per cent of their ESRD patients to be accounted for by diabetes or hypertension. This discrepancy can be explained by the fact that the diagnoses in the series listed in *Table 21.7* were for the most part made on clinical grounds, and were not biopsy proven. Thus, many small end-stage kidneys were called 'chronic glomerulonephritis', 'chronic interstitial nephritis' or 'other', without a biopsy. As discussed earlier, our results have demonstrated the poor correlation between clinical and pathologic diagnoses in the elderly population. We therefore believe our results to depict more accurately the incidence of various aetiologies of ESRD in the elderly population, since our study was based on tissue diagnosis.

Evaluation of the elderly patient

The diagnosis and documentation of the aetiology of ESRD in the elderly should be as thorough as in any age group. However, there are certain points which need to be emphasized in the elderly that are not necessary in the younger population. A careful history should be taken in regards to exposure to toxic substances, especially antibiotics, non-steroidal anti-inflammatory agents (see Chapters 14 and 20), anti-hypertensive medications, sedatives, etc. The elderly are frequently taking a variety of diuretics, mood-altering drugs and other pharmacologic agents. The decreased filtering ability, glomerular alterations, attenuated blood supply, change in immune responsiveness, and other factors dealt with elsewhere and in this text, clearly make the elderly patient at greater risk than the younger patient to the potential side effects of various toxic substances (Davies and Shock, 1950; Wesson, 1969; Friedman *et al.*, 1972; Takazakura *et al.*, 1972; Darmady, Offer and Woodhouse, 1973; Papper, 1973; Hollenberg *et al.*, 1974; Kaplan *et al.*, 1975; Griffiths *et al.*, 1976; Rowe *et al.*, 1976; McLachlan *et al.*, 1977; Bolton, 1984a). Thus, acute allergic interstitial nephritis and nephropathy related to non-steroidal agents, as well as other iatrogenic causes, should be carefully sought. Pre-renal causes of decreased function in the elderly should also be carefully examined. Apparent 'chronic renal failure' may actually be on the basis of a cardiovascular origin. We are very thorough in examining the patient for possible malignancy. The risk of malignancy is greatly increased in the elderly and may be associated with various types of glomerulopathies. Solid malignancies, as well as cryoglobulinaemia, macroglobulinaemia, other monoclonal gammopathies and light chain disease should also be sought. Collagen vascular disease should be considered with tests for anti-nuclear factor, rheumatoid factor, anti-DNA, immune complexes and serum complement. Although systemic lupus erythematosus *per se* is less common in the elderly than in the young, nevertheless, a variety of auto-immune diseases do indeed increase with age and may present in an atypical way in the elderly.

Routine laboratory examination thus should include chest roentgenogram, examination of the kidneys by ultrasonography to determine that obstruction is not present (see Chapter 19), to determine the size and echogenicity of the kidneys, and to determine if a mass or cyst is present (Chapter 17). Routine biochemical studies should be obtained as well as those noted above. One of the most valuable tests, although quite non-specific, is the erythrocyte sedimentation rate. While this may be elevated to some degree in many elderly, a marked elevation in patients with a normal serum albumin could be a clue that an underlying inflammatory process is present and further emphasize the need for diagnostic approaches.

Renal biopsy in elderly patients

Table 21.8 presents our indications for renal biopsy in the elderly patient. We have used quotes around ESRD, since it is apparent from our study and from the literature that patients who appear to have end-stage disease may not necessarily have it. The items in *Table 21.8* obviously need to be considered relative to the actual clinical presentation of the patient. If a patient has nephrotic syndrome and

Table 21.8 Indications for renal biopsy in the elderly patient

1. Proteinuria, nephrotic syndrome
2. Acute renal failure without clear aetiology
3. Rapidly decreasing renal function
4. Active urinary sediment with decreased function
5. Apparent chronic renal disease with an accelerated phase
6. Diabetic patient with atypical presentation
7. Atypical chronic renal failure — 'end-stage renal disease'

proteinuria >700 mg/24 h, an aetiology should be sought as it may be potentially treatable. A large number of possible aetiologies fall into this category, as described in our results section, and the diagnosis of nephrotic syndrome and proteinuria has previously been dealt with in detail (Bolton, 1984b). If the elderly patient does not have small shrunken kidneys and does not have a clearly defined known aetiology for heavy proteinuria and nephrotic syndrome, i.e. amyloidosis or typical diabetes, then a renal biopsy is indicated. A number of these patients will have lipoid nephrosis which responds well to therapy, some will have membranous nephropathy, which may also respond favourably to steroid therapy, and others will clearly have aetiologies which should not be treated.

Acute renal failure without clear aetiology is also an indication for biopsy. In the hospital setting, elderly patients not infrequently have acute renal failure secondary to hypotension, toxic drugs, etc., but those with proteinuria appear to be at much greater risk of developing acute renal failure. As shown in the present study, acute renal failure on presentation results from a variety of histologic subtypes which may have treatable aetiologies. We also consider that rapidly decreasing renal function is an indication for biopsy. This is obviously a factor which relies upon the judgement of the primary physican. External causes, such as non-steroidal anti-inflammatory agents and drugs associated with allergic interstitial nephritis, should be sought and corrected prior to obtaining a biopsy. The biopsy should be procured if none of these factors is present and if the renal function continues to deteriorate. Urinary sediment as well as laboratory data on the patient should be carefully examined, as decreasing renal function with an active sediment is a clear indication for renal biopsy.

Crescentic glomerulonephritis is much more common in the elderly population, with or without vasculitis, both in our series and others (Moorthy and Zimmerman, 1980), and it may progress to ESRD in a period of weeks if untreated. We have had very good success in the treatment of this cause of decreased function in the elderly patient and are very aggressive in diagnosing its process in the elderly patient with an active sediment and decreasing function (Bolton and Couser, 1979; Bolton, 1984a, 1984b, 1984c). We also obtain biopsies on those patients who appear to have chronic renal disease but who have a precipitous change in their reciprocal serum creatinine curves without apparent cause. This may occur because of a superimposed acute process on the original underlying disease, such as acute interstitial nephritis or crescentic nephritis. It should be noted that those patients in our present series with acute interstitial nephritis were not diagnosed clinically.

The diabetic patient, even with long-standing diabetes, who has an atypical presentation should receive confirmation of the diagnosis to be certain to rule out treatable aetiologies. Atypical findings in the diabetic include duration of disease of <10 years, the concomitant presence of another disease known to cause renal disease such as vasculitis, an active urinary sediment with red cell casts, hypocomplementaemia, the presence of serologic parameters of collagen vascular disease such as a positive anti-nuclear factor and rheumatoid factor, the absence of retinopathy and neuropathy (J.L. Glickman, W.K. Bolton and B.C. Sturgill, 1984, personal communication).

Lastly, but importantly, patients with apparent chronic renal failure which is atypical in its presentation, manifestations or course should be biopsied. This category depends in large degree upon the attending physician and may include chronic renal failure with enlarged kidneys, chronic renal failure with kidneys that are non-echo dense, selective proteinuria or the presence of a gammopathy and exposure to toxic substances. It should be remembered that in the patient with proteinuria and nephrotic syndrome, the results of the biopsy will play a role in determining the likelihood of various types of associated malignancy. We routinely look closely for lymphoma in those elderly patients with lipoid nephrosis and for adenocarcinoma in those patients with membranous nephropathy, but in practice in most patients with malignancy-associated membranous nephropathy the tumour is obvious and appears simultaneously with the nephrotic syndrome. The diagnosis of an underlying malignancy in a patient presenting with proteinuria or nephrotic syndrome and consequent resection of the malignancy with cure of the patient is certainly a classic example of preventive medicine. It is also our philosophy that the patient should not receive a biopsy if the findings are going to have no bearing on the subsequent therapy.

One should consider that, in the elderly patient, the type of underlying disease responsible for decreased renal function and end-stage nephropathy is somewhat different from that seen in the younger population, and may not present with many of the physical findings and symptoms of the younger patient. The elderly patient needs to be approached not only with thoroughness provided for the younger patient, but also with an eye to the differences in the types of disease, their presentation, and the fact that therapy can be successful in preventing the development of ESRD in many patients.

Treatment

Little information is available about the therapy of chronic renal disease in the elderly. Current knowledge of treatment of various types of renal disease in the aged is carefully and thoroughly dealt with in other chapters of this text. Our own experience in treatment of elderly patients with renal disease suggests that many patients, if appropriately diagnosed and treated, will have a favourable response to therapy and be maintained or show an improvement such that they will not progress to end-stage disease and require dialysis (Bolton, 1984, 1986).

The approach to the patient with apparent ESRD or decreasing function which appears to be progressing to ESRD should be individualized. The attending physician and the patient should carefully consider the risk of diagnosis for the purpose of intervention compared with the benefits of the studies required. It is clearly established that dialysis in the elderly population is associated with a higher mortality rate relative to younger individuals (see Chapter 22) and should be considered in deciding whether or not to be aggressive in diagnosing an underlying and potentially treatable process. It is the philosophy at our institution aggressively to seek out any potentially treatable aetiology for functional abnormality in the aged. It is our feeling that patients should not be discriminated against on the basis of their age, and that satisfactory results of treatment can be obtained in the elderly as well as in the young.

Acknowledgements

The authors appreciate the excellent technical assistance of R. Berry and secretarial expertise of B. Rogers. This work was supported in part by USPHS Grant AM 32530 from the NIADDKD and Clinical Research Center Grant RR 00847.

References

BAILEY, G.L., MORELIN, A.J., GRIFFITH, H.J.L., ZSCHAECK, D., GHANTOUS, W.N., HAMPERS, C.L. *et al.* (1972). Hemodialysis and renal transplantation in patients of the 50–80 age group. *Journal of the American Geriatric Society,* **20,** 421–429

BOLTON, W.K. (1984). The role of high dose steroids in nephritic syndromes: the case for aggressive use. In *Controversies in Nephrology and Hypertension,* edited by R.G. Narins, pp. 421–459. New York; Churchill Livingstone

BOLTON, W.K. (1986). Nephrotic syndrome in the aged. In *The Nephrotic Syndrome,* edited by R.G. Glassock and J.S. Cameron. New York; Dekker (in press)

BOLTON, W.K. (1984c). Treatment of glomerular diseases: pulse methylprednisolone in primary and multisystemic diseases. In *Nephrology,* edited by R.R. Robinson, pp. 1464–1473. New York; Springer

BOLTON, W.K., BENTON, F.R., MACLAY, J.G. and STURGILL, B.C. (1976). Spontaneous glomerular sclerosis in aging Sprague–Dawley rats. I. Lesions associated with mesangial IgM deposits. *American Journal of Pathology,* **85,** 277–302

BOLTON, W.K. and COUSER, W.G. (1979). Intravenous pulse methylprednisolone therapy of acute crescentic rapidly progressive glomerulonephritis. *American Journal of Medicine,* **66,** 495–502

BOLTON, W.K. and MESNARD, R.M. (1982). New technique of kidney tissue processing for immunofluorescence microscopy: formol sucrose/gum sucrose/paraffin (FSGSP). *Laboratory Investigation,* **47,** 206–213

BOLTON, W.K. and STURGILL, B.C. (1980). Spontaneous glomerular sclerosis in aging Sprague–Dawley rats. II. Ultrastructural studies. *American Journal of Pathology,* **98,** 339–350

BOLTON, W.K. and STURGILL, B.C. (1981). Ultrastructure of the aging kidney. In *Aging and Cell Structure,* edited by J.E. Johnson, Jr., pp. 215–250. New York; Plenum

CHESTER, A.C., RAKOWSKI, T.A., ARGY, W.P., GIACALONE, A. and SCHREINER, G.E. (1979). Hemodialysis in the eighth and ninth decades of life. *Archives of Internal Medicine,* **139,** 1001–1005

DARMADY, E.M., OFFER, J. and WOODHOUSE, M.A. (1973). The parameters of the aging kidney. *Journal of Pathology,* **109,** 195–213

DAVIES, D.F. and SHOCK, N.W. (1950). Age changes in glomerular filtration rate, effective renal plasma flow, and tubular excretory capacity in adult males. *Journal of Clinical Investigation,* **29,** 496–507

DEPARTMENT OF HEALTH AND HUMAN SERVICES, HEALTH CARE FINANCING ADMINISTRATION, BUREAU OF DATA MANAGEMENT AND STRATEGY (1984). *End-stage Renal Disease Patient Profile Tables, 1982.* U.S. Government Printing Office, p. 7

FRIEDMAN, S.A., RAIZNER, A.E., ROSEN, H., SOLOMON, N.A. and SY, W. (1972). Functional defects in the aging kidney. *Annals of Internal Medicine,* **76,** 41–45

GHANTOUS, W.N., BAILEY, G.L., ZSCHAECK, D., HAMPERS, C.L. and MERRILL, J.P. (1971). Long term hemodialysis in the elderly. *Transactions of the American Society of Artificial Internal Organs,* **17,** 125–128

GRIFFITHS, G.J., ROBINSON, K.B., CARTWRIGHT, G.O. and McLACHLAN, J.S.F. (1976). Loss of renal tissue in the elderly. *British Journal of Radiology,* **49,** 111–117

HOLLENBERG, N.K., ADAMS, D.F., SOLOMON, H.S., RASHID, A., ABRAMS, H.L. and MERRILL, J.P. (1974). Senescence and the renal vasculature in normal man. *Circulation Research,* **34,** 309–316

KAPLAN, C., PASTERNACK, B., SHAH, H. and GALLO, G. (1975). Age-related incidence of sclerotic glomeruli in human kidneys. *American Journal of Pathology,* **80,** 227–234

KJELLSTRAND, C.M., SHIDEMAN, J.R., LYNCH, R.E., BUSELMEIER, T.J., SIMMONS, R.L. and NAJARIAN, J.S. (1976). Kidney transplants in patients over 50. *Geriatrics,* **31,** 65–73

MALLINSON, W.J.W., FLEMING, S.J., SHAW, J.E.H., BAKER, L.R. and CATTELL, W.R. (1984). Survival in elderly patients presenting with uraemia. *Quarterly Journal of Medicine,* **53,** 301–307

McLACHLAN, M.S.R., GUTHRIE, J.C., ANDERSON, C.K. and FULKER, M.J. (1977). Vascular and glomerular changes in the aging kidney. *Journal of Pathology,* **121,** 65–78

MOORTHY, A.V. and ZIMMERMAN, S.W. (1980). Renal disease in the elderly: clinicopathologic analysis of renal disease in 115 elderly patients. *Clinical Nephrology,* **14,** 223–229

PAPPER, S. (1973). The effects of age in reducing renal function. *Geriatrics,* **28,** 83–87

ROWE, J.W., ANDRES, R., TOBIN, J.D., NORRIS, A.H. and SHOCK, N.W. (1976). The effect of age on creatinine clearance in man: a cross-sectional and longitudinal study. *Journal of Gerontology,* **31,** 155–163

SAMIY, A.H. (1983). Renal disease in the elderly. *Medical Clinics of North America,* **67,** 463–480

TAKAZAKURA, E., SAWABU, N., HANDA, A., TAKADA, A., SHINODA, A. and TAKEUCHI, J. (1972). Intrarenal vascular changes with age and disease. *Kidney International,* **2,** 224

TAUBE, D.H., WINDER, E.A., OGG, C.S., BEWICK, M., CAMERON, J.S., RUDGE, C.J. *et al.* (1983). Successful treatment of middle aged and elderly patients with end stage renal disease. *British Medical Journal,* **286,** 2018–2020

WALKER, P.J., GINN, H.E., JOHNSON, H.K., STONE, W.J., TESCHAN, P.E., LATOS, D. *et al.* (1976). Long-term hemodialysis for patients over 50. *Geriatrics,* **31,** 55–61

WESSON, L.G. Jr. (1969). Renal hemodynamics in physiological states. In *Physiology of the Human Kidney,* pp. 96–108. New York; Grune and Stratton

Chapter 22

Dialysis treatment of end-stage renal disease in the elderly

Claudio Ponticelli, Giorgio Graziani, Alberto Cantaluppi and Richard Moore*

Introduction

Until a few years ago many uraemic patients were excluded from maintenance dialysis programmes. Due to the scarcity of resources, replacement therapy was reserved for patients under 50 years, who were considered more able to continue their professional activity and less prone to serious complications than older people. More recently, however, increasing facilities and experience has allowed the extension of regular dialysis treatment, and several reports have shown the benign course and the satisfying rehabilitation in chronic dialysis patients older than 50 (Figueroa, 1968; Cohen, Comty and Shapiro, 1970; Ghantous *et al.*, 1971; Da Porto *et al.*, 1975; Alloatti *et al.*, 1976; Garini *et al.*, 1976; Walker *et al.*, 1976; Taube *et al.*, 1983; Mallinson *et al.*, 1984).

Thus, today, with the relevant exception of Britain (Berlyne 1982), in the Western world an age of over 50 is no longer a leading consideration in selecting patients for maintenance dialysis. More controversy exists about the indications for chronic dialysis in the elderly over the age of 65. The problem is of considerable size. About 11 per cent of the total population in Western countries are older than 65 (Summer, 1979), and elderly patients are particularly liable to terminal renal failure (Rostand *et al.*, 1982) (see the Preface to this volume). In countries with no limit to available facilities, such as the USA and Japan, there is now a tendency to offer dialysis to all-comers, independently of their age or their expected quality of life. But in countries with restricted facilities, age is still considered either as an absolute indication of non-acceptability or as a criterion for selection (Mathew, D'Apice and Kincaid-Smith, 1983).

According to the Registry of the European Dialysis and Transplant Association, on 31 December, 1983, 7428 patients older than 65 at the start of treatment were alive on renal replacement therapy in Europe. Their current mean age was 72.6 years, they comprised 8.7 per cent of all registry patients and amounted to 12.8 patients per million population. The number of elderly patients alive on replacement therapy was quite different in the various European countries (*Figure 22.1*), reflecting great differences in the resources allocated to the treatment of end-stage renal failure in the elderly by different governments. Comparing the different types of replacement therapies between patients older than 65 and the whole uraemic population in Europe, it appears that only a negligible minority of elderly patients receive a renal transplant (see Chapter 23) or can tackle home haemodialysis. Most older patients are treated by hospital haemodialysis; however, peritoneal dialysis is more often used in older than in younger patients (*Figure 22.2*).

*On behalf of the EDTA–European Renal Association Registry.

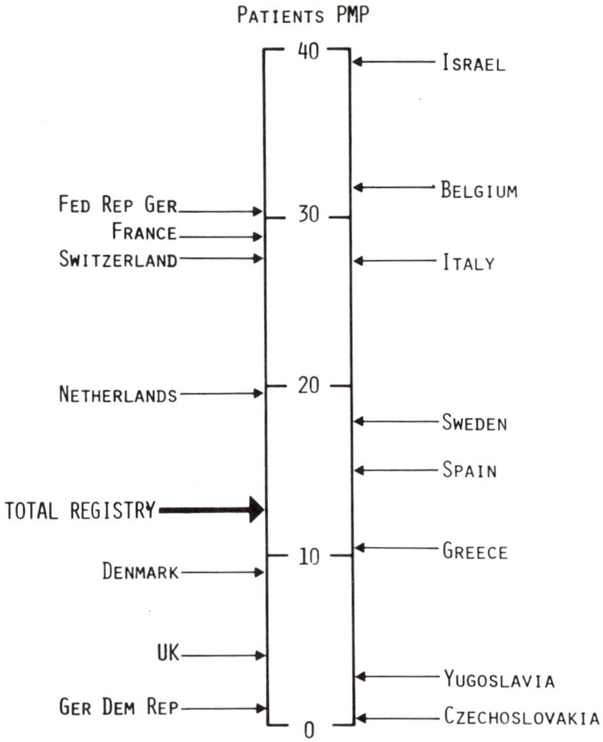

Figure 22.1 Number of patients older than 65 years, per million population, alive on renal replacement therapy in various European countries on 31 December, 1983

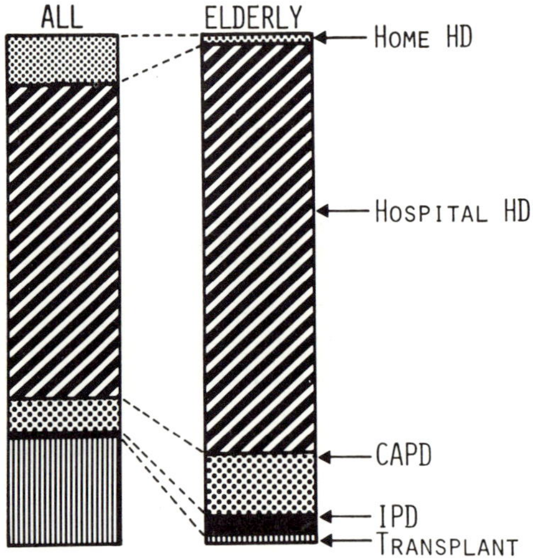

Figure 22.2 Proportion of patients alive on 31 December, 1983 according to different modes of therapy. Patients older than 65 years are compared with all patients on the European Registry

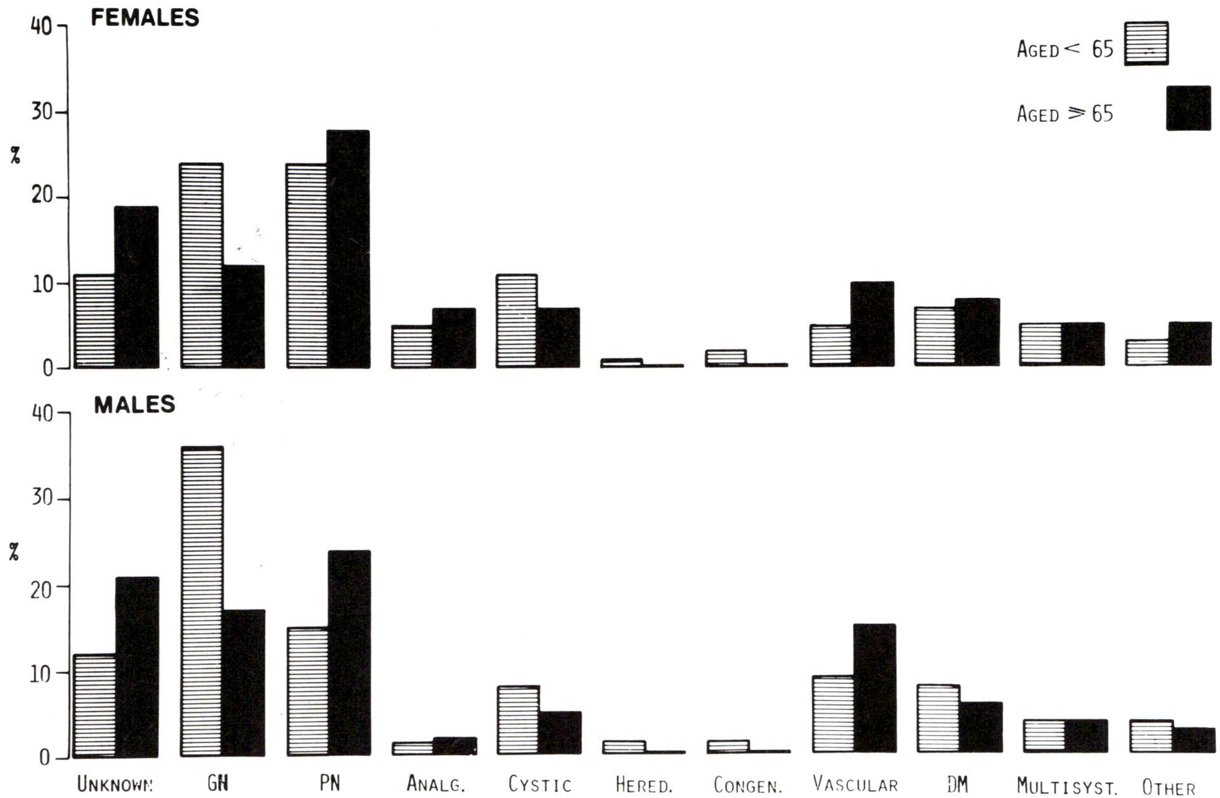

Figure 22.3 Primary renal disease distribution in patients older and younger than 65 years who commenced renal replacement therapy in Europe 1980–83. Unknown = chronic renal failure, aetiology uncertain; GN = glomerulonephritis; PN = pyelonephritis; Analg. = drug-induced nephropathy; Cystic = cystic kidney disease; Hered. = hereditary diseases; Congen. = congenital diseases; Vascular = vascular causes of renal failure, including hypertension; DM = diabetes mellitus; Multisyst. = multisystem disease involving the kidney; Other = other renal diseases

The distribution of primary renal diseases leading to uraemia in these patients is rather different from those responsible for uraemia in younger people (*Figure 22.3*): diseases of unknown origin, pyelonephritis and renovascular diseases are more common in elderly patients, whereas glomerulonephritis and cystic diseases are more common in younger patients. However, although one cause of renal failure was assigned as the cause in this analysis, renal failure in the elderly may often be multifactorial, involving for example a combination of diabetes, hypertension, obstructive nephropathy, atherosclerosis and urinary tract infection (Parsons, 1977; Chester *et al.*, 1979).

General problems in older dialysis patients

The underlying disease and the physiological deterioration in the physical and physiological condition may complicate dialytic treatment, and may impair full rehabilitation in elderly uraemic patients. Bone disease, malnutrition, neurological disorders, cardiovascular disease and psychosocial problems are the most relevant factors which can complicate chronic dialysis in the elderly.

Bone disease

The complex skeletal abnormalities of advanced renal failure can be aggravated in older uraemic patients by the physiological progressive osteopenia which follows the menopause in woman, and appears after 65 years of age in man. Bone mineral density, cortical thickness and the total quantity of calcium are all inversely related to the age of the subject (Riggs *et al.*, 1982). It has been calculated that total body calcium reduces in women at a rate of 1.1 per cent per year (about 7.6 g per year) after the menopause, and at a rate of 0.7 per cent per year (about 7 g per year) in men older than 50. Therefore, at 80 years of age women have lost about 28 per cent and men about 20 per cent of the calcium contained in their skeleton when they were aged 30. In the elderly, there is also a progressive and linear reduction of bone trabecular volume. At 80 years, men have lost some 27 per cent and women some 41 per cent of the bone trabecular volume they had at 20 years of age (Malluche *et al.*, 1982; Gruber *et al.*, 1984). Moreover, in older women the low plasma levels of oestrogens can *per se* produce a reduced activity of 1α-hydroxylase in the kidney (Gallagher *et al.*, 1976; Heaney *et al.*, 1978). Thus, even in normal elderly persons, especially in women, an osteoporosis can develop and worsen over the years.

The occurrence of uraemic osteodystrophy, the frequent protein malnutrition, the lack of exposure to solar radiation and the reduced levels of physical activity further complicate and aggravate the bone disease in older patients on maintenance dialysis. It is often difficult to separate the respective role of age, uraemia or other factors in the pathogenesis of skeletal disorders which can affect these patients. A high incidence of spontaneous fractures (13.7 per cent) and of vascular or metastatic calcifications (17.2 per cent) has been reported in elderly dialysis patients (Alloatti *et al.*, 1976). Skeletal pain, muscular hypotrophy and a slowing of nerve conduction velocity are more frequent in older than in younger uraemic patients. These disorders, which are often caused by the bone and nerve changes of the elderly (Garini *et al.*, 1976), can impair the physical activity and the degree of rehabilitation.

The objectives of management in bone disease of older uraemic patients are to suppress secondary hyperparathyroidism, to prevent protein malnutrition, and to prevent vascular calcification which can aggravate the atherosclerotic lesions. An adequate protein intake (at least 1 g/kg per day), administration of aluminium hydroxide to prevent hyperphosphataemia and hyperparathyroidism, dietary supplements of calcium, use of an appropriate calcium concentration in the dialysis bath and prophylactic treatment with vitamin D derivatives (Ken-Sung *et al.*, 1984) are mandatory to prevent the development of severe bone disease in older uraemic patients. The therapy of osteoporosis is still controversial. In women with severe bone pain and/or high risk of vertebral fractures, ethinyl oestradiol, at least 25 μg/day, associated with vitamin D and/or sodium fluoride (50 μg/day) proved to be efficacious (Riggs *et al.*, 1982). In elderly uraemic men, a course of vitamin D and/or calcitonin may be tried.

Malnutrition

Malnutrition is one of the most important complications of dialysis in the elderly. In some series, cachexia accounted for about one-third of the deaths in older uraemics (Quarello, Ramello and Piccoli, 1984). In normal subjects, the nutritional status, as assessed by upper arm anthropometry (Bishop, Bowen and Ritchey, 1981), tends to be progressively impaired after 45–60 years (Tuttle, Swendseid and Basset, 1960). In older patients on maintenance dialysis, the combination of physiological decrease in muscular mass due to age, together with the abnormalities of endogenous amino acid pool caused by uraemia, loss of amino acids during dialysis and the possible occurrence of hypercatabolic states (i.e. infection, stress, etc.), can lead to protein malnutrition. Moreover, because of the frequent episodes of intradialytic cardiovascular instability and/or cardiac arrhythmias, low dialyser blood flow rates are often necessary during haemodialysis in older patients. This can result in an inadequate dialysis and consequent asthenia, thirst, anorexia and psychic depression, leading to insufficient calorie and protein intake. On the other hand, in chronic peritoneal dialysis, the combination of protein loss and decreased appetite may be responsible for decreased serum albumin levels and negative nitrogen balance (Williams *et al.*, 1981).

To prevent malnutrition, protein intake should be higher than 1 g/kg body weight for haemodialysis patients (Kluthe *et al.*, 1978) and more than 1.2 g/kg body weight for continuous ambulatory peritoneal dialysis (CAPD) patients (Blumenkrantz, 1981), with at least 6.3 g/day of essential amino acids (Giordano, 1978). With a similar dietetic regimen and adequate dialysis, we did not find any difference between a group of older patients (mean age 55.6 ± 2.3) and another group of younger patients (mean age 42 ± 5.1) in upper arm anthropometry and intracellular composition of muscle (Graziani *et al.*, 1984).

Neurological disorders

The combination of cerebral atherosclerosis, electrolyte disturbances, acidosis and the reduction of brain metabolism (Scheinberg, 1954), probably related to the inhibition of cerebral enzyme activities by unknown toxins, can result in manifold and frequent neurological disorders in older uraemic patients.

Wernicke's syndrome, characterized by changes in ocular motility and ataxia associated with defective recent memory and mental confusion, may develop in malnourished dialysis patients, such as the elderly (Faris, 1968).

Multi-infarct dementia is a widespread decline of intellectual capacities with pseudobulbar palsy, dysphagia and dysarthria that can result from occlusion of the arteries supplying basal ganglia, thalamus, internal capsule, pons, cerebellum and the sensorial centre (Jennekens and Jennekens-Schinkel, 1983). The syndrome is related to the presence of multiple small infarcts and is one of the major causes of mental deterioration in the elderly (Hachinsky, Lassen and Marshall, 1974).

Binswanger's encephalopathy may develop in early senescence as a result of long-term hypertension and atherosclerosis. There is a loss of spontaneity with sluggishness and perseveration. Aphasia, unilateral neglect, memory loss, motor and sensory dysfunctions develop gradually, with periods of progression alternating with periods of stabilization (Jennekens and Jennekens-Schinkel, 1983). Transient ischaemic attacks are frequent in older dialysis patients and can also occur during intradialytic hypotensive episodes. Cerebral thrombosis or embolism, intracerebral haemorrhage and subdural haematoma are among the major causes of death in dialysis patients. These complications are particularly frequent in older patients with atherosclerosis and a long history of arterial hypertension.

Polyneuropathy is one of the most principal manifestations in chronic uraemia. In older dialysis patients, the nerve conduction velocity is even slower than in younger patients. This probably reflects a physiological decrease in conduction velocity which occurs after 50 years of age, when the number of fibres with large diameter progressively reduces, and vascular and connective tissues in the peripheral nerves are rearranged (Brown, 1972).

Cardiovascular disease

Although the initial belief that the hyperlipidaemia of dialysis can accelerate atherosclerosis (Lindner *et al.*, 1974; Lazarus *et al.*, 1975) has been recently challenged both by experimental (Kamstrup, Tredegaard and Stender, 1980; Horsch *et al.*, 1981) and clinical studies (Burke *et al.*, 1978), there is no doubt that cardiovascular disease is the major cause of death in dialysis patients. The risk of coronary artery complications is particularly elevated in older patients (Rathaus, Kortzes and Bernheim, 1980; Rostand *et al.*, 1982; Rostand, Kirk and Rutsky, 1982) and in patients with a history of ischaemic heart disease (Comty and Shapiro, 1983; Rostand, Kirk and Rutsky, 1984).

Preventive measures are probably of little benefit in elderly patients as they already have established atherosclerosis. Nevertheless, since sporadic cases suggesting the possibility of reversing atherosclerosis with medical therapy have been reported (Basta *et al.*, 1976), correction of hypertension (Vincenti *et al.*, 1980) and of hyperlipidaemia (Haire *et al.*, 1978; Ponticelli *et al.*, 1978) and withdrawal of smoking (Haire *et al.*, 1978), which have been found to be related to atherosclerosis in dialysis patients, may be tried.

Since the finding of abnormal ventricular wall motion is an important predictor of the presence of coronary heart disease (Rostand, Kirk and Rutsky, 1984), non-invasive techniques such as echocardiography or scintiscan studies should be performed in symptomatic patients in order to decide which patients should be studied by angiography. In fact, older patients with significant coronary artery narrowing, in whom survival or quality of life are threatened, can be successfully submitted to coronary bypass surgery (Crawford *et al.*, 1977; Byrd and Sullivan, 1978).

On the other hand, dialysis may benefit uraemic patients with congestive heart failure or cardiomyopathy by improving global and resting left ventricular function and exercise tolerance (Kramer *et al.*, 1984). Left ventricular function, which is generally related to hyperhydration, is the major prognostic factor in coronary artery disease. Thus, older patients with left ventricular dysfunction and exertional angina not only require early institution of antianginal therapy, but also need careful volume restriction and shorter interdialytic periods (Kramer *et al.*, 1984).

Psychosocial problems

The numerous problems of renal disease and dialysis are exaggerated in the elderly by a series of problems related to the age. According to McKevitt and Kappel (1978) they include:

(1) *Physical deterioration.* More than 85 per cent of non-uraemic older subjects have at least one medical condition such as joint disease, cardiovascular disease, visual or hearing loss.
(2) *Reduced mental functioning.* As a part of the aging process, slowed intellectual function and memory occur in many patients.
(3) *Poverty.* At retirement, income usually drops by 50 per cent or more and during the years that follow it deteriorates even further.
(4) *Problems of transportation.* Elderly patients are often unable to drive. Many of them live in the centre of cities, and in large cities with poor public transit service the high cost of private transportation can limit access to recreational opportunities and isolate the patient from family and friends.
(5) *Psychological problems.* Anxiety often becomes chronic in old age, recurrent episodes of depression appear and the suicide rate is increased in the elderly. The loss of their social role, dependence on their families, reactive depression to poor prognosis, fear of abandonment by care-givers and death of relatives and friends can further complicate the psychological problem (Rife *et al.*, 1979).

Thus, an older person needing regular dialysis must face several limitations and problems. Some patients show an impressive capacity to adapt to their diminishing capabilities and multiple physical problems, and are able to cope with the rigours of dialysis. However, some patients react with excessive dependence, while others resist what they consider intrusive care, refuse to adhere to schedules and do not maintain personal hygiene and nutrition.

In order to minimize the problems of these patients, the approach of dialysis staff is critical. Flexibility in the arrangement of dialysis stations, well-planned composition of the dialysis group and regular psychological support during the hours of haemodialysis can be helpful (Jenneckens and Jenneckens-Schinckel, 1983). Fair discussion of clinical problems, encouragement of interest in current events and the participation in unit projects can provide a major sense of security. Physical exercise to maintain strength should also be recommended. Social workers can alleviate loneliness, anticipate specific problems and aid patients with problems regarding transportation, medication and finances. The organization of meetings with participation of patients, their families, social workers and doctors can remove some sources of concern and reduce depression and anxiety.

Problems related to haemodialysis

About 83 per cent of treated uraemic patients in Europe older than 65 are treated by haemodialysis. Haemodialysis can pose special problems in older patients, which will be briefly discussed in this section.

Vascular access

The internal arteriovenous fistula is the best available access for maintenance haemodialysis. However, in many elderly patients peripheral arteriosclerosis and/or insufficient dilatation of the venous system can impair the good functioning of the fistula. In a recent investigation it has been found that 25 per cent of hospitalizations in older patients were caused by problems related to vascular access (Schaefer, 1985). In order to allow a gradual thickening and arterialization of the venous walls, an arteriovenous fistula should be prepared early in the difficult cases, some 4–6 weeks prior to haemodialysis. It is preferable to use an end-artery fistula instead of a side-artery fistula, at least in the distal extremity, to avoid a 'steal syndrome' and digital necrosis (Buselmeier *et al.*, 1973).

In patients with short-lived fistula, a conduit can be placed subcutaneously between an artery and a vein. The types of material most commonly used are autogenous saphenous veins, bovine carotid arteries, Hemasite and expanded polytetrafluoroethylene grafts (Goretex). They can be placed in the forearm, in the anterior upper thigh and, in desperate cases, between the axillary artery on one side and the axillary vein on the other side, and tunnelled subcutaneously across the anterior chest. There are no data on the survival of these internal arteriovenous shunts in aging patients. In diabetic patients, who usually have major problems of vascular access, bovine or polytetrafluorethylene graft survive longer than arteriovenous fistulas (Kjellstrand *et al.*, 1983). On the other hand, these grafts have a higher incidence of infections, so that in difficult patients the choice between fistula and heterologous grafts must be individualized. It seems reasonable to assume that patients with considerable peripheral arteriosclerosis or strictures and fibrosis of peripheral veins will have short-lived fistula, and therefore probably will benefit from a heterologous graft as the primary access (Kjellstrand *et al.*, 1983).

In patients who have exhausted any possible vascular access, repeated intermittent femoral vein cannulation by the Seldinger technique has been used for up to several years (Nidus and Neusy, 1981; Catizone and Zucchelli, 1982). Another approach is the introduction of a subclavian catheter which can be left *in situ* for several weeks or months and then substituted (Uldall, 1981). Laceration of great vessels, pleura or heart can occur as a result of catheter placement. To minimize these life-threatening complications, medical staff should be properly trained and supervised. The long-term presence of the catheter in the subclavian vein can result in thrombosis and infection. These complications are relatively frequent and potentially serious (Huffman, Sherertz and Mattern, 1983).

Intradialytic complications

In our experience, only 20 per cent of hospital dialyses performed in 40 patients older than 65 were completely free from symptoms. In 60 per cent of cases, patients complained of mild and rapidly reversible symptoms such as moderate hypotension, headache, nausea, weakness, etc. In about 25 per cent of dialyses, older patients suffered from more severe symptoms including cardiac arrhythmias, severe cardiovascular instability and angina pectoris episodes.

Cardiac arrhythmias

Some 16 to 50 per cent of patients suffer from disturbances of cardiac rhythm during dialysis (Avram *et al.*, 1978; Morrison *et al.*, 1980; Blumberg *et al.*, 1983; Ramirez,

Brueggemeyer and Newton, 1984; Weber *et al.*, 1984). Cardiac arrhythmias are particularly frequent in patients with underlying heart disease. Therefore, although these disorders can develop at any age and even in children, they are particularly frequent in older patients (Jacobs *et al.*, 1985) who have often cardiac hypertrophy, amyloid infiltration, metastatic calcification, coronary heart disease, electrocardiographic changes and/or hypertension. The rapid correction of extracellular volume, acidosis and hyperkalaemia may act synergistically with the disturbed myocardial function in inducing supraventricular and ventricular arrhythmias, which occur most frequently during the first and second hours of haemodialysis (Morrison *et al.*, 1980).

Digitalis administration has also been recognized as one of the most important causes of arrhythmias and conduction defects during haemodialysis (Del Greco and Grumer, 1962; Ferrier, Saunders and Mendez, 1973; Morrison *et al.*, 1980; Blumberg *et al.*, 1983). Changes in K^+ and Ca^{2+} can account for the elevated rate of cardiac arrhythmias in digitalized patients. Potassium is a competitive inhibitor of digitalis binding to cardiac Na^+–K^+ ATPase. Thus, when K^+ is reduced, digitalis binding rates to membrane sites are enhanced. The dramatic drop in serum potassium concentration, which occurs with conventional dialysis bath potassium concentrations during the first 2 h of haemodialysis, has a direct membrane effect, and can increase cardiac excitability, so potentiating the arrhythmogenic stimulus of cardiac glycosides. A rise in serum calcium concentration (Ferrier and Moe, 1973) and a too rapid reduction in magnesium during dialysis may also precipitate cardiac arrhythmias (Del Greco and Grummer, 1962). Many elderly uraemic patients are given digitalis (Chester *et al.*, 1979). They are particularly sensitive to the changes of volaemia, serum potassium, calcium and magnesium during hemodialysis and therefore are prone to develop intradialytic arrhythmias.

A judicious use of digitalis and elevated bath potassium concentration are the best preventive measures of cardiac arrhythmias. Whenever possible, it is preferable to treat cardiac failure with adequate ultrafiltration and with good control of hypertension instead of using digitalis (Blumberg *et al.*, 1983). In patients with serious cardiac disease requiring digitalis, it is justifiable to perform Holter monitoring in order to identify atrioventricular dissociation, supraventricular tachycardia or ventricular premature beats. Since supraventricular arrhythmias are particularly frequent in hypokalaemic patients dialysed with low potassium solution, increasing the potassium bath concentration to 4–4.5 mmol/l and maintaining pre-dialytic potassium serum levels below 5–5.6 mmol/l, by oral ionic exchange resin, is the best preventive approach. In our experience, preliminary results with this policy seem encouraging.

The administration of 400 mg of quinidine sulphate 45 min prior to haemodialysis, together with increased potassium bath concentration, is effective in eliminating both frequent and complex ventricular arrhythmias (Morrison *et al.*, 1980). On the other hand, in the presence of hypokalaemia anti-arrhythmic agents are not only ineffective but also may exacerbate arrhythmias. We have achieved good results in managing cardiac arrhythmias with intravenous canrenone (Soldactone), an aldosterone antagonist which inhibits ouabain-sensitive Na^+ efflux and has a positive inotropic effect. In ventricular arrhythmias, mexiletine, 250 mg intravenously followed by 200 mg by mouth 2–3 times per day, can be effective. Different from other antiarrhythmic agents, this drug does not have negative ionotropic activity, does not induce arterial hypotension and is almost totally insensitive to the presence of hypokalaemia.

Cardiovascular instability

Arterial hypotension, often associated with nausea, vomiting, cramps and/or headache, occurs in some 20–30 per cent of all haemodialyses. Hypotension is generally triggered by the acute reduction in blood volume caused by sodium and fluid depletion during dialysis. In haemodialysis patients, several factors can impair a prompt adaptation of the vascular bed to hypovolaemia: (1) uraemic autonomic neuropathy (Kersch *et al.*, 1974); (2) intradialytic hypoxaemia (Hunt *et al.*, 1984); (3) intradialytic fall of plasma osmolality caused by low sodium dialysis solutions (Redaelli *et al.*, 1979), with consequent shift of water into the intracellular compartment; (4) the peripheral vasodilating and cardiodepressant effects of acetate used as a buffer in the dialysis solution (Aizawa *et al.*, 1977); and (5) the slower response of adrenergic arteriolar receptors either due to the loss of catecholamines during dialysis (Zucchelli *et al.*, 1978), or to a reduction of the sodium pool in patients dialysed with low sodium dialysis baths (Locatelli *et al.*, 1978).

Older patients are particularly prone to cardiovascular instability. In fact, the atherosclerotic lesions further interfere with the vascular adaptation to hypovolaemia, and the nervous dysautonomia progressively worsens with age. In elderly patients, hypotensive episodes can be complicated by transient ischaemic attacks, angina pectoris and/or cardiac arrhythmias. Thus, every effort should be made in order to prevent cardiovascular instability in these patients. Good results have been reported with sequential ultrafiltration–diffusion dialysis (Bergstrom *et al.*, 1976), haemofiltration (Chen, Chaignon and Omvi, 1978), isonatric haemodialysis with a bath sodium concentration the same as the patient's plasma water (Locatelli *et al.*, 1978), substitution of bicarbonate for acetate in dialysate (Graefe, Milutinovich and Faltette, 1978) and recirculating dialysis with bicarbonate (Citterio *et al.*, 1982). These modifications of the standard technique can prevent in many patients the fall of peripheral vascular resistance which occurs during dialysis. They seem, therefore, particularly indicated in elderly patients with intradialytic cardiovascular instability. However, due to the potential risks of hypotension in the elderly, older patients with intractable dialysis intolerance should be switched to chronic peritoneal dialysis.

Angina pectoris

Older patients, who have an increasing prevalence of coronary artery disease, are particularly exposed to the risk of dialysis-related cardiac death. Indeed, the severity of myocardial ischaemia may be enhanced by anaemia and left ventricular hypertrophy which are generally present in uraemic patients. Moreover, a number of haemodialysis-induced events may precipitate symptoms of ischaemic heart disease. Haemodialysis may be associated with reduction in blood pO_2 (Burns and Scheinhorn, 1982), alterations in haemoglobin–oxygen affinity (Hirszel *et al.*, 1975), reduced myocardial oxygen balance, and an increased myocardial contractility causing myocardial under-oxygenation (Nixon *et al.*, 1983; Pedersen, Rasmussen and Cleeman-Rasmussen, 1983). Hypotension and increased heart rate are also common. Thus, haemodialysis may simultaneously reduce coronary artery perfusion pressure, coronary artery filling time and myocardial oxygen demands (Rostand, Kirk and Rutsky, 1984), leading to the danger of angina pectoris and even myocardial infarction in older patients with underlying heart disease. In order to reduce this risk, it has been suggested that the haematocrit should be maintained above 25 per cent by regular blood transfusions (Walker *et al.*, 1976), since the correction of anaemia can restore the cardiac output to normal in dialysis patients. In patients with repeated episodes of angina during the latter hours of haemodialysis, shorter dialysis may be required. However, refractory patients should be considered for chronic peritoneal dialysis.

Problems related to peritoneal dialysis

Peritoneal dialysis removes fluid and metabolic wastes slowly so that patients can tolerate better the fluid shift. For this reason many authors (Tenckhoff, 1974; Mion *et al.*, 1981; Oreopoulos, 1983) consider peritoneal dialysis as the treatment of choice for the elderly patient with cardiovascular disease, problems of vascular access and/or dialytic intolerance.

About 15 per cent of uraemic patients older than 65 are treated by peritoneal dialysis in Europe, versus 7 per cent in the general dialysis and transplant population. Two forms of peritoneal dialysis are used today: intermittent peritoneal dialysis (IPD) and CAPD, with its modifications of continuous cycling peritoneal dialysis (CCPD), and combined peritoneal dialysis (CPD).

Although peritoneal dialysis is generally assumed to be safe, it may be associated with significant morbidity and mortality. Most of the complications can be prevented and, when they do develop, can be brought under control by appropriate measures. Units with an experienced staff can handle the technical problems and rarely are forced to discontinue peritoneal dialysis. Nevertheless, older patients can pose special problems.

Dialysate leakage

Even in the elderly the most popular dialysis catheter is the Tenckhoff peritoneal dialysis catheter. The insertion technique is similar to that used for younger patients. However, special care must be taken to prevent dialysate leakage. Indeed, the risk of external leak through the incision and catheter exit site is higher in elderly patients who have lax abdominal wall (Ponce *et al.*, 1982). To avoid this complication, the best technique is to postpone the start of peritoneal dialysis for 2 weeks after catheter insertion, performing catheter flushing with heparinized saline on a daily or alternate day basis.

Hernia formation

One of the most common surgical complications of IPD, and CAPD in particular, is hernia formation. With instillation of dialysis fluid into the peritoneal cavity, the intra-abdominal pressure rises. In elderly patients who often have poor abdominal wall muscle tone, the likelihood of hernia formation is increased. The types of hernias which develop during peritoneal dialysis include incisional, inguinal, diaphragmatic and umbilical hernias. These hernias can sometimes be complicated by partial or complete bowel incarcerations. Women can develop rectocystocele, with or without uterine prolapse. Other consequences of persistently raised intra-abdominal pressure include worsening of symptoms of hiatus hernia and haemorrhoids (Oreopoulos *et al.*, 1982).

Musculoskeletal complication

Most of the elderly patients on CAPD complain of mild backache, but severe backache is uncommon. This complaint is probably related to the increased lordotic posture which these patients adopt while carrying 2 litres of dialysate intraperitoneally. CAPD may aggravate pre-existing lumbar disc disease, and it is becoming evident that severe backache in elderly patients with pre-existing disc disease may constitute a contraindication to CAPD (Oreopoulos and Khanna, 1981).

Hypotension

Patients on CAPD may develop symptomatic orthostatic hypotension, probably as a result of excessive sodium removal via the dialysate relative to the dietary sodium intake, leading to the gradual development of sodium depletion (Leenen *et al.*, 1983). Depression of aldosterone secretion secondary to hypokalaemia may also contribute to this phenomenon. Hypotension usually responds readily to sodium replacement, but some patients remain hypotensive with consequent hampered rehabilitation and risk of precipitation or aggravation of peripheral ischaemic symptoms (Brown *et al.*, 1981).

Peripheral vascular disease

In patients with generalized vascular disease, particularly that involving the iliac and femoral vessel, reduced perfusion as a result of systemic hypotension, which frequently complicates CAPD, can precipitate or aggravate peripheral ischaemic symptoms (Brown *et al.*, 1981). Whether the physical pressure of dialysate on the vessels, especially in the supine position, can induce or contribute to these symptoms is uncertain. Corrective or palliative surgery may become necessary in such patients to relieve the symptoms.

Diverticulosis

Diverticula are common in older patients, and may predispose to development of diverticulitis with secondary faecal peritonitis. However, to date there is not enough evidence to exclude patients with extensive diverticulosis from peritoneal dialysis (Wu *et al.*, 1983). If such patients are accepted into the peritoneal dialysis programme, prevention of constipation is of utmost importance.

Peritonitis

A higher incidence of peritonitis could be expected in elderly patients as a consequence of impaired immunological defences, reduced motor skills and visual acuity, and increased incidence of diverticulosis. However, published reports indicate that the incidence of peritonitis is similar or only marginally worse than that observed in younger patients (Kaye, Pajel and Somerville, 1983; Nissenson *et al.*, 1984; Cutler *et al.*, 1984). In our CAPD experience with the use of a Y-connector with disinfectant (Maiorca *et al.*, 1983) which greatly reduces the contamination risk, even in the presence of motor and visual problems, the incidence of peritonitis in 16 patients older than 65 years was even lower than that observed in 61 younger patients (1/80 patient-months versus 1/50 patient-months).

Other complications and hospitalizations

The frequency of catheter skin exit-site infection requiring antibiotic treatment is not different between patients over and under 65 years of age (Kaye, Pajel and Somerville, 1983). In a large series by Nissenson *et al.* (1984), which compared 183 patients over 60 years with 592 younger patients, the technique survival (excluding death and transplantation) and the peritoneal catheter longevity of older patients was not different from that seen in the 21–60-year-old patients.

The number of days of hospitalization per patient per year, both in the Nissenson *et al.* (1984) and the Mion *et al.* (1983) series, was only slightly higher in older than in younger patients.

Results

The cumulative actuarial survival curve for patients treated by regular *haemodialysis* in Europe is presented in *Figure 22.4*. The data clearly show a progressively increasing mortality rate with age. The 2-year survival rate is 61 per cent for patients older than 65 and 56 per cent for those older than 70 years.

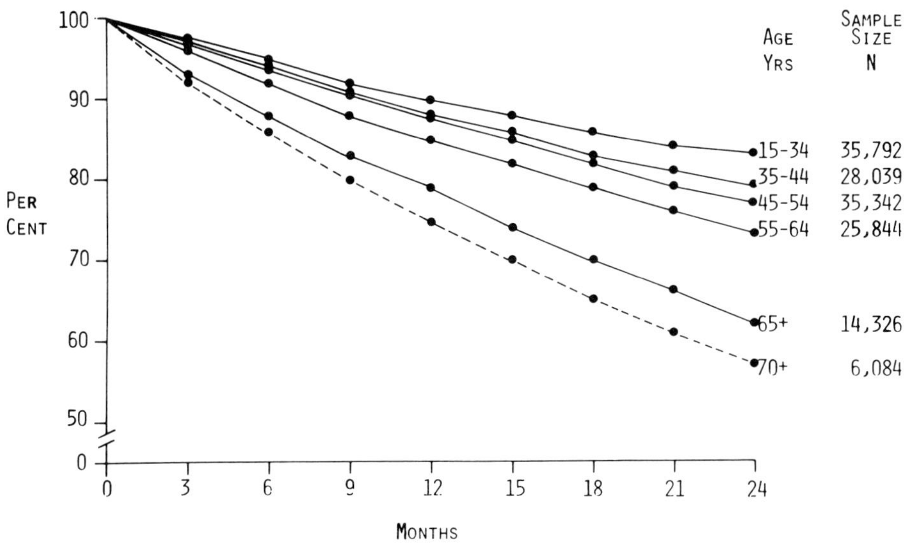

Figure 22.4 Patient survival after starting regular haemodialysis, according to age group. The number of patients (*N*) is shown by the sample size on the right of the figure

The results for *CAPD* are similar, the 2-year survival rate being 56 per cent for patients over 65 and 50 per cent for patients over 70 years (*Figure 22.5*). Cardiac and vascular diseases accounted for most of the deaths in the elderly patients. In a far from negligible number of patients, 'social problems' (i.e. interruption of treatment and suicide) were registered as the cause of death (*Figure 22.6*). Interruption of treatment accounted for an impressive 22 per cent of deaths in the series of Neu and Kjellstrand (1986). The decision to stop treatment was particularly frequent in patients over 60 years of age, amongst whom 1 in 6 stopped dialysis.

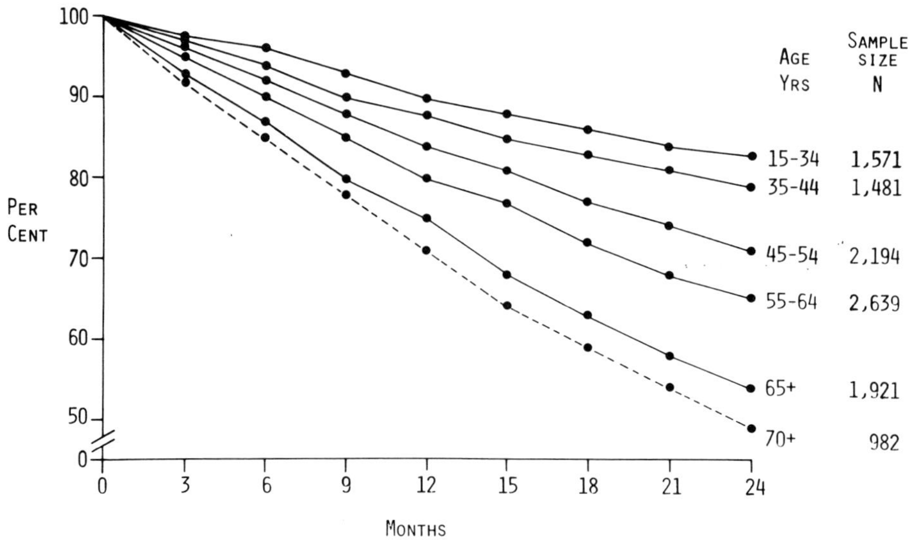

Figure 22.5 Patient survival after starting CAPD, according to age group. The number of patients (*N*) is shown by the sample size on the right of the figure

Haemodialysis *versus* peritoneal dialysis

The results in terms of survival in older patients treated by chronic dialysis are clearly worse than those obtained in younger patients. Nevertheless, taking into account the limited life expectancy of older people with normal renal function, regular dialysis treatment can allow a reasonable proportion of the expected life to be achieved by older uraemic patients. This can justify the progressively increasing number of elderly patients submitted to chronic dialysis. Indeed, in Europe, older patients accounted for 7 per cent of new dialysis patients in 1975, 8.6 per cent in 1978 and 15 per cent in 1982 (Brunner *et al.*, 1979; Wing *et al.*, 1983). On the basis of the cumulative results observed from European centres, it appears that the life expectancy of older uraemic patients is similar whether using haemodialysis or peritoneal dialysis. It is therefore difficult to indicate what is the 'best' dialysis treatment in the elderly.

However, some relative indications can be given. Patients with severe hypertension, cardiovascular problems and difficult vascular access are probably better candidates for peritoneal dialysis. Moreover, haemodialysis patients with severe intradialytic cardiac arrhythmias, angina and/or cardiovascular instability should be switched to CAPD. On the other hand, in patients with lower limb obliterative arteriopathy, previous extensive abdominal surgery, a history of diverticulitis and/or intractable hernia, haemodialysis is preferable. CAPD patients with severe orthostatic hypotension or frequent peritonitis episodes should be transferred to haemodialysis.

However, it should be pointed out that in the elderly, most haemodialyses have to be performed in the hospital. Indeed, in Europe, only 2 per cent of elderly patients are treated by home haemodialyis (*Figure 22.2*). This is due both to the frequent intradialytic complications and to the difficulty in organizing home haemodialysis

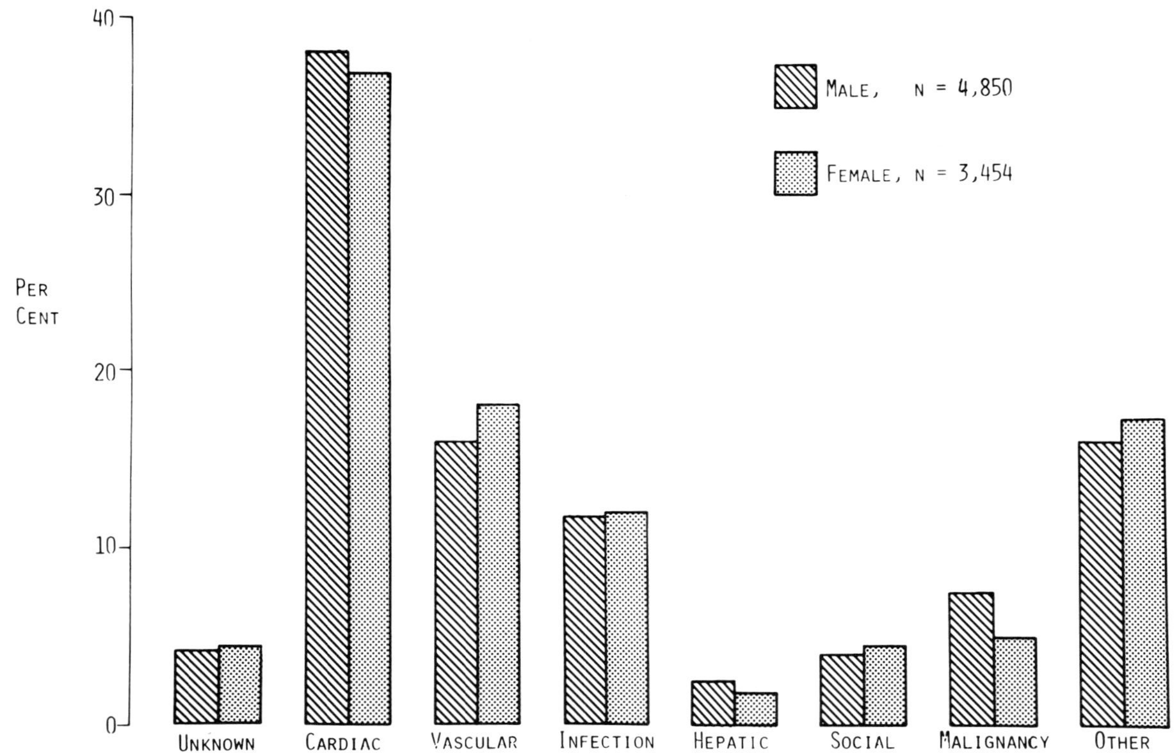

Figure 22.6 Causes of death in patients older than 65 years at start of treatment. Note: vascular includes cerebrovascular accident and pulmonary embolus, social includes suicide and discontinuation of therapy

because of the physical and psychological limitations of the patients and their partners. Considering the shorter life expectancy of older patients, the quality of life is particularly relevant. Home treatment performed with relative ease and comfort in a familiar environment is certainly the best treatment (Marai *et al.*, 1983). Since peritoneal dialysis is easy to organize at home, and CAPD in particular is a home treatment exclusively, we tend to recommend CAPD as the treatment of choice for the elderly patient suffering from end-stage renal failure, whenever the social and family situation is favourable. However, considering the frequent complications both of haemodialysis and CAPD in elderly patients, an integrated dialysis programme, more than a definitive choice between the two techniques, is probably the best approach.

Conclusions

Selecting patients for maintenance dialysis programmes is often more a political than a medical problem. If the health policy of a country is to give unrestricted resources for dialysis, one can adhere to the principle that a doctor has to provide care for all ages. As a consequence, if a person has renal failure he must have dialysis, regardless of age and clinical conditions. However, if financial or political restrictions limit the number of patients that can be treated, it is necessary to design arbitrary selection criteria, which should be endorsed and promulgated by the funding authority (Mathew, D'Apice and Kincaid-Smith, 1983).

Although older patients have a higher mortality rate, more frequent and severe clinical and psychological problems, and a poorer degree of rehabilitation, calendar age *per se* should not be considered as a contraindication. Indeed, many older patients have a good tolerance to dialysis and achieve satisfying rehabilitation; moreover, the mean survival of patients aged over 65 is considerably better than that of patients with carcinoma of the bronchus and carcinoma of the colon (Taube *et al.*, 1983), who are not refused treatment in any country.

The predicted quality of life should be the main consideration in selecting patients for regular dialysis. The expectancy of a poor quality of life, and the impossibility of rehabilitation in severely disabled patients, seems to us to justify fully the refusal of a stressing and expensive treatment. Unfortunately, assessing the possible future adaptation of the patient to dialysis is not at all easy, and this is especially the case for elderly patients. It may happen that patients who had been judged not fit for dialysis show good compliance to the treatment, and good rehabilitation. On the other hand, some older patients, active and lively before dialysis, can progressively develop apathy, dementia and/or cachexia on dialysis. The most difficult choice concerns the dependent elderly patient. In our own experience, no rehabilitation can be expected in these patients without adequate family support. But in many cases, for economic or family reasons, the relatives in practice cannot spend their time to run a home dialysis programme, or to assist the patient. The choice between a vital treatment for an older patient and the risk of destroying the harmony of a family is a very difficult one. Only a comprehensive and realistic exposure of the problems with the family may help in reaching a decision which always remains difficult.

Acknowledgements

Data referring to the European experience and the data reported in the illustrations have been especially provided from the computer files of the European Dialysis and

Transplant Association-European Renal Association Registry. The authors wish to thank Dr A.J. Wing and the Registry committee for their assistance in providing the data.

References

AIZAWA, Y., OHMORI, T., IMAI, K., MATSUOKA, M. and HIRASAWA, Y. (1977). Depressant action of acetate upon the human cardiovascular system. *Clinical Nephrology,* **8,** 477–481

ALLOATTI, S., SEGOLONI, G., MARTINI, P.F., QUARELLO, F., COPPO, R., GROTT, G. *et al.* (1976). La dialisi nel paziente anziano. *Minerva Nefrologica,* **23,** 379–384

AVRAM, M.M., EDSON, J., GAN, A. and EDSON, J.N. (1978). Continuous monitoring of cardiac rhythm in hemodialysis patients. *Dialysis and Transplantation,* **7,** 516–517

BASTA, L.L., WILLIAMS, C., KLOSCHOS, J.M. and SPECTOR, A.A. (1976). Regression of atherosclerotic stenosing lesions of the renal arteries and spontaneous cure of systemic hypertension through control of hyperlipidemia. *American Journal of Medicine,* **61,** 420–423

BERGSTROM, J., ASABA, H., FÜRST, P. and OULES, R. (1976). Dialysis, ultrafiltration and blood pressure. In *Proceedings of the European Dialysis and Transplant Association* (Hamilton, 1976), edited by B.H.B. Robinson, P. Veerestraeten and J.B. Hawkins, pp. 293–300. London; Pitman

BERLYNE, G. (1982). Over 50 and uremic = death (Editorial). *Nephron,* **31,** 189–190

BISHOP, C.W., BOWEN, P.E., RITCHEY, S.J. (1981). Norms for nutritional assessment of American adults by upper arm anthropometry. *American Journal of Clinical Nutrition,* **34,** 2530–2539

BLUMBERG, A., HÄNSERMANN, M., STRUB, B. and JENZER, H.R. (1983). Cardiac arrhythmias in patients on maintenance hemodialysis. *Nephron,* **33,** 91–95

BLUMENKRANTZ, M.J. and SCHMIDT, R.W. (1981). Managing the nutritional concerns of the patient undergoing peritoneal dialysis. In *Peritoneal Dialysis,* edited by K.D. Nolph, pp. 275–308. The Hague; Nijhoff

BROWN, P.M., JOHNSTON, K.W., FENTON, S.S.A. and CATTRAN, D.C. (1981). Sympatomatic exacerbation of peripheral vascular disease with chronic ambulatory peritoneal dialysis. *Clinical Nephrology,* **16,** 258–261

BROWN, W.F. (1972). A method for estimating the number of motor units in thenar muscles and changes in motor unit count with ageing. *The Journal of Neurology, Neurosurgery and Psychiatry,* **35,** 845–849

BRUNNER, F.P., BRYNGER, H., CHANTLER, C., DONCKERWOLCKE, R.A., HATHAWAY, R.A., JACOBS, C. *et al.* (1979). Combined report on regular dialysis and transplantation in Europe, IX 1978. In *Proceedings of the European Dialysis and Transplant Association* (Amsterdam, 1979), edited by B.H.B. Robinson, J.B. Hawkins and R.B. Naik, p.p.2–69, London; Pitman

BURKE, J.F., FRANCOS, G.C., MOORE, L.L., CHO, S.Y. and LASKER, N. (1978). Accelerated atherosclerosis in chronic dialysis patients. Another look. *Nephron,* **21,** 181–185

BURNS, C.B. and SCHEINHORN, D.J. (1982). Hypoxemia during hemodialysis. *Archives of Internal Medicine,* **142,** 1350–1353

BUSELMEIER, T.J., NAJARIAN, J.S., SIMMONS, R.L., RATTAZZI, L.C., VON HARTITZSCH, B., CALLENDER, C.O. *et al.* (1973). A–V fistulas and the diabetic; ischemia and gangrene may result in amputation. *Transactions of the American Society of Aritifical Internal Organs,* **19,** 49–52

BYRD, L.H. and SULLIVAN, J.F. (1978). Successful coronary artery bypass in a hemodialysis patient. *Journal of Dialysis,* **2,** 33–37

CATIZONE, L. and ZUCCHELLI, P. (1982). Catheterization of the femoral vein for chronic hemodialysis. *Dialysis and Transplantation,* **11,** 1088–1093

CHEN, W.T., CHAIGNON, M. and OMVI, K.P. (1978). Hemodynamic studies in chronic hemodialysis patients with hemofiltration/ultrafiltration. *Transactions of the American Society of Artificial Internal Organs,* **24,** 682–685

CHESTER, A.C., RAKOWSKI, T.A., ARGY, W.P., GIACALONE, A. and SCHREINER, G.E. (1979). Hemodialysis in the eighth and ninth decades of life. *Archives of Internal Medicine,* **139,** 1001–1005

CITTERIO, A., CASATI, S., GRAZIANI, G., CANTALUPPI, A., LORENZANO, E. and PONTICELLI, C. (1982). La tolleranza dialitica: confronto fra emodialisi con acetato in passo singolo e bicarbonato in passo singolo e recircolo. In *Nefrologia Dialisi e Trapianto,* edited by D. Brancaccio, A. Lupo, L. Oldrizzi, C. Rugiu and E. Valvo, pp. 287–290. Milan; Wichtig

COHEN, S.L., COMTY, C.M. and SHAPIRO, F.L. (1970). The effect of age on the results of regular hemodialysis treatment. In *Proceedings of the European Dialysis and Transplant Association* (Barcelona, 1970), edited by J.S. Cameron, D. Fries and C.S. Ogg, pp. 254–260. London; Pitman

COMTY, C.M. and SHAPIRO, F.L. (1983). Cardiac complications of regular dialysis therapy. In *Replacement of Renal Function by Dialysis,* edited by W. Drukker, F.M. Parsons and J.F. Maher, pp. 595–610. The Hague; Nijhoff

CRAWFORD, F.A., SELBY, J.H., BEWER, J.P. and LEHAN, P. (1977). Coronary revascularization in patients maintained on hemodialysis. *Circulation*, **56**, 684–687

CUTLER, S.J., STEINBERG, S.M., NOVAK, J.M. and NOLPH, K.D. (1984). Report of the National CAPD Registry of the National Institutes of Health. Characteristics of Participants and Selected Outcome Measures for the Period January 1, 1981 through December 31, 1983. A publication of the National CAPD Registry of the National Institute of Arthritis, Diabetes, and Digestive and Kidney Diseases (July, 1984)

DA PORTO, A., BOCCI, C., ANTONUCCI, F., BERTOLONE, G., ADAMI, A., CASCONE, C. *et al.* (1975). Emodialisi nell'anziano. *Minerva Nefrologica*, **22**, 14–21

DEL GRECO, F. and GRUMMER, H. (1962). Electrolyte and electrocardiographic changes in the course of hemodialysis. *American Journal of Cardiology*, **9**, 43–50

FARIS, A.A. (1968). Wernicke's encephalopathy a complication of chronic hemodialysis. *Archives of Neurology*, **4**, 101–109

FERRIER, G.R. and MOE, G.K. (1973). Effect of calcium on acetylstrophanthidin induced transient depolarizations in canine Purkinje tissue. *Circulation Research*, **33**, 508–515

FERRIER, G.R., SAUNDERS, J.H. and MENDEZ, C. (1973). A cellular mechanism for the generation of ventricular arrhythmias by acetylstrophanthidin. *Circulation Research*, **32**, 600–609

FIGUEROA, J.E. (1968). Management of uremia in older patients: hemodialysis and renal transplantation. *Journal of the American Geriatric Society*, **16**, 1323–1330

GALLAGHER, J., RIGGS, B.L., EISMAN, J., ARNAUD, S.B. and DE LUCA, M.F. (1976). Impaired production of 1,25-dihydroxyvitamin D in post-menopausal osteoporosis. *Clinical Research*, **24**, 580–585

GARINI, G., CAMBI, V., ARISI, L., BIGNARDI, L., ROSSI, E., SAVAZZI, G. *et al.* (1976). La dialisi breve nell'anziano. *Minerva Nefrologica*, **23**, 371–378

GHANTOUS, W.N., BAILEY, G.L., ZSCHAECK, D., HAMPERS, C.L. and MERRILL, J.P. (1971). Long-term hemodialysis in the elderly. *Transactions of the American Society of Artificial Internal Organs*, **17**, 125–128

GIORDANI, C. (1978). Nutrizione e metabolismo proteico nei pazienti in dialisi. In *Il Rene Artificiale*, edited by W. Drukker, F.M. Parsons and J.F. Maher, pp. 745–751. Rome; Capozzi

GRAEFE, U., MILUTINOVICH, J. and FALTETTE, W.C. (1978). Less dialysis induced morbidity and vascular instability with bicarbonate in dialyzate. *Annals of Internal Medicine*, **88**, 332–337

GRAZIANI, G., CANTALUPPI, A., CASATI, S., CITTERIO, A., PONTICELLI, C., TRIFIRO, A. *et al.* (1984). Branched chain and aromatic free aminoacids in plasma and skeletal muscle of uremic patients undergoing hemodialysis and CAPD. *International Journal of Artificial Organs*, **7**, 85–88

GRUBER, H.E. and NACHMAN, B. (1984). Metabolic bone disease and the elderly: current approach to diagnosis and therapy. *Nephron*, **38**, 76–86

HACHINSKY, V.E., LASSEN, B.A. and MARSHALL, J. (1974). Multi-infarct dementia. A cause of mental deterioration in the elderly. *Lancet*, **2**, 207–210

HAIRE, H.M., SHERRARD, D.J., SCARDAPANE, D., CURTIS, E.K. and BRUNZELL, J.D. (1978). Smoking, hypertension and mortality in a maintenance dialysis population. *Cardiovascular Medicine*, **3**, 1163–1168

HEANEY, R.P., RECKER, R.R. and SAVILLE, P.D. (1978). Menopausal changes in bone remodeling. *Journal of Laboratory and Clinical Medicine*, **92**, 964–970

HIRSZEL, P., MAHER, J.F., TEMPEL, G.E. and MENGEL, C.E. (1975). Effect of hemodialysis on factors influencing oxygen transport. *Journal of Laboratory and Clinical Medicine*, **85**, 978–986

HORSCH, A., RITZ, E., HENCK, C.C., HOFFMAN, W., KUHNE, E. and BISSON, M. (1981). Atherogenesis in experimental uremia. *Atherosclerosis*, **40**, 279–289

HUFFMAN, K.A., SHERERTZ, R.J. and MATTERN, W.D. (1983). An appraisal of the subclavian dialysis catheter. *International Journal of Artificial Organs*, **6**, 176–177

HUNT, J.M., CHAPPELL, T.R., HENRICH, W.L. and RUBIN, L.J. (1984). Gas exchange during dialysis. *American Journal of Medicine*, **77**, 255–260

JACOBS, C., DIALLO, A., BALAS, E.A., NECTOUX, M. and ETIENNE, S. (1985). Maintenance hemodialysis treatment in patients aged over 60 years. Demographic profile, clinical aspects and outcome. In *Proceedings of the European Dialysis and Transplant Association*, edited by A.S. Davison and P. Guillou, pp. 447–489. London; Pitman

JENNEKENS, F.G.I. and JENNEKENS-SCHINKEL, A. (1983). Neurological aspects of dialysis patients. In *Replacement of Renal Function of Dialysis*, edited by W. Drukker, F.M. Parsons and J.F. Maher, pp. 724–741. The Hague; Nijhoff

KAMSTRUP, O., TREDEGAARD, E. and STENDER, S. (1980). Effect of chronic uremia on plasma lipids and the aortic accumulation of cholesterol in hypercholesterolemic rabbits. *Nephron*, **26**, 280–285

KAYE, M., PAJEL, P.A. and SOMERVILLE, P.J. (1983). Four years' experience with continuous ambulatory peritoneal dialysis (CAPD) in the elderly. *Peritoneal Dialysis Bulletin*, **3**, 17–19

KEN-SUNG, T., MEATH, M. III, KUMAR, R. and RIGGS, B.L. (1984). Impaired vitamin D metabolism with aging in women. Possible role in pathogenesis of senile osteoporosis. *Journal of Clinical Investigation*, **73**, 1668–1672

KERSH, E.S., KRONFIELD, S.J., UNGER, A., POPPER, R.W., CANTOR, S. and COHN, K. (1974). Autonomic insufficiency in uremia as a cause of hemodialysis-induced hypotension. *New England Journal of Medicine,* **290,** 650–653

KJELLSTRAND, C.M., WHITLEY, K., COMTY, C.M. and SHAPIRO, F.I. (1983). Dialysis in patients with diabetes mellitus nephropathy. *Diabetic Nephropathy,* **2,** 5–17

KLUTHE, R., LÜTTGEN, F.M., CAPETIANU, T., HEINZE, V., KATZ, N. and SÜDHOFF, A. (1978). Protein requirements in maintenance hemodialysis. *American Journal of Clinical Nutrition,* **31,** 1812–1820

KRAMER, W., WIZEMANN, V., KINDLER, M., THORMANN, J., GREBE, S.F., SCHÜTTERLE, G. *et al.* (1984). Influence of fluid removal rate during hemodialysis on left ventricular performance and exercise tolerance in patients with coronary heart disease. *Clinical Nephrology,* **21,** 280–286

LAZARUS, J.M., LAWRIE, E.G., HAMPERS, C.L. and MERRILL, J.P. (1975). Cardiovascular disease in uremic patients on hemodialysis. *Kidney International,* **2S,** S167–S175

LEENAN, F.H.H., SHAH, P., BOER, W.H., KHANNA, R. and OREOPULOS, D.G. (1983). Hypotension on CAPD: an approach to treatment. *Peritoneal Dialysis Bulletin,* **3S,** S33–S35

LINDER, A.L., CHARRA, B., SHERRARD, D.J. and SCRIBNER, B.H. (1974). Accelerated atherosclerosis in prolonged maintenance hemodialysis. *New England Journal of Medicine,* **290,** 697–701

LOCATELLI, F., COSTANZO, R., DI FILIPPO, S., PEDRINI, L., MARAI, P. *et al.* (1978). Ultrafiltration and high sodium concentration dialysis: pathophysiological correlation. In *Proceedings of the European Dialysis and Transplant Association* (Istanbul, 1978), edited by B.H.B. Robinson and J.B. Hawkins, pp. 253–259. London; Pitman

McKEVITT, P. and KAPPEL, D. (1978). Psychosocial needs and concerns of the elderly on dialysis. *Dialysis and Transplantation,* **7,** 435–441

MAIORCA, R., CANTALUPPI, A., CANCARINI, G.C., SCALAMOGNA, A., BROCOLI, R., GRAZIANI, G. *et al.* (1983). Prospective controlled trial of a Y-connector and disinfectant to prevent peritonitis in continuous ambulatory peritoneal dialysis. *Lancet,* **2,** 642–644

MALLINSON, W.J.W., FLEMING, S.J., SHAW, J.E.H., BAKER, L.R.I. and CATTELL, W.R. (1984). Survival in elderly patients presenting with uraemia. *Quarterly Journal of Medicine,* **210,** 301–307

MALLUCHE, M., MAYER, W., SHERMAN, D. and MASSRY, S.G. (1982). Quantitative bone histology in 84 normal American subjects. Micromorphometric analysis and evaluation of variance in iliac bone. *Calcified Tissue Research,* **34,** 449–455

MARAI, A., RATHAUD, M., GIBOR, Y. and BERNHEIM, J. (1983). Chronic dialysis in the elderly: intermittent peritoneal dialysis or hemodialysis? *Peritoneal Dialysis Bulletin,* **3,** 183–186

MATHEW, H., D'APICE, A.J.F. and KINCAID-SMITH, P. (1983). Selection of patients and the integration between dialysis and transplantation, the quality of life of the patients. In *Replacement of Renal Function by Dialysis,* edited by W. Drukker, F.M. Parsons and J.F. Maher, pp. 280–289. The Hague: Nijhoff

MION, C., SLINGENEYER, A., CANAUD, B., MOURAD, G., CHONG, G., BRANGER, B. and OULÉS, R. (1983). Review of a 4-year experience of continuous ambulatory peritoneal dialysis. In *Nephrology 83,* edited by G. D'Amico and G. Colasanti, pp. 175–187. Milan; Wichtig

MION, C., SLINGENEYER, A., CANAUD, B. and ELIE, M. (1981). A review of seven years' home peritoneal dialysis. In *Proceedings of the European Dialysis and Transplant Association* (Paris, 1981), edited by B.H.B. Robinson, J.B. Hawkins and A.M. Davison, pp. 91–107. London; Pitman

MORRISON, G., MICHELSON, E.L., BROWN, S. and MORGANROTH, J. (1980). Mechanism and prevention of cardiac arrhythmias in chronic hemodialysis patients. *Kidney International, 17,* 811–819

NEU, S. and KJELLSTRAND, C.M. (1986). Stopping long-term dialysis: an empirical study of withdrawal of life-supporting treatment. *New England Journal of Medicine,* **314,** 14–19

NIDUS, B.D. and NEUSY, A.J. (1981). Chronic hemodialysis by repeated femoral vein cannulation. *Nephron,* **29,** 195–197

NISSENSON, A.R., GENTILE, D.E., SODERBLOM, R., BRAX, C. and THE MEDICAL REVIEW BOARD NCC/4 (1986). CAPD in the elderly—regional experience. In *Frontiers in Peritoneal Dialysis,* edited by J.F. Maher and J.F. Winchester, pp. 312–317. New York; Field Rich

NIXON, J.V., MITCHELL, J.H., McPHAUL, J.J. Jr. and HENRICH, W.L. (1983). Effect of hemodialysis on left ventricular function: dissociation of changes in filling volume and in contractable state. *Journal of Clinical Investigation,* **71,** 377–384

OREOPULOS, D.G. (1983). Peritoneal dialysis. In *Textbook of Nephrology,* edited by S.G. Massry and R.J. Glassock, pp. 8.30–8.37. Baltimore; Williams and Wilkins

OREOPULOS, D.G. and KHANNA, R. (1981). Complications of peritoneal dialysis other than peritonitis. In *Peritoneal Dialysis,* edited by K.D. Nolph, pp. 309–343. The Hague; Nijhoff

OREOPULOS, D.G., KHANNA, R., WILLIAMS, P. and VAS, S.I. (1982). Continuous ambulatory peritoneal dialysis—1981. *Nephron,* **30,** 298–303

PARSON, V. (1977). What decreasing renal function means to aging patients. *Geriatrics,* **32,** 93–100

PEDERSEN. T.,, RASMUSSEN, K. and CLEEMAN-RASMUSSEN, K. (1983). Effect of hemodialysis on cardiac performance and transmural myocardial perfusion. *Clinical Nephrology,* **19,** 31–36

PONCE, S.P., PIERRATOS, A., IZATT, S., MATHEWS, R., KHANNA, R., ZELLERMAN, G. *et al.* (1982). Comparison of the survival and complications of three permanent peritoneal dialysis catheters. *Peritoneal Dialysis Bulletin*, **2**, 82–86

PONTICELLI, C., BARBI, G.L., CANTALUPPI, A., DONATI, C., ANNONI, G. and BRANCACCIO, D. (1978). Lipid abnormalities in maintenance dialysis patients and renal transplant recipients. *Kidney International*, **8S**, S72–S78

QUARELLO, F., RAMELLO, A. and PICCOLI, G. (1985). La dialisi nell'anziano. *Giornale Italiano di Nefrologia*, **2**, 29–34

RAMIREZ, G., BRUEGGEMEYER, C.D. and NEWTON, J.L. (1984). Cardiac arrhythmias on hemodialysis in chronic renal failure patients. *Nephron*, **36**, 212–218

RATHAUS, M., KORZETS, Z. and BERNHEIM, J. (1980). Results of regular hemodialysis treatment in the elderly. *Dialysis and Transplantation*, **9**, 1015–1018

REDAELLI, B., SFORZINI, S., BONOLDI, G., DADONE, C., DI FILIPPO, S., FILORAMO, F. *et al.* (1979). Hemodialysis with 'adequate' sodium concentration in dialysate. *International Journal of Artificial Organs*, **2**, 133–140

RIFE, M., BLEEKER, N., BURLEY, J., GELLMAN, A., GILMORE, B., HICKERSON, M. *et al.* (1979). The dependent elderly on dialyis. *Dialysis and Transplantation*, **8**, 867–878

RIGGS, B.L., WAHNER, H.W., SEERMAN, E., OFFORD, K., DUNN, K., MAZESS, R. *et al.* (1982). Changes in bone mineral density of the proximal femur and spine with aging. Differences between postmenopausal and senile osteoporosis syndromes. *Journal of Clinical Investigation*, **70**, 716–723

ROSTAND, S.G., KIRK, K.A. and RUTSKY, E.A. (1982). Relationship of coronary risk factors to hemodialysis-associated ischemic heart disease. *Kidney International*, **22**, 304–308

ROSTAND, S.G., KIRK, K.A. and RUTSKY, E.A. (1984). Dialysis-associated ischemic heart disease: insights from coronary angiography. *Kidney International*, **25**, 653–659

ROSTAND, S.G., KIRK, K.A., RUTSKY, E.A. and PATE, B.A. (1982). Racial differences in the incidence of treatment for end-state renal disease. *New England Journal of Medicine*, **306**, 1276–1279

SCHAEFFER, K. (1985). Optimum dialysis treatment for patients over 60 with primary renal disease. Survival and clinical results from 244 patients treated with either haemodialysis or haemofiltration. In *Proceedings of the European Dialysis and Transplant Association*, **21**, 510–517

SCHEINBERG, P. (1954). Effects of uraemia on cerebral blood flow and metabolism. *Neurology*, **4**, 101–106

SUMMER, C.R. (1979). The Methuselah syndrome. *Dialysis and Transplantation*, **8**, 866

TAUBE, D.H., WINDER, E.A., OGG, C.S., BEWICK, M., CAMERON, J.S., RUDGE, C.J. *et al.* (1983). Successful treatment of middle aged and elderly patients with end stage renal diseases. *British Medical Journal*, **286**, 2018–2020

TENCKHOFF, H. (1974). Peritoneal dialysis today: a new look. *Nephron*, **12**, 406–436

TUTTLE, S.G., SWENDSEID, M.E. and BASSETT, S.M. (1960). Methionine requirements of men over sixty. *Federation Proceedings*, **19**, 11–16

ULDALL, P.R. (1981). Subclavian cannulation for hemodialysis. *International Journal of Artificial Organs*, **4**, 213–214

VINCENTI, F., AMEND, W.J., ABELE, J., FEDUSKA, N.J. and SALVATIERRA, O. (1980). The role of hypertension in hemodialysis-associated atherosclerosis. *American Journal of Medicine*, **68**, 363–369

WALKER, P.J., GINN, H.E., JOHNSON, H.K., STONE, W.J., TESCHAN, P.E., LATOS, D. *et al.* (1976). Long-term hemodialysis for patients over 50. *Geriatrics*, **31**, 55–61

WEBER, H., SCHWARZER, C., STUMMVOL, H.K., JOSKOWICS, G., WOLF, A., STEINBACH, K. and KAINDL, F. (1984). Chronic hemodialysis: high risk patients for arrhythmias? *Nephron*, **37**, 180–185

WILLIAMS, P., KAY, R., HARRISON, J., McNEIL, K., PETTIT, J., KELMAN, B. *et al.* (1981). Nutritional and anthropometric assessment of patients on CAPD over one year: contrasting changes in total body nitrogen and potassium. *Peritoneal Dialysis Bulletin*, **1**, 82–87

WING, A.J., BROYER, M., BRUNNER, F.P., BRYNGER, H., CHALLAH, S., DONCKERWOLCKE, R.A. *et al.* (1983). Combined report on regular dialysis and transplantation in Europe, XIII, 1982. In *Proceedings of the European Dialysis and Transplant Association* (London, 1983) edited by A.M. Davison and P.S. Guillou, pp. 2–71. London; Pitman

WU, G. and THE UNIVERSITY OF TORONTO COLLABORATIVE DIALYSIS GROUP (1983). A review of peritonitis episodes that caused interruption of CAPD. *Peritoneal Dialysis Bulletin*, **3S**, S11–S13

ZUCCHELLI, P., CATIZONE, L., DEGLI ESPOSTI, E., FUSAROLI, M., LIGABUE, A. and ZUCCALA, A. (1978). Influence of ultrafiltration on plasma renin activity and adrenergic system. *Nephron*, **21**, 317–324

Chapter 23

Renal transplantation in older patients

David Taube, J. Stewart Cameron and Sabri Challah*

Introduction

There is little doubt that the most effective, successful and cheapest form of treatment of patients with end-stage renal failure (ESRF) is renal transplantation. Recently, with the introduction of the immunosuppressive agent, cyclosporin A, this form of treatment has become even more successful and safe, with overall 1-year allograft survival and patient survival rates of approximately 90 per cent and 95 per cent, respectively, reported by individual centres (Taube *et al.*, 1985; Vanrenterghem *et al.*, 1985). In 1983–84, the 1-year first cadaver graft survival for the whole of Europe was 80 per cent, even including patients treated with azathioprine rather than cyclosporin.

Traditionally, however, transplantation of patients with ESRF over the age of 50 years has been viewed with anxiety. Fifteen years ago this may have been justified, with high mortality rates due to infectious and cardiovascular complications. Simmons and colleagues stated that the only truly 'high risk' group of transplant patients were those over the age of even 45 receiving cadaver transplants, with a 1-year allograft survival of 20 per cent in a small number of patients (Simmons *et al.*, 1971). The transplantation of these 'elderly high risk' patients has greatly improved both in terms of allograft and patient survival over the past 15 years. The purpose of this chapter is to review the transplantation of 'elderly' (defined as over the age of 50 years) patients with ESRF, and to present recent data from our own and other centres describing the use of cyclosporin A in these patients. This chapter is much shorter than many of its predecessors in this book, as relatively few older patients were transplanted until recently.

Transplantation of elderly patients in Western Europe and the USA

Of the patients receiving transplants in Western Europe during 1983, 6.5 per cent were 55 or older. During a similar period in the USA from January 1982 to June 1984, 6 per onset of the total number of cadaveric renal transplants were performed on patients aged 55 or more (Sommer *et al.*, 1986).

In Western Europe (*Table 23.1*), the performance of transplantation in the older patient in renal failure varies greatly from country to country. In general, it is those countries with a high proportion of their patients with ESRF bearing successful allografts which show the highest proportion of patients over the age of 55 bearing

*On behalf of the EDTA–European Renal Association Registry.

Table 23.1 Transplantation of patients aged 55 and above in Europe

Country	*'Stock' of existing patients at 31 December 1983* All patients over 55 years (p.m.p.)*	>55 with functioning graft (p.m.p.)	Tx deaths as % of total on treatment >55		*Activity during 1983* All new patients over 55 years (p.m.p.)	Tx>55 (p.m.p.)	Died >55
Norway	187 (197)	81 (88)	43.3	High	70 (72)	27 (36)	52
Finland	151 (162)	48 (55)	31.8	High	63 (63)	7 (14)	38
Sweden	407 (260)	93 (66)	22.9	High	163 (104)	19 (18)	115
UK	1259 (97)	222 (18)	17.6	High	485 (40)	100 (8)	242
Denmark	206 (174)	27 (20)	13.1	High	56 (46)	10 (8)	58
Ireland	35 (59)	3 (6)	8.5	Medium	14 (23)	1 (2)	5
Switzerland	589 (396)	38 (27)	6.6	Medium	151 (108)	12 (13)	80
Netherlands	822 (287)	15 (6)	1.8	Low	248 (91)	9 (4)	127
Israel	334 (571)	3 (10)	0.9	Low	89 (68)	0 (0)	61
Spain	1968 (316)	16 (3)	0.8	Low	621 (98)	11 (3)	261
Austria	386 (205)	3 (3)	0.8	Low	173 (88)	2 (2)	88
France	3845 (327)	24 (2)	0.6	Low	950 (81)	3 (5)	714
FRG	4658 (277)	30 (2)	0.6	Low	1391 (81)	10 (1)	23
Belgium	833 (377)	5 (3)	0.6	Low	278 (22)	1 (1)	144
Italy	4208 (382)	12 (1)	0.3	Low	1167 (106)	3(0.2)	679
Portugal	282 (195)	1 (1)	0.3	Low	124 (90)	2 (3)	30
Yugoslavia	392 (123)	1 (1)	0.25	Low	167 (50)	0 (0)	75
All Europe	21 453	630	2.9		6637	225	3791

Notes: (a) Data in this and subsequent tables refer to data from patients transplanted having commenced treatment over the age of 55; patients who commenced treatment before this age and were transplanted after 55 are therefore *not* included.
(b) *p.m.p. = patient per million population *over the age of 55*, i.e. age-specific transplantation rates. In the countries in the table, from 19 to 23 per cent of the total population are over 55 years.
(c) Tx = transplanted.

allografts (left) and the highest transplantation rates per year (right), in relation to new patients taken on. The Scandinavian countries and the UK use transplantation liberally in the over-55 age group. In Italy, France and West Germany, however, where transplantation is less popular, the transplantation of patients 55 or older is even less frequent, this age group contributing less than 1 per cent of the total number of transplants performed in Italy and France in 1983. This depressing state of affairs is magnified by the fact that the incidence of renal failure increases with age (see Preface and Chapter 22) and in the USA, for example, 50 per cent or more of the treated ESRF population is now aged over 50 (Sommer *et al.*, 1986). The UK, which has a notoriously poor record for the treatment of elderly patients with ESRF (Berlyne, 1982), comes out quite well from these statistics. About one-tenth of the transplants performed in the UK during 1983 were performed in patients aged 55 or more. The more cynical explanation for this statistic is one of financial expediency rather than enlightened altruism, as transplantation in the UK is known to be the cheapest form of treatment for ESRF.

Allograft and patient survival in Western Europe

We have previously postulated that one of the reasons in the UK why patients with ESRF aged 55 or over may be refused treatment is anticipation of a poor prognosis (Taube *et al.*, 1983). *Table 23.2* analyses the patient and allograft survival in Western Europe over recent years and compares them with results obtained in younger age groups.

Table 23.2 Patient and graft survival in older patients, Europe 1974–83

Cadaver donor	*Recipient survival**	(a) *Patient survival** *over 55 at CD Tx*	*0*	*1 yr*	*2 yr*	*3 yr*	*4 yr*	*5 yr*
		No. of patients at risk at time stated	1431	879	651	505	332	214
		Actuarial survival (%)	100	71.3	62.3	54.7	48.5	44.4
		±s.e.	0	3.6	3.9	4.2	4.4	4.4
		(aged 45–54	100	90	80	72)		
	Graft survival	(b) *Graft survival* *over 55 at CD Tx*	*0*	*1 yr*	*2 yr*	*3 yr*	*4 yr*	*5 yr*
		No. of grafts at risk at time stated	1425	636	465	364	244	156
		Actuarial survival (%)	100	51.4	44.9	40.1	35.1	32.4
		±s.e.	0	4.4	4.2	4.2	4.1	4.0
		(aged 45–54	100	65	60)	(1979–81 only)		
Live donor	*Recipient survival**	(c) *Patient survival** *over 55 at LD Tx*	*0*	*1 yr*	*2 yr*	*3 yr*	*4 yr*	*5 yr*
		No. of patients at risk at time stated	111	74	54	46	36	23
		Actuarial survival (%)	100	73.5	65.5	61.3	54.4	51.9
		±s.e.	0	6.9	7.4	7.6	8.1	8.1
	Graft survival	(d) *Graft survival* *over 55 at LD Tx*	*0*	*1 yr*	*2 yr*	*3 yr*	*4 yr*	*5 yr*
		No. of grafts at risk at time stated	111	60	44	36	29	17
		Actuarial survival (%)	100	57.4	52.8	52.8	43.8	41.3
		±s.e.	8.2	8.0	8.0	8.4	8.3	

* *Patient survival* includes subsequent survival on other modes of treatment after graft failure, i.e. it represents the *real* survival of the patients following Tx.

Patient and cadaver allograft survival during this period, *before* the widespread use of cyclosporin A, in patients aged 55 or over, is generally 10–15 per cent less than that of the younger age groups (*Table 23.2,* (a) and (b)). This is not an enormous difference, and some 5–10 per cent depend solely upon the greater age of the group. In our view, these data do not justify the low rate of transplantation of elderly patients in Western Europe.

Causes of allograft loss and death in patients aged 55 or over in Western Europe

The major cause of allograft loss in this age group of patients was, not unexpectedly, rejection (*Table 23.3*). The next most common cause of allograft loss was technical problems (vascular or ureteric). *Table 23.3* also shows that cardiac or vascular causes were the most common reasons why patients with functioning allografts died. Sepsis was the next most common cause.

Live-related transplantation in Western Europe in patients aged 55 or more

Live-related transplantation is understandably an unpopular form of transplantation in Western Europe in elderly patients. During the 10-year period

Table 23.3 Causes of death or allograft loss in older patients: Europe 1974–83 (Data from the EDTA–ERA Registry)

Causes of allograft loss	*No. of allografts lost*	*Causes of death post-transplant*	*No. of complications*
Rejection	387	Cardiac	103
Technical	45	Other vascular	82
Recurrent disease	17	Infections	187
Infection	16	Other	80
Other	21		
	486	No. of patients	395
Out of 1068 grafts, 968 CD, 92 LD			

1974–83, only 111 live-related transplantations in patients over 55 had been reported to the EDTA–ERA Registry. The patient and allograft survivals are not substantially different from those experienced with cadaveric transplants (*Table 23.2,* (c) and (d)).

Transplantation of elderly patients in individual centres

The data presented above are gathered from a wide variety of disparate sources, and an alternative way of assessing the status of transplantation in these patients is to look at the results obtained from individual selected centres. We have selected the data to reflect the periods 1975–80 and 1981–83, both of which involve the use of prednisolone and azathioprine, and have then compared them with data from 1983

Table 23.4 Patient and allograft survival rates in individual series

CADAVER RENAL TRANSPLANTATION IN ELDERLY PATIENTS (1975–80) USING AZOTHIOPRINE

Year of report	*Centre and author*	*No. of patients*	*Percentage survival at 1 yr* Patient	Allograft
1975	Delmonico	26*	57.4	Not available
1976	Kjellstrand	33	66	Not available
1978	Golper	30	75	58
1980	Wedel	38†	60	60
1980	Kock	38†	66	62
1980	Ost	34†	60	49

CADAVER RENAL TRANSPLANTATION IN ELDERLY PATIENTS (1981–83) USING AZATHIOPRINE

Year of report	*Author*	*No. of patients*	*Percentage survival at 1 yr* Patient	Allograft
1981	Sommer	62	60	57
1983	Okiye	29	78	61
1983	Taube	38	73	67

CADAVER RENAL TRANSPLANTATION IN ELDERLY PATIENTS (1983–86) USING CYCLOSPORIN A

Year of report	*Author*	*No. of patients*	*Percentage survival at 1 yr* Patient	Allograft
1983	Ringdén	29	85	73
1985	Taube	60	88	84
1986	Sommer	52	92	86

*Includes 3 live-related transplants.
†Patients aged 60 or over

to the present time, involving the use of cyclosporin A and prednisolone as immunosuppressive agents.

Table 23.4 shows that patient and allograft survival, as judged by the data gathered from these selected centres over the past 10 years, has clearly improved. This improvement is not only attributable to the use of cyclosporin A, as the results obtained using conventional immunosuppression with azathioprine during the period 1981–83 are 5–10 per cent better than the period 1975–80. However, the greatest apparent improvement coincides with the use of cyclosporin A, and it is important to note that, in the two largest and most recent series involving the use of cyclosporin A, patient and allograft survival are not substantially different. Sommer *et al.* (1986) have collected data on 680 older patients receiving cadaver renal allografts in the USA in 1982–84, 482 using azathioprine and 198 using cyclosporin. Patient survivals were excellent and not improved by cyclosporin, but there was modest improvement in allograft survival (*Table 23.5*). Our own study is reported briefly below.

Table 23.5 Patient and graft survival in elderly patients transplanted in the USA (Health Care Finance Authority) — percentage 1-year survivals in elderly patients treated with prednisolone/azathioprine or cyclosporin A

Age (yr)	*Prednisolone/azathioprine* No.	*Percentage survival* Patients	Grafts	*Cyclosporin A* No.	*Percentage survival* Patients	Grafts
55–60	339	84	59	130	89	55
60–65	115	85	67	59	79	67
>65	28	63	43	9	100	75
	482			198		

(Data collected by Sommer *et al.*, 1986)

Use of cyclosporin A in elderly patients receiving renal allografts at Guy's and Dulwich hospitals, London

Although we used cyclosporin A initially in our centre during 1983, we became reasonably familiar with its use by the beginning of 1984. For this reason we report here the results of 60 recent cadaveric transplants performed during the period January 1984 to July 1985 using cyclosporin A in recipients aged 50 years or more at the time of transplantation.

Patients

Fifty-nine patients (45 males, 14 females) received 60 cadaveric allografts. The oldest patient was 76 years at the time of grafting.

Immunosuppression

At Guy's Hospital (29 patients), cyclosporin A 7 mg/kg was given orally preoperatively. Postoperatively, the patients in this study received cyclosporin A 14 mg/kg/day for the first 2 weeks, tapering rapidly to 6 mg/kg/day at 3 months post-transplantation. Prednisolone 15 mg/m^2 body surface area (BSA)/day was given from day one, reducing to 7.5 mg/m^{2}BSA/day at 1 year.

The immunosuppressive regimen at Dulwich Hospital was similar. Cyclosporin A 8 mg/kg was given orally preoperatively followed by 16 mg/kg/day for the first 3 postoperative days, before being reduced to 10 mg/kg/day for a further 4 days. The dose was then altered to keep trough whole blood cyclosporin A concentrations between 400 and 800 ng/ml. Prednisolone 20 mg/day was given for the first month, then 15 mg/day for the next month and 10 mg/day or less thereafter. The diagnosis of allograft rejection or cyclosporin A nephrotoxicity was based on allograft biopsy, as previously described. Allograft rejection was treated with high dose steroids or if judged to be particularly severe, a course of anti-lymphocyte or anti-thymocyte globulin was administered. Cyclosporin A nephrotoxicity was managed by 2 mg/kg/day reduction in cyclosporin A (Guy's Hospital) or as a 20 per cent reduction of the total dose (Dulwich Hospital).

Results

One-year patient and allograft survival was 87.8 per cent and 83.8 per cent, respectively. There was no difference in patient or allograft survival when the patients were divided into a 50–60 year old group (35 patients) and a 61 or greater year old group (24 patients). Of the 60 allografts, a total of 8 were lost as a result of irreversible rejection and 9 patients died (15 per cent), 6 of them with functioning allografts. Death with a functioning allograft was considered using the life table method (Cutler and Ederer, 1958) as 'lost to follow-up'. The causes of patient death are given in *Table 23.6.*

Table 23.6 Causes of patient death in those over 50 in Guy's/Dulwich hospitals (UK) — cyclosporin A study

Cardiovascular or cerebrovascular disease		5
Malignancy		1
Infection		2 (interstitial pneumonitis, pelvic peritonitis)
Chronic pancreatitis		1
	Total	9/60 (15%)

In our 1983 study using azathioprine and steroids as immunosuppression, the most common cause of death among our transplanted patients was sepsis. Interestingly, our current study using cyclosporin A shows that sepsis is now less common than cardiovascular or cerebrovascular disease as a cause of death. Although fortunately the numbers are small, these results suggest that we are not over-immunosuppressing our patients, and that the cardiovascular or cerebrovascular deaths are part of the normal aging process. However, cyclosporin A has been reported to be associated with an increased incidence of thromboembolic complications (Vanrenterghem *et al.*, 1985), although we (Choudhury *et al.*, 1985) have not been able to confirm this observation, along with other units. It is possible nevertheless that this contributes to the vascular deaths. These results are similar also to the data of Sommer *et al.* (1986), in which the commonest cause of death was cardiovascular accidents.

It would therefore appear from our own and other studies that cyclosporin A is associated with a marked improvement in patient and allograft survival. The results are obviously preliminary, and clearly more time is required to evaluate the full advantages and perhaps disadvantages of cyclosporin A. However, based on our data and that of Sommer *et al.* (1986), we can no longer justify the use of prednisolone and azathioprine in the treatment of patients over 50 or more. Preliminary data from the EDTA–ERA Registry suggest that the beneficial effects of cyclosporin A are not restricted to single centres. In a small number of patients the 6-month allograft and patient survivals in 1983 were approximately 85 per cent and 90 per cent, respectively. Thus at present the use of cyclosporin A is most encouraging in elderly patients and we hope that the long-term results remain as good.

The current role of transplantation in the management of elderly patients with ESRF

Chapter 22 shows that the 1-year survival of patients aged 55–64 on dialysis alone is approximately 85 per cent and 75 per cent at 1 and 2 years, respectively. The data for CAPD are similar. *Table 23.2*, spanning the years 1974–83 and all patients over the age of 55, shows that the survival of patients after their first cadaveric allograft is 71 per cent and 62 per cent at 1 and 2 years, respectively. It is therefore clear that during this period of time the mortality of elderly patients with ESRF was greater after transplantation during the first year. However, by the second year after the initiation of treatment, the mortality rates were similar. These data are similar to those in our 1983 azathioprine study (Taube *et al.*, 1983) (*Table 23.7*) which shows that patient survival on different modes of therapy becomes similar after 3 years.

Table 23.7 Survival of patients aged 55 or more on different forms of therapy at Guy's/ Dulwich hospitals (UK)

	Percentage survival				
	1 yr	2 yr	3 yr	4 yr	5 yr
Haemodialysis (patients never transplanted)	80.4	80.4	61.6	61.5	61.5
Transplantation (azathioprine, –1982)	73	68.8	61.9	61.9	61.9
Transplantation (cyclosporin A, 1983–85)	87.8	------ Not yet available ------			

With the use of cyclosporin A, as *Table 23.7* demonstrates, patient mortality may be similar to that experienced with haemodialysis or CAPD even during the first year post-transplantation.

What mode of treatment therefore should be offered to patients aged 55 or more with ESRF? We suggest that elderly patients should be encouraged to select transplantation as their primary mode of therapy, at least up to the age of 75. As with patients under the age of 55, we avoid transplantation in those patients with malignancy or active, chronic infections such as bronchiectasis. We believe that transplantation is an excellent form of therapy for those patients with ischaemic heart disease, as a good functioning kidney is a constantly effective form of after-load reduction. A further point is poor cardiac performance and instability in the elderly uraemic patient (see Chapter 22). We have been impressed, clinically, in many patients with the improvement in wellbeing and cardiac performance after a transplant, with a normal haemoglobin concentration and without uraemic cardiomyopathy. Thus, poor cardiac performance may actually be one indication *for* transplantation, rather than a contraindication. Furthermore, in the UK where there are increasing financial constraints in the National Health Service, the question of cost–benefit also arises. Clearly, transplantation is the choice of therapy for ESRF in these elderly patients in our centres. Vascular disease affecting the iliac vessels may be a problem, but an endarterectomy can be performed first, and we have placed grafts successfully on to aorto-iliac bypass prostheses. So far, we have had no problems of 'steal' from the lower limbs.

This policy presupposes that an adequate supply of cadaver kidneys is available to permit their use in the older patients; the greater the shortage of organs, the less keen will physicians be to use up the 'valuable' organ for an older, rather than a younger, patient. Fortunately, this is not at the moment a problem in the South-East of England, with a transplantation rate of just over 40/million/yr during 1984, for a population of just over 7 million (South-East and South-West Thames Regions).

Conclusions

Patients aged 55 or more are rarely transplanted in most parts of Western Europe or the USA. The reasons for this are not clear, as review of the evidence and data from individual centres reveals that patient survival, particularly with the use of cyclosporin A, is similar to that on haemodialysis or CAPD. Probably shortage of donor kidneys determines their use in younger patients. We suggest that more elderly patients with ESRF should be transplanted, as this form of therapy offers the best rehabilitation in this age group at a cheaper cost, and with a similar survival to other modes of ESRF treatment.

Acknowledgements

The authors would like to thank the physicians and surgeons and nursing staff of the Guy's and Dulwich hospitals renal units for their help and encouragement.

References

BERLYNE, G.M. (1982). Over 50 and uremic = death. *Nephron,* **31,** 189–190

CHOUDHURY, N., NEILD, G.H., BROWN, Z. and CAMERON, J.S. (1985). Thromboembolic complications in cyclosporin-treated kidney allograft recipients (Letter). *Lancet,* **ii,** 606

CUTLER, S.J. and EDERER, F. (1958). Maximum utilization of the life-table method in analyzing survival. *Journal of Chronic Diseases,* **8,** 690–712

DELMONICO, F.L., COSIMI, A.B. and RUSSEL, P.S. (1975). Renal transplantation in the older age group. *Archives of Surgery,* **110,** 1107–1109

GOLPER, T.A., BARRY, M.J. and BENETT, W.M. (1978). Primary cadaver kidney transplantation in older patients: survival equal to dialysis. *Transactions of the American Society for Artificial Internal Organs,* **24,** 282–287

KJELLSTRAND, C.M., SHIDEMAN, J.R., LYNCH, R.E., BUSELMEIER, T.J., SIMMONS, R.L. and NAJARIAN, J.S. (1976). Kidney transplants in patients over 50. *Geriatrics,* **31,** 65–73

KOCK, B., KUHLBÄCK, B., AHONEN, J., LINDFORS, O. and LINDSTROM, B.L. (1980). Kidney transplantation in patients 60 years and older. *Scandinavian Journal of Urology and Nephrology,* **54** (Suppl.), 103–105

OKIYE, S.E., ENGEN, D.E., STERIOFF, S., JOHNSON, W.G., FROHNERT, P.P., OFFORD, K.P. and ZINCKE, H. (1983). Primary renal transplantation in patients 50 years of age and older. *Transplantation Proceedings,* **15,** 1046–1052

OST, L., GROTH, C.G., LINDHOLM, B., LUNDGREN, G., MAGNUSSON, G. and TILLEGARD, A. (1980). Cadaveric transplantation in patients of 60 years or above. *Transplantation,* **30,** 339–340

RINGDEN, O., OST, L., KLINTMALM, G., TILLEGARD, A., FAIRMAN, I., WILCZEK, H. and GROTH, C.G. (1983). Improved outcome in renal transplant recipients above 55 years of age treated with cyclosporine and low doses of steroids. *Transplantation Proceedings,* **15** (Suppl.), 2507–2512

SIMMONS, R.L., KJELLSTRAND, C.M., BUSELMEIER, T.J. and NAJARIAN, J.S. (1971). Renal transplantation in high risk patients. *Archives of Surgery,* **103,** 290–298

SOMMER, B.G., FERGUSON, R.M., DAVIN, T.D., KJELLSTRAND, C.M., FRYD, D.S., SIMMONS, R.L. and NAJARIAN, J.S. (1981). Renal transplantation in patients over 50 years of age. *Transplantation Proceedings,* **13,** 33–35

SOMMER, B.G., MANDELBAUM, D.M., MITCHELL, H.L. and FERGUSON, R.M. (1986). Renal transplantation in the middle aged and elderly uremic patients. In *Geriatric Nephrology,* edited by D.G. Oreopolous, pp. 157–168. Dordrecht; Nijhoff

TAUBE, D.H., WILLIAMS, D.G., NEILD, G.H., CAMERON, J.S., HARTLEY, B., OGG, C.S., RUDGE, C.J. and WELSH, K.I. (1985). Differentiation between allograft rejection and cyclosporin nephrotoxicity in renal transplant recipients. *Lancet,* **ii,** 171–174

TAUBE, D.H., WINDER, E.A., OGG, C.S., BEWICK, M., CAMERON, J.S., RUDGE, C.J. and WILLIAMS, D.G. (1983). Successful treatment of middle aged and elderly patients with end stage renal failure. *British Medical Journal,* **286,** 2018–2020

VANRENTERGHEM, Y., ROELS, L., LERUT, T., GRUWEZ, J., MICHIEWEN, P., GRESELE, P., DECKMYN, H., COLUCCI, M., ARNOUT, J. and VERMYELN, J. (1985). Thromboembolic complications and haemostatic changes in cyclosporin-treated cadaveric allograft recipients. *Lancet,* **i,** 999–1002

WEDEL, N., BRYNGER, H. and BLOHME, L. (1980). Kidney transplantation in patients 60 years and older. *Scandinavian Journal of Urology and Nephrology,* **54** (Suppl.), 106

Index

[Note: For the effect of aging on specific renal functions, see the entry Aging, effect on.]